DATE DUE

D0769080

HANDBOOK OF
GROUP PSYCHOTHERAPY

Recent titles in the

Wiley Series on Personality Processes

Irving B. Weiner, *Editor*

University of South Florida

Handbook of Group Psychotherapy

An Empirical and Clinical Synthesis

Edited by

Addie Fuhriman

Gary M. Burlingame

A WILEY-INTERSCIENCE PUBLICATION

JOHN WILEY & SONS, INC.

New York • Chichester • Brisbane • Toronto • Singapore

Dedicated with affection
to
the creators and architects of our first and primary group

Nona and Wendell

Ruth and Leroy

This text is printed on acid-free paper.

Copyright © 1994 by John Wiley & Sons, Inc.

All rights reserved. Published simultaneously in Canada.

This publication is designed to provide accurate and
authoritative information in regard to the subject
matter covered. It is sold with the understanding that
the publisher is not engaged in rendering legal, accounting,
or other professional services. If legal advice or other
expert assistance is required, the services of a competent
professional person should be sought.

Library of Congress Cataloging in Publication Data:

ISBN: 0-471-55592-4

Printed in the United States of America

10 9 8 7 6 5 4 3 2 1

Editorial Advisory Board

Contributors

Sally H. Barlow, Ph.D.
Associate Professor of Psychology
Brigham Young University
Provo, Utah

Richard L. Bednar, Ph.D.
Professor of Psychology
Brigham Young University
Provo, Utah

Sidney Bloch, M.B.Ch.B., Ph.D.
Associate Professor and Reader
Department of Psychiatry
University of Melbourne and
Senior Psychiatrist
St. Vincent's Hospital
Fitzroy, Victoria
Australia

Virginia Brabender, Ph.D.
Associate Professor and
Director of Internship Training
Institute for Graduate Clinical Psychology
Widener University
Chester, Pennsylvania

Simon H. Budman, Ph.D.
Harvard Community Health Plan
Assistant Professor of Psychology
Harvard University Medical School
Boston, Massachusetts

Gary M. Burlingame, Ph.D.
Associate Professor of Psychology
Brigham Young University
Provo, Utah

Eric C. Crouch, F.R.C.Psych.
Consultant Psychiatrist and Clinical
Director of Mental Health
South Buckinghamshire NHS Trust
Amersham Hospital
Amersham, Buckinghamshire
England

John C. Dagley, Ph.D.
Associate Professor and Director of
Counseling Psychology Program
University of Georgia
Athens, Georgia

Annette Demby, M.S.W.
Assistant Director of Mental Health
Research and Training Department
Harvard Community Health Plan
Boston, Massachusetts

Robert R. Dies, Ph.D.
Professor of Psychology
University of Maryland
College Park, Maryland

Stephanie J. Eppinger, M.A.
Counseling Psychology Program
University of Georgia
Athens, Georgia

April Fallon, Ph.D.
Assistant Professor and Associate
Director of Outpatient Division
Department of Psychiatry
Medical College of Pennsylvania
Philadelphia, Pennsylvania

Addie Fuhriman, Ph.D.
Dean of Graduate Studies and
Professor of Psychology
Brigham Young University
Provo, Utah

George M. Gazda, Ed.D.
Research Professor and
Associate Dean for Research
College of Education
University of Georgia
Athens, Georgia

Gerald Goodman, Ph.D.
Associate Professor of Psychology
University of California Los Angeles
Los Angeles, California

Marion K. Jacobs, Ph.D.
Adjunct Professor of Psychology and
Coordinator of Psychology Clinic
University of California Los Angeles
Los Angeles, California

Theodore J. Kaul, Ph.D.
Associate Professor of Psychology
Ohio State University
Columbus, Ohio

John C. Kircher, Ph.D.
Associate Professor
Department of Educational Psychology
University of Utah
Salt Lake City, Utah

Robert H. Klein, Ph.D.
Clinical Associate Professor of
   Psychiatry
Albert Einstein College of Medicine
Bronx, New York and
Yale University School of Medicine
New Haven, Connecticut

Morton A. Lieberman, Ph.D.
Professor of Psychology
University of California
San Francisco, California

K. Roy MacKenzie, M.D.
Clinical Professor of Psychiatry
University of British Columbia
Var.couver, British Columbia
Canada

J. Kelly Moreno, Ph.D.
Assistant Professor
Department of Psychology and Human
   Development
Cal Poly State University
San Luis Obispo, California

Patricia L. Owen, Ph.D.
Director of Butler Center for Research
   and Learning
Hazelden Foundation
Center City, Minnesota

William E. Piper, Ph.D.
Professor and Co-Director
Psychotherapy Research Center
Department of Psychiatry
University of Alberta
Edmonton, Alberta, Canada

Richard Reilly, Ph.D.
Coordinator of Group Psychotherapy
Harvard Community Health Plan,
   Somerville Center
Somerville, Massachusetts

Paul G. Simeone, Ph.D.
Harvard Community Health Plan
Clinical Instructor of Psychology
Harvard University Medical School
Boston, Massachusetts

Elizabeth A. Stewart, M.Ed., J.D.
Counseling Psychology Program
University of Georgia
Athens, Georgia

Randy Stinchfield, Ph.D.
Associate Director of Center for
   Adolescent Substance Abuse
Department of Pediatrics
University of Minnesota
Minneapolis, Minnesota

Shawn Taylor, B.A.
Clinical Psychology Program
Brigham Young University
Provo, Utah

Ken C. Winters, Ph.D.
Director of Center for Adolescent
   Substance Abuse
Department of Pediatrics
University of Minnesota
Minneapolis, Minnesota

Janine Wanlass, Ph.D.
Assistant Professor and Chair
Department of Psychology
Westminster College
Salt Lake City, Utah

Preface

We thought it was an "idea whose time had come!" In fact, given the evolutionary state of the field, in both research and practice, the idea of a book devoted solely to the empirical bases for group psychotherapy was past due. The prevalent and prolific use of group therapy across disciplines, populations, treatment foci, and settings certainly demands accountability in terms of its conceptual and procedural efficacy. The abundance of empirical work by both researchers and practitioners warrants such consideration as well.

We are aware that much is in print regarding the use of the group format in the therapeutic enterprise. Texts abound that narrate theoretical propositions, describe conceptual models, and detail intervention strategies. Some are more conceptually driven, others more empirically driven. Less apparent are substantial reviews that represent the empirical nature of group therapy. More typical are reviews of group research in singular chapters nested within a text or handbook, intended to highlight significant results as they relate to clinical practice or methodological direction. Given the volume of empirical work and the diversity of focus, the number of articles referred to in a single work have been substantially limited, the scope notably narrowed. A few reviews have critiqued specific topics (e.g., leadership) or populations (e.g., schizophrenics). Prevailing over all these are repeated major calls for a "research focus" in both clinical and empirical matters.

In the past two decades, there has been a substantial increase in published studies across the entire gamut of group application; literally hundreds of group psychotherapy outcome and process studies have been conducted and reported. The resulting articles appear not simply in journals devoted to the cause of group psychotherapy and behavior change, but in those that represent a wide range of general and specific interests in psychotherapy as well. We were struck not only by the amount of conceptual and empirical work that has been accomplished, but also by the increased refinement in methodology that accompanies it. Indeed, it appeared to us that the field had moved far beyond what a single chapter could capture in terms of the breadth and depth of what we know clinically and what we are studying empirically. Thus, the time seemed right.

In their preface to the first edition of *The Handbook of Psychotherapy and Behavior Change,* Allen Bergin and Sol Garfield noted that it was intended to "fill a gap." That same gap continues to exist in the group psychotherapy literature; this effort was crafted to respond to that lacuna and to bring together and "bin" the extant literature into a single, comprehensive empirical display of how group therapy works and what it does. The individual chapters in all sections represent central theoretical and clinical concerns that have a sufficiently developed body of empirical literature from which to draw substantive conclusions. The intent is to provide a comprehensive review of each area and thus a foundation for practice and a springboard for future research.

We followed Bergin and Garfield's lead in the conceptual framework of the layout of the book, specifically as reflected in the first, second, and fourth sections. In Part One, the conceptual and methodological foundations, it seemed important to trace and bring together the two historically influential lines of inquiry of small group psychology and group psychotherapy, reflecting their sometimes separate, sometimes interwoven, and at times, disparate contributions. In examining the efficacy of group therapy, it seemed important to draw from the existing reviews. It would be difficult for the interested reader to pull together the "state of the art" literature, because studies appear in very diverse journals—some 160—across various disciplines; the intent here is to understand what they have to say in total.

Part Two, structural entities, includes the main parameters that are considered when assessing outcome as it occurs within group formats. These are the units created by the players (i.e., client-members, therapist, subgroups) and constitute the structural boundaries of the group. Missing in the discussion is attention to that unique structural component of group therapy, composition. Although the significant implications of composition loom large, the past empirical investment in isolating and studying the effect of composition on both process and outcome is scant.

Part Three, therapeutic components of the group ecosystem, relates to the features of psychotherapy that are unique to or relate substantially to the functional ecology and dynamics of a group. These peculiar properties center on the interpersonal nature of small group functioning—in essence, the driving force of a therapeutic group. The interpersonal and group dynamics are found nested within the group's interaction, its therapeutic factors, and its developmental growth as a functional entity. Not only are these three properties found in all groups, but they are also relevant across theoretical models and treatment groups. In total, they represent the longest trail and greatest volume of empirical effort in understanding group process.

Selecting the specific areas for the special application section presented its own challenge. Without doubt, there exists a wide range of foci and populations from which to select, but the choice is complicated by the minimal effort or amount of empirical work in a single area. For example, until most recently, the heterogeneity of client characteristics used in group composition resulted in a broad base of classification (i.e., inpatient or out-patient groups), without specific disorder designation or assignment to group treatment by disorder classification. Thus, there are fewer studies that focus on group treatment for specific disorders. In some areas, there has been a recent flurry of research activity, but it is predominately characterized by anecdotal and single case descriptions. In the final analysis, topics in the special application section were selected on assorted criteria, such as the volume of existing empirical evidence, the currency of clinical attention, group as the primary treatment mode, and the lack of either a previous or recent review.

When we began this venture, we gave the authors the general charge to provide a review of the empirical record of outcome and process in a designated area of group psychotherapy and counseling. If previous reviews were not in existence, then they were to track the entire empirical trail; if the area had received previous consideration by way of a comprehensive review, attention was to be given to more recent research, emphasizing in particular the past decade. In some instances, the extant literature warranted the exposure of some conceptual and theoretical work. The chapters were to provide the scientific foundation for group therapy and were to speak to both the clinician and the researcher, providing implications to both parties, when appropriate. Finally, if it were substantiated and seemed timely, the authors were encouraged to describe some conceptual modeling that could serve as a springboard for future inquiry.

We feel fortunate to have had a thoughtful and knowledgeable advisory board who provided assurance as to the direction of the book. We were also fortunate to have the quality of individual contributors that are represented herein. All in their own right are clinicians and researchers; many have years of extensive involvement with inquiry into the process and outcome of group treatment. We are grateful for what they have given and believe their work and perspectives hold promise for future practice and research. Finally, we are appreciative of the unsung heroines and heroes whose work is woven within each chapter—those *individuals* who carry their curiosity about what "works" in group psychotherapy to fruition by designing, conducting, and publishing group studies.

ADDIE FUHRIMAN
GARY M. BURLINGAME

Acknowledgments

We are grateful to the many individuals who contributed to the completion of this Handbook. In addition to the advisory board and the contributing editors, several individuals were called upon to review specific chapters: Ariadne P. Beck, Allen E. Bergin, Don E. Norton, Joseph Olsen, Scott R. Woodward, and Irvin D. Yalom. We are indebted to them for their input and assistance. Appreciation is also extended to Kurt Graham, Analee Munsey, and Karl Barnum for their extensive efforts in the preparation of the final manuscript; and gratitude to Linda Adams for the preparation of the indexes and Nancy Marcus Land and Denise Netardus at Publications Development Corporation for their help in the production process. Once again, the "whole" was highly dependent on its parts.

Contents

PART ONE

Conceptual and Methodological Foundations

CHAPTER 1

Group Psychotherapy: Research and Practice

ADDIE FUHRIMAN and GARY M. BURLINGAME

HISTORICAL ROOTS

The realization of group influence goes back hundreds of years, and although the structure, purpose, and definition of "group" have been, and continue to be modified, evidence that the group and its processes influence social, psychological, and behavioral change persists. The subset of "group psychotherapy" finds its roots in more recent times, specifically the 20th century. Group psychotherapy is reported to have existed in "disguised forms" since the turn of the century (Ruitenbeek, 1969). There are similarities between today's theory and practice of group psychotherapy and the more obscure forms of the past.

Group psychotherapy has evolved in neither a linear nor unified fashion. In fact, one historian of group therapy described its past as "conglomerate, complex, confabulatory, and conflictual" (Anthony, 1971). Methods and theories originating in diverse disciplines (medicine, sociology, psychology, theater) have contributed to the conglomerate nature of group therapy's history. Its complexity is nested in the acceptance of humans as social beings with interpersonal influence as a central feature of therapy and, in a more extreme sense, in the notion that the group is a more fundamental unit than the individual (Foulkes & Anthony, 1957). The history of group psychotherapy is conflictual and, to a degree, confabulatory in its determination of the significance of various "who" and "what" and "when" occurrences.

The Early Years: People and Processes

It is generally agreed that group psychotherapy is a product of 20th-century America, and from some perspectives, its beginning here represents a natural outgrowth of what was "essentially a free group culture" (Sadock & Kaplan, 1983). Input from European quarters is evident in the early theory and practice of group psychotherapy, both by the transplant of individuals to America (i.e., Moreno) or by singular European contributors. Some (Dreikurs, 1969a; 1969b) report that the innovation of group

3

was simultaneously active in Europe, but went unnoticed because of the lack of reporting.

Pratt, Moreno, Marsh, Lazell, Burrow, and Adler represent individuals who are consistently recognized for their contribution to the initial definition, theory, and practice of group psychotherapy and to its subsequent movement. Each presented a specific perspective or practice. As early as 1905, Joseph Pratt began seeing his tuberculosis patients within a class format, primarily as a labor-saving device, expecting them to commit to a specified normative behavior deemed crucial to the cure of tuberculosis. He attributed the success of the classes to patients' sense of identification with one another, their hope of recovery, and their faith in the class, the methods, and the physician. Some years later, Pratt changed to a more psychotherapeutic approach, believing from his experience that if the mind improved the body would follow.

In the meantime, in Europe, Jacob Moreno was theorizing therapy based on interpersonal and group influence and spontaneous expression and acting-out, resulting in form as psychodrama. To the unwashed, Moreno's primary contribution is psychodrama, but by his own words and intent, core to all he did, both early and later on, was the treatment of patients within the interpersonal context of the group; the dynamics of the group were his focus.

The second decade found others applying therapeutic concepts within a group format. Both Cody Marsh and E. W. Lazell began to treat institutionalized mental patients in a group setting, for the most part bringing patients together in a class structure and applying psychoeducational methods. Marsh is credited with the beginning of "milieu" therapy; he used the classes to stimulate group emotion and to facilitate more active involvement by the patients in their own treatment, believing that individual dignity was important and better maintained in a class than in therapy. He espoused a social-emotional orientation both as an explanation of, and treatment for, mental disease, vividly represented in his statement, "By the crowd they have been broken, by the crowd they shall be healed." This expression best illustrates the shift in emphasis from the content to the interactive, dynamic process of the group class.

During the same decade, Lazell was treating hospitalized schizophrenics in a group setting using lectures and other psychoeducational methods. He attributed the success of the class format to the patients' getting to know one another and thus being able to share the universalities of individual experiences. Some consideration was given to the effectiveness of the group format even this early, as evidence of positive outcome was noted by Lazell's nursing staff, who observed in patients a decreased need for nightly sedatives.

There are those who credit Alfred Adler and his co-workers with being the first to conduct group psychotherapy. Adler never acknowledged being a group therapist, although his theories contributed to group therapy's initial conceptualizations. His philosophy described humans as social, goal-directed, motivated by a desire to belong, and able and willing contributors. In this context, the group becomes a highly suitable setting to uncover and influence maladaptive and conflictual behavior. Social and cultural adaptation were viewed as a purpose of group treatment and were facilitated by therapeutic factors of encouragement, optimism, and intermember support. Many followers of Adler implemented his ideas into the practice of group therapy. Most notably was Rudolf Dreikurs, who treated alcoholics as well as his private practice psychiatric patients within a group format. He thought the group was a natural setting, whether it was limited to family members or was inclusive of others. He used individual sessions to collect detailed history, then relied on the dynamics of the group to facilitate change. Specifically, Dreikurs conceptualized the therapeutic aspects of group treatment to be the interaction among the patients, cohesion, universality, and confrontation. From his point-of-view, member influence was different than therapist influence and should be utilized. Hans Syz believed the social situation of the group offered factors and opportunities that coincided with the social situation outside of the group. His belief was highlighted by the treatment use of the "here and now" as an intervention strategy in the group.

Freud is also among the originators of group psychotherapy, though he never conducted group psychotherapy per se (although some describe his "Wednesday Night" Vienna discussion group as a form of group practice). Nevertheless, he was aware that the inclusion of others in therapy quantitatively and qualitatively influenced the processes of analysis, sometimes to an advantage, other times to a disadvantage. The consideration of the group as a whole that has dynamics and experiences of its own was also part of his thinking.

During the early 1920s, Trigant Burrow developed group analysis, in part because he was concerned that individual dynamics were being emphasized in therapy while the individual's relationship to social forces remained neglected. He designed an intensive residential setting, worked with neurotic disorders, and described self-disclosure, consensual validation, and a here-and-now focus as factors facilitating change. He, too, considered the group as an entity with dynamics of its own.

Both Louis Wender and Paul Schilder applied a psychoanalytic approach to psychotic, hospitalized adult patients in groups. For them, the re-creation of the family was a central curative mechanism. Schilder also thought the sense of universality that was created within the group was a mediating factor in the patient's recovery. Samuel Slavson, considered by some as the father of modern group therapy, maintained an individual focus in the group and underscored the importance of transference. His main concentration and contribution was in the application of group therapy to a child population. Further evidence of the establishment of a field is the credentialing of practitioners; group therapy ventured into this area through Alexander Wolf, who first initiated a certification program in group therapy. Wolf was also recognized for his classical work on psychoanalysis in group therapy, and was innovative as well in his use of alternate group sessions: one session with the leader, one without.

The naming of group therapy and its entrance into the framework of empirical science came at the hands of Moreno in 1932 with the first book published on group psychotherapy (and his first book in America). Moreno came to America in part with the intent of introducing his ideas concerning "group." Whereas previous group experiences simply addressed the group members, the orientation was now focused on working with the individuals and the ensuing interaction. Indeed, in the 1930s the group "came of age" as a therapeutic entity and professionals whose primary focus was psychotherapy were heavily involved. Although most treatment foci originated from a psychoanalytic orientation, varying perspectives were brought to bear on the purpose, process, and populations. By the late 1930s, psychotherapists (albeit mostly psychiatrists) were conceptualizing group therapy and practicing it among several clinical populations.

Conglomerate and Complex

Conglomerate and complex were terms used to describe the history of group psychotherapy. They are also relevant terms to the evolved theory, practice, and research of group therapy. An examination of their applicability provides some insight into the current empirical evidence and perhaps gives us some promise for research as well as clinical endeavors in the future.

The field suffers with and is blessed by multiple origins. In describing group therapy, we have noted on other occasions that those who theorize, conceptualize, and practice group treatment have "begged, borrowed, and bilked" from many areas. On the other hand, the contributors themselves came from diverse origins. Traces of theory emanate from such diverse areas as personality theory, field theory, and systems theory, thus influencing our intra-, inter-, and contextual focus. Theoretical orientations also left their mark at various times and to differing degrees, but with lingering influence. Traces of psychoanalytic, group dynamics, existential-experiential, and behavioral theories can be found today in the way group therapy is defined, conceptualized, implemented, and evaluated. Current theory and practice contain threads from multiple disciplines, including psychiatry, psychology, education, social work, and organizational behavior. Ultimately, group therapy stands to gain a richness from its past and present conglomerate nature, particularly if the separate contributions are understood, tracked, and evaluated in terms of the meaning of the whole enterprise of group.

For both the clinician and the researcher, the complexity involved in group therapy is problematic and is something to be dealt with at a variety of levels. At first blush, we are faced with an entity comprised of multiple, interactive parts: clients, therapist(s), and the group as a whole. At any one time, individual, subgroup, and total group properties are operating, whether we are treating or measuring them. At the same time, the focus may simultaneously be on the interpersonal relationships as well as the psychological problems of individual members. Additionally, while the therapist, individual clients, and the group each has singular influence, the interactive influence must also be considered.

As they are evident and occur within the group, core constructs in psychotherapy are extremely intricate, with implications for practice and research. Take, for example, the therapeutic relationship that in group treatment encompasses multiple relationships: therapist to client, clients to clients, and clients and therapist to the group as a whole. Identifying the sources, processes, and influences of the mechanisms of change becomes exponentially complex in group. Tracking the significance of therapeutic interventions is also extremely involved, related in part not only to the designated focus but also to the unpredictable impact on the secondary participants and observers of the action. Transference, a key construct in the individual therapeutic relationship and one which most agree is difficult to define and measure, is certainly no less difficult to understand and assess in the context of a group. Its origins and possibilities are nested not only in the therapist-client relationship, but in the client-client and client-group affiliation.

Borrowed constructs from various theoretical orientations also add their intrigue and difficulty, particularly in their relationship to, and recognition of, the group structure. For example, what differences occur when we implement a cognitive-behavioral model in a group setting? Certainly the dynamics of the therapeutic relationship are altered; the potency of the clients' interaction may be impacted, and the vicarious learning of observing clients affected. Regrettably, all three are more than likely diminished. But do we know?

Perhaps, though, the "coup de grâce" in the residing complexity of group therapy is that we have a system in which diverse categories of phenomena have the potential to develop simultaneously, and in which there is always a concern as to what constitutes a singular, cumulative, or collective phenomenon. Adding to this multiplicity, the group is a moving, evolving system, comprised of interlocking parts from which, predictably, emerges a catalytic process. The finality of this complexity is that the process and the group can never go back.

DOES GROUP PSYCHOTHERAPY WORK?

The past teaches us that longevity of a treatment does not necessarily insure effectiveness (blood letting). Even though the practice of group psychotherapy has existed on two continents for nearly a century in various forms, one must still ask: What is the cumulative empirical evidence regarding group psychotherapy's overall efficacy? Appraisal of the effectiveness of group psychotherapy requires one to first address another question: Effective in comparison to what? It is evident that reviewers have responded to this question in different ways over the past 45 years and that the method of addressing this question often seems to affect the answer derived.

Early reviewers (Burchard, Michaels, & Kotkov, 1948; Thomas, 1943) address the question of effectiveness by independently cataloging studies rather than making collective statements from the literature. One of the earliest reviews was Burchard and his colleagues (1948), who reviewed 15 scientifically oriented studies of group psychotherapy. They developed a seven-factor descriptive framework to handle the wide diversity of orientation, goals, techniques, and methods found across studies. This schema not only displayed the lack of uniformity in data reported across studies, but also demonstrated the difficulty in formulating general conclusions regarding group therapy. For instance, their evaluation dimension, which addressed the success of treatment, has the least amount of information of any dimension, and the data reported were so diverse that comparative statements are impossible to derive. After attesting to their belief in the value of group psychotherapy, these authors conclude that it was "extremely difficult to draw clear-cut distinctions between group 'therapy' and [sic] many endeavors to modify the behavior, personality, and character of human beings through group participation" (pp. 257–258). As will become evident, this remark seems to be prophetic when one considers subsequent reviews of group psychotherapy.

From the 1960s forward, reviews included more composite statements of overall efficacy and less individual cataloging of studies. Twenty-two extend from the early 1960s into the 1990s (Table 1.1). While not exhaustive of all reviews published in the last three decades, these are representative of the general trends in how group psychotherapy has been viewed. Table 1.1 highlights the treatment orientation, the number of studies examined in a single review, what group treatment was compared with to determine its overall effectiveness, the population being treated, and finally, general outcome conclusions drawn from the review.

Group Therapy Outcome in the 1960s

Several important characteristics illustrate the reviews of the 1960s. First, there is a great deal of diversity in the treatment orientations of the various studies, ranging from large group milieu and nondirective therapies to traditional analytic models of treatment (Table 1.1). In addition to the traditional case studies and anecdotal reports that characterized most of the group literature in the first half of this century, there was an emergence of investigations that empirically compared group therapy with other experimental conditions, such as control groups (no-treatment conditions), group treatment alternatives, individual therapy, and combined treatment conditions (e.g., conjoint individual and group).

Nonetheless, most comparative studies reviewed in the 1960s were field studies that relied on captive populations and nonequivalent comparison groups. Specifically, comparison groups were often groups of convenience (e.g., two wards in the same hospital) and hence regarded as nonequivalent (Cook & Campbell, 1979). An important common factor to note across most of the studies reviewed in the 1960s is the high proportion of institutionalized subjects. Research subjects included a high number of inpatients as well as incarcerated adults and adolescents. Anderson's (1968) review stands out as the exception in reviewing counseling groups composed primarily of students.

The first three reviews in the 1960s provided only tentative support for the efficacy of group treatment. For instance, Rickard (1962) echoed a conclusion uttered 15 years earlier (Burchard et al., 1948): the tremendous variability in patients, therapists, and measures leads to an inadequate empirical test of the efficacy of group treatments. Pattison (1965) concluded that there was some behavioral support (e.g., soiling, hospital incidents, ward behavior scales) for group treatment success with institutionalized patients, but cautioned that these criteria could only loosely be related to the effect of group therapy. He reports disappointing results when psychological tests were used as dependent measures and calls for measures that match the changes targeted in group treatment. Stotsky and Zolik (1965) recommended group therapy as a helpful adjunctive treatment when combined with individual or pharmacological therapy but gave minimal support for its having an independent effect. An optimistic summary of these and contemporary conclusions (e.g., Krieger & Kogan, 1964) is that group therapy provides a strong complementary role to other more robust therapies, but it is not a robust independent treatment and should be examined by future controlled research to determine its effect.

Two later reviews (Mann, 1966; Anderson, 1968) during this decade espouse conclusions that are far more positive than the first three. The most complete review comes from Mann (1966) who critiqued more than 40 diversely conceived and executed studies and concluded that:

> regardless of the group psychotherapeutic method being tested or the instruments used to test it, the results were uniform. Change was found in approximately 45% of the studies. Thus, the present review clearly substantiates the fact that group psychotherapy does, indeed, produce objectively measurable changes in attitude, personality, and behavior. But this review does not indicate the clear superiority of one method of group psychotherapy over another; nor does it support the notion that group psychotherapy in general tends to produce only certain types of change in the patients who participate in it. (pp. 145–146)

Exactly 50% (11) of the studies used by Rickard (1962) in his inconclusive review were included in Mann's paper, yet the two authors arrived at

TABLE 1.1. Group Psychotherapy Review Articles

Author	Treatment Orientation	# of St.	WLC	OT/LT	I	COM	Sample	Conclusions
			Comparison					
Rickard (1962)	Nondirective, psychoanalytic, psychodrama	22	X	X	X	X	Mixed inpatient & outpatient	Too much variability among patients, therapists, and measures for comparisons to be more than tentative. Efficacy of group remains to be empirically validated.
Pattison (1965)	Psychodrama, milieu, analytic	U					Inpatient, prison, addict, delinquent	Group activity is therapeutic using behavioral criteria, disappointing with psychometric criteria and promising with construct criteria. Notes that the research on individual psychotherapy and small group research has yet to be effectively incorporated into group psychotherapy research.
Stotsky & Zolik (1965)	Psychodrama, round table, & heterogeneous group	U	X	X	X	X	Psychotics	The results of controlled experimental studies do not offer clear support for using group therapy as an independent modality, but they do support group as an adjunctive or helpful intervention when combined with other treatments (drugs, individual, etc.).
Mann (1966)	Psychodrama, nondirective	41	X	X		X	Mixed diagnosis, adult & children, most institutionalized	Group therapy produces change in behavior, attitude, and personality regardless of orientation, method of comparison, or instruments.
Anderson (1968)	Counseling groups	6	X	X		X	Primarily students	Group counseling associated with higher GPA and personality change when compared to control. No differences when compared to other treatment or combined.

Study	Type of therapy	N				Population	Findings
Meltzoff & Kornreich (1970)	Heterogeneous, expressive, nondirective, systematic desensitization, behavior, analytic	6		X	X	Hospitalized adults, adult outpatients, children	80% of adequately controlled studies reviewed showed primarily positive results with both individual and group therapy. Six studies which made direct comparisons between group and individual found equivalent outcome with a slight tendency for individual to be more effective.
Bednar & Lawlis (1971)	Heterogeneous, group psychotherapy, self-help, activity, milieu, work, insight	38	X	X	X	Mixed inpatient & outpatient, delinquents, alcoholics, sex offenders, students	Group therapy is valuable in treating neurotics, psychotics, and character disorders. It is a two-edged sword that can facilitate client deteriotation.
Luborsky et al. (1975)	Heterogeneous	12	X		X	Unspecified	Most of the 13 comparisons showed no significant differences between group and individual treatment. There was a tie in nine comparisons, group was better in two comparisons, and individual was better in two comparisons. One study had two comparisons.
Grunebaum (1975)	Unspecified	U		X		Heterogeneous	Only meager data exist comparing group and individual therapy and the evidence suggests that they are equally effective in most instances. Some findings suggest that benefits may be disorder specific, such as phobias better treated by individual therapy, and group more effective for schizophrenic outpatients.
Emrick (1975)	Heterogeneous	384	X		X	Alcoholics	Found a general trend for both individual and group to be effective in treating alcoholism.
Lieberman (1976)	Heterogeneous, psychotherapy, & personal growth groups	47	X		X	College students, adults	Group consistently produced favorable outcome over controls. Reported no outcome differences in studies that compared group with individual format. Noted that the indices used to measure outcome are relatively insensitive to the potentialities of different treatment contexts such as group and individual psychotherapy.

TABLE 1.1. (Continued)

Author	Treatment Orientation	# of St.	Comparison WLC	Comparison OT	Comparison IOM	Sample	Conclusions
Parloff & Dies (1977)	Heterogeneous, psychotherapy groups	39	X	X	X	Psychoneurotic, schizophrenic, addiction, legal offenders	Group has no unique advantage over other treatments with schizophrenic patients, no firm conclusions can be drawn with psychoneuroses, and limited support for effectiveness with addicts.
Bednar & Kaul (1978)	Heterogeneous, behavioral, TA, unspecified group therapy, & encounter groups.	21		X	X	College students, delinquents, prisoners, psychiatric patients	Group treatments have been more effective than no treatment, placebo, and other recognized psychological treatments.
Solomon (1983)	Psychodynamic, aversion	2		X	X	Alcoholics	Combined individual and group related to poorest outcome while individual and group as independent Tx showed equivalent outcomes.
Kanas (1986)	Heterogeneous	40	X	X		Outpatient & inpatient schizophrenics	Group therapy proved to be superior to controls in 67% of inpatient and 80% of outpatient studies with long-term therapy being the best.
Kaul & Bednar (1986)	Experimental psychotherapy groups	17	X	X		Primarily adult mixed diagnosis	Mixed but favorable outcomes for the efficacy of group psychotherapy.
Toseland & Siporin (1986)	Heterogeneous	32	X		X	Heterogeneous	Results of this review indicated that group treatment was as effective as individual treatment in 75% of the studies included, and was more effective in 25%. In the 32 studies reviewed, there was no case in which individual treatment was found to be more effective than group treatment.
Bostwick (1987)	Unspecified	13		X	X	Unspecified	Individual treatment had less premature termination than group while combined individual and group treatment proved superior in reducing drop-outs over either modality.

Study	Treatment type	N	WLC	COM	OT	I	Population	Findings
Oesterheld et al. (1987)	Heterogeneous, (e.g., behavioral, insight, cognitive-behavioral, dynamic)	18	X	X	X		Bulimia	Group seems to be helpful but methodological limitations preclude robust conclusions.
Zimpfer (1987)	Heterogeneous: (e.g., group counseling, multi-modal, growth, insight)	19	X	X			Elderly	Group has no significant advantage over other therapies.
Freeman & Munro (1988)	Cognitive-behavioral, eclectic, supportive, didactic	13	X	X	X	X	Bulimia	Neither drug or group as effective as individual but all are more effective than placebo. Group most cost-effective and combined group and individual most effective of all treatments.
Cox & Merkel (1989)	Heterogeneous	32	X		X	X	Bulimia	In a review of 15 groups and 17 individual studies (only one study provided a comparison between the two modalities, the rest were inferential) it was concluded that there was no support for the two treatments having any differential effectiveness.
Zimpfer (1990)	Cognitive-behavioral, psychoeducational behavior	31	X	X			Bulimia	Regardless of treatment type and outcome criteria, group was shown to be an effective treatment.
Piper & McCallum (1991)	Self-help, consciousness, cognitive restructuring, behavioral skills, dynamic	5	X	X	X		Grief	Group treatment has not been adequately tested to determine its efficacy.
Vandorvoort & Fuhriman (1991)	Cognitive-behavioral, psychodynamic, cognitive	12	X	X			Outpatient, depression	Group efficacious in treating depressions with little evidence for differences between individual and group.

Note: WLC = wait list control or comparable control group, OT = other group treatment comparison including pharmacotherapy, I = individual therapy comparison groups, COM = combined treatment group, e.g. group plus individual or group plus ward treatment.

divergent conclusions. A charitable explanation resides in Mann's mettle in simply counting the number of positive findings and essentially ignoring the fact that they came from different comparison groups, measures, and patient populations. In short, he embraced a 45% improvement rate as a respectable criterion for successful improvement.

Outcome Studies in the 1970s

The major reviews that followed in the next decade were based on studies that met more rigorous experimental criteria. Many of these reviewers proffered substantially different conclusions than their predecessors (Table 1.1). Across these seven reviews, group therapy not only consistently demonstrated its effectiveness when compared to control groups (Bednar & Kaul, 1978; Emrick, 1975; Lieberman, 1976; Luborsky, Singer, & Luborsky, 1975), but also produced comparable results to individual and alternative psychological treatments (Bednar & Kaul, 1978; Emrick, 1975; Lieberman, 1976; Luborsky et al., 1975; Meltzoff & Kornreich, 1970). These more encouraging conclusions, in contrast to those from the 1960s, may be the result of the increased rigor in investigations, movement from inpatient to diverse outpatient settings, and the emerging conceptual maturity of the field (e.g., Yalom, 1975, 1985).

Nevertheless, circumspection is warranted before one wholeheartedly adopts these conclusions. Some reviewers (Grunebaum, 1975; Parloff & Dies, 1977) during this decade still suggested that other treatment formats might be more efficacious with certain disorders. For instance, Grunebaum recommended individual treatment for phobias while Parloff and Dies deemed the treatment literature on psychoneuroses to be too embryonic to arrive at any firm conclusion. Other reviewers (Bednar & Lawlis, 1971) considered group therapy as less effective in treating patients with thought disorders, although this conclusion was challenged by later writers (e.g., Grunebaum, 1975; Kanas, 1986). An additional reason for circumspection is the lack of specificity regarding curative forces operative in group treatment that would causally account for patient improvement (Bednar & Kaul, 1978; Parloff & Dies, 1977).

Outcome Findings from the 1980s

A favorable development in the reviews of the 1980s was an increased specificity of focus. In contrast to many of the global reviews of earlier decades, in which group therapy was dealt with as an all inclusive generic treatment modality, more recent reviews concentrate on either specific treatment models or populations related to specific disorders. For the most part, group therapy as a treatment format has many variations and forms. This trend is manifested in the reviews that focus on group therapy's effectiveness in treating depression, eating disorders, bereavement, schizophrenics, and the elderly, rather than heterogeneous in- or outpatient populations found in earlier review periods. Another important refinement in this decade is the nearly uniform inclusion of multiple comparison groups, including both inert and active treatment conditions; this enables reviewers to make statements regarding both general and differential efficacy of the group format.

The conclusions of the past 12 years are parallel to those of the 1970s. Group therapy demonstrated significant improvement over inert comparison groups (Freeman & Munro, 1988; Kanas, 1986; Kaul & Bednar, 1986; Vandervoort & Fuhriman, 1991; Zimpfer, 1990) and proved comparable or superior to other active treatment conditions (Cox & Merkel, 1989; Oesterheld, McKenna, & Gould, 1987; Solomon, 1983; Toseland & Siporin, 1986; Zimpfer, 1987). In a few cases, conclusions regarding the effectiveness of the group format varied from these positive conclusions. For instance, group effectiveness in dealing with clients recovering from grief could not be determined given the limited and flawed investigations (Piper & McCallum, 1991), and a higher rate of premature termination was found for clients in group over the individual format (Bostwick, 1987). Nevertheless, the general conclusion to be drawn from some 700 studies that span the past two decades is that the group format consistently produced positive effects with diverse disorders and treatment models.

Special Issues and Concerns

This literature provides a respectable foundation upon which to build confidence in the overall effectiveness of the group treatment format. However, two concerns sully the sanguine viewpoint regarding the potency of the group format. The first concern stems from recent meta-analyses in which group therapy was shown to be inferior to other active treatments and to produce effects that were only comparable to inactive treatment conditions. The second concern lies in the frequent practice of combining group therapy with other treatments, subsequently clouding the picture in determining the independent effect of group treatment.

Meta-Analysis

In the late 1970s, Smith and Glass (1977) applied a new review strategy to psychotherapy outcome research: meta-analysis. Briefly, meta-analysis quantifies the effectiveness of a particular form of treatment by using a common measuring standard called an *effect size*. The effect size is an estimate derived from a large number of studies that quantifies the average amount of change one could expect with a particular treatment. A primary advantage of meta-analysis is this single index of "likely" client change. This is in contrast to reporting X number of studies that demonstrate a positive or negative effect, that is, the box score method.

The past decade has produced two meta-analyses with contradictory conclusions. That is, treatment offered in a group was shown to be inferior when compared to individual therapy. Seven meta-analyses published during the past ten years all compare the relative effectiveness of group versus individual format; some compare the group format with inert treatment conditions (Table 1.2). Careful inspection of these meta-analyses reveals that four of the seven state conclusions that parallel the aforementioned reviews from this decade—no reliable differences were found between individual and group treatment (Miller & Berman, 1983; Robinson, Berman, & Neimeyer, 1990; Smith, Glass, & Miller, 1980; Tillitski, 1990). One of the remaining three meta-analyses (Shapiro & Shapiro, 1982) reports a slight but nonsignificant difference between the two modalities. However, the last two (Dush, Hirt, & Schroeder, 1983; Nietzel, Russel, Hemmings, & Gretter, 1987) not only report significant superiority for individual over group treatment, but also equivalent improvement profiles for patients treated in placebo control and group therapy conditions.

A comparative analysis of the individual studies that comprise these two disparate meta-analyses (Dush et al., 1983; Nietzel et al., 1987) leads to the following explanation. In contrast to the majority of the meta-analyses in Table 1.2, the Dush and Nietzel meta-analyses rely exclusively on cognitive behavioral investigations. Moreover, careful inspection of several of the individual studies used in these two meta-analyses suggest that the majority of investigations used group as a *convenient* format to deliver predetermined treatment interventions (e.g., self-statement modification). That is, in those studies in which group treatment fared poorly, it appears that no attempt was made to incorporate or capitalize on unique properties deemed therapeutic to the group format (cf. Yalom, 1975; Bloch & Crouch, 1985). The typical investigation made no mention of attempts to facilitate traditional therapeutic factors (e.g., cohesion, universality) or to use the group-as-a-whole. Instead, the group format seems to be a convenient, cost-effective vehicle for the delivery of a treatment package originally designed for use in individual therapy. This does not necessarily suggest that such treatment orientations cannot actively utilize unique therapeutic or interpersonal factors associated with group treatment, nor does it suggest that such factors cannot naturally emerge in more structured treatments. What these studies suggest is that the treatments used in these investigations did not appear to attend to or facilitate group properties, rather they can best be described as individual treatment in the presence of others.

In contrast to the group investigations found in the Dush and Nietzel meta-analyses, most of the investigations that support the comparable efficacy of group therapy appear to highlight one or more of the unique properties of the group format. That is, rather than considering group as a *convenient and economical* format, these investigations selected group as *the* format to treat a distinct clientele or deliver a particular model of therapy based upon clinical or conceptual grounds. Thus, when group is used as *the* format to capitalize on unique therapeutic factors operative in a group environment, it is associated with larger effects than when it is considered as a format to deliver a *singular, specific* type of treatment (e.g., cognitive-behavioral).

Group Therapy Combined with Other Treatments

The question of differential efficacy when group therapy is combined with other treatment models (e.g., individual, milieu, and drug therapy) has existed for decades. Many early writers considered group therapy appropriate only when it was combined with some other form of treatment. For instance, in an early primer for group therapy, Lewis (1947) declared that "experts in group therapy do not claim that it is a substitute for individual treatment, but feel that it is indicated in special, carefully chosen cases" (p. 10).

While many of these early writers expressed convictions based on clinical practice, a few empirical investigations were published that provided parallel support. Baehr (1954), in a study of 66 WWII hospitalized veterans, found that patients who received both individual and group therapy achieved the greatest gains on a self-report scale of discontentment than those patients who were treated solely with either individual or group therapy. It is important to note that these overall gains were stable when the absolute amount of time a patient spent in treatment was controlled. In a similar contemporary investigation, Powdermaker and Frank (1953) addressed the larger effect for combined therapy by trying to tease apart the independent effects of individual and group therapy. Patients treated in combined individual and group therapy were thought to derive their primary benefit first from individual therapy (57% of patients), then from group (27%), and finally equally from both modalities (13%). It is important to note that there was no direct comparison of the two modalities in this study and that the breakdown was based on a subjective estimate of psychiatrists who were more familiar with individual treatment and hence might have been biased against the overall efficacy of group therapy.

A number of the reviews in Table 1.1 extend these early findings regarding the comparative efficacy of uniting the two formats. A robust finding from the last three decades of research is that combined individual and group treatment results in superior outcomes when compared to the independent effects of either modality (Bostwick, 1987; Freeman & Munro, 1988; Pattison, Brissenden, & Wohl, 1967). A few reviewers (Stotsky & Zolik, 1965; Anderson, 1968) have arrived at less positive conclusions, but overall, the empirical research has regarded the combined format as an effectual strategy for a wide variety of patients.

In recent years, the literature trail has moved beyond papers that attempt to determine the comparative efficacy of combining group therapy with other treatments. Rather, specific attention has focused on developing the clinical and pragmatic issues of how best to combine group with other treatments (e.g., Clarkin, Marziali, & Munroe-Blum, 1991; Lipsius, 1991; Rutan & Alonso, 1982). A harbinger of this shift was a text written by Ormont and Strean (1978) that provided a clinical treatise on how to combine individual

TABLE 1.2. Group vs. Individual Meta Analyses

Author	Treatment Orientation	Group Characteristics	Sample	Conclusions
Smith et al. (1980)	Heterogeneous	Variable	Heterogeneous	The mode in which therapy was delivered made no difference in its effectiveness. Indeed, the average effects for group and individual therapy are remarkably similar. The average effect size was 0.87 for individual therapy and 0.83 for group therapy. Of the studies reviewed, 43% were individual and 49% were group.
Shapiro & Shapiro (1982)	Heterogeneous	Average time spent in therapy was 7 hours	Heterogeneous	This refined meta-analysis of the one conducted by Smith and Glass (1977) reported that although individual therapy appeared the most effective mode ($M = 1.12$), it was closely followed by the predominant group mode ($M = 0.89$), and the only striking Tx mode finding was for couple/family therapy ($M = 0.21$).
Miller & Berman (1983)	Cognitive behavioral	Duration of treatment relatively short	Adolescents and adults, student/community volunteers & outpatients, anxious and/or depressed	This meta-analysis of 48 studies reported that cognitive behavior treatment was equally effective in group and individual formats when compared to a non-treatment group (indiv. 0.93/group = 0.79), and when compared with other treatment controls (indiv. = 0.31/group = 0.18); it should be noted that none of the studies in the review directly compared individual with group treatment within a single study.
Dush et al. (1983)	Cognitive behavioral self-statement modification	Mean weeks of treatment were 5.9 with a range of 1–26	Approximately ¼ of studies used outpatients, ¼ used community volunteers, & ½ used undergraduate depressed and anxious volunteers	Treatment modality was highly influential, with the mean effect for individual therapy nearly double that of group therapy, across all comparisons. When compared to no-treatment controls, the effect size was 0.93 for individual and 0.58 for group, and when compared to placebo controls was 0.71 for individual and 0.36 for group.

Study	Treatment	Details	Population	Findings
Nietzel et al. (1987)	Cognitive, behavioral, & other	Mean number of hours in treatment was 16.3, with a range of 3–69 (distribution between group and individual hours not made)	Individuals with unipolar depression, adults	Reports a reliable difference between individual and group treatment, with group treatment being less effective. Clients treated with group ($M = 12.47$) reported more depressive symptoms than clients, receiving individual treatment ($M = 10.06$).
Robinson et al. (1990)	Included treatments with a prominent verbal component (i.e., cognitive, cognitive-behavioral, behavioral, & general verbal therapy)	Number of clients per group ranged from 3 to 12 ($M = 7$)	Depressed individuals	Analysis indicated that both group and individual therapy produced more improvement than no treatment, and that the effects of the two approaches were comparable. The 16 studies which compared individual/group therapy with a waitlist control, and the 15 studies which compared group with a waitlist control produced nearly equal effect sizes (0.83 and 0.84 respectively).
Tillitski (1990)	Therapy, counseling, psychoeducational	Heterogeneous	Adults, adolescents, children diagnostically heterogeneous	In this re-examination of a subset of the studies looked at by Toseland and Siporin (1986), Tillitski reports finding the same average effect size for both group and individual treatment (1.35), and states that this effect was consistently greater than that of controls (0.18). Also, counseling was found to be almost twice as effective as either therapy or psychoeducation, recent studies produced larger effect sizes, and group tended to be better for adolescent and individual tended to be better for children.

and group therapy within a psychoanalytic framework. Porter (1980) further documents this shift by citing a dozen papers published over 14 years that chronicle both case study and conceptual support for the growing acceptance of the combined treatment format. He clarifies the difference between *combined* therapy in which the client is in both formats with the same therapist and *conjoint* therapy in which there is simultaneous treatment in both formats by different therapists.

Several additional conceptual advancements have appeared during the last decade. An excellent example is Slavinsky-Holy's (1983) application of an object relations perspective to the combined treatment of borderline patients. She argues that the use of both modalities facilitates individuation and splitting off from the therapist and that group therapy specifically enables the therapist to make context-relevant boundary issue interpretations. Gans (1990) provides a complementary contribution by tabulating the complex interplay of unconscious factors that occurs within patients in combined individual and group treatment. Amaranto and Bender (1990), in a fascinating reversal, explore how individual therapy can be used as a helpful adjunctive format to group therapy. With group as the primary treatment, infrequent individual therapy sessions are used to focus on members' ongoing group work and resistances that are inhibiting a productive use of the group. If significant resistances develop, more frequent individual sessions are available to assist members in the efficient use of group therapy.

A great deal of heuristically valuable conceptual material has developed over the last decade in this area. With some confidence, one can conclude that a combined approach can often be more efficacious than an independent application of one format or another. However, little understanding exists regarding the complex interplay between psychotherapeutic processes generated by combining treatments. Nevertheless, preliminary comparative process findings portend fascinating results. For instance, Brykczynska (1990), by means of a creative design, uncovered variations in the therapeutic relationship offered by the same therapist as a function of modality. Specifically, patients treated by the same therapist in either individual or group therapy systematically reported a different therapeutic relationship. More importantly, evidence from symptom reduction measures of outcome suggested that these relationship differences account for client improvement in very different ways, depending upon the modality with which the patient is being treated. Although only suggestive, these findings support some of the conceptualization just reviewed and await further empirical exploration.

EVOLUTIONARY THEMES

Topical Tales from Two Fields

Given the half-life of psychological knowledge, it makes little sense to reflect on or deduce meaning from group studies spanning 90 years of this century. On the other hand, perusal of the content or topical foci of the two lines of inquiry, small group psychology and group psychotherapy, lends some understanding to the state of research in group psychotherapy today and a modicum of insight into its conceptual roots. A topical overview also lends insight into what not only defines group process but what potentially influences it.

The phenomenon of small group process can be traced over the last 90 years through two lines of fairly independent thought and inquiry. The empirical contributions to small group psychology came largely from social psychology; the empirical evidence of group psychotherapy relied for the most part on theory transferred from the individual therapeutic tradition. It was not until the early 1970s that researchers in the two fields acknowledged the conceptual overlap and began to consider the relevancy of one field to the other (Dies, 1979).

The two endeavors are also distinguished by their overriding perspective. In the case of small group psychology, the focus is on the study of the "group," its characteristics and dynamics, and what aspects of its functioning facilitate the accomplishment of a task. On the other hand, the predominant perspective underlying group psychotherapy research is individual change and how change is facilitated within a group setting.

In the pursuit of discovering therapeutic outcome, and in the more recent venture into therapeutic process, group psychotherapy scientists and practitioners have made modest use of small group psychology and what it conceptually offers regarding the process that is birthed and developed within the context of a group. Nevertheless, an examination of the topical themes of group psychology reveals some theoretical and behavioral interconnections as they have evolved over the years.

Small Group Psychology Themes

The empirical trail of small group psychology records a steady growth in the number of studies published throughout this century. The early years (1900–1940) went from 1 to 30 per year; although prior to 1935, few were scientifically based (Zander, 1979). The following decades showed a dramatic increase both in quantity and quality, although a nagging concern persisted that the field lacked an integration of empirical findings. For the most part, the thematic content of small group psychology centers on the functioning of the group, specifically the structure of the group, its ability to accomplish the task at hand, and the interpersonal climate that facilitates task performance (Table 1.3).

Until the 1940s, issues of concern regarding the structure of the group focused mainly on reference group influence, norms, membership effect, and leadership, specifically leadership styles. Since then, the focus has broadened to include not only norms and leadership, but member roles, development, and group composition. Probably the most consistent and well-developed inquiry has been that of leadership, producing overarching

TABLE 1.3. Small Group Psychology: Thematic Evolution

	1900–1910	1911–1920	1921–1930	1931–1940	1941–1950	1951–1960	1961–1970	1971–1980	1981–1991
Models/Approaches									
Interpersonal influence	X					X	X	X	X
Problem-solving/Decision making	X		X	X	X			X	X
Group structure				X	X	X	X	X	X
Group climate				X	X	X	X	X	X
Leadership						X	X	X	X
Components						X	X	X	X

theories and describing the effectiveness of varying leader styles and techniques. Problem solving and decision making dominate the emphasis on group task, a record that is more sporadic than other themes. This effort has concentrated on identifying the kind of problems best solved by a group, the group's impact on individual problem-solving behavior, and the behaviors best suited to solve problems.

Interpersonal influence and focus span a wide range of topics from attention on conformity to the organization and effect of coalitions, social pressure, and balanced relations within a group. The core aspect of a group is its interpersonal nature and is clearly seen in studies describing the group climate. Here issues surrounding communication styles and patterns, conflict presence and resolution, and cooperative/competitive theories and behaviors are specifically addressed. Although not labeled such, process components of interest to group psychology investigators also reflect the interpersonal focus: cohesion, feedback, interaction and communication, and member participation.

The small group movement reached its height during the 1960s and 1970s. It is during this period that most of the theory and model building occurred. The focus of such activity centers generally on group dynamics and sociometry, and largely proposes models and processes for T-groups (sensitivity training) and personal growth groups.

Curiously, in the 1930s and later in the 1970s, the matter of overlap between the two fields or their relationship to one another became evident, in that some group psychologists were interested in social interaction as an aspect of mental illness treatment. It would be safe to say that this interest probably was part of the small group personal growth movement and represents in content the "coming together" of the two fields. The contribution of small group psychology to group psychotherapy is clearly evident in its empirical focus on the interpersonal and interactive nature of groups. As well, its inquiry into the group as a whole and the dynamical properties governing the group's development, functional characteristics and climate, and influence on individual change loom as significantly important to group psychotherapy. Regrettably, group psychotherapy has made but modest application of either the conceptual or empirical work of small group psychology, and has expended little effort to replicate or relate such theory and findings in therapeutic settings or situations.

Group Psychotherapy Themes

Categories of empirical study in group psychotherapy appear substantially different from those in small group psychology and perhaps stand as a testament to the separation of the two fields until the early 1970s (Table 1.4). In some cases, the general categories appear similar (e.g., structure, formats), in most cases, the specific listings are distinctively dissimilar. During the early years (1900–1940), the main lines of inquiry were topically focused on models and approaches, the therapeutic relationship, the ecosystem,

TABLE 1.4. Group Psychotherapy: Thematic Evolution

	1900–1910	1911–1920	1921–1930	1931–1940	1941–1950	1951–1960	1961–1970	1971–1980s
Formats/Theories/Models	X	X	X	X	X	X	X	X
Patient/Client populations	X	X	X	X	X	X	X	X
Therapeutic relationship			X	X	X	X	X	X
Therapist variables							X	X
Therapeutic factors	X	X	X	X	X	X	X	X
Structure							X	X
Interaction analysis							X	X
Client outcomes						X	X	X
Eco-system	X	X	X		X			X

curative factors, and interest in the physically ill, the mentally ill (as a generic category), and ultimately the child, adolescent, familial, and elderly patient. The topical focus expanded during the following 40 years. The specificity of empirical concern in the 1980s (Table 1.4) is even more heartening, in that investigators are not only examining the broad scope impacting a group (e.g., theoretical orientation, selection, relationship), but are also applying more precision to the inquiry (e.g., client by therapeutic factor by time in treatment; cognitive-behavior model by adolescent client by substance abuse treatment).

Two theoretical orientations or models of group therapy dominated the early years and continued until the late 1930s: psychodrama and psychoanalytic/dynamic. From these beginnings, interest broadened to apply models of group therapy into diverse populations and settings (family, play therapy, activity group, Tavistock, theme-centered group), some of which paralleled current interest in individual therapy (Gestalt, Transactional Analysis, counseling and personal growth group). There was also some interest in pursuing concurrent or combined individual and group treatment. The changing focal orientation waxed and waned over these years and in part can be seen in the various models and theories as they emerged. Theorists appeared to value one of three orienting perspectives: intrapersonal, interpersonal, or integral. In other words, the mechanisms of change, the intervention focal point, or the conceptual framework undergirding therapeutic effectiveness were attributed or applied to the individual's personal dynamics, the member-to-member dynamics, or the group as a whole. It is not until the 1980s that it becomes clear that all three perspectives are critical and that it is the interaction of these three dynamical components that is central to the understanding of group process. To this end, inquiry into specificity is a virtue.

The client populations studied in group therapy also reflect an evolutionary theme, clearly one of general diagnosis to more specific classifications and descriptions. Initially patients were the medically or physically ill; clearly the group was adjunctive treatment to the medical problems. Subsequently, the generic "mentally ill" inpatients were seen in groups for emotional or mental relief. Finally, closer to the 1940s, clinicians and investigators were specifying treatment to disturbed children and adolescents, elderly, and families. From the 1940s through the 1970s further delineation occurred, with treatment and inquiry focusing on inpatients (specifically chronics, psychotics, and schizophrenics), outpatients, neurotics, addicts (alcoholics), criminal offenders, juvenile delinquents, and children and adolescents. Nevertheless, to a large measure, these more distinctive patient categories were rather general in nature. The study of precise populations in a group setting (e.g., substance abuse criminal offenders, substance abuse adolescent inpatient offenders, cancer recovery patients, caregivers to the elderly) was to be left to the 1980s.

With the focus on the individual within the group, it is not surprising that writers during the first two decades had little to say regarding the therapeutic relationship. It was not until the 1920s and 1930s that the relationship gained much attention, and when it did much of it related to the client's transference relationship to the therapist (perhaps another reflection of the influence of psychodynamic thought during this period). During the 1930s, the therapeutic relationship was considered in terms of a client-to-client, client-to-therapist, or a group-as-a-whole relationship. Inquiry into the relationship was in evidence from the 1940s through the 1980s, although it is rather surprising that the effort is so modest, given the interpersonal nature of the group endeavor. It may be that what focus did occur was in fact a transfer from research in individual treatment (during the 1950s and 1960s). The client-therapist and the client-client relationships were examined far more than the client-group relationship. Member expectations and transferences occurring between clients were also specific considerations. One factor lending insight into the relative paucity of relationship inquiry may be the fact that a number of writers in the 1970s and 1980s were identifying the therapeutic factor of cohesion as being the equivalent of the therapeutic relationship; in the case of group therapy this is a tripartite representation (client-client, client-therapist, client-group) with all three dimensions contributing to the overall therapeutic relationship. As is well-documented (Bednar & Kaul, 1978; Kaul & Bednar, 1986), cohesion has one of the most extensive records of inquiry during these past two decades.

In the early years, patients and therapists identified selective factors deemed important to growth and change in patients in group settings. In the first two decades, hope (Pratt, Marsh), identification (Pratt), catharsis (Marsh), insight (Lazell, March), universality (Lazell), and interpersonal or social factors (Lazell) drew attention. Added to these in the following two decades were cohesion (Adler, Dreikurs, Horney), identification (Burrow), and re-creation of the family (Wender). Although not conceptualized as curative factors, these characteristics were considered important aspects of the therapeutic process occurring within the group.

The greatest concentration and expansion of inquiry into therapeutic factors came during the 1970s and 1980s; more than likely this emergence was due to the conceptual framework formulated by previous writers and investigators during the 1950s and 1960s, and the development of instruments designed to measure such properties. Most of the research in these decades centers on the factors articulated by Yalom (1975, 1985): altruism, catharsis, cohesion, family re-enactment, hope, identification, insight, interpersonal learning, self-disclosure, universality, and vicarious learning. Additional, more recently articulated, factors have also received empirical attention (e.g., feedback, here and now focus, reality testing, role flexibility, and consensual validation). As an area of inquiry, therapeutic factors stand as almost a singular contribution of group therapy to the therapeutic process literature. This research appears to be driven by the core assumption that client change results from the interpersonal or interactional nature of group, at least as it is manifested by the majority of specific therapeutic factors. The findings of the past three decades reveal that some factors (cohesion, interpersonal learning, catharsis) are universally valued across diverse clientele, while others have differential value depending on the specific populations.

While inquiry into client variables records a continuous effort throughout this century, therapist or leader variables drew little attention until the 1960s. Group psychotherapy relied, to a large measure, on the leadership findings from small group research. The "borrowing" of results from small group psychology is probably most evident in the leadership literature (e.g., leadership styles, leader centrality). Studies originating from group therapy during the 1960s and 1970s highlight nonspecific factors and specific intervention strategies. Confrontation, interpretation, self-disclosure, reinforcement, modeling, and overall style head the list of therapeutic interventions, followed by investigations into interventions aimed at guiding group process (e.g., implementing structured techniques, focusing on the individual or the group, determining the centrality of the leader). The function and influence of the leader received some attention, evidenced, for example, in the effect of alternating leader-attended, leader-absent sessions, and leaderless groups. Of importance is the distinction of the unique therapist roles in a group setting when compared to an individual format. These roles respond to the need for the group therapists to be flexible in the application of intervention strategies, to balance power and influence, to facilitate multiple relationships, aim the focus on either content or process, and select an individual, interpersonal, or group focus.

The 1960s saw inquiry initiated into the interactional aspect of the group and the conceptualization of the structural properties. The focus on interpersonal dialogue exemplifies the coming together of the two fields, with interactional analysis drawing on communication analysts in small group psychology and group psychotherapy. In the 1970s and 1980s, this line of inquiry continued in the therapeutic field, and currently is experiencing an increased attention focused on defining group process through the interactional dialogue of the group members (clients and therapists).

Group therapy studies that define the structural properties of the group represent an acknowledgment by investigators of the reality and influence of the group as an entity. The most conceptualized and studied structural component is that of group development. Although development was initiated and amplified by the small group theorists, therapeutic process investigators continue to explore the phenomenon, particularly in its relationship to individual processes and behavior change.

Beginning in the 1970s and continuing through the 1980s, selected investigators directed attention to the study of group norms and their relationship to the interpersonal functioning of the group (another evidence of the relationship of the two fields of inquiry). Additional attention focused on structuring components that might be related to the overall effectiveness of the group, specifically, pre-group interviews, instruction, and training.

How clients are individually and collectively selected for group certainly is a key mechanism that structurally defines the nature of the group. Given the importance of client variables in individual therapy, and the presumed importance of client composition on the group, it is indeed unfortunate that only modest empirical attention exists in the area of selection and composition. Although conceptual frameworks for the formation of a group exist, with the exception of a few investigators, what is primarily studied is composition as it is manifested by homogeneity of a specific population or theme.

At the end of this topical tirade lies a small body of research relating to the group as an ecosystem. During the first three decades (and later to be resurrected during the 1980s), consideration was given to the group as a whole, milieu therapy, and residential treatment; in other words, attention focused on the social context of the group. The group-as-a-whole construct was only sporadically addressed until the 1960s, due in part to the inherent difficulty of measuring the complex group, particularly as it relates to the individual components and their interaction, and to the influence of the group as an entity. It is more customary to track singular issues or components and to presume that process is linear, rather than track a component in context and assume that the process is dynamic.

Methodological Themes in Group Psychotherapy

Paralleling the topical evolution is an aggregate analysis of the predominant methodologies relied upon by group psychotherapy researchers. A prevailing conception in research methodology (Bednar, Burlingame, & Masters, 1988; Rosenthal & Rosnow, 1984) is that the scientific methods used in the social sciences can be ordered on the basis of rigor from descriptive (case study and survey), through relational (correlational), to more controlled methods of investigation (quasi-experimental and experimental).

Ordering investigations along a continuum of research methodology, to some degree, communicates the level of rigor and clinical relevance associated with investigations. Thus, when one catalogs the type and frequency of particular methodologies employed in an area of inquiry, it generates a rough estimate of the rigor inherent in the conclusions being made in the field. For instance, while experiments establish the necessary control to make firmer empirical conclusions regarding the efficacy of a particular treatment, they often lack the descriptive richness found in case studies. Whereas case studies provide the descriptive detail to better the understanding of "what treatment looked like," they lack the empirical stamp of approval required in our increasingly cost-effective and accountable zeitgeist.

A primary supposition underlying the ordering of investigations by methodology is that a knowledge base generated from a variety of methods has a greater potential for meeting both rigor and relevance criteria. While not axiomatic, group research that carefully incorporates descriptive research (case studies and surveys) along with rigorous experimentation will paint a better picture of the phenomena of interest. Hence, the interest in evaluating the group literature by the type of methodology used.

Given this rationale, the aforementioned literature (articles published from 1980–1992) was cataloged using five general method types: (1) experimental designs, (2) quasi-experimental designs, (3) correlational, (4) survey, and (5) descriptive case studies. If an investigation manipulated an independent variable and used random assignment into two or more treatment conditions, it was classified as an experiment. Those studies that manipulated a variable but did not use random assignment were classified as quasi-experimental investigations. Studies that focused primarily on exploring the relationship between treatment, therapist, and/or client variables, or concentrated primarily on measurement issues (reliability, validity) were classified under the correlational rubric. Studies based on survey methods were classified as such with the final category, case study, reflecting an assorted menagerie of investigations relying on pseudo-experimental or pre-experimental methods (Huck, Cormier, & Bounds, 1974), including not only case studies, but one-group pretest-post-test designs, and nonequivalent static-group comparisons.

Overall, very few topical areas of group research used all five method types over the past 12 years. The only research topic in which studies were evenly dispersed across all five methods was group therapy investigations of addictive disorders. Research on children/adolescents, personality disordered patients, and criminal populations had sparse representation in the correlational to experimental range and tend to rely more heavily on case study and survey methods. Alternatively, group research with eating disorder populations was more likely to use experimental designs to test treatment efficacy, although several descriptive case studies are evident.

A significant number of research themes appear to place a heavy emphasis on quasi-experimental and experimental methods, with most investigations focusing on treatment efficacy questions. Studies that fell into these categories include research that focused on treating victims of incest, inpatient and medical populations, depressive disorders, and the elderly. The few studies that explored patient characteristics (e.g., locus of control) and the impact of structuring treatment also tend to rely primarily on these types of designs.

Understandably, those investigations that utilized correlational methods include process studies involving both outpatient and inpatient (e.g., schizophrenia) populations. Additionally, studies focusing on interactional analysis and therapeutic factors also were more likely to be found in the correlational category. Finally, research involving less conventional group applications (dance, movement, drama, dream, fixed role) for the most part rely exclusively on case study methods, while more traditional applications (person centered, cognitive-behavioral, etc.) use quasi-experimental to experimental methods.

It is impossible to divine the goals or motives of a group psychotherapy researcher. However, after one reviews more than 400 articles on group psychotherapy spanning the past 12 years, a perspective begins to develop on both the substantive and methodological level. During the past decade, the group psychotherapy literature has been substantively dominated by treatment directed at depression, children/adolescents, criminal offenders, patients with physical or medical disorders, eating disorders, and assorted inpatient populations. The principal methodology driving this research has been comparative designs (quasi-experimental and experimental) that address the efficacy of specific treatments (e.g., cognitive-behavioral).

In an ideal empirical world, one would like to see a systematic progression of descriptive, relational, and experimental methods applied to different patient populations and treatment approaches. The knowledge base generated from this systematic empirical endeavor would undoubtedly produce the best understanding. Unfortunately, the group literature does not fit this ideal scenario, as evidenced by the brief description of methods used over the past decade.

One of the best strategies in accommodating to our variegated knowledge base is exemplified in a recent review of group therapy for bulimics (Zimpfer, 1990). In this review, conclusions and recommendations were generated after a careful collation of all descriptive, correlational, and experimental findings. This strategy contrasts the more typical reviews in which investigations that meet only the most stringent experimental criteria are reviewed. The latter approach not only gives the reader a restricted view of the literature, but also bypasses an often large and clinically meaningful group of articles.

THE 1980s: CONGLOMERATE AND
COMPLEXITY REVISITED

In an attempt to unravel the conglomerate and complex nature of the research literature from the 12 years, the substantive themes were crossed by the principal characteristic of members that comprised each study. While not exhaustive, this summary of more than 400 articles published during 1980–1992 reflects major thematic thrusts and client populations (Table 1.5).* For example, nearly 30 distinct client populations were identified in these studies. Only a dozen are highlighted, with less frequently investigated populations (e.g., pathological gamblers, Vietnam veterans, stutterers) eliminated for comparative purposes. In a similar vein, only those thematic areas that had a sizeable number of studies were included. For

---

* The topical and methodological themes of the 1980s (1980–1992) were derived from the noted 400 articles on group psychotherapy. A bibliographic listing of the selected literature may be obtained from the editors.

TABLE 1.5. Substantive Themes by Clinical Populations

	Child/ Adolescent	Medical	Depressed	Eating Disorder	Substance Abuse	Criminal	In- Patient	Family/ Marital	Elderly	Out- Patient	Schizophrenic	Sexual Abuse	Personality Disorder	Not Specified	Other*
Models/Approaches															
Cognitive-behavioral	X	X	X	X	X	X	X	X	X	X		X	X	X	X
Short-term	X	X	X				X	X	X	X		X	X	X	
Rogerian										X					X
Gestalt											X			X	
Personal growth						X	X							X	
Psychodrama	X					X	X								
Therapist variables	X	X	X	X	X	X	X	X	X	X	X		X	X	X
Directiveness			X							X	X				X
Interpretation												X		X	
Therapeutic factors	X	X	X	X	X	X	X	X	X	X	X			X	X
Structure	X	X	X	X	X	X		X	X	X		X	X	X	X
Development						X		X		X				X	
Pregroup training								X		X				X	
Interaction	X		X		X	X	X	X	X	X	X	X		X	X

*Various nontherapeutic designations.

instance, although more than thirty treatment models were identified, most appeared so infrequently in the sample of studies that they did not warrant inclusion for comparative analysis (e.g., Tavistock groups, clinical sociology groups, validation therapy, sex role differentiation groups, phenomenological therapy), resulting in only six being highlighted. While such infrequency does not lend itself to comparative analysis, it nevertheless underscores the increased specificity of approach and population that is occurring in the research.

On the one hand, the information detailed in Table 1.5 might be viewed as another conglomerate of empirical toil. With each tally representing from one to dozens of published studies, one can begin to note the diversity of themes and populations encompassed in recent investigations. An alternative perspective is that contemporary group research is attempting to tease apart the complexity of group psychotherapy by carefully dissecting its component parts. If one accepts the recurrent observation that interaction rather than main effects characterize findings in most psychological investigations, the findings in Table 1.5 can be seen as a promising harbinger. That is, the diversity of focus and population may not be a conglomerate, but rather an answer to the seasoned call for specificity regarding precise treatments being offered to distinct client populations with salient therapist characteristics either measured or controlled. If so, it once again calls our attention to the need for replication across populations and settings.

Models and Approaches

The number of investigations focusing on cognitive behavioral group treatment by far outweigh the application of any other model. Although more frequently applied to depressed, eating disordered, and outpatient populations, this approach was systematically employed in the reviewed studies with every patient population listed, except one (schizophrenics). Unfortunately, what is not portrayed by Table 1.5 is the multifarious nature of many investigations, such as factorial investigations that simultaneously examine several dimensions (e.g., treatment model by therapist variables). These design practices will undoubtedly lead to a clearer understanding of the model by patient by therapist interaction.

In contrast to structured approaches such as cognitive behavioral treatment, interpersonal models of group therapy (e.g., Yalom, Rogerian) that emphasize interactive-interpersonal treatment do not frequently occupy the primary focus of the studies reviewed. More often, these traditional groups serve a comparative-treatment condition function. The diminishing use of interactive-interpersonal models is disconcerting, given the aforementioned differences reported regarding the effect sizes between these two applications of group therapy. That is, cognitive behavioral group treatment studies seem to be associated with smaller effect sizes than those derived from more traditional interactive-interpersonal models. A final observation regarding models lies with the short-term approaches. Although the vast majority of the group literature can be considered brief in duration (Burlingame & Fuhriman, 1990), only those studies using a model that was clearly designated as a conceptually based short-term approach was coded under the short-term category. Despite this more restrictive definition, conceptually planned models of short-term therapy were applied with nearly two-thirds of the patient populations citing a more expansive realm of influence from previous decades.

Therapist Variables

A similar pattern of diversity is reflected within the therapist variable dimension. Studies coded into this category had to manipulate or measure some therapist attribute directly or report on a unique therapist effect in the result section, including post hoc findings. In spite of the frequency of studies addressing therapist effects that spanned nearly every patient category, conclusions regarding therapist variables appear to be consistently based on secondary or discovered (post hoc) findings. Studies that single out and systematically study therapist variables are rare, with only a handful focused on the primary effect of interventions or therapist attributes.

Therapeutic Factors

Studies coded into the therapeutic factors category include the traditional "curative" factors as well as investigations that measure some aspect of the group process that was considered restorative. This thematic focus area is one of the most robust spheres within the group literature reviewed. Not only were there a large number of studies that fell within this category, but the studies also evenly span each patient population category. The combined effect of a large number of studies crossed with diverse patient populations is a requisite to unraveling the complexity of how therapeutic factors operate across diverse settings and clientele.

Despite these strengths, an important refinement much needed in the therapeutic factor or change mechanism area of research is the inclusion of multiple sources and methods for their assessment. The majority of studies within this category rely on a single client self-report measure to evaluate the therapeutic qualities of the group. While single-point assessments are helpful, complexity is best unraveled when multiple perspectives and measures are used.

Structure and Interaction

The structure category tallies the investigations that explore the effects of structured versus unstructured group treatments, group development, and the influence of pre-group training on group process and outcome. A paucity of studies focuses attention on the latter two groupings, with most investigations falling into the unspecified patient population category. As evidenced in Table 1.5, what we can know regarding group development and pre-group training is circumscribed by the lack of diversity of populations used in such investigations.

A similar, though less restricting pattern, is noted in studies that focus on structured versus unstructured treatments. A greater number of studies fall into this category and reflect a relatively broad spectrum of clientele as well. However, the vast majority of structure studies use either unspecified or adolescent and child populations. That is, although the relative number of populations studied within this theme is nearly comparable to those found in the therapeutic factors theme, the absolute number of studies is far smaller.

Finally, the interaction category reflects investigations that concentrate on the interplay between members and leaders. Usually such studies rely on behavioral observation systems that categorize and plot aspects of group verbalizations. Studies centered on interaction analyses seem to have increased during the 1980s. While investigated less than therapeutic factors, it is heartening to see the diversity of clientele in which interactional patterns are being studied and detailed.

Concluding Comment

An analysis of the emergent patterns across all thematic dimensions gives rise to a few general observations. First, in contrast to earlier decades, research often seems to be driven by specific client population concerns, rather than more general theoretical or conceptual issues. As with congress, it seems that the "special interest groups" wield a great deal of influence in what is being investigated and published. Although this is not necessarily an unsatisfactory state of affairs, it does have a tendency to decrease the generalizability of the knowledge base.

Second, research that is based on viewing the group as a dynamic therapeutic ecosystem is noticeably underemphasized. The shortage of studies that focus on composition, group development, and interaction illustrate such inattention. That is, the less one highlights the importance of the group as an entity above and beyond the individual members, the less interest generated in factors that describe the group's evolution (e.g., group development) and dynamic properties (e.g., interaction).

The de-emphasis on the interactive ecosystem is disconcerting, given that group therapy's unique contribution to the psychotherapy literature lies within the distinctive properties of the ecosystem. Although the aforementioned increase in factorial designs may shed light on the interplay between individual client, therapist, and group factors, our hope is that the shortage of research on ecosystem dimensions (composition, development, and interaction) is temporary and does not portend a long-term future trend.

A concluding perspective to this historical and empirical overview lies in an examination of previous solicitations and observations from past reviewers of the group literature. Inspection of the research "calls" from successive reviews reveals an emerging maturity in ensuing decades that often entails more complex and obstinate conceptual and empirical problems. For instance, in a review of studies conducted during the 1960s, Anderson's (1968) general conclusion was that there was still no body of theoretically related knowledge upon which to found the practice of group psychotherapy. Nearly a decade later, Lieberman (1976) proposed that one way to increase the relevancy of research for the practice of group psychotherapy was to conduct collaborative investigations that link process with outcome. A key element for success in responding to such requests would be a collaboration between researchers and practitioners. Such collaborative efforts would not only alleviate the logistical difficulties in carrying out robust group investigations, but would also insure relevancy to group practice.

Two reviews of the same vintage suggested additional refinements. Parloff and Dies (1977) called for explicit definitions and descriptions of varying techniques and forms of group therapy. Such specificity could then be used to stimulate the development of treatment manuals for different classes of patients being treated in the group format. Specificity was seen as a necessary step in separating out the conceptual identity of the group discipline from other treatment modalities (e.g, individual). In a contemporary review, Dies (1979) also envisioned greater specificity as requisite to delineating salient group parameters and understanding the group in the larger context of a client's life.

A few years later, Hartman (1979) suggested that the complexity of the group experience might be better mirrored by content analysis systems rather than by single process variables. The increasing recognition of the complexity of studying group psychotherapy is extended into the 1980s with the observation that research designs should consider and test intervening group process variables in order to explain differential client outcome, rather than relying on simple main effects as a primary explanatory variable (Kaul & Bednar, 1986). These authors still considered the primary and unique characteristics of group to be undefined. However, other contemporary reviewers (Klein, 1985) concluded that enough was known to suggest the need for group leaders to develop specific skills, including system diagnostic, individual, subgroup, and large group intervention strategies.

Reviewing these observations brings us full circle to the description of group therapy as conglomerate and complex. Nearly every reviewer, to one degree or another, bemoans the inability to link one group study with another in a manner that makes integrated conclusions possible and practice coherent: conglomerate revisited. There is an increasing level of sophistication in recommendations not only concerning the who, what, and how in therapeutic investigations, but also the understanding of their relationships and dynamics: complexity revisited. It is this interplay between the conglomerate and complex that makes the study and practice of group psychotherapy a challenge—one that is exciting, stimulating, and well worth the effort.

REFERENCES

Amaranto, E., & Bender, S. (1990). Individual psychotherapy as an adjunct to group psychotherapy. *International Journal of Group Psychotherapy, 40*(1), 91–101.

Anderson, A. (1968). Group counseling. *Review of Educational Research, 33,* 209–226.

Anthony, E. J. (1968). Reflections on twenty-five years of group psychotherapy. *International Journal of Group Psychotherapy, 18,* 277–301.

Anthony, E. J. (1971). The history of group psychotherapy. In H. Kaplan and B. Sadock (Eds.), *Comprehensive group psychotherapy* (1st ed.). Baltimore, MD: William & Wilkins.

Back, K. W. (1979). The small group: Tightrope between sociology and personality. *The Journal of Applied Behavioral Science, 15*(3), 283–294.

Baehr, G. (1954). The comparative effectiveness of individual psychotherapy, group psychotherapy, and a combination of these methods. *Journal of Consulting Psychology, 13,* 179–183.

Bednar, R., Burlingame, G., & Masters, K. (1988). Systems of family treatment: Substance or semantics? In R. Rosenweig & L. Porter (Eds.), *Annual Review of Psychology, 39,* 401–434. Palo Alto, CA: Annual Reviews, Inc.

Bednar, R., & Kaul, T. (1978). Experiential group research: Current perspectives. In S. Garfield & A. Bergin (Eds.), *Handbook of psychotherapy and behavior change* (2nd ed.). New York: Wiley.

Bednar, R., & Kaul, T. (1979). Experiential group research: What never happened! *The Journal of Applied Behavioral Science, 15*(3), 311–319.

Bednar, R., & Lawlis, G. (1971). Empirical research in group psychotherapy. In A. Bergin & S. Garfield (Eds.), *The handbook of psychotherapy and behavior change.* New York: Wiley.

Bloch, S., & Crouch, E. (1985). *Therapeutic factors in group psychotherapy.* Oxford: Oxford University Press.

Bostwick, G. (1987). Where's Mary? A review of the group treatment dropout literature. *Social Work with Groups, 10*(3), 117–132.

Brykczynska, C. (1990). Changes in the patient's perception of his therapist in the process of group and individual psychotherapy. *Psychotherapy and Psychosomatics, 53*(1), 179–184.

Burlingame, G. M., & Fuhriman, A. (1990). Time-limited group therapy. *The Counseling Psychologist, 18*(1), 93–118.

Burchard, E., Michaels, J., & Kotkov, B. (1948). Criteria for the evaluation of group therapy. *Psychosomatic Medicine, 10*(3), 257–274.

Clarkin, J., Marziali, E., & Munroe-Blum, H. (1991). Group and family treatments for borderline personality disorder. *Hospital and Community Psychiatry, 42*(10), 1038–1043.

Cook, T., & Campbell, D. (1979). *Quasi-Experimentation: Design and analysis issues for field settings.* Boston, MA: Houghton Mifflin.

Cox, G., & Merkel, W. (1989). A qualitative review of psychosocial treatments for bulimia. *The Journal of Nervous & Mental Disease, 177*(2), 77–84.

Dies, R. (1978). Introduction: Therapy and encounter group research. *Small Group Behavior, 9*, 163–172.

Dies, R. (1979). Group psychotherapy: Reflections on three decades of research. *The Journal of Applied Behavioral Science, 15*(3), 361–374.

Dies, R. (1993). Research on group psychotherapy: Overview and clinical applications. In A. Alonso & H. Swiller (Eds.), *Group therapy in clinical practice.* Washington, DC: American Psychiatric Press.

Dreikurs, R. (1950). Psychotherapie de groupe. Paper read at the *International Congress on Psychiatry,* Paris, France.

Dreikurs, R. (1969a). Early experiments with group psychotherapy: A historical review. In H. Ruitenbeek (Ed.), *Group therapy today.* New York: Atherton Press.

Dreikurs, R. (1969b). Group psychotherapy from the point of view of Adlerian psychology. In H. Ruitenbeek (Ed.), *Group therapy today.* New York: Atherton Press.

Dush, D., Hirt, M., & Schroeder, H. (1983). Self-statement modification with adults: A meta-analysis. *Journal of Consulting and Clinical Psychology, 94*, 408–422.

Emrick, C. (1975). A review of psychologically oriented treatment of alcoholism. *Journal for the study of alcoholism, 36*(1), 88–108.

Foulkes, S. H., & Anthony, E. J. (1957). *Group psychotherapy: The psychoanalytic approach.* London: Penguin Books.

Freeman, C., & Munro, J. (1988). Drug and group treatments for bulimia/bulimia nervosa. *Journal of Psychosomatic Research, 32*(6), 647–660.

Fuhriman, A., & Barlow, S. (1982). Cohesion: Relationships in group therapy. In M. Lambert (Ed.), *Psychotherapy and patient relationships.* Homewood, IL: Dorsey Professional Series.

Fuhriman, A., & Burlingame, G. (1990). Consistency of matter: A comparative analysis of individual and group process variables. *The Counseling Psychologist, 18*(1), 6–63.

Gans, J. (1990). Broaching and exploring the question of combined group and individual therapy. *International Journal of Group Psychotherapy, 40*(2), 123–137.

Gazda, G. M. (1989). An analysis of the group counseling research literature. In G. M. Gazda (Ed.), *Group counseling: A developmental approach* (4th ed.). Boston, MA: Allyn & Bacon.

Grunebaum, H. (1975). A soft-hearted review of hard-nosed research on groups. *International Journal of Group Psychotherapy, 25*(2), 185–197.

Hartman, J. (1979). Small group methods of personal change. *Annual Review of Psychology, 30*, 453–476.

Huck, S., Cormier, W., & Bounds, W. (1974). *Reading statistics and research.* New York: HarperCollins.

Kanas, N. (1986). Group psychotherapy with schizophrenics: A review of controlled studies. *International Journal of Group Psychotherapy, 36*, 339–351.

Kanzer, M. (1983). Freud: The first psychoanalytic group leader. In H. Kaplan & B. Sadock (Eds.), *Comprehensive group psychotherapy* (2nd ed.). Baltimore, MD: Williams & Wilkins.

Kaul, T., & Bednar, R. (1986). Experiential group research: Results, questions & suggestions. In S. Garfield & A. Bergin (Eds.), *Handbook of psychotherapy and behavior change.* New York: Wiley.

Klein, E. B. (1985 May). Group work: 1985 and 2001. *Journal for Specialists in Group Work,* 108–111.

Krieger, M., & Kogan, W. (1964). A study of group processes in the small therapeutic group. *International Journal of Group Psychotherapy, 14,* 178–188.

Lakin, M. (1979). Introduction: What's happened to small group research? *The Journal of Applied Behavioral Science, 15*(3), 265–270.

Lewis, N. (1947). Foreward in S. Slavson (Ed.), *The practice of group therapy.* New York: International Universities Press.

Lieberman, M. (1976). Change induction in small groups. *Annual Review of Psychology, 27,* 217–250.

Lipsius, S. (1991). Combined individual and group psychotherapy: Guidelines at the interface. *International Journal of Group Psychotherapy, 4*(3), 313–327.

Luborsky, L., Singer, B., & Luborsky, L. (1975). Comparative studies of psychotherapy. *Archives of General Psychiatry, 32,* 995–1008.

Mann, J. (1966). Evaluation of group psychotherapy. In J. Moreno (Ed.), *The international handbook of group psychotherapy.* New York: Philosophical Library.

McGrath, J., & Kravitz, D. (1982). Group research. *Annual Review of Psychology, 33,* 195–230.

Meltzoff, J., & Kornreich, M. (1970). *Research in psychotherapy.* New York: Atherton Press.

Miller, R., & Berman, J. (1983). The efficacy of cognitive behavior therapies: A quantitative review of research evidence. *Psychological Bulletin, 94,* 39–53.

Moreno, J., & Whitin, E. (1932). *Application of the group method to classification.* New York: National Commission on Prison and Prison Labor.

Neiberg, N. A. (1980). Group psychotherapy: Retrospect, current status, and prospects. *International Journal of Group Psychotherapy, 30*(3), 259–271.

Nietzel, M., Russel, R., Hemmings, K., & Gretter, M. (1987). Clinical significance of psychotherapy for unipolar depression: A meta-analytic approach to social comparison. *Journal of Consulting and Clinical Psychology, 55*(2), 156–161.

Oesterheld, A., McKenna, M., & Gould, N. (1987). Group psychotherapy of bulimia: A critical review. *International Journal of Group Psychotherapy, 37*(2), 163–184.

Ormont, L., & Strean, H. (1978). *The practice of conjoint therapy: Combining individual and group treatment.* New York: Human Science Press.

Parloff, M., & Dies, R. (1977). Group psychotherapy outcome research. *International Journal of Group Psychotherapy, 27,* 281–319.

Pattison, E. (1965). Evaluation studies of group psychotherapy. *International Journal of Group Psychotherapy, 15*(3), 382–397.

Pattison, E., Brissenden, A., & Wohl, T. (1967). Assessing specific effects of inpatient group psychotherapy. *International Journal of Group Psychotherapy, 17,* 283–297.

Piper, W., & McCallum, M. (1991). Group interventions for persons who have experienced loss: Description and evaluative research. *Group Analysis, 24,* 363–373.

Porter, K. (1980). Combined individual and group psychotherapy: A review of the literature. *International Journal of Group Psychotherapy, 30*(1), 107–114.

Powdermaker, F., & Frank, J. (1953). *Group psychotherapy: Studies in methodology of research and therapy.* Cambridge, MA: Harvard University Press.

Rickard, H. (1962). Selected group psychotherapy evaluation studies. *Journal of General Psychology, 67,* 35–50.

Robison, F., & Ward, D. (1990). Research activities and attitudes among ASGW members. *Journal for Specialists in Group Work, 15,* 215–224.

Robinson, L., Berman, J., Neimeyer, R. (1990). Psychotherapy for the treatment of depression: A comprehensive review of controlled outcome research. *Psychological Bulletin, 108*(1), 30–49.

Roller, B. (1986). Group therapy marks fiftieth birthday. *Small Group Behavior, 17*(4), 472–474.

Rosenthal, R., & Rosnow, R. (1984). *Essentials of behavioral research: Methods and data analysis.* New York: McGraw-Hill.

Ruitenbeek, H. (1969). *Group therapy today.* New York: Atherton Press.

Rutan, J., & Alonso, A. (1982). Group therapy, individual therapy, or both? *International Journal of Group Psychotherapy, 32*(3), 267–282.

Sadock, B., & Kaplan, H. (1983). History of group psychotherapy. In H. Kaplan & B. Sadock (Eds.), *Comprehensive group psychotherapy* (2nd ed.). Baltimore, MD: Williams & Wilkins.

Schaffer, J. B., & Galinsky, M. D. (1974). *Models of group therapy and sensitivity training.* Englewood Cliffs, NJ: Prentice Hall.

Schiedlinger, S. (1984). Group psychotherapy in the 1980's: Problems and prospects. *American Journal of Psychotherapy, 38*(4), 494–504.

Shapiro, D., & Shapiro, D. (1982). Meta-analysis of comparative therapy outcome studies: A replication and refinement. *Psychological Bulletin, 92,* 581–604.

Slavinsky-Holy, N. (1983). Combining individual and homogenous group psychotherapies for borderline conditions. *International Journal of Group Psychotherapy, 33*(3), 297–312.

Smith, M., & Glass, G. (1977). Meta-analysis of psychotherapy outcome studies. *American Psychologist, 32,* 752–760.

Smith, M., Glass, G., & Miller, T. (1980). *The benefits of psychotherapy.* Baltimore, MD: Johns Hopkins University Press.

Solomon, S. (1983). Individual versus group therapy: Current status in the treatment of alcoholism. *Advances in Alcohol and Substance Abuse, 2*(1), 69–86.

Spitz, H. (1984). Contemporary trends in group psychotherapy: A literature survey. *Hospital and Community Psychiatry, 35*(2), 132–142.

Stotsky, B., & Zolik, E. (1965). Group psychotherapy with psychotics. *International Journal of Group Psychotherapy, 15*(3), 321–344.

Thomas, G. (1943). Group psychotherapy: A review of recent literature. *Psychosomatic Medicine, 5,* 166–180.

Tillitski, L. (1990). A meta-analysis of estimated effect sizes for group versus individual versus control treatments. *International Journal of Group Psychotherapy, 40*(2), 215–224.

Toseland, R., & Siporin, M. (1986). When to recommend group treatment. *International Journal of Group Psychotherapy, 36,* 172–201.

Vandervoort, D., & Fuhriman, A. (1991). The efficacy of group therapy for depression. *Small Group Research, 22*(3), 320–338.

Vriend, J. (1985). We've come a long way group. *Journal for Specialists in Group Work, 10*(2), 63–67.

Yalom, I. D. (1975/1985). *The theory and practice of group psychotherapy* (2nd/3rd ed.). New York: Basic Books.

Zander, A. (1979). The psychology of group processes. *Annual Review of Psychology, 30,* 417–451.

Zander, A. (1979). The study of group behavior during four decades. *Journal of Applied Behavioral Science, 15*(3), 272–282.

Zimet, C., & Fine, H. (1955). Methodology and evaluation in group psychotherapy. *Group Psychotherapy, 11,* 186–196.

Zimpfer, D. (1987). Groups for the aging: Do they work? *Journal for Specialists in Group Work, 12*(2), 85–92.

Zimpfer, D. (1990). Group work for bulimia: A review of outcomes. *Journal for Specialists in Group Work, 15*(4), 239–251.

CHAPTER 2

Methodological Considerations in Group Psychotherapy Research: Past, Present, and Future Practices

GARY M. BURLINGAME, JOHN C. KIRCHER, and SHAWN TAYLOR

A recurrent observation made by reviewers of group psychotherapy research is that investigators often seem to be unaware of others' work and thus fail to build on past knowledge and mistakes (cf. Kaul & Bednar, 1986; Rickard, 1962). It seems that such historical myopia has led to a research and methodology literature that is neither cumulative nor integrated. In preparing for this chapter, we reviewed nearly 50 years of methodological critiques and recommendations for conducting group psychotherapy research. Not only did it seem that many group therapy investigators declined to attend to the methodological recommendations predating their research, but also that reviewers who offered methodological commentary were relatively unaware of preceding or contemporary methodological recommendations.

Perhaps this inattention is related to the uneasiness and antipathy that is often generated when clinicians confront methodological and statistical issues. Such apprehensive emotional responses were documented more than 30 years ago by Luchins (1960) and are still present for many. Perhaps we have forgotten the longstanding adage that the "scientific method is simply the way in which we test impressions, opinions, or surmises by examining the best available evidence" (Cohen & Nagel, 1934, p. 192), and that "experimental and statistical methods do not create insight, they merely verify them" (Frank, 1950, p. 200). Perhaps we are reluctant to confront the inherently complex task of quantifying the dynamic properties of the small group, an effort that was recently branded as having an astronomical number of methodological difficulties (Salvendy, 1991).

The intent of this chapter is to provide a guide to methodological issues confronted in group psychotherapy research. Our strategy centers first on collating and reviewing methodological recommendations raised during the last 50 years. This historical documentation not only establishes the field's methodological heritage, but also serves to identify recurrent methodological criteria. These criteria are also used to describe and evaluate the methodological practices used during the past 12 years of group therapy research. We conclude with several prescriptive recommendations that address the strengths and weaknesses delineated during the past decade of empirical toil.

PREVIOUS METHODOLOGICAL REVIEWS AND RECOMMENDATIONS

It is a reasonably simple task for a methodologist to construct an ideal set of criteria based on standard research design and methods texts (e.g., Cook & Campbell, 1979; Kirk, 1982), and then employ these criteria to judge a body of research. While this practice may be defensible on scientific grounds, it fails to consider the relative maturity of a particular area of inquiry. By necessity, scientific inquiry must often emphasize descriptive and pre-experimental methods over pure experimental strategies as a means of avoiding research reports that are methodologically sound, but largely without substance or relevance. At worst, indifference to the developmental stage of knowledge in constructing and applying review criteria leads to the creation of a straw man that will unquestionably find research strategies wanting; at best, it culls robust studies with solid methodologies, yet offers a narrow perspective on findings of a particular body of research.

To avoid a strict purist stance in selecting methodological criteria from which to evaluate the past decade of group research, we examined nearly 60 major reviews and methodology papers from 1948–1992. This literature provided a content-relevant context from which to compile an inventory of methodological issues, recommendations, and criteria. Two major trends emerge in these review articles. First, publications from the 1940s through the 1970s tend to treat group psychotherapy as a specific treatment applied in diverse settings with varied diagnostic groups. Hence, reviews from this period are likely to be global, focusing on several types of treatment orientations and patient groups. In comparison, reviews published during the 1980s and 1990s, as a group, tend to be far more limited and specific in their coverage. They approach group therapy as a format, and focus on a specific treatment orientation (e.g., cognitive-behavioral, interpersonal, psychodynamic) or patient population (bulimia, depression, sex offenders, etc.).

A second trend, occurring in more than half of the papers (36), is the reviewers' efforts to highlight specific methodological issues or suggestions. During the early years, these recommendations were globally aimed at group psychotherapy investigations, whereas later comments and suggestions often centered on specific treatment, population, or format issues. These issues and recommendations are summarized in three tables addressing: (a) global research design issues (Table 2.1), (b) characteristics of measures and variables typically used in group investigations (Table 2.2), and (c) specific issues that relate to the observation and analysis of group treatment, therapists, group members, and the group-as-a-whole (Table 2.3). The numeric entries in each table represent the number of papers that raise a particular issue during a given decade.

Design

Not surprisingly, the global design considerations summary contains the largest number of entries. As shown in Table 2.1, the most frequent and long-standing recommendation is a call for reliance on careful observation of group events as a means of discovering salient relationships. In earlier years, this recommendation took the form of criticism of the amount of energy

TABLE 2.1.   Design Recommendations and Issues

	Number of Articles Published					
	1940s	1950s	1960s	1970s	1980s	1990s
Designs rely on careful observation of group events to discover relationships	1	2	3	2	1	
Need greater control, specification of independent variables, and randomization of subjects		1	4	1	1	1
Antagonism between researcher and practitioner exists		1	2	3	1	
Controlled, complex large factional designs needed for comparative conclusions			3	1	2	1
Designs should focus on process-outcome relationships		2	1	1	2	
Pre/post and follow-up testing and replication is needed			2	3		
Specify (or avoid) concurrent treatments to tease out specific effects of inpatient group therapy			2		1	2
Search for interaction rather than main effects; global effectiveness not meaningful			2	1	2	
Research should be naturalistic field and not laboratory or experimental			1	2		
Checks on experimenter bias and impact of research on client is recommended			1	1		
Need designs that test for intervening variables				1	1	
Design should remain at level of clinical hypothesis testing		1	1			
Patients in comparative studies should be comparable on outcome measures at pretreatment			1			1
Quasi-experiments posed as alternative to naturalistic and experimental methods			1			
Group therapists operate from particular not general theories—these particular postulates need study			1			

devoted to devising adequate controls, rather than to accumulating and documenting the clinical observations essential to the discovery of significant relationships (Burchard, Michaels, & Kotkov, 1948; Frank, 1950). During the 1960s, writers (Bennis, 1960; Pattison, Brissenden, & Wohl, 1967) continued to emphasize the importance of descriptive research. For instance, Stotsky and Zolik (1965) suggested that descriptive studies provide the fodder necessary to nourish focused experimental studies. Twenty years later, Kaul and Bednar (1986) re-emphasized this position by admonishing group investigators to remember that "step one in science is careful observation and description," and that group research can benefit from understanding "that while explanation is the crown of science, description is its base" (p. 710–711).

The second most frequent recommendation can be viewed as counterpoint to the above, because it underscores the need for greater experimental control and specification of independent variables. While much of the group research conducted between 1940 and 1960 involves meager description, ineffectual comparisons, and anecdotal reports (cf. Luchins, 1960; Mann, 1966; Rickard, 1962), the beginnings of a move toward increasing rigor can be found in an early paper by Frank (1950) in which he discussed the importance, yet infeasibility of randomizing subjects in group investigations. Frank considered matching as an alternative, but concluded that the field lacked the information necessary to identify the variables on which subjects should be matched.

A relatively greater emphasis on rigor in group investigations began to emerge in the early 1960s. For example, Bennis (1960) stressed the importance of controlling experimenter bias, and Rickard (1962) called for large-scale factorial designs as a means of reaching firm comparative treatment conclusions. One of the most eloquent and useful early deliberations on rigor in group psychotherapy research was provided in a symposium in which each member of the panel addressed a different set of methodological problems in group therapy research (Bennis, 1961; Gundlach, 1967; Parloff, 1961). As can be seen in Table 2.1, the emphasis on rigor seemed to propel many of the recommendations generated by subsequent reviewers during the 1960s and into the 1970s. Suggestions included how to create equivalent treatment conditions, the importance of using pre- and post-testing along with follow-up, specification, or avoidance of concurrent treatments that might contaminate the specific effects under study, and the significance of developing designs that could test for interaction rather than main effects. In essence, these suggestions parallel the recommendations one finds in standard experimental design textbooks.

From the late 1970s into the 1980s, a fascinating shift in methodological recommendations began to emerge. For example, Parloff and Dies (1977) suggested that group research methodology suffered more from a clinical-conceptual malaise than from technical or methodological shortcomings. They suggested that researchers should focus less on methodological precision, and more on the relevancy of research to the practice of group therapy. Other writers also began to adopt and expand this position. For instance, Fuhriman, Drescher, and Burlingame (1984) argued that group psychotherapy process research needed to place methodological consider-ations within a group-specific conceptual paradigm, and proposed such a model (Burlingame, Fuhriman, & Drescher, 1984). Kaul and Bednar's (1986) recommendations also echoed this theme by suggesting that re-search designs conceptually and methodologically recognize and clarify the numerous sources of influence in group research.

The design recommendations in Table 2.1 reveal a circuitous course across the decades, with bids for clinical and conceptual relevancy dominat-ing the early research, a call for greater methodological rigor moving into the forefront during the 1960s and 1970s, followed by a return to an empha-sis on the importance of methodological rigor within a conceptually rele-vant framework. The process-outcome research during the last 40 years is a good example of how design recommendations in group therapy have evolved. In the 1950s, Sherwood (1956) and Cartwright and Zander (1953) asserted that the relationship between group functions and their associated outcomes is the most contextually relevant and important group research that can be conducted. Writers in the 1960s and 1970s (Anderson, 1968; Hartman, 1979; Lieberman, 1976) echoed this view, but also pointed out that rigorous process research consistently used analogue or laboratory set-tings with manipulation of process variables that often do not parallel the mechanisms of change in actual group therapy (Bednar & Kaul, 1978; Dies, 1979). The emerging consensus of reviewers during the 1980s and 1990s is perhaps best typified by Dies (1985), who argued that it may be neces-sary to compromise methodological rigor if one is to study natural process-outcome relationships. A promising methodological endnote for the late 1980s and early 1990s was the introduction of specific strategies and de-signs for conducting small-n research in group therapy (Husle-Killacky, Robison, & Morran, 1991; Robison, Morran, & Hulse-Killacky, 1989).

Measures and Variables

If the guidance outlined in Table 2.1 regards *how* researchers might go about observing group therapy, then the suggestions contained in Table 2.2 are more descriptive as to *what* investigators should observe in group therapy investigations. That is, the table summarizes reviewers' advice concerning what measures should be included in research on group psychotherapy.

As might be expected, early reviewers (Bennis, 1960; Frank, 1950; Rickard, 1962) declared that our knowledge was too limited to measure the salient aspects of group therapy adequately. One group of writers during this time frame suggested that substantive group phenomena operate on an indirect, symbolic level and consequently cannot be measured objectively (e.g., Stock & Lieberman, 1962). This claim of limited knowledge and few measures is consistent with the aforementioned early design recommendation for careful descriptive/observational research.

The group literature moved from a paucity of measures in the 1950s and early 1960s, into a 15-year period in which it was inundated with diversely conceived and seemingly unrelated measures. This era of measurement proliferation is reflected in the consensual assertion of reviewers in the late 1970s who declared that it was impossible to compare group psychotherapy studies adequately because too many instruments were being used (Hartman, 1979; Lieberman, 1976; Parloff & Dies, 1977). To remedy this problem, these same reviewers and others (Bednar & Kaul, 1978; Zander, 1979) called for the conceptual and methodological development of a parsimonious set of variables that would describe the dynamic properties of group change. Comments from the mid-to-late 1980s describe a recalcitrant state of definitional imprecision and ambiguity in the variables being studied in group psychotherapy (Erickson, 1982; McGrath & Kravitz, 1982; Scheidlinger, 1984; Kaul & Bednar, 1986). This review demonstrates that the situation has changed little. Perhaps we could have averted our present predicament had we adopted Bennis' (1960) advice that conceptual clarification precede efficient experimentation.

Several recommendations directed at group psychotherapy variables and measures persistently reappeared as each decade passed (Table 2.2). For instance, the importance of using individualized measures of change as opposed to global measures of change was raised nearly 40 years ago (Zimet & Fine, 1955), and was re-emphasized by reviewers during each ensuing decade (Dies, 1979; Hartman, 1979; Kaul & Bednar, 1986; Pattison, 1965; Rickard, 1962; Rosenvinge, 1990). An equally persistent recommendation has been to match measures of change with the unique goals of treatment, the patients being treated, and the research question (Harman, 1991; Kaul & Bednar, 1986; Luchins, 1960; Pattison, 1965). Finally, issues surrounding the measurement of change and therapy process have been discussed at various times in the group literature (Burchard et al., 1948; Pattison et al., 1967; Hartman, 1979; Kaul & Bednar, 1986; Rosenvinge, 1990).

Observation and Analysis Issues

Table 2.3 summarizes specific recommendations regarding how investigators have reported and analyzed their findings across four different observational units: treatment, group, therapist, and member. The most frequent issue raised across all four categories is the need for greater specificity on the particulars of each observational unit. For example, 12 reviewers across five decades point out that the precise goals and strategies used in treatment are often missing in the research report. This consistent lack of precision explains, in part, the frequent call for treatment standardization and development of manuals (Kaul & Bednar, 1986; Parloff & Dies, 1977; Piper & McCallum, 1991). Recommendations for greater specificity regarding the

TABLE 2.2.   Measure and Variable Recommendations and Issues

	Number of Articles Published				
	1940s/1950s	1960s	1970s	1980s	1990s
Match outcome measures with unique goal of treatment, patient, and research question; develop context and treatment specific measures		4	1	1	1
Measure outcome in a quantifiable fashion (reliable, valid)	1	1	2	1	2
Definitional imprecision and ambiguity exist; group therapy borrows identity from individual			2		
Suggest individualized measures of change instead of global objective measures	1	3	2		1
Existing knowledge too limited to test and measure abstract constructs in group. Knowledge too limited to match subject variables	2	2	1		
Multiple outcome measures from different domains		3	1	1	
Develop small set of variables to describe group change; need clinical-conceptual development			1		
Too many outcome measures render it impossible to compare studies			3		1
Develop interactional process measures		2			
Measures should be developed at different levels of inference				2	
The most salient factors in group treatment cannot be manipulated		1			
Group phenomena operate on indirect, symbolic levels and cannot be measured		1			
Specify criteria for improvement		1			
Integrate variables/constructs from social psychology to group therapy			1		

duration, setting, and management of treatment dropped off in the late 1970s, suggesting improved reporting in these areas.

In the early literature, specificity as it relates to the group as a unit of observation includes more straightforward issues such as composition, degree of attrition, developmental stage of the group, and open or closed membership criteria (Burchard et al., 1948; Gundlach, 1967; Pattison, 1965). In later years, reviewers raise more complex observational issues, such as describing the interactional style and climate of the group members (Dies, 1979; Harman, 1991; Kaul & Bednar, 1986; Lieberman, 1976; Parloff & Dies, 1977).

Increased precision in describing the therapist's treatment orientation and rationale, leadership style, and relationship with group members is a

TABLE 2.3.   Observational Units of Analysis Recommendations and Issues

	Number of Articles Published				
	1940s	1960s	1970s	1980s	1990s
Treatment					
Greater specificity on goals and strategies of treatment	1	5	4	2	
Greater specificity on duration and management of sessions	1	2	1		
Greater specificity on setting and aids used by therapist	1	3			
Treatment standardization: develop manuals with specific techniques for specific patients			2	1	1
Quantitative and qualitative description and manipulation of treatment intervention		1		1	
Link intervention to therapeutic process to change					
Group					
Specify: composition, open-closed group, degree of turnover, interaction styles and climate of group members, group parameter (interactual climate, member characteristic, leader investment)	2	4	4	1	1
Therapist					
Specification of leadership style and relationship developed with group members	1	2	2	1	
Specification of therapist treatment orientation/rationale	1	1	2	1	
Control for therapist effects by multiple or crossed therapist/condition		1	1	1	1
Equivalent matched therapist characteristics/experience, orientation, skill, intervention, and relationship		2	1	1	
Use more experienced therapists			2		
Train leaders to a specified level of treatment competence			1	1	
Member					
Specification of patient characteristics	1	3	3	1	1
Patient populations should be comparable on age, diagnosis, sex		2			

recommendation spanning five decades. Later years find reviewers making suggestions for control of specific leader effects, including the need to have multiple therapists per condition, crossing therapists, and equivalence in therapist treatment competence, training, experience, delivery of intervention, and salient personality characteristics (Dies, 1977; Kaul & Bednar, 1986; Lieberman, 1976; Rosenvinge, 1990). Calls for specificity in describing salient patient characteristics extend from 1948 to the present, and include age, sex, socioeconomic status, diagnosis, severity of disorder, and salient personality characteristics.

COMPOSITE REVIEW CRITERIA

The indisputable convergence of reviewer exhortations for careful observation and description across the past five decades is difficult to disregard. Accordingly, descriptive specificity on therapist, patient, group, and treatment factors is the primary criteria in the methodological review that follows. These factors include therapist and client age, gender, and ethnic status as well as client diagnosis, the theoretical orientation, and experience level (low < 2 years, medium 2–5 years, high > 5 years) of the therapist. Group and treatment factors were coded according to (1) whether the study was field (actual clients) or analogue (recruited nonclinical population), (2) mean size and number of groups, (3) number, frequency, and duration of sessions, and (4) whether the treatment was driven by a specific manual (e.g., cognitive-behavioral), general treatment model (e.g., interpersonal approaches), or an unspecified "natural" approach.

Another focus area is the issue of the rigor and clinical relevance in both research design and the examined measures and variables. Instead of establishing criteria that might be unduly harsh or lenient on research representing different levels of developmental maturity, we generated a rigor-relevance continuum by which each study was classified into one of four general categories: descriptive research, correlational, quasi-experimental, and experimental. We then developed methodological review criteria that matched the rigor and relevance expected in a particular type of design and its associated measures and variables. For instance, one would expect more descriptive richness and contextual integrity from a case study, but an accompanying inability to rule out alternative explanations for statistically or clinically "significant" results. On the other hand, the precision and internal validity associated with a randomized block experiment enables one to rule out alternative explanations; however, the descriptively rich recording of unplanned therapeutic events is often sacrificed.

The descriptive research category includes case studies and clinical illustrations in which data were collected, reported, and analyzed in some fashion. Although the definition of data collection was liberal, spanning from archival inquiry to direct observation, only those studies that engaged in actual measurement of patients or therapists were included in the descriptive category. This type of research is often seen as a primary source for generating clinical hunches and insights into the change mechanisms of therapy. Descriptive or qualitative research is viewed as discovery-oriented and serendipitous (Neimeyer & Resnikoff, 1982) and eschews the confirmation aims of the hypothetico-deductive method (Manicas & Secord, 1983). Accordingly, review criteria minimize rigor and emphasize the clinical relevance of procedures and measures.

The correlational category includes basic measurement studies that assess the reliability, validity, or dimensionality of process or outcome instruments. Additionally, correlational methods explore relations among

client and therapist characteristics (e.g., age, sex, race, theoretical orientation, clinical diagnosis), or between subject characteristics and measures of
group process or outcome. Although it is difficult to draw strong causal inferences when variables are measured rather than manipulated, correlational methods can be evaluated on both the rigor and relevance of measures
being investigated (Pedhazur, 1982).

Whereas correlational studies may or may not compare two or more
groups of subjects, quasi-experimental research invariably compares two or
more groups of subjects. Furthermore, independent variables are manipulated in such investigations. We considered a study a quasi-experiment if one
or more variables were manipulated rather than measured.

To qualify for inclusion in the experimental category of this review,
a study had to meet two criteria. The first requirement was that one or more
of the independent variables was manipulated by the investigator and not
merely measured. The second criterion was that subjects were randomly
assigned to treatment conditions. What distinguished between these experiments and quasi-experiments was the presence or absence of random assignment. In the discussion that follows, we sometimes refer to experiments and
quasi-experiments collectively as comparative group studies.

LITERATURE BASE: 1980–1992

The literature base was established by a computer-assisted search of the
"psycinfo database." Any published article that dealt with group psychotherapy, counseling, or treatment was retrieved in abstract form. A total
of 2,025 abstracts were recovered from the database. Each abstract was read
by an advanced clinical psychology graduate student, or a faculty member
with approximately 10 years of experience teaching graduate research
methods in psychology. Research reports that appeared to involve data collection (801) were retrieved for this review.

A team of five research assistants and two faculty from two graduate psychology programs independently reviewed each article to determine whether
it met the minimal criteria for an empirical study (i.e., actual data collection). Reviews, position papers, clinical illustrations, and models (approximately 360) were discarded leaving 400 research reports. These studies were
then rated on: (a) design type (descriptive, correlational, quasi-experimental
and experimental), (b) the aforementioned therapist, patient, group, and
treatment factor criteria, and (c) sample, measures, and analyses used. In addition, several design-specific criteria that are described in subsequent sections were rated.

Study Features

Of the 400 research reports in our literature base, 149 (37%) are descriptive studies, 59 (15%) use correlational designs, 90 (23%) are considered

quasi-experimental, and 102 (26%) meet our criteria for experimental designs. A small number (<40) of reports became available after the review process was complete and are not included in this report. Nevertheless, this pool of studies represents possibly the largest sample of group psychotherapy studies reviewed in a single report.

Therapist Characteristics

The most striking feature of the therapist variables is the degree to which nominal descriptive characteristics are absent from the reports: therapist age (96%), race (94%), sex (62%), and level of training or experience (77%). Even therapist treatment orientation is unspecified in approximately half (48.5%) of the research reports. While the available data are insufficient to draw firm, general conclusions about the therapists who administered the treatments during the last 12 years of research, a few cautious conclusions may be justified. For instance, in the studies that report therapist characteristics, the majority of the groups were led by both male and female therapists (61%) with either 2 to 5 years (33%) or more than 5 years (43%) of clinical experience.

Therapist treatment orientation is the most frequently reported therapist characteristic (51.5%). Theoretical approaches include psychodynamic (31%), cognitive-behavioral (21%), behavioral (11%), eclectic (7%), psychodrama (5%), Rogerian (3%), interpersonal-existential (3%), and psychoeducational (3%). The remaining 15% fall into a miscellaneous category (e.g., dance, movement, rational-emotive).

Given the dearth of reported data, comparisons across study type are, for the most part, unwarranted. However, a few cursory trends are proffered. Interestingly, descriptive studies report therapist information more often than pre-experimental and experimental investigations. In addition, descriptive and quasi-experimental studies tend to use more experienced therapists than the experimental or correlational studies. Finally, psychodynamic groups are more frequently studied using descriptive, case-study methods (50%), whereas behavioral and cognitive-behavioral groups are more commonly studied by pre-experimental or experimental methods (78%).

Client Characteristics

The reporting percentages that pertain to client characteristics are considerably higher than those for therapist characteristics. The bulk of studies have groups composed of both male and female adults (Table 2.4). Client ethnicity is rarely reported (25%). When it is, the groups are often described as ethnically diverse (72%).

While client diagnoses at times follow the general guidelines of the *Diagnostic and Statistical Manual of Mental Disorders* (DSM-III-R; American Psychiatric Association 1987), reported diagnoses (e.g., neuroses) or subject groupings often do not fall clearly within a DSM-III-R category. In many studies, there is either no specified DSM psychopathology (e.g., victims of sexual abuse, persons in need of stress reduction), or the report is unclear as to the particular nature or range of presenting problems (e.g., psychiatry inpatients or outpatients at a mental health clinic). Thus, a more accurate descriptive label for this category might be "presenting problem."

As evident in Table 2.4, the client problem categories most heavily emphasized during the last decade include stress reduction (13%), mood disorders

TABLE 2.4.   Frequencies of Client Variables for Descriptive, Correlational, Quasi-Experimental, and Experimental Studies

Client Variable	Descriptive (n = 149)	Correlational (n = 59)	Quasi-Experimental (n = 90)	Experimental (n = 102)
Age				
Child (< 13)	13	2	1	3
Adolescent (13–18)	16	3	7	2
Young adult (19–30)	15	7	8	9
Adult (31–60)	79	29	55	64
Older adult (> 60)	3	2	2	6
Unreported	23	16	17	18
Sex				
Male only	23	3	11	5
Female only	35	4	14	19
Mixed	78	29	52	57
Unreported	13	23	13	21
Race				
White only	7	4	7	5
Nonwhite only	5	0	0	2
Mixed	23	9	19	18
Unreported	114	46	64	77
Client problem				
Normal	23	10	7	6
Outpatient	25	10	4	7
Mood disorder	7	8	10	13
Stress	0	6	11	17
Inpatients	8	6	12	6
Medical (cancer, pain, etc.)	16	0	3	11
Anxiety disorders	7	1	4	11
Substance abuse	10	2	6	5
Thought disorder/dementia	11	2	6	4
Eating disorders	7	0	6	10
Criminal behavior	7	4	8	2
Sexually abused	4	3	2	3
Personality disorder	6	3	3	0
Neurotic	0	1	4	6
Behavioral/Development disorder	6	0	0	0
Speech/Language disorder	2	0	0	0
Retardation	1	0	1	0
Sleep disorders	0	0	1	0
Unreported	9	3	2	1

Note: The sample was classified as adult when the subjects' ages were either limited to 30–60 years or contained a heterogeneous mixture of younger, middle–aged, and older adults.

(12%, typically depression), "normal" clients (9%, e.g., battered women, individuals with low self-concept, and special interest groups), unspecified inpatient populations (9%), unspecified outpatient populations (8%), eating disorders (6%), and anxiety disorders (6%). More rigorous designs (experimental and quasi-experimental) are commonly used to study general medical populations (e.g; pain reduction, cancer patients), group therapy for stress reduction, as well as mood, anxiety, and eating disorders.

Group and Treatment Characteristics

The typical group averages about twelve 90-minute sessions (Table 2.5). Very few investigations focus on groups that continue more than one year, although quasi-experimental investigations are more likely to examine groups of longer duration. Predictably, most groups meet on a once-per-week basis with higher ranges representing monthly extrapolations of more intense meeting schedules of inpatient or marathon-like settings. A small percentage (8%) of the investigations are carried out under analogue conditions (Table 2.6).

In an attempt to ascertain the degree of treatment integrity, the level of treatment structure was coded for each study (Table 2.6). The highest level of structure consists of treatments that are guided by a specific manual. This methodological tactic increases the likelihood of understanding what intervention and strategies are being used as well as decreasing the variability due to idiosyncratic therapist effects. Treatment manuals are used in only 13% of the studies. Predictably, experimental investigations rely more heavily on manuals (23%) to guide treatment delivery than do other study types.

TABLE 2.5. Medians, Means, and Ranges for Selected Group Structure Variables for Descriptive, Correlational, Quasi-Experimental, and Experimental Studies

Structure Variable	Descriptive (n = 149)	Correlational (n = 59)	Quasi-Experimental (n = 90)	Experimental (n = 102)
Number of groups				
Median	1	3.0	3.0	4
Mean	3	9.7	4.9	5.3
Range	1–75	1–72	1–54	1–54
Session duration (min)				
Median	90	90	90	90
Mean	92	109.7	92	95
Range	40–300	45–210	40–240	25–210
Total # of sessions				
Median	10	13.5	12	10
Mean	21.4	14.7	18.4	13
Range	1–200	4–75	1–150	3–52
Session frequency (month)				
Median	4	4	4	4
Mean	4.9	10.8	6.7	5.2
Range	1–20	4–60	1–30	2–30

TABLE 2.6.   Frequencies of Case Study, Pre-Experimental, and Experimental
Studies Conducted in Actual (Field) or Analogue Settings, and Treatment
Structure (Manual, Model, and Natural)

Structure Variable	Descriptive (n = 149)	Correlational (n = 59)	Quasi-Experimental (n = 90)	Experimental (n = 102)
Field setting	145	51	84	90
Analogue setting	4	8	6	6
Manual	0	3	6	23
Model	78	17	46	35
Natural	68	29	32	34
Unratable	3	10	6	10

Treatment manuals are predominantly used in conjunction with cognitive-behavioral (59%), behavioral (18%); and psychodynamic (12%) therapies.

Investigators who simply refer to a particular model of treatment that informally guided the course of group treatment are coded as model-driven. In these cases, authors typically state, "group therapists followed a Yalom model of group treatment" or "therapists followed the Tavistock model of group treatment." Overall, the model-driven level of treatment specificity is reported in 39% of the studies. The lowest level of treatment specificity is coded as natural. This occurs in 38% of the reviewed studies. In these studies, no attempt is made to specify a model of group treatment. Rather, investigators describe treatment as *"outpatient open therapy groups"* or *"group psychotherapy."*

Sample and Variable Characteristics

The typical study uses four therapists and 43 subjects with median values not varying significantly across the pre-experimental and experimental studies reviewed (Table 2.7). Predictably, correlational studies use significantly larger samples on average (approximately 150% larger) than either quasi-experimental or experimental studies. Nearly two-thirds (60%) of the experimental studies and one-third of the quasi-experimental studies compare treated groups to an inactive control group (e.g., waitlist). A high percentage of both experimental (40%) and quasi-experimental (29%) studies employ active control groups (e.g., placebo-attention); a smaller number include both active and inactive control groups (27% and 17%, respectively).

Overall, 422 psychological tests were used as sources of dependent measures for statistical analysis. There is significant variability in the average number of dependent variables used in an investigation across study type. More than two-thirds of the dependent measures are used only one time in the 400 studies! Only thirteen (5.8%) measures are employed more than five times. Symptom-based measures such as the Beck Depression Inventory (52 studies), the Symptom Checklist 90 (34 studies), the Minnesota Multiphasic

TABLE 2.7.   **Study Characteristics Including Number of Therapists, Sample Size, Active, or Inactive Control Group**

Study Characteristics	Correlational (n = 59)	Quasi-Experimental (n = 90)	Experimental (n = 102)
Number of therapists			
Median	2	2	3
Mean	5.1	3.6	4.2
Range	1–30	1–36	1–18
Sample size			
Median	42	43	45
Mean	90.8	62.3	62.7
Range	3–523	8–502	10–261
Active control group	2	26	41
Missing	55	30	7
Inactive control group	1	30	60
Missing	55	30	7

Personality Inventory (14 studies), and the State-Trait Anxiety Inventory (15 studies) have the highest frequency of use.

The majority of the instruments are client self-report questionnaires (81%). Thirteen percent of the instruments are behavioral coding systems in which one or more observers monitor group sessions and record the behavior of group members. With few exceptions (e.g., Hill Interaction Matrix), most behavioral observations measures are used only once. Of the 422 instruments, 18 (4%) are designed to be completed by a psychologist or physician based on a structured interview. The Hamilton Psychiatric Rating Scale for Depression (17) and the Social Adjustment Scale (12) are the most frequently used structured interviews. Together, they represent nearly half (44%) of the structured interviews in the reviewed literature.

In addition to using standard psychometric instruments, investigators often created their own questionnaires or behavioral coding systems. Investigators generated homemade self-report measures in 101 (23%) of the studies and behavioral measures in 75 (17%) of the studies. Physical measurements (e.g., weight or physical strength) and physiological data (e.g., heart rate) serve as dependent variables in only 18 (4%) of the studies (Table 2.8).

Statistical Analyses

Although investigators used a variety of inferential statistical techniques, traditional univariate methods of data analysis based on parametric models (e.g., ANOVA, t-tests, Pearson correlation, ANCOVA, multiple regression) are relied on more often than nonparametric methods (e.g., chi-square, Spearman rank-order correlation, Mann-Whitney, Wilcoxin, sign ranks). At times, investigators report only descriptive statistics, such as means, standard deviations, frequencies, and percentages.

TABLE 2.8.   Dependent Variable Characteristics

	Correlational (n = 59)	Quasi-Experimental (n = 90)	Experimental (n = 102)
Number of dependent variable			
Median	10.5	11.5	8
Mean	19.2	17.1	10.2
Range	1–178	1–178	1–178

	Descriptive (n = 149)	Correlational (n = 59)	Quasi-Experimental (n = 90)	Experimental (n = 102)
Type of dependent variable				
Self-report	85	46	72	90
Behavioral observation	94	25	37	41
Physical/Physiological	3	1	5	12
Strucured interview	11	11	10	23

Note: The percentages do not sum to 100 because the categories were not mutually exclusive (i.e., more than one type of outcome measure may have been analyzed in a given study).

There were few attempts by investigators to assess the psychometric properties of the selected instruments. Of the 400 studies summarized in Table 2.9, only 15 (4%) use psychometric or factor analytic methods to assess the dependability and dimensionality of measured variables. In view of the frequency with which investigators develop their own self-report and other behavioral measures, this finding is particularly unsettling. The development and use of instruments in the group literature far exceeds the extant basic research on their reliability and validity.

DESCRIPTIVE GROUP RESEARCH

The descriptive category was initially created to assemble and evaluate qualitative group research against a set of standards derived from the qualitative methodology literature (e.g., Polkinghorne, 1991). The central goal was to conduct a parallel review for qualitative, pre-experimental, and experimental group studies using contextually and developmentally appropriate review criteria.

As a means of cataloging the qualitative methods that characterize recent group psychotherapy research, a detailed coding sheet was created based on criteria culled from the qualitative literature. Unfortunately, this coding scheme proved to be rather superfluous because of the limited number of authentic qualitative studies. After eliminating all non-empirical articles (including clinical models, illustrations, and position papers), what remained was not a collection of qualitative research efforts, but an assortment of 149 investigations that do not clearly fit into any of the predetermined categories

TABLE 2.9. Frequency of Studies Reporting the Use of Various Statistical Techniques

Statistical Analysis	Descriptive (n = 149)	Correlational (n = 59)	Quasi-Experimental (n = 90)	Experimental (n = 102)
ANOVA	8	15	37	57
t-test	14	13	27	30
Other	40	4	7	7
Pearson correlation	11	19	7	9
Chi-square	5	3	18	18
MANOVA	0	4	13	21
ANCOVA	1	1	15	19
Multiple regression	1	14	2	6
Post hoc	0	1	9	13
Rank-order correlation	2	5	3	2
Mann-Whitney	2	1	4	4
Factor analysis	0	4	1	3
Psychometric	0	4	1	2
Wilcoxin	3	1	1	2
Sign ranks	1	0	1	0
Path analysis	0	1	0	0

Note: Other includes primarily descriptive statistics such as percentages, frequencies, and measures of central tendency.

(qualitative, correlational, quasi-experimental, or experimental). The majority of these studies consist of therapist case reports, single group evaluative reports, and one-group (pretest/post-test) investigations. In some instances, the studies report on several intact psychotherapy groups that use either post-treatment observation or patient surveys as a basis for drawing conclusions. In general, these research efforts do not correspond to the characteristics of the prototypic qualitative investigation; more appropriately, they can be grouped under the relatively diffuse and less exclusive heading of "descriptive studies." Rosenthal and Rosnow's (1984) use of the term "descriptive inquiry" may be helpful here, because it refers to any method of inquiry that seeks to map out what happens behaviorally.

While it is unreasonable to evaluate these descriptive studies on the basis of standard qualitative or empirical criteria (Cook & Campbell, 1979; Strauss & Corbin, 1990), it does not make sense to dismiss 40% of the group literature. Thus, the initial criteria were revised to delineate and evaluate three primary dimensions of descriptive investigations (cf. Kazdin, 1980; Rosenthal & Rosnow, 1984): (1) basic study parameters, (2) data collection and analysis procedures, and (3) reliability and validity of conclusions.

Basic Study Parameters

Given that an important organizing principle for most descriptive research is to provide a comprehensive and integrated portrayal of process phenomena

(Rosenthal & Rosnow, 1984), it is surprising to discover that 45% of the studies in this category are primarily concerned with evaluating the outcome of a particular group treatment. Less than one-third (31%) examine therapy process or treatment strategies; 16% explore both process and outcome dimensions, and 8% address specific client, therapist, and group characteristics.

In recognition that a capacity for discovery and exploration can be a primary advantage associated with small-n descriptive studies, reports were coded on whether the research was guided by exploration as opposed to hypothesis confirmation orientation. More than half (53%) of the investigations maintain a clear goal of hypothesis confirmation with most hypotheses addressing treatment efficacy. Conversely, 43% of the descriptive studies are rated as pursuing a discovery, descriptive, or exploratory orientation (4% were mixed or unratable). Within this latter grouping, numerous types of research questions exist, suggesting a widespread effort to apply exploratory and descriptive orientations.

The final study parameter examined is the method used to generate the sample under investigation. More than half (56%) of the studies employ samples of convenience (e.g, ill-defined groups already in existence), which is further complicated by the fact that little or no information is provided regarding client selection or composition. The next most common method for generating samples involves therapist clinical judgment (21%), followed by client self-referral (7%), both of which rely on unspecified criteria for inclusion. Only 5% of the studies systematically select subjects who meet clearly specified criteria according to well-established clinical assessment batteries.

The heavy reliance on samples of convenience is disappointing, given the relative ease of obtaining a well-defined and homogeneous sample of subjects in small-n research. For instance, it is far easier to find 7 or 8 borderline, personality-disordered patients who meet specific criteria for inclusion in a descriptive study than to find 50 such patients for a larger comparative treatment investigation.

Data Collection and Analysis Procedures

Descriptive research stresses the importance of careful observation and description (Bednar, Burlingame, & Masters, 1988; Rosenthal & Rosnow, 1984) and often results in data collection and analytic strategies that are strikingly different from studies that utilize relational or causal designs (Rosenthal & Rosnow, 1984; Strauss & Corbin, 1990). In the 149 descriptive studies, the most frequent method of generating or collecting data is through the use of subjective measures and evaluations of therapy process or change. Nearly two thirds (62%) of the articles report data-gathering strategies in which at least half of the measures are subjective; approximately 50% of the studies rely solely on subjective methods. Such methods typically take the form of therapists or clients offering their impressions of the therapy experience. Although portions of transcribed material are sometimes used as markers or "measures" of change, case description and participant impressions are the dominant format for communicating a therapeutic strategy or demonstrating client response to treatment. Other data collection strategies, such as the use of unstandardized questionnaires, formal behavioral observation (including audio/videotapes and live observation), and more objective measures (e.g., structured interviews, standardized self-report scales) are used at roughly equivalent rates.

In two-thirds of the studies (65%), data are collected from a single source. Of these, the therapist, client, and an independent rater provide the data in 48%, 40%, and 11% of the studies, respectively. Data are collected from two or more sources in 30% of the studies. Typically, the client and therapist are measured on the same or similar dimensions.

A single global assessment of therapy is made in 37% of the studies—two measurement occasions (pre- and post-treatment) are used 16% of the time, and three or more repeated measurements over the course of the investigation occur in about 25% of the studies. Continuous observation protocols occur infrequently (7%). The remaining 15% of the studies are unratable. Nine studies (6%) attempt to observe, record, and discuss critical change incidents during the course of treatment.

Approximately one-third (51) of the studies rely exclusively on the results of standard statistical analyses to reach conclusions (ANOVA, t-test, Pearson correlation), with a quarter of the studies (n = 35) relying exclusively on descriptive statistics (percentages, frequencies). A second third (51) employ subjective analyses, usually involving clinical judgments by a therapist or independent rater. Interestingly, subjective or "ocular" analysis is often performed irrespective of whether a subjective, objective, or behavioral measure is used to plot or track therapeutic variables. A combination of quantitative and subjective analysis is used in 13% of the studies, while formal content analysis is rarely utilized (4%). No analysis of any sort is undertaken in 15% of the studies.

Reliability and Validity of Conclusions

Although it is nearly impossible to determine the accuracy of inferences drawn from descriptive research, it is possible to assess the likelihood of unbiased conclusions. Bias is greatest when therapist and researcher roles overlap, when subjective measures are used, and when analyses are informal. It was possible to determine the identity of the therapist and the researcher in more than half of the publications (93). In two-thirds (62) of these cases, the researchers/authors also serve as the therapists. Although this condition does not guarantee that bias exists, it does raise concern. One standard method for countering such concern, especially in situations in which the data are subjective in nature, is to conduct reliability checks on data collection procedures. Unfortunately, only a small percentage (13%) of the descriptive studies report on the reliability of data collection protocols.

As a means of further addressing the confidence that can be placed in findings and conclusions, the descriptive investigations were evaluated on two further dimensions. First, consideration was given to the degree to which results were triangulated by independent sources or measures. The process of triangulation, which complements the notion of reliability checks, suggests that if descriptive findings are independently corroborated with two or more measures, or by two or more individuals, then greater confidence can be placed in the findings (Miles & Huberman, 1984). Approximately one-fifth (18%) of the total number of studies under scrutiny contain findings that are triangulated by multiple sources.

The number of investigations in which researchers made an effort to verify conclusions with study participants is also evaluated. This strategy is often employed to increase confidence in the reliability and validity of results in descriptive research and can be accomplished through a variety of means, ranging from debriefing to eliciting additional information from clients after the formal study is completed. Unfortunately, only four studies (3%) use these methods to bolster the integrity of findings.

EVALUATIVE OBSERVATIONS

The potpourri of studies found in the descriptive category makes it difficult to generate equitable evaluative comments on extant methodological practices. While it is unfair to judge this body of research on either quantitative (Cook & Campbell, 1979) or qualitative criteria (Strauss & Corbin, 1990), the absolute number of descriptive studies (40%) requires a thoughtful response as to apparent strengths and weaknesses.

The goal of outcome evaluation and hypothesis confirmation exhibited in approximately one half of the descriptive investigations deserves some comment. Although it is generally accepted that outcome studies are better addressed through the use of pre-experimental or experimental designs (Cook & Campbell, 1979), it is also likely that future group investigators, because of logistical constraints, will continue using small-n designs to explore treatment efficacy. Given this reality, a few recent methodological practices should be considered before small-n investigations are undertaken.

Although single subject designs have been employed for decades in behavioral research (Hersen & Barlow, 1976), Robison et al. (1989) recently provided an example of how such designs can be used in group psychotherapy investigations. Application of such models could address (through repeated measurement) the ill-conceived practice of global, end-of-session evaluation of outcome seen in more than a third of the reviewed studies. A second, equally important, methodological advancement to consider is the Reliable

Change Index (RCI)(Jacobsen, Follette, & Rivensdorf, 1984). The RCI was developed to plot change of individual patients using standardized objective measures of change. It enables researchers to display the percentage of individuals who improve, deteriorate, or show no change as a result of treatment. Such reporting would be a substantial improvement over the subjective evaluations of improvement that abound in the literature. However, it is important to note that neither one of these strategies handles the vital concerns addressed by a comparison group. In the absence of a control/comparison group in outcome evaluation studies, treatment effects uncovered by small-n studies are always susceptible to alternative explanations (e.g., maturation, third variables) and should be replicated.

Since a primary goal of descriptive research is to generate hypotheses for more focused experimental inquiry, the fact that less than half of the studies incorporate a discovery or exploratory orientation with a well-specified population is disappointing. Even when discovery-oriented aims were espoused, they were often associated with haphazard data collection procedures and subjective analyses. An exploratory orientation is not a license to use unstandardized or poorly described methods of data collection or analysis. Incorporation of well-defined qualitative research models (Berg, 1989; Miles & Huberman, 1984; Polkinghorne, 1991; Strauss & Corbin, 1990) into future small-n group therapy studies would undoubtedly improve such investigations. These models are particularly well suited for the sizable number of reports (47%) that explore treatment strategy or process-outcome questions.

PRE-EXPERIMENTAL AND EXPERIMENTAL GROUP RESEARCH

The quality of inferences drawn from group research may be evaluated on a number of dimensions. One dimension typically employed to rate the quality of an inference involves the rigor of methods relied on to generate the data from which one makes conclusions. As mentioned earlier, methods can be evaluated on both rigor and relevance dimensions. However, given the higher levels of rigor characteristic of pre-experimental and experimental designs, the criteria selected for evaluating the methodologies herein are based on Cook and Campbell's (1979) authoritative text. Threats to four types of validity are examined: (1) statistical conclusion validity, (2) internal validity, (3) construct validity, and (4) external validity.

These criteria were selected because: (a) they approximate our only "gold standard" for evaluating research methodologies in general, (b) details regarding each type of validity are familiar and readily available to most researchers, and (c) evaluating the presence or absence of a threat, in many cases, involves objective ratings using published procedure sections of research reports.

Statistical Conclusion Validity

Statistical conclusion validity refers to the extent to which conclusions regarding a statistical relationship (covariation) between independent and dependent variables can be considered valid and relates to the risks of Type I and Type II decision errors. For instance, if group therapy (independent variable) is an effective treatment for depression (dependent variable), a valid statistical relationship will exist between the two variables. The issues concerning statistical conclusion validity involve procedures that would spuriously hide or inflate statistical relationships. They include: compounding Type I error rate problems, violations of statistical assumptions, design specification errors, and statistical power.

Compounding Type I Error Rate

If several statistical tests are performed at the same nominal alpha level (e.g., .05), the cumulative risk of a Type I error proportionately increases with the number of statistical tests performed. Since the cumulative risk of Type I errors depends, in part, on the number of dependent measures in a study, the number of outcome variables per investigation excluding descriptive and demographic variables were examined. As can be seen in Table 2.8, there are nearly twice as many dependent variables in the correlational and quasi-experimental studies (19.2, 17.1, respectively) as in the experimental investigations (10.2). If the number of statistical tests performed roughly parallels the number of dependent variables, the cumulative risk of Type I error is substantially lower in the experimental investigations.

The cumulative risk of Type I error can also be estimated by reviewing the subject-to-variable ratio. The mean subject-to-variable ratios for correlational, quasi-experimental, and experimental are 4.8, 3.6, and 6.1, respectively. These values correspond to the relative degree of rigor one might expect; that is, experimental studies tend to be more focused and are probably less susceptible to Type I errors. However, the absolute value of these ratios falls below rule-of-thumb conventions suggested by some authors (e.g., Keppel, 1991; Pedhazur, 1982).

Violations of Statistical Assumptions

Many statistical techniques, including ANOVA and t-tests, require that the observations be normally and independently distributed. When observations are not independent, the statistical tests are positively or negatively biased, depending on the sign of the correlation among observations (Kenny & Judd, 1986). Positively biased tests may indicate that a relationship exists when it does not (Type I error) and also spuriously inflate the estimated magnitude of treatment effects. Negatively biased tests can actually diminish or completely mask a valid statistical relationship.

Of 192 comparative group studies, 170 (89%) treat observations from members of therapy groups as though they were independent and make no attempt to evaluate the degree of dependency between member observations. Whether observations within therapy groups were correlated in these studies is unknown; however, even weak associations among observations can seriously compromise the validity of such statistical tests. For instance, in a study in which two groups of six clients receive one treatment and another two groups of six clients receive another treatment, and null conditions prevail (no treatment effects), a positive correlation of only 0.20 among observations within individual psychotherapy groups more than doubles the expected value of F, and a moderate correlation of 0.40 nearly quadruples F.

The likelihood of correlated observations in the aforementioned group studies seems high. The clients within a psychotherapy group share a common history and typically interact with the same therapist over a period of several weeks. Under these conditions, it is reasonable to believe that the self-reports or behavioral observations of clients within the same therapy group will be correlated. For example, if cohesion begets cohesion, positive correlations among cohesion scores for individual members can be expected. Negatively correlated observations are also possible. If speech is dominated by one or two individuals, and speech is related to a variable of interest (e.g., a verbally-based indicator of insight), a negative correlation would exist among members of the group.

It should be noted that positive or negative correlations among observations within groups can be easily assessed with intraclass correlation coefficients (Strout & Fleiss, 1979). The statistical test for positive or negative dependency involves computing a "two-tailed" F-ratio that compares the variance among therapy group means to the variance within groups (Kenny & Judd, 1986).

Related problems of dependency in group research arise in repeated measures ANOVA (assumption of sphericity) and ANCOVA (homogeneity of regression) designs which are used in 98 of the studies reviewed. These problems can be particularly problematic when group researchers rely on temporally contiguous repeated observations (sphericity) or have treatment groups that demonstrate nonequivalent relationship (heterogeneity) between the dependent variable and a covariate. Only 1 (2%) of 55 studies in which repeated measures ANOVA are reported employs the appropriate correction (Geisser-Greenhouse or Huynh-Feldt adjustment), and 1 of 43 studies in which ANCOVA is used tests the assumption of homogeneity.

Together, these findings suggest that investigators are almost universally insensitive to the assumptions that underlie the statistical techniques they use to draw inferences regarding treatment effects. For example, if the assumption of homogeneity of regression is untenable, the results of the ANCOVA are usually uninterpretable. Violations of the assumption of independence are particularly problematic in group research, and the widespread inattention to these assumptions seriously compromises the statistical validity of conclusions derived from group therapy investigations.

Design Specification Errors

A common practice in group psychotherapy research is to assign clients to therapy groups, and therapy groups to either a control or experimental condition. If multiple groups are assigned to a condition, and a different therapist leads each group, then clients are nested under therapists, and therapists are nested under treatment conditions. Under these conditions, the appropriate ANOVA test for treatment effects involves treating the therapy group or therapist as the unit of analysis rather than the individual client.

If therapist as a factor is ignored in the design (Crits-Christoph & Mintz, 1991), the F-ratio for treatment effects may be positively biased, increasing the probability of Type I error. In the studies reviewed, 176 have multiple groups nested under treatments. Of these, only 15 (9%) consider therapist effects in their data analysis. The worst case scenario resulting from this nearly uniform inattention to testing for differences among therapists is that more than 90% of the group research may have positively biased F-tests that can spuriously indicate an effect for group treatment when none exists. A more favorable interpretation is that a sizable, yet indeterminate number of studies are overestimating the effect of treatment. These overestimates impact the effect size estimates derived from extant meta-analyses on group psychotherapy (see Fuhriman & Burlingame, Cahpter 1 this volume), resulting in a serious problem.

For instance, if the differences among therapists in the same treatment condition are significant, the test (F-ratio) for the effectiveness of treatment will invariably be significant, irrespective of whether or not there are treatment effects. This occurs because the differences among therapists become a component of the overall estimate of treatment. If differences among therapists are negligible, there is no need to treat therapist as a factor in the design (Kirk, 1982). Therapist effects are considered "negligible" when they are not significant when tested with a liberal alpha of 0.20 or 0.30 (Kirk, 1982; Winer, 1971).

Statistical Power

The power of a statistical test relates to its sensitivity in detecting treatment effects when they exist. If group researchers are going to invest a great deal of time and money in a particular study, they would ideally want to have an 80% to 90% chance of finding a difference if one is there (power of 0.80 to 0.90). Additionally, post hoc estimation of power can be very useful in interpreting the results of completed studies (Stevens, 1986). That is, nonsignificant results may be the result of a treatment that makes no difference or of poor power from small sample size or effect size.

Given these considerations, the median sample sizes reported in Table 2.7 were used to compute global estimates of the power of statistical tests used in the group literature to detect small, medium, and large treatment effects (Cohen, 1988). The probabilities of rejecting the null hypothesis (power) for the different study types are rather revealing (Table 2.10). Predictably, the power is considerably greater for large treatment effects ($M = 0.65$) than for small effects ($M = 0.09$), with all observed power values falling well below the value of 0.80 recommended by Cohen (1988), especially for small- and medium-size effects. Since these results are based on median sample sizes, the values represent the power of a typical group study. A more sobering thought is that the power achieved in 50% of the reviewed literature is less than the values shown in Table 2.10.

Inconsistent treatment delivery decreases the reliability of the independent variables (treatment) and curtails statistical power. Treatment reliability can be reduced when treatment is administered inconsistently over multiple sessions because of therapist drift or variable clinician skill (Kazdin, 1986). The use of treatment manuals is one method for maximizing the reliability of treatment implementation, thereby reducing differences among therapists and the risk of Type I errors (Crits-Christoph & Mintz, 1991; Crits-Christoph et al., 1991). Unfortunately, fewer than 1 in 6 of the comparative group studies rely on treatment manuals (Table 2.6). Inconsistent treatment delivery can also be minimized through periodic reviews of therapy sessions over the course of treatment. This occurs in fewer than 1 in 7 of the comparative group studies.

Low reliability of dependent measures also adversely affects statistical power. Although a comprehensive psychometric analysis of the 447 instruments used in the literature extends beyond the scope of this chapter, a number of conditions exist that create concern regarding the reliability of dependent variables for group psychotherapy research. Most measures are used in only one study, and reliability data are rarely reported. Altogether, 20% of the instruments can be classified as unstandardized behavioral or self-report measures, with more than half (52%) of the behavioral observations being "homemade," investigator-generated coding systems. Of the 103 studies that rely on raters to measure subject behaviors, only 27 (26%) report interrater reliability data. Finally, fewer than half of the instruments cited by the authors of the comparative studies are referenced in the *Mental Measurements Yearbook* (Buros, 1965–1989). This reliance on diverse and

TABLE 2.10. Power to Detect Small, Medium, and Large Treatment Effects Based on Median Sample Sizes for Correlational and Comparative Group Studies

	Effect Size			
	Small (.2)	Medium (.5)	Large (.8)	1.0
Study type				
Correlational (n = 59)	.08	.28	.60	.79
Comparative group (n = 192)	.09	.34	.70	.88

Note: Values are standard deviations.

unstandardized measures makes it virtually impossible to evaluate the dependability of data obtained in the group therapy literature.

Internal Validity

Internal validity refers to the extent to which changes (variance) in the dependent variable can be causally attributed to the independent variable rather than to an uncontrolled factor. The preferred procedure for ruling out threats to internal validity is the random assignment of subjects to different treatment conditions—the hallmark of experimental designs. It is assumed that when subjects are randomly assigned to conditions, they should experience the extraneous influences in the same manner (e.g., history), irrespective of their treatment condition. When subjects are not randomly assigned to treatment conditions, they may respond in different ways to a variety of factors over which the investigator has little control. The percentage of studies using random assignment is reflected in the relative frequency of experimental (40%) versus quasi-experimental and correlational (60%) studies presented earlier. Since random assignment is absent in the majority of studies, both positive and negative findings may be the result of pre-existing differences among treatment conditions or other third-variable problems (Cook & Campbell, 1979).

Even when subjects are randomly assigned to treatment conditions, attrition over the course of a study can undermine internal validity. Subjects who prematurely drop out of treatment may differ in important respects from those who remain, raising the possibility of selection bias (Cook & Campbell, 1979). Data concerning attrition are not reported in 60 of the 192 (31%) comparative group studies. In the remaining 132 studies, attrition rates range from 0% (n = 25) to 63% (n = 1), with the mean attrition being 18% (SD = 15.2) across studies. This average attrition is nearly double the 9% to 10% value reported by Shapiro and Shapiro (1983) in their meta-analysis. Tests for differential attrition or obvious differences on demographic and pretest measures between those who dropped out and those who completed the study are performed in 24 (22%) of the 107 studies in which attrition rates exceeded 0%. Attrition complicates interpretation of the results in one third (8 of 24) of these studies.

A final issue in ruling out alternative causes concerns assessing the effect of maturation, nonspecific effects, and the durability of change. If such effects can be ruled out, or quantified, the confidence in the putative cause of group treatment is increased. Approximately half (47%, n = 90) of the comparative group studies use an inactive comparison group (e.g., waitlist) to provide a check on changes over time that might be unrelated to treatment (maturation). Another third (35%, n = 67) use active control groups (e.g., placebo) to reduce the risk that nonspecific effects might explain client change. Only 8% (n = 16) of the studies employ both methods as a means of ruling out alternative causes. Last, the use of follow-up assessment to ascertain the durability of treatment effects occurs in nearly half (46%, n = 88) of the comparative studies reviewed. Although the time frames vary from several weeks to several years, it is an encouraging note that durability of treatment effects are being more regularly considered.

In regard to internal validity, the above data reveal both negative and positive characteristics of the methods used in group therapy studies. On the one hand, internal validity is compromised by infrequent tests for attrition, differential attrition, and infrequent use of random assignment. On the other hand, the logistical difficulties of randomly assigning subjects to therapy groups are sizable, especially since the majority of studies (90%) are carried out in naturalistic settings. Indeed, the fact that 40% of the studies employ random assignment can be viewed as a strength, and clearly demonstrates improvement over previous decades of group research. Confidence in the growing rigor of group investigations is further substantiated by noting that nearly half of the studies use some type of follow-up assessment, and that 136 of the 192 (72%) comparative studies incorporate a comparison group to control for the effects of factors other than those manipulated by the investigator.

Construct Validity

Construct validity refers to the extent to which independent and dependent variables selected by the investigator adequately represent the theoretical constructs that the research purports to investigate. Several factors can limit construct validity (Cook & Campbell, 1979); nevertheless, this review focuses on (1) the extent to which the treatments are adequately described and implemented, (2) the specificity of outcome measurement procedures, and (3) the extent to which multiple measures and methods of measurement are used in the assessment of outcome.

The construct validity of a cause-effect relationship in group treatment cannot be established by a single investigation. Indeed, years of programmatic research are needed to isolate the specific components of treatment that produce positive outcomes in clients (Kazdin, 1986). Thus, it is essential that investigators adequately describe the treatment under scrutiny, and maintain reliable implementation so that knowledge can accumulate across different time periods and investigative teams. The use of treatment manuals is one method of explicating relevant features of the treatment and facilitating attempts by other investigators to replicate findings. Unfortunately, this was the least prevalent tactic. In the vast majority of studies (87%), treatments are so poorly specified (i.e., rated as model or natural), that it would be impossible for future investigators to understand the specific components of treatment required for replication. A similar problem is noted in Shapiro and Shapiro's 1983 meta-analysis of comparative individual therapy outcome research.

A complementary method to ensure reliable treatment delivery is to check treatment implementation periodically across sessions. In this procedure, treatment integrity is evaluated both within and across conditions to ascertain if multiple therapists are delivering the same basic treatment components. Unfortunately, this practice is followed in only 13% of the comparative group studies.

The construct validity of the outcome or process being measured is greatest when the data closely approximate salient attributes of the problem targeted for treatment. The further a measure strays from being a direct assessment of a targeted problem, the greater the potential threat to construct validity for a particular investigation. Several observations can be made regarding the construct validity of measures used to study the effects of group psychotherapy. More than half of the dependent measures (56%) are self-report (Table 2.8), and while these measures can be precise estimates of psychological constructs (Mischel, 1968), they are more commonly viewed as indirect estimates with inherent construct validity limitations (Shapiro & Shapiro, 1983).

Approximately 32% (n = 92) of the correlational, quasi-experimental, and experimental studies include two modes of assessment in their measurement of effects; 7% (n = 19) use three or more modes of assessment. Although the degree of convergence across modalities is not coded, the observed frequency of multi-modal assessment is an encouraging sign.

Notwithstanding the benefits of multimodal assessment, the diversity of measures employed in recent years is a source of grave concern. A total of 361 different instruments are used in the 251 pre-experimental and experimental studies. The authors of the descriptive studies introduce an additional 61 instruments. If one considers that many instruments provide scores on several subscales, the number of different measures used to capture the effects of group psychotherapy during the last 12 years greatly exceeds the number of studies published during the same time period! It might be argued that the diversity of outcome measures suggests that investigators are using group psychotherapy in a wide variety of settings to treat heterogeneous clinical populations. However, it is inconceivable that there are even one-tenth as many salient dimensions of client or therapist behaviors as there are instruments for measuring them. Together, these data suggest that the literature is replete with single-shot explorations of poorly specified treatments and theoretical constructs.

External Validity

External validity refers to the extent to which the findings of a study may be generalized to and across populations of therapists, clients, settings, and times. The ability to generalize depends on the amount of information reported in the original investigation. If salient facts regarding the therapists, clients, treatments, and settings are missing in the original report, generalization is limited.

The absence of descriptive data across the 251 reports reviewed severely compromises external validity. Even the most nominal therapist characteristics, such as age, sex, race, and experience, are missing in most publications, leaving little that can be said about the group therapists who have administered the group treatments studied during the past 12 years. While a higher proportion of studies adequately describes their clients (Table 2.4), specificity of client problems remains low. Investigators who use a recognizable standard to determine the diagnosis or targeted problem are the exception and not the rule. A significant proportion of studies also fail to report basic treatment characteristics, such as session duration (37%), frequency (35%), and total number of sessions (26%). Surprisingly, even the number of groups that participated in the investigation is not reported in 17% of the studies.

On the one hand, the high proportion of studies using actual clients with real problems (92%) and the heterogeneous compositions of groups both argue for a high rating on external validity. On the other hand, the failure of most investigators to report basic therapist, client, and treatment characteristics makes it difficult to know how to generalize the results.

CONCLUSIONS AND PRESCRIPTIVE THOUGHTS

As compared to earlier decades (1940s to 1980), the past 12 years of group literature appear to have higher levels of rigor in both design and analysis. For instance, several previous reviewer directives seem to have been heeded in reports published during the past decade. The evidence for increased experimental control includes the use of comparison or control groups, random assignment, factorial designs, multiple measures, treatment manuals, and multiple assessments (e.g., pre, post, and follow-up), all of which strengthen the internal validity of group investigations. In addition, the studies often demonstrate a high level of relevancy for the practice of group therapy (external validity) on several dimensions. Research is predominantly conducted in naturalistic clinical settings using experienced clinicians instead of graduate students or trainees. In addition, a high percentage of outcome studies employ specific clinical populations. These improvements in rigor and relevance are promising harbingers for the development of a robust empirical foundation for group therapy so essential in today's increasingly accountable health care environment.

While the aforementioned practices are certainly favorable, we hasten to add that future investigators ought to address important weaknesses that threaten the soundness of research on therapy groups. The most serious threat involves the construct validity of causes and effects in group psychotherapy (Cook & Campbell, 1979). Although there is improvement in reporting the general parameters of group therapy (duration, number of sessions, context, etc.), nearly 90% of the studies still describe group treatment with a single word or phrase. From most investigations, little or nothing is learned about the characteristics or leadership style of the therapists or the properties of the group interaction. In the absence of such information, it is impossible to articulate what is meant by group psychotherapy. In technical language, these practices limit the construct validity of the putative cause of client improvement. This means that although changes in clients are observed, there is no idea how or why they occur. Unpacking the potentially efficacious aspects of composite interventions is an important first step in understanding and specifying causal mechanisms for treatment effects, requiring thoroughly described treatment strategies in the reports. In time, such reports might facilitate the development of theories of the therapeutic process and agents of change.

Another major problem concerns the construct validity of effects. The sheer volume of measures being used in the group literature makes it virtually impossible to delineate the nature of reliable effects to be expected. A favorable interpretation of the proliferation of measures may be that investigators are attempting to match outcome measurement with the unique goals of treatment. That is, as investigators conduct group therapy outcome studies with more diverse populations (e.g., schizophrenics to divorce adjustment groups), they may be forced to select or develop widely disparate measures that are closely aligned with unique treatment goals for these populations. While the use of measures that are targeted to specific treatment goals is laudable and certainly conforms to previous methodological suggestions, it does not absolve the investigator from using measures with adequate psychometric properties. Plotting change on a measure with unknown reliability and validity does little to support the efficacy of group treatment. In fact, the proliferation of untested measures, may, in fact, be counterproductive if poor measurement obscures therapeutic change.

Statistical conclusion validity is the second most serious area of weakness noted. The bad news is that the combined impact of low statistical power, untested dependency between observations, design specification errors, and unknown reliability of treatment implementation raise serious concerns regarding the group literature's ability to detect reliable treatment effects. The good news is that most of these threats to statistical conclusion validity can be readily rectified by conscientiously applying established design and analysis procedures. Our collective judgment is that many, but not all, of the aforementioned threats could have been addressed without undue cost (time or money) to the research protocol.

Prescriptive Model

To culminate this review, we address a few of the major problems in the group literature by organizing a series of questions in the form of a flowchart (Figure 2.1). The flowchart is designed to point out design or analysis considerations for the researcher who faces a given set of conceptual and logistical constraints. This model is heuristic rather than prescriptive, with the order of decisions based on deficiencies in the recent group literature

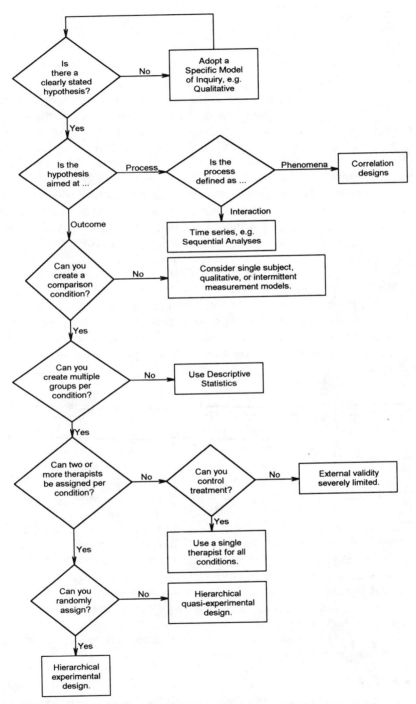

Figure 2.1. Design considerations for group psychotherapy research.

rather than the absolute value of one design consideration over another. It is an idealized structure that serves as a basic guide and may need to be adapted or modified in practice.

Hypothesis Clarity

A problem that frequently emerges in the more than 400 group psychotherapy articles is that of determining what the investigator was actually studying, that is, understanding the research hypothesis. It is commonly accepted that the value of a body of research is directly related to the quality of its hypotheses, with quality being determined by the clarity of the constructs and relationships examined. In general, hypotheses can be thought of as "if-then" propositions: If a particular type of group psychotherapy is effective, then patients who receive this treatment will improve. At a minimum, the generation of clearly stated if-then propositions from inexact questions such as "Does group treatment work?" or "How does group treatment work?" involves the ability to (a) specify the most simple and basic elements of treatment (the presumed cause or the *if* clause) and (b) reliably measure variables associated with treatment (e.g, the presumed change or *then* clause). If the investigation fails on either count, then a clearly stated hypothesis does not exist and the adoption of an alternative model of inquiry is more appropriate (Figure 2.1). When hypotheses are unclear or poorly formulated, the application of rigorous experimental and quasi-experimental designs is premature and not likely to foster better understanding of group process and therapeutic factors.

One alternative model of inquiry might be a specific qualitative research strategy (e.g, Berg, 1989; Miles & Huberman, 1984; Polkinghorne, 1991; Strauss & Corbin, 1990). Careful observation and description—a hallmark of qualitative inquiry—is a process that can lead to greater clarity regarding both the elements of treatment and their purported effects. Such research is essential given the aforementioned construct validity problems and will undoubtedly lead to more clearly articulated research objectives that will be of long-term benefit to the group psychotherapy literature.

The emphasis on adopting a specific alternative model discourages the continued reporting of anecdotal information that lacks heuristic value. Application of sound alternative protocols can generate clearer hypotheses that may at a later time be subjected to more traditional research methods. This reciprocal process is reflected in the feedback loop between hypothesis clarity and alternative models. The placement of qualitative research as a method of achieving hypothesis clarity is not meant to limit qualitative methods to this single function or to suggest that qualitative methods are the only alternative to achieving hypothesis clarity.

Process Hypotheses

If the hypothesis is clearly stated, the next decision is to determine whether the research focuses primarily on treatment outcome or process. The ideal scenario is to consider process and outcome simultaneously in treatment research. However, for the sake of simplicity, process and outcome have been arbitrarily separated for independent consideration.

If the hypothesis concerns group process, it is necessary to pose another question: "How is process defined?" Fuhriman et al. (1984) propose that a key feature in defining group psychotherapy process is how time is handled. They suggest that process be defined in terms of discrete phenomena or as a continuous flow of events (interaction). The process as phenomena perspective is represented in the vast majority of group process research. In these studies, process is typically captured by the intermittent administration of a self-report or behavioral observation instrument over the course of several weeks of treatment. In studies in which the researcher measures rather than manipulates a variable of interest, and then relates one measured variable to another, the design recommendation is to consider correlation, regression, and split-plot (repeated measures ANOVA) design standards. Typical issues in such designs include reliability of the instrument, sample size, and appropriate measures of association (Cohen & Cohen, 1983; Pedhazur, 1982).

If a study fits the "process as interaction definition," the research protocol relies on the continuous, moment-to-moment measurement of one or more variables of interest to provide across-time summaries. Such protocols typically rely on methods of behavioral observation, using measures such as the Hill Interaction Matrix (Hill, 1965) or continuous physiological measures (e.g., skin conductance, heart rate). If the goal of a study is to measure the continuous flow of a variable, or the relationship between one such continuous variable and another, the use of time-series analyses such as sequential analysis (Bakeman & Gottman, 1986; Gottman & Roy, 1990) or split-plot designs is recommended.

Outcome Hypotheses

The majority of group therapy studies test the efficacy of treatment. Outcome studies are not only the most frequent type of investigation, but also have the undesirable distinction of having the most design flaws. The majority of the remaining decisions in Figure 2.1 are developed around the most frequent and severe design flaws.

The first issue under consideration is whether the investigator can create an adequate comparison group. Kazdin (1980) describes the advantages and disadvantages of several types of control groups for comparative group designs. These include the traditional no-treatment, waitlist, and placebo control groups. However, he also describes options such as the no-contact and yoked control groups, which are essentially nonexistent in the group literature. This is unfortunate in that such procedures often prove to be less costly and intrusive than the more traditional methods. In the absence of a control group, an alternative strategy is to compare patients treated in group therapy with those being treated with a therapy that has an empirically substantiated level of effectiveness.

Without a comparison group, it is virtually impossible to design an adequate test of treatment efficacy. Single group pretest/post-test studies cannot establish the efficacy of a treatment; there are far too many plausible rival explanations for significant change over the course of treatment. However, in the absence of an adequate comparison group one can adopt several alternatives. Both qualitative and single-subject (group) designs can be used to explore individual patient change on a case-by-case basis. Finally, outcome studies without comparison groups can use all of the intermittent measurement designs discussed in the process hypothesis section. The difference is that outcome would be repeatedly measured (instead of process) and examined for changes over time using a conventional standard statistical model.

Multiple Groups per Condition

When one is testing the efficacy of a particular form of group psychotherapy, it is essential to have two or more therapy groups per treatment condition. When a treatment condition is represented by a single group, that treatment condition and the psychotherapy group are completely confounded. Moreover, it is likely that the F-test will be biased (positively or negatively) due to dependency among the scores for individual members of the psychotherapy groups. Unfortunately, when there is a single group per treatment condition, there is no way to assess the degree of dependency among individual group members. Thus, when treatment is administered to a single psychotherapy group, descriptive statistics such as the mean or median should be used to summarize the data, since tests for statistical significance are likely to be misleading.

Multiple Therapists/Condition

In general, it is preferable to have two or more therapists for each treatment condition. For example, if investigators are interested in comparing group treatment X to group treatment Y, there should be at least two therapists conducting two comparable groups in which treatment X is being delivered, and another two therapists and two groups nested under treatment Y. In situations in which one therapist administers one treatment, the therapist and treatment are hopelessly confounded. This type of confounding occurs in a sizable percentage of the studies. Under these conditions, it is impossible to determine whether client change is affected by a particular therapist, a specific treatment strategy, or a combination of both. Since it is impossible to isolate the cause of therapeutic effects when treatments and therapists are confounded, such designs should be avoided.

When several therapists administer a given treatment, it is possible to form an error term (mean square for therapist) to test for treatment effects. However, since the degrees of freedom for the error term depend on the number of therapists, the power of the test for treatment effects is likely to be extremely low unless the number of therapists is large. If a test for differences among therapists is nonsignificant, there is more justification for using the individual client as the unit of analysis, with a substantial gain in the degrees of freedom and power to detect treatment effects (Kirk, 1982). However, this practice still does not dismiss the observational dependency among group members. Attempts at modeling the potentially correlated error using techniques from other areas of research (e.g., social network analysis) have yet to be applied in the group psychotherapy literature.

Control of Treatment

In a recent meta-analysis (Crits-Christoph et al., 1991), the impact of therapist effects was skillfully documented using several well-known psychotherapy outcome studies. In brief, the meta-analysis suggests that outcome studies that employ a manualized treatment approach demonstrate negligible variability among therapists in the same treatment condition. However, significant between-therapist variability is evident in studies that were unable to control treatment implementation through manuals or other structured treatment guidelines.

Although it is problematic to pursue a study that uses a single therapist, these findings suggest that if treatment implementation can be controlled and monitored, it may be possible to conduct an adequate single therapist study on the relative effectiveness of two or more group treatments. As indicated in Figure 2.1, when an investigator can control treatment implementation, and the same therapist conducts all groups, the therapist is a constant and is no longer a factor in the design. However, this approach is problematic unless one can be certain that other therapists would implement the treatment in the same manner. Otherwise the generalizability of any observed effects is severely limited. An investigator who uses a single therapist and is unable to control or monitor treatment delivery faces virtually insurmountable generalizability problems.

Random Assignment

If a comparison group can be created, and multiple groups and therapists can be allocated for each treatment condition, the next question, then, is whether subjects can be randomly assigned to treatment and comparison conditions. Random assignment rules out most serious threats to internal validity. When random assignment is possible, one should apply the standards associated with hierarchical experimental designs (Keppel, 1991; Kirk, 1982).

In the absence of random assignment, the design is quasi-experimental (Cook & Campbell, 1979). In quasi-experiments, pre- and post-test measures are commonly obtained from control and experimental treatment groups. The data are then typically analyzed with ANCOVA or a mixed design (split-plot) ANOVA to determine if the change from pretest to post-test for one treatment condition differs significantly from the change exhibited by the other treatment condition(s). By analyzing change, these procedures control for pre-existing differences between treatment conditions at pretest (selection bias).

However, the aforementioned analysis of change is not immune from threats to internal validity. For example, the subjects in different conditions may mature at different rates or undergo different histories that could affect their post-test scores and thereby bias the results. A consideration of potential threats to internal validity is often required when interpreting the results of quasi-experiments. Moreover, the analysis of repeated measures does not solve the problem of nonindependence among the scores from clients nested in the same psychotherapy group. The (residualized) change scores from the members of each psychotherapy group may be correlated, and this must be taken into account.

Concluding Thought

The tedium associated with collecting, collating, and reviewing the group therapy literature of the past decade was a task that generated mixed emotions. On the one hand, it is discouraging to see the mistakes pointed out in one decade repeated in the following one! On the other hand, it is rewarding to note important improvements in methodology, thus raising our hopes regarding the potential for significant change in the practice of group researchers. The heuristic model, herein, is proffered in hopes of making a small contribution to continued methodological improvements as we move into the next century of group psychotherapy research.

REFERENCES

American Psychiatric Association. (1987). *Diagnostic and statistical manual of mental disorders* (3rd ed., rev.). Washington, DC: American Psychiatric Association.

Anderson, A. (1968). Group counseling. *Review of Educational Research, 33,* 209–226.

Bakeman, R., & Gottman, J. (1986). *Observing interaction: An introduction to sequential analysis.* Cambridge, MA: Cambridge University Press.

Bales, R. (1950). *Interaction process analysis: A method for the study of small groups.* Cambridge, MA: Addison-Wesley.

Bednar, R., Burlingame, G., & Masters, K. (1988). Systems of family treatment: Substance or semantics? In R. Rosenweig & L. Porter (Eds.), *Annual Review of Psychology, 39,* 401–434. Palo Alto, CA: Annual Reviews Inc.

Bednar, R., & Kaul, T. (1978). Experiential group research: A current perspective. In S. Garfield & A. Bergin (Eds.), *Handbook of Psychotherapy and Behavior Change.* New York: Wiley.

Bennis, W. (1960). A critique of group therapy research. *International Journal of Group Psychotherapy, 10,* 63–77.

Bennis, W. (1961). Three research approaches to a question in the field of group psychotherapy: A case study in research formulation. *International Journal of Group Psychotherapy, 11,* 272–283.

Berg, B. (1989). *Qualitative research methods for the social sciences.* Boston, MA: Allyn & Bacon.

Burchard, E., Michaels, J., & Kotkov, B. (1948). Criteria for the evaluation of group therapy. *Psychosomatic Medicine, 10*(3), 257–274.

Burlingame, G., Fuhriman, A., & Drescher, S. (1984). Scientific inquiry into small group process: A multidimensional approach. *Small Group Behavior, 15*(4), 441–470.

Buros, O., & The Buros Institute of Mental Measurement. (1965–1989). *Mental measurements yearbook* (6th, 7th, & 8th eds.). Highland Park, NJ: Gryphon Press. (9th & 10th eds.) Lincoln, NE: The University of Nebraska—Lincoln.

Cartwright, D. & Zander, A. (1953). *Group dynamics.* White Plains: Row-Peterson.

Cohen, J. (1988). *Statistical power analysis for the behavioral sciences* (2nd ed.). New York: Academic Press.

Cohen, J., & Cohen, P. (1983). *Applied multiple regression/correlation analysis for the behavioral sciences.* Hillsdale, NJ: Lawrence Erlbaum.

Cohen, M., & Nagel, E. (1934). *An introduction to logic and scientific method.* New York: Harcourt Brace & Co.

Cook, T., & Campbell, D. (1979). *Quasi-Experimentation: Design and analysis issues for field settings.* Boston, MA: Houghton Mifflin.

Crits-Christoph, P., Baranackie, K., Kurhias, J., Beck, A., Carroll, K., Perry, K., Luborsky, L., McLellan, T., Woody, G., Thompson, L., Galkigher, D., & Zitrin, C. (1991). Meta-analysis of therapist effects in psychotherapy outcome studies. *Psychotherapy Research, 1*(2), 81–91.

Crits-Christoph, P., & Mintz, J. (1991). Implications of therapist effects for the design and analysis of comparative studies of psychotherapies. *Journal of Consulting and Clinical Psychology, 59,* 20–26.

Dies, R. (1977). Pragmatics of leadership in psychotherapy and encounter group research. *Small Group Behavior, 8,* 229–248.

Dies, R. (1979). Group psychotherapy: Reflections on three decades of research. *The Journal of Applied Behavioral Science, 15,* 361–374.

Dies, R. (1985). Research foundation for the future of group work. *Journal for the Specialist in Group Work, 10,* 68–73.

Erickson, R. (1982). Inpatient small group psychotherapy: A survey. *Clinical Psychology Review, 2,* 137–151.

Frank, J. (1950). Group psychotherapy in relation to research. *Journal of Group Psychotherapy, 3,* 197–203.

Fuhriman, A., Drescher, S., & Burlingame, G. (1984). Conceptualizing small group process. *Small Group Behavior, 15*(4), 427–440.

Gottman, J., & Roy, A. (1990). *Sequential analysis: A guide for behavioral researchers.* Cambridge, MA: Cambridge University Press.

Gundlach, R. (1967). Three research approaches to a question in the field of group psychotherapy: To convert a clinical judgment into a research design. *International Journal of Group Psychotherapy, 11,* 265–271.

Harman, M. (1991). The use of group psychotherapy with cancer patients: A review of recent literature. *The Journal of Specialists in Group Work, 16*(1), 56–61.

Hartman, J. (1979). Small group methods of personal change. *Annual Review of Psychology, 30,* 453–476.

Hersen, M., & Barlow, D. (1976). *Single-case experimental designs: Strategies for studying behavior change.* New York: Pergamon.

Hill, W. (1965). *Hill interaction matrix.* Los Angeles: University of Southern California.

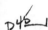

Hulse-Killacky, D., Robison, F., & Morran, D. (1991). Reporting group research: Conceptual and technical considerations for preparing manuscripts. *The Journal for Specialists in Group Work, 16*(2), 101–108.

Jacobsen, J., Follette, W., & Rivensdorf, D. (1984). Psychotherapy outcome research: Methods for reporting variability and evaluating clinical significance. *Behavior Therapy, 15,* 336–352.

Kaul, T., & Bednar, R. (1986). Experiential group research: Results, questions & suggestions. In S. Garfield & A. Bergin (Eds.), *Handbook of Psychotherapy and Behavior Change.* New York: Wiley.

Kazdin, A. (1980). *Research design in clinical psychology.* New York: Harper & Row.

Kazdin, A. (1986). The evaluation of psychotherapy: Research design and methodology. In S. Garfield & A. Bergin (Eds.), *Handbook of Psychotherapy and Behavior Change.* New York: Wiley.

Kenny, D., & Judd, C. (1986). Consequences of violating the independence assumption in analysis of variance. *Psychological Bulletin, 99,* 422–431.

Keppel, G. (1991). *Design and analysis: A researchers handbook.* Englewood Cliffs: Prentice Hall.

Kirk, R. (1982). *Experimental design: Procedures for the behavioral sciences,* (2nd ed.). Monterey: Brooks/Cole.

Lieberman, M. (1976). Change induction in small groups. *Annual review of psychology, 27,* 217–250.

Luchins, A. (1960). An approach to evaluating the achievements of group psychotherapy. *Journal of Social Psychology, 52,* 345–353.

Manicas, P., & Secord, P. (1983). Implications for psychology of the new philosophy of science. *American Psychologist, 38,* 399–413.

Mann, J. (1966). Evaluation of group psychotherapy. In J. Moreno (Ed), *The international handbook of group psychotherapy.* New York: Philosophical Library.

McGrath, J., & Kravitz, D. (1982). Group research. *Annual Review of Psychology, 33,* 195–230.

Miles, M., & Huberman, A. (1984). *Qualitative data analysis.* Beverly Hills, CA: Sage.

Mischel, W. (1968). *Personality and assessment.* New York: Wiley.

Neimeyer, G., & Resnikoff, A. (1982). Qualitative strategies in counseling research. *The Counseling Psychologist, 10*(4), 75–85.

Parloff, M. (1961). Three research approaches to a question in the field of group psychotherapy: Rigor by design. *International Journal of Group Psychotherapy, 11,* 255–283.

Parloff, M., & Dies, R. (1977). Group psychotherapy outcome research. *International Journal of Group Psychotherapy, 27,* 281–319.

Pattison, E. (1965). Evaluation studies of group psychotherapy. *International Journal of Group Psychotherapy, 15*(3), 382–397.

Pattison, E. (1966). Evaluation of group psychotherapy. *Current Psychiatric Therapies, 6,* 211–218.

Pattison, E., Brissenden, A., & Wohl, T. (1967). Assessing specific effects of inpatient group psychotherapy. *International Journal of Group Psychotherapy, 17,* 283–297.

Pedhazur, E. (1982). *Multiple regression in behavioral research.* New York: Holt, Rinehart and Winston.

Piper, W., & McCallum, M. (1991). Group interventions for persons who have experienced loss: Description and evaluative research. *Group Analysis, 24,* 363–373.

Polkinghorne, D. (1991). Qualitative procedures for counseling research. In C. Watkins Jr. & L. Schneider (Eds.), *Research in Counseling.* Hillsdale, NJ: Lawrence Erlbaum.

Rickard, H. (1962). Selected group psychotherapy evaluation studies. *Journal of General Psychology, 67,* 35–50.

Robison, F., Morran, D., & Hulse–Killacky, D. (1989). Single subject research designs for group counselors studying their own groups. *The Journal for Specialists in Group Work, 14*(2), 93–97.

Rosenvinge, J. (1990). Group therapy for anorexic and bulimic patients. *Acta Psychiatrica Scandinavica, 82*(361), 38–43.

Rosenthal, R., & Rosnow, R. (1984). *Essentials of behavioral research: Methods and data analysis.* New York: McGraw-Hill.

Salvendy, J. (1991). Group psychotherapy in the late twentieth century: An international perspective. *Group, 15*(1), 3–13.

Scheidlinger, S. (1984). Group psychotherapy in the 1980's: Problems and prospects. *American Journal of Psychotherapy, 38*(4), 494–504.

Shapiro, D., & Shapiro, D. (1983). Comparative therapy outcome research: Methodological implications of meta-analysis. *Journal of Consulting and Clinical Psychology, 51,* 42–53.

Sherwood, C. (1956). Some recommendations for research in the field of group psychotherapy. *Group Psychotherapy, 9,* 126–132.

Stevens, J. (1986). *Applied multivariate statistics for the social sciences.* Hillsdale, NJ: Lawrence Erlbaum.

Stock, D., & Lieberman, M. (1962). Methodological issues in the assessment of total-group phenomena in group therapy. *International Journal of Group Therapy, 12,* 312–325.

Stotsky, B., & Zolik, E. (1965). Group psychotherapy with psychotics. *International Journal of Group Psychotherapy, 15*(3), 321–344.

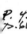

Strauss, A., & Corbin, J. (1990). *Basics of qualitative research.* Newbury Park, NY: Sage Publishing.

Strout, P., & Fleiss, J. (1979). Intraclass correlations: Uses in assessing rater reliability. *Psychological Bulletin, 86,* 420–428.

Winer, B. (1971). *Statistical principles in experimental design* (2nd ed.). New York: McGraw-Hill.

Zander, A. (1979). The study of group behavior during four decades. *The Journal of Applied Behavioral Science, 15,* 272–282.

Zimet, C., & Fine, H. (1955). Methodology and evaluation in group psychotherapy. *Group Psychotherapy, 11,* 186–196.

PART TWO

Structural Entities in Group Psychotherapy

CHAPTER 3

Client Variables

WILLIAM E. PIPER

Characteristics of the client (or patient) have always occupied a central place in the formulations of clinicians and researchers who are invested in group therapy. It is the client who is usually the prime mover in what turns out to be a complex sequence of clinical events. He or she is initially interested in finding out whether therapy is recommended and, if so, what particular kind. These decisions have a profound impact on how the client invests time and emotional energy for a significant, even if limited, period of time. Ultimately it is the client who must be satisfied if the clinician and the form of therapy are to remain viable. For the therapist, selection decisions affect how he or she spends professional time and whether the investment is satisfying. In the case of group therapy, the number of people who are affected by each selection decision is multifold. The fate of all clients in the group is in part determined by each member.

For the researcher, the client provides a wealth of variables to be studied. Either singly or in combination, client variables can be investigated regarding their relationships with important clinical events such as whether clients remain, work, and benefit in therapy groups. Due to their sheer number, client variables provide a formidable challenge to the researcher in regard to the issue of control. Through methods of research design or statistics, researchers frequently attempt to control (or balance) the effects of client characteristics, while the effects of other variables (e.g., technique) are being investigated. Researchers also face increasing demands to describe their samples carefully. That includes providing standard information about the demographic, diagnostic, and pathologic features of their sample and its relationship to larger samples of which it is a subset. Such information allows clinicians to determine whether the sample is comparable to their practice caseloads and researchers to generalize and carry out replications. Because of the natural tendency of client characteristics to occupy a central place in the experience and formulations of clinicians and researchers, the question has sometimes been raised as to whether their effects have been overestimated (i.e., whether they have been oversold as influential variables, particularly when they are considered by themselves). Determining their unique and combined effects with other variables has become an intriguing and complex challenge.

At the practical level of making a decision about the suitability of a particular patient for a specific group, the clinical decision may appear deceptively simple. The complexity quickly becomes apparent with the questions, Is this patient suitable compared to other patients? Is this group appropriate compared to other therapy groups? Is this group appropriate compared to other types of treatment (e.g., individual therapy or medication)? These are questions that researchers and clinicians routinely address.

In this chapter, I review the research evidence for the importance of client characteristics to significant events in group therapy. First, a consideration of the conclusions of a number of previous reviews will be made. Second, the evidence from research studies conducted during the past 40 years will be reviewed. Third, the evidence will be considered in terms of the previous conclusions. Finally, implications for future work in the area of client characteristics and selection will be considered.

During the past 15 years, a number of authors have reviewed or summarized the research literature concerning client characteristics in group therapy (Bednar & Kaul, 1978; Bond & Lieberman, 1978; Hawkins & White, 1978; Kaul & Bednar, 1986; Power, 1985; Rutan & Stone, 1984; Woods & Melnick, 1979; Yalom, 1985). Most of these authors have concluded that there are relatively few methodologically sound studies where the investigation of client characteristics was a primary objective. In many studies, the exploration of client characteristics was a secondary or post hoc endeavor. Because of the lack of strong studies, some authors (e.g., Rutan & Stone, 1984; Yalom, 1985) have based their reviews on a mixture of research studies, clinical reports, and their own clinical experience. While that has been necessary in order to provide a more coherent and complete narrative that is meaningful and potentially useful to practitioners, one must remember that the research base for many conclusions about patient selection is unfortunately small.

In addition to sharing the impression that there are too few methodologically strong selection studies, reviewers have identified a number of common themes concerning the (1) limitations associated with previous research and (2) recommendations for future research.

In regard to limitations, from the studies that have been conducted, each with its own set of client characteristics, it is not difficult to find evidence of statistically significant predictive relationships. Many of the findings make conceptual and clinical sense (e.g., a relationship between motivation and desirable therapy process or between social skills and favorable outcome). However, if one attempts to formulate an overall impression, one faces a dilemma akin to the question, "Is the glass half empty or half full?" Most of the reviewers have not been impressed. The quotations of three of the reviewers convey the tone: Yalom (1985), "to date, empirical research has failed to deliver"; Rutan & Stone (1984), "there is a dearth of data to provide specific guidelines"; and Bond & Lieberman (1978), "Although a vast clinical and empirical literature testifies to an impressive effort to locate salient predictors, directly practical information promising even the most modest level of confidence is seldom evident or implicit." What is the problem? First, the number of nonsignificant relationships far outweigh the significant ones. As might be expected, the latter tend to be highlighted. However, the possibility of chance findings, or what statisticians refer to as Type I error, is real. Second, many of the correlations, although statistically significant, are small in magnitude and therefore of questionable clinical importance. Most researchers are pleased if they find a correlation of 0.50 between a predictor and a dependent variable. While such a finding signifies that 25% of the variation of the dependent variable can be explained, it also indicates that 75% cannot. Third, there is a lack of replication or cross-validation of findings. The urge to discover new predictor variables rather than verify previously identified ones seems to resemble the familiar urge to find new group therapies that has characterized the field during the last several decades.

Despite this unsatisfying state of affairs, reviewers have *not* suggested that researchers should stop investigating client characteristics as predictors. Instead, they have made a number of recommendations which are summarized in Table 3.1. Probably the two that have been made most strongly and that have appeared in almost every review are (1) to use a multivariate approach with a set of predictors and (2) to examine their interactions. The set would likely include two or more client characteristics and other types of predictors. In the past, most researchers have behaved as if they believed that single client predictors were so powerful that they could override variation and the combination of other influential variables, such as type of group, technique or therapist. One set of reviewers, Roback and Smith (1987) stated, "We believe that dropping out of treatment is usually a complex interaction between patient, group, and therapist factors, but much of the literature tends to focus on only one of these dimensions." The desirability of a multivariate approach is evident. The overall strength of predictions, or in statistical terms the total amount of variation accounted for, can generally

TABLE 3.1.   Recommendations for Future Research Investigating the Impact of Client Characteristics

1. Use a multivariate approach with more than one client characteristic and more than one type of predictor (e.g., client, group and therapist characteristics).

2. Examine the interactions among predictors.

3. Use a conceptual rationale as a basis for prediction.

4. Use interpersonal and behavioral client characteristics as predictors.

5. Calculate improvement over base rates.

6. Include more than one type of group therapy in each study.

7. Attempt to replicate and cross-validate the findings of previous studies.

be increased by including multiple predictors. Additionally, the ability of each predictor to independently and significantly contribute to the prediction can be determined. This is not a trivial issue since overlap among various predictors is a common phenomenon.

A third recommendation is to make predictions on the basis of theory or a conceptual rationale rather than blindly running correlations between available predictors and dependent variables. This has been a major theme of Bednar and Kaul (1978, 1986) in their reviews of the literature. It has also been made by Bond and Lieberman (1978) who emphasized the importance of conceptualizing the intervening group process that links client characteristics to outcome. They correctly point out that without an understanding of the intervening processes, a significant predictor may have little relevance for the specific form of therapy being studied. That is, it might simply represent a general predictive indicator that applies to many therapies.

A fourth recommendation, which has been particularly championed by Woods and Melnick (1979), is to use interpersonal variables, particularly behavioral ones, as predictors. In their view, the traditional, dyadic intake interview has been one of the least useful but most commonly used methods of obtaining predictor scores. In the same vein, they argue that it is not surprising that formal diagnostic categories, which are not meant to represent interpersonal behavior, and demographic characteristics have seldom provided significant correlations. The frequent investigation of such variables seems much more attributable to their easy availability.

A fifth recommendation, which has been made by Garfield (1986), concerns the issue of base rates. For any particular sample of clients and their therapy groups, a certain percentage will be found to remain, work, and benefit over a period of time. For example, the base rate for remainers may be 67% (i.e., about a third of the clients drop out prematurely). As a result of conducting a study, an investigator may discover that a particular client characteristic is significantly associated with remaining. Despite the significant correlation, if the client characteristic were used to make selection/rejection decisions, the retention rate for the groups might only increase to 70%. That would hardly be regarded as an important improvement in the retention rate. Very few selection studies have compared the effects of their predictors to base rates.

A sixth recommendation involves the experimental design of selection studies. Quite simply it advocates the inclusion of more than one type of therapy group in each study. As Hollon (1984) has argued, if only a single treatment is studied, one cannot be sure that a significant association between a predictor and outcome has anything to do with the particular treatment. That is, it may predict improvement for a variety of treatments or even the case of no treatment. If so, the meaning and implications of the findings are very different. The predictor would be regarded as a general prognostic indicator rather than a selection criterion for a particular treatment. Finally, the seventh recommendation concerns the need for replication and cross-validation of findings. Given the multitude of variables capable of influencing outcome, little confidence can be placed in one-shot selection discoveries.

In summary, there is strong consensus among those who have carefully reviewed the literature about what is desirable in future research investigating client characteristics. Researchers should use a multivariate approach that explores interactions among different types of predictors. More than one type of group therapy should be studied. The approach should be theoretically based and use interpersonal and behavioral measures. Multivariate statistical procedures such as multiple regression or discriminant function analysis should be used to maximize prediction and determine the unique contribution of individual predictors. Comparisons with base rates should be made. Finally, there is an important need to replicate and cross-validate the findings of previous investigators.

RESEARCH LITERATURE

In surveying the research literature of the past 40 years concerning client characteristics in group therapy, four primary inclusion criteria were used: (1) The study included a client characteristic that varied as an independent variable, (2) the clients in the study participated in an interactive group of at least three or more clients and a therapist, (3) the purpose of the group included bringing about change in regard to personal problems, and (4) the study included more than one therapy group. The intent of these inclusion criteria was to base the review on therapy groups, not experiential training groups, or dyadic or triadic entities from social-psychological research. Previous reviews often included research findings concerning these latter types of groups, the rationale being that therapy and nontherapy groups have many dynamic processes in common and that clients with personal problems participate in nontherapy groups. While therapy groups and nontherapy groups share some characteristics, an examination of their objectives, techniques, and compositions reveals that they are far from identical. The present review restricted itself to therapy groups in the interest of maximizing the clinical relevance of the findings. In addition, requiring variation of the client characteristics and more than one group insured exclusion of therapist reports of their experience with a single type of client or a single therapy group. Although interesting, such reports tend to be highly impressionistic and idiosyncratic.

The method of discovering research studies included conducting computerized literature reviews (Medline, PsychLit), examining the contents of major group therapy and other professional journals, and examining previous reviews and chapters that discussed client characteristics. This method identified 83 studies that met the inclusion criteria. They span the period from 1952 to 1992. The earlier 20-year period (1952–1971) included 24 studies or about one per year, while the later 20-year period (1972–1992) included 59 studies or about three per year, a three-fold increase. The number of studies that investigated interpersonal variables as client characteristics during the earlier period (6) compared to the later period (16) resembled the overall pattern. An even more dramatic difference involved the number of studies that investigated the interaction between client characteristics and other types of variables (usually different types of group therapy) during the earlier period (1) compared to the later period (22). The differences between the two time periods reveal not only growth in the number of studies conducted, but growth in the number of more sophisticated studies.

The 83 studies are diverse in terms of the types of client characteristics, therapy groups, and dependent variables studied. Approximately 74% of the studies involved outpatients and 26% involved inpatients or incarcerated clients. Because of the diversity, there are many ways to categorize the studies. Client characteristics can be divided into demographic, diagnostic, pathologic, personality, expectancy, intellectual/cognitive, and other types of variables. Therapy groups represent a variety of technical and theoretical orientations. Dependent variables can be divided into areas of attendance, remaining, therapy process, and treatment outcome. Additional methods of categorization include the type of client (e.g., inpatient, partial hospitalization patient, outpatient) and the type of measure (e.g., self-report questionnaire, psychological test score, interview rating, group behavior rating). Individual investigators differ in how they categorize variables. For example, MMPI profiles (as client characteristics) have been regarded as diagnostic, pathologic, or personality variables by different investigators.

Thus, the potential ways to categorize variables are numerous and without fixed boundaries. Because of these difficulties and due to space limitations, the present review will be selective in its method of categorization of the studies. Given the recommendations of previous reviewers, major emphasis will be given to studies that have investigated interaction effects. Such studies represent many of the most sophisticated studies. In addition to examining interactions, they often incorporate several of the other desirable qualities summarized in Table 3.1 (e.g., a multivariate approach, a conceptual rationale, more than one type of group therapy). Given the unique relevance of interpersonal variables to group therapy, a major emphasis will also be given to studies that have investigated them as client characteristics. Lesser emphasis will be given to other types of client characteristics (e.g., demographic characteristics).

There are also different ways of reviewing and summarizing studies. Smith, Glass, and Miller (1980) distinguished among the approaches of narrative integration, box scores, and meta-analysis. The present review primarily used a box score approach. Thus, each study was examined to see whether it provided evidence of a statistically significant association between client characteristics and dependent variables. Because of the period of time covered and the statistical information that was not available, a meta-analytic approach was not attempted.

STUDIES INVESTIGATING INTERACTION EFFECTS

These studies reflect the complexity of the group situation. Each investigated the combined effect of a client characteristic and some other type of variable (e.g., type of therapy or type of therapist). The 23 interaction studies will be considered chronologically (Table 3.2). Nineteen of the studies (83%) reported significant results, which attests to the promise of exploring interaction effects in group therapy. The earliest study was Meichenbaum, Gilmore, and Fedoravicius (1971). Time-limited short-term therapy groups were used with speech-anxious students. As part of a post hoc exploration, the investigators found that desensitization group therapy was more effective with students whose speech anxiety was confined to formal speech-giving situations, while insight group therapy was more effective with students whose anxiety occurred in a variety of social situations.

In two related studies with a large sample of alcoholic inpatients, McLachlan (1972, 1974) investigated two different types of interactions. In each study, the predictor variable was the client's conceptual level defined by the developmental theory of Harvey, Hunt, and Schroder (1961). After detoxification, clients were treated with 26 hours of client-centered group therapy. There was greater improvement for clients whose conceptual level was matched with the conceptual level of their therapists (i.e., high-high or low-low),than for mismatched client-therapist pairings. The finding held up 12 to 16 months after the clients participated in aftercare. In addition to the client-therapist interaction, an interaction effect was found between client conceptual level and the type of aftercare program. High conceptual level clients did better in low structure aftercare programs, while low conceptual level clients did better in high structure aftercare programs. In another study that examined the match between clients and therapists, Beutler, Jobe, and Elkins (1974) focused on attitude similarity in a number of different areas that varied in their centrality, to the client. Both outpatients and inpatients were included in the research sample. For attitudes of medium centrality, the greater the similarity between the client and the therapist, the better the outcome according to patient ratings.

In 1974, two studies were published that investigated the treatment of maladjusted college students with time-limited short-term group therapy (Abramowitz & Abramowitz, 1974; Abramowitz, Abramowitz, Roback, & Jackson, 1974). In the first report, students high in psychological mindedness improved more in insight-oriented groups, while students low in psychological mindedness improved more in noninsight-oriented groups. In the second report, students high in internal locus of control improved more in nondirective therapy, while students high in external locus of control improved more in directive therapy. The locus of control variable was also investigated by Kilmann and Howell (1974). A large sample of institutionalized female drug addicts was treated with either structured (directive) or unstructured (nondirective) marathon group therapy. In this study, addicts high in internal locus of control improved more than high externals

TABLE 3.2.   Studies Investigating the Interaction of Client Characteristics and Other Variables

Investigators	Client Characteristics	Types of Interacting Variables (Therapy or Therapist)
Meichenbaum et al. (1971)	Focality of speech phobia	Desensitization group, insight group
McLachlan (1972)	Conceptual level	Therapist conceptual level
McLachlan (1974)	Conceptual level	High structure aftercare, low structure aftercare
Beutler et al. (1974)	Attitudes	Therapist attitudes
Abramowitz et al. (1974)	Internal-external locus of control	Directive group, nondirective group
Abramowitz & Abramowitz (1974)	Psychological mindedness	Insight-oriented group, noninsight-oriented group
Kilmann & Howell (1974)*	Internal-external locus of control	Structured marathon group, unstructured marathon group
Kilmann et al. (1975)	Internal-external locus of control	Unstructured marathon group, structured traditional group
Hargreaves et al. (1974)	Motivation, shyness-upsetness	Group, individual, minimal contact group
Covi et al. (1976)	Interpersonal sensitivity	Group, minimal supportive individual
Finney & Moos (1979)*	Social-competence	Residential programs
Annis & Chan (1983)		Intensive group, routine institutional care
Pilkonis et al. (1984)	Age, chronicity of problems, social class	Group, individual, conjoint (couple)
Simons et al. (1985)	Learned resourcefulness	Cognitive group, pharmacotherapy
MacKay & Liddell (1986)	Cognitive response	Cognitive group, noncognitive group
Stoppard & Henri (1987)	Conceptual level	High structure group, low structure group
de Carufel & Piper (1988)	Object relations, likability, etc.	Short-term individual, short-term group, long-term individual, long-term group
Kadden et al. (1989)	Psychopathology, sociopathy, neuroimpairment	Interactional group, coping skills group
Neimeyer & Weiss (1990)*	Depression, demographics, etc.	Cognitive group, interactional group
Sexton et al. (1990)*	Ego strength, diagnosis	Interactional group, handicraft group
Beutler et al. (1991)	Coping style, (externalization), defensiveness, (resistance potential)	Cognitive-behavioral group, focused-expressive group, supportive individual
Cooney et al. (1991)	Psychopathology, sociopathy, neuroimpairment	Interactional group, coping skills group
Follette et al. (1991)	Previous treatment	Interpersonal transaction group, process group

*No significant interaction effect.

regardless of the type of therapy. Thus, there was no evidence for an interaction effect. A third publication relevant to the investigation of locus of control was authored by Kilmann, Albert, and Sotile (1975), although the clients—undergraduate volunteers—may not have represented a clinical sample. Kilmann et al. reported finding interaction effects in two substudies, one involving marathon groups and one involving "traditional group therapy." In both, clients high in internal locus of control showed greater positive change in unstructured groups, while clients high in external locus of control showed greater positive change in structured groups. The variation in findings across the studies investigating interaction effects for locus of control suggests that higher order interaction effects may be involved. For example, whether or not interactions between locus of control and the structure of therapy are found may depend on other patient features (e.g., whether the sample is comprised of mildly maladjusted students or drug addicts). A final study conducted in 1974 was reported by Hargreaves, Showstack, Flohr, Brady, and Harris (1974). Two client characteristics within a sample of male alcohol and drug clients were studied—motivation and the degree to which clients were shy and upset. A series of significant interaction effects between the two client characteristics and type of therapy (individual, group, minimal contact) were found for participation, remaining, and outcome.

Significant interaction effects were also reported by Covi, Lipman, Alarcon, and Smith (1976) in a large-scale study involving chronically ill, mostly female, depressed outpatients treated with combinations of group psychotherapy and medication or minimal supportive psychotherapy and medication. Clients high in interpersonal sensitivity on the SCL-90 did well in minimal supportive psychotherapy, while clients low in interpersonal sensitivity did well in group psychotherapy. However, it must be noted that interpersonal sensitivity was the only significant predictor out of 22 variables investigated in the study. In another large-scale study involving over 300 alcoholics involved in five different residential treatment programs that utilized group techniques, Finney and Moos (1979) were unable to detect significant patient (social competence)-program interaction effects. In contrast, however, Annis and Chan (1983) found significant interaction effects for male offenders with alcohol and drug problems between positive self-image and type of therapy on criteria of recidivism. Offenders with a positive self-image did better with intensive group therapy, while offenders with a negative self-image did better with routine institutional care.

Pilkonis, Imber, Lewis, and Rubinsky (1984) conducted a well-designed comparative outcome study involving individual, group, and conjoint (couple) psychotherapy. Using a comprehensive battery of outcome measures, evidence of main effects for the type of therapy was negligible. In contrast, a number of significant interaction effects between certain patient characteristics (age, chronicity of problems, socioeconomic status) and type of therapy were found. For example, older clients evidenced greater symptomatic improvement in group therapy and conjoint therapy, while younger clients evidenced greater symptomatic improvement in individual psychotherapy. The investigators emphasized the importance of the fit between client characteristics and type of therapy. A similar conclusion was reached by Simons, Lustman, Wetzel, and Murphy (1985) who studied the comparative outcomes of very different types of therapy, combinations of group cognitive therapy and nortriptyline/placebo among depressed outpatients. Clients high in learned resourcefulness did better with cognitive therapy, while clients low in learned resourcefulness did better with pharmacotherapy. MacKay and Liddell (1986) also studied the effects of cognitive group therapy among a small sample of agoraphobic clients. Cognitive responder clients did better in cognitive group therapy, while noncognitive responder clients did better in noncognitive therapy.

Stoppard and Henri (1987) focused on the same client conceptual level variable that McLachlan had studied using, however, a sample of unassertive women. The two types of therapy utilized were high-structure-behavioral training and low-structure-cognitive training. For one of the central outcome variables, role-play assertive behavior, low conceptual level clients improved more in the high-structure training, while high conceptual level clients did equally well in both types of training. Thus, partial evidence for the predicted interaction effect was found. However, for another outcome variable, anxiety during the role-play, high conceptual level clients did better in high-structure training, which was contrary to the prediction. The findings of the study suggest the presence of higher order interaction effects involving client conceptual level, type of therapy, and type of outcome variable.

Following a comparative outcome study that investigated four forms of time-limited psychotherapy (short-term individual, short-term group, long-term individual, long-term group) with a sample of psychiatric outpatients (Piper, Debbane, Bienvenu, & Garant, 1984), de Carufel and Piper (1988) searched for client characteristics that were differentially related to the individual vs. group forms of psychotherapy. This has long been an issue of keen interest by clinicians and researchers. The measures of the client characteristics came from ratings of the client by an interviewer prior to the onset of therapy. Although they did not find any "hard" differentiators (i.e., single predictors that were significantly related to improvement for one form of therapy and significantly related to worsening for the other form of therapy), they did find a number of "soft" differentiators (i.e., single predictors that were significantly related to improvement for one form of therapy but not significantly related to improvement for the other form of therapy). The investigators reasoned that for a particular patient a pattern of scores on a number of "soft" differentiators might favor one form of therapy over the other. For example, according to the findings, a high score on the variable object choice and low scores on the variables motivation for group therapy, object type, and psychodynamic formulation would favor short-term individual psychotherapy over short-term group psychotherapy. The investigators emphasized the importance of replicating their findings with a larger sample and greater range of scores on the predictor variables.

Kadden, Cooney, Getter, and Litt (1989) studied the effects of two types of six-month, time-limited group therapy for a large sample of alcoholic clients who had completed a 21-day inpatient program. Coping skills training involved a structured cognitive-behavioral approach and interactional group therapy involved an unstructured, here-and-now approach. No overall significant differences in outcome were found for the two types of group therapy. The three primary client characteristics investigated were global psychopathology, sociopathy, and neuropsychological impairment. Clients high in psychopathology or sociopathy improved more in coping skills training, while clients low in sociopathy improved more in interactional therapy. These findings confirmed the investigators' hypothesis that poorer functioning clients would benefit more from a structured therapy while higher functioning clients would benefit more from an unstructured therapy that demanded greater social skills. However, contrary to the investigators' prediction, clients high in neuropsychological impairment improved more in interactional therapy. The study is a good example of an investigation where some of the theory-based hypotheses were supported while others were not, thus requiring a revised explanation for the latter. In a two-year follow-up assessment of the clients, the investigators reported that the original pattern of findings were maintained (Cooney, Kadden, Litt, & Getter, 1991).

Neimeyer and Weiss (1990) studied a number of client characteristics (symptomatic, cognitive, demographic/background) as predictors of outcome for two very different types of group therapy (cognitive/behavioral, psychodynamic/process-oriented) for a large sample of depressed outpatients. Symptomatic and cognitive characteristics emerged as significant predictors while demographic/background characteristics did not. To their surprise, they found no significant differentiators of improvement for the two different types of therapy. Sexton, Fornes, Kruger, Grendahl, and Kolset (1990) similarly found no significant evidence for a predicted client-therapy interaction. The primary client characteristic was ego strength and the two types of group treatment were an emotionally demanding interactional therapy and a nondemanding handicraft activity for psychiatric inpatients.

In contrast to the previous two studies, Beutler et al. (1991) found considerable evidence for client-therapy interactions in a sample of clients with major depressive disorder. The two primary client characteristics were coping style (externalization) and defensiveness (resistance potential), which were operationalized by combining scales from the MMPI. The three, time-limited short-term treatments were cognitive-behavioral group therapy, focused expressive (gestalt) group therapy, and supportive individual therapy conducted by telephone. Clients high in externalization improved more in group cognitive therapy, while clients low in externalization improved more in supportive therapy. Clients high in resistance potential improved more in supportive therapy, while clients low in resistance potential improved more in the two group therapies. These interaction effects were found for the Hamilton Rating Scale for Depression, but not for the Beck Depression Inventory, which again highlights the fact that client-therapy interactions are further dependent on particular outcome variables. Finally, in another recent study that involved the treatment of sexually abused (incest) women with two types of group therapy (structured interpersonal transaction therapy, unstructured process therapy), Follette, Alexander, and Follette (1991) found a trend for an interaction with client history of previous treatment. Clients with previous treatment did better in the process therapy, while clients without previous treatment did well in both types of group therapy.

As indicated earlier, the evidence for significant interaction effects in the 23 studies is considerable. The general implication for the clinician is to continually think in terms of matching clients and therapies when assessing clients. If the clinician does not offer different therapies within his own practice or clinic, arrangements for referrals to other therapies must be established. Forming conclusions about specific matches from the literature is problematic, however. As soon as one focuses on specific client characteristics or therapies, the number of relevant studies shrinks to only a few. Nevertheless, it is the responsibility of the clinician to become familiar with the relevant literature. The potential benefits to the clinician and clients are substantial. The use of relatively inexpensive assessment tools may significantly improve selection decisions.

Some client characteristics (e.g., internal/external locus of control or conceptual developmental level), which appeared in several earlier studies, seem to have come into and gone out of fashion over the years. Interestingly, their absence in more recent studies cannot be attributed to nonproductivity in earlier studies. A promising feature of some of the more recent studies is that the hypotheses appear to be more a function of theory-based a priori formulations rather than post hoc explorations of available variables. Another conclusion that can be reached from surveying the studies is that the findings probably reflect only part of higher order, more complex interactions. There are definite suggestions from several of the studies that therapist characteristics and types of outcome variables must be taken into consideration in generating predictions about client characteristics and types of therapy.

STUDIES INVESTIGATING INTERPERSONAL VARIABLES AS PREDICTORS

A number of different types of measures of interpersonal behaviors can be differentiated. They include: ratings of group behavior from direct observation, ratings of dyadic interview behavior from direct observation, ratings of interpersonal traits from interview information, ratings of interpersonal problems from interview information, scores for interpersonal traits from psychological tests and scores for interpersonal problems from psychological tests. Each of these types will be considered.

Direct Observation of Group Behavior

Despite the fact that all therapy groups require certain types of group behavior from their clients, only four of the studies reviewed used ratings of group behavior from direct observation as predictors. Giedt (1961) studied nurses' ratings of chronic psychiatric inpatients' ward behavior. The nurses rated patients on the Motility, Affect, Cooperation, and Communication (MACC) scales of Ellsworth (1957). Patients then participated in short-term therapy groups. Several desirable behaviors in the therapy groups were combined to create a suitability score for group therapy. Giedt found significant associations between the communication, cooperation, motility, and total adjustment scales of the MACC and the suitability composite. Thus, behavior on the wards was predictive of subsequent group therapy process. In a similar type of study, although with a small sample of severe emphysema patients, Pattison and Rhodes (1974) studied nurses' ratings using the Nurses' Observation Scale for Inpatient Evaluation (NOSIE; Honigfeld & Klett, 1965). Although the NOSIE ratings were not significantly related to group therapy process, they were significantly related to treatment outcome.

In a third study, Piper and Marrache (1981) focused upon client behavior in four, one-hour group pretraining (preparation) sessions that preceded the onset of dynamically oriented, long-term group psychotherapy for psychiatric outpatients. A process analysis of the pretraining behavior provided client scores for participation, on-task behavior, responsivity to the leader, and on-task responsivity to the leader. A process analysis of the clients' group therapy behavior during the first four months, using a modification of the Hill Interaction Matrix (Hill, 1965), provided an analogous set of client scores. Significant correlations were found between each of the pretraining scores and the analogous group therapy scores. The study provided strong confirmation of the predictive ability of previous client group behavior for subsequent client group therapy behavior. In contrast, ratings of client characteristics that were based on a dyadic interview conducted prior to the onset of therapy were poor predictors of client group therapy behavior. Also, neither the pretraining scores nor the interview scores were significantly related to client attendance or remaining in the therapy groups.

In a fourth study, which provided an opportunity to replicate the findings of Piper and Marrache (1981), Connelly and Piper (1989) also focused upon client behavior in group pretraining sessions that preceded long-term group psychotherapy for psychiatric outpatients. The investigators focused on two of the client variables (participation, on-task behavior) during the first two of the four pretraining sessions. In addition to using the process analysis method of the previous study to derive the client pretraining scores, the leaders of the pretraining sessions, who were not the therapists of the subsequent therapy groups, also rated each client on participation and on-task behavior. Similar to the findings of the previous study, significant correlations were found between participation in pretraining and participation in group therapy, and between on-task behavior in pretraining and on-task behavior in group therapy using the process-analysis scores. In addition, however, significant correlations with the group therapy scores were also found using the leader-rated scores. Evidence was also found for significant correlations between the pretraining scores (process analysis generated or leader rated) and some of the outcome variables in the study. Using leader-rated scores is a considerable saving of time. Process analysis-generated scores require several hours of work for trained raters, while leader-rated scores require only a few minutes of the leader's time. The study of Connelly and Piper thus provided a replicated confirmation of the predictive ability of client group behavior that is rated from direct observation. As a set, all four of the studies that used this type of measure of interpersonal variables yielded significant findings, three with therapy process and two with treatment outcome.

Direct Observation of Dyadic Behavior

There were also four studies that used ratings of dyadic interview behavior from direct observation. Given the frequency of initial interview assessments, it is surprising that more investigators have not used ratings of the client's actual interview behavior. Among a sample of male psychiatric outpatients participating in short-term, dynamically oriented group therapy, Kotkov (1958) found that patients who had been more friendly and less composed in their initial interviews tended to be remainers rather than dropouts. Levine, Levin, Sloan, and Chappel (1972) studied a sample of black, male heroin addicts who participated in a methadone maintenance program that included a weekly, two-hour group meeting. Interview ratings of capacity for object relatedness were not significantly related to improvement in the program. The third study was that of de Carufel and Piper (1988), which was cited above among the interaction studies. Two of the variables (interaction with the interviewer, response to interpretation) were rated directly from the client's interview behavior. Neither were significantly related to improvement for the short-term and long-term forms of group psychotherapy. The fourth study was conducted by Hoberman, Lewinsohn, and Tilson (1988). Depressed adults were treated with Lewinsohn's time-limited Coping with Depression Course. The initial assessor's rating of the client using the Barrett-Lennard Relationship Inventory (Barrett-Lennard, 1962) was actually inversely related to improvement in depression. Overall, the results from using direct ratings of dyadic behavior are entirely different from those using direct ratings of group behavior. None of the studies yielded a significant direct relationship with treatment outcome.

Interview Information

It has been somewhat more common to use the initial interview to assess interpersonal traits or problems from the historical report of the client. Seven of the studies reviewed provided information about such variables. Findings were excluded when the predictor variable was measured in the same way as the outcome variable (e.g., the Social Ineffectiveness Scale), since pre- and postmeasures usually are highly correlated. Frank, Gliedman, Imber, Nash, and Stone (1957) reported no significant relationship between ratings of social ineffectiveness and remaining in a large sample of psychiatric outpatients that were treated with group or individual therapy; although Nash, Frank, Gliedman, Imber, and Stone (1957), using a subsample of the larger study and more differentiated definitions of remainers and dropouts, did report a significant inverse relationship between social ineffectiveness and remaining. In the previously cited study by Levine et al. (1972), the rating for object relatedness was partly based on historical information provided by the client. It was not significantly related to outcome. Mintz, O'Brien, and Luborsky (1976) attempted to predict the outcome of group therapy for schizophrenic patients who had recently been discharged from the hospital. However, their social effectiveness scale was not significantly related to outcome. As indicated previously, the interview-based ratings in the Piper and Marrache (1981) study were poor predictors of client group therapy behavior, attendance, and remaining. In the previously cited study by de Carufel and Piper (1988), two of the three object relations ratings were significantly related to improvement in both short-term and long-term forms of group psychotherapy. Finally, in the previously cited study by Hoberman et al. (1988), a global social adjustment rating was significantly related to improvement in depression. Overall, the results involving ratings of interpersonal traits or problems from the historical report of the client have been mixed. Four of the seven studies reported significant findings; two involved treatment outcome.

Psychological Test Scores

The most frequent measures of interpersonal variables in the studies reviewed are psychological test scores. Typically they are the easiest and most economical to measure, which may explain their popularity. Contrary to what one might expect, they are not limited to the older studies. Nine of the eleven studies were published between 1973 and 1992. Yalom, Houts, Zimerberg, and Rand (1967) found a significant relationship between the client's interpersonal compatibility with other group members using the FIRO-B (Schutz, 1958) and client popularity in an outpatient sample. However, no significant relationship was found with outcome. Another significant relationship with therapy process (verbal participation) was found in outpatient group therapy by Aston (1970) using a projective measure of client-object relations. Koran and Costell (1973) also used the FIRO-B to measure interpersonal compatibility in an attempt to predict remaining in outpatient group therapy. However, neither compatibility nor scores from the HIM-B, a questionnaire derivative of the Hill Interaction Matrix, was significantly related to remaining. A successful predictor of remaining, for which the study is often cited, was client compliance in completing the questionnaires for the study. Also searching for questionnaire interpersonal predictors of remaining Connelly, Piper, de Carufel, and Debbane (1986) were successful while McCallum, Piper, and Joyce (1992) were not.

In their study of alcoholic patients treated in residential programs, Finney and Moos (1979) found a significant relation between a composite measure of social competence, which was based on a background questionnaire, and treatment outcome. In a study of outpatients treated in time-limited group therapy, Budman, Demby, and Randall (1980) also found a significant relationship between a questionnaire measure of interpersonal relations and outcome. Steinmetz, Lewinsohn, and Antonuccio (1983), however, did not find a significant relationship between an initial measure of social adjustment and improvement in a sample of depressed outpatients. The original study by Kadden et al. (1989) and the two-year follow-up study by Cooney et al. (1991) involving the aftercare treatment of alcoholics were described in the section concerning interaction effects. Sociopathy was measured by the Socialization Scale of the California Psychological Inventory (Megargee, 1972). As indicated, clients high on sociopathy did better with coping skills training, while clients low in sociopathy did better with interactional therapy. A rather complex relationship (curvilinear) between a measure of interpersonal distress and outcome was also reported by Mohr et al. (1990) in a study of time-limited group therapy for depressed outpatients. Both positive responders and negative responders had high levels of interpersonal distress while nonresponders had a moderate level of interpersonal distress, according to the Inventory of Interpersonal Problems (Horowitz, Rosenberg, Baer, Ureno, & Villasenor, 1988).

Similar to the results for interpersonal interview variables, the results for psychological test scores include a mixed pattern of significant and nonsignificant relationships. One of three studies yielded significant relationships with remaining, two of two studies for process variables and five of seven studies for outcome variables. Although mixed, the results were not barren as some reviewers have concluded. What is clearly lacking are attempts to replicate and cross-validate the significant findings. In summary, the most promising measures of interpersonal variables involve ratings of group behavior from direct observation; the least promising involve ratings of dyadic behavior from direct observation, and in between are measures of interpersonal traits and problems from interview information or psychological test scores.

The clinical implications associated with these findings are relatively clear. Clinicians should carefully consider the patient's group behavior. Many patients who are referred to group therapy have had previous experience in therapy groups. A description of the patient's behavior from the perspectives of the referring source and the patient may prove to be very informative. Even better would be an opportunity to observe the patient directly in a group. When forming a new group, a procedure that is common in some clinics is to conduct a "group screen." This involves meeting with several potential group therapy patients at the same time. Such a procedure, which is not inconceivable for private practice, can sometimes capitalize on combining the tasks of assessment and preparation. It provides both the patient and therapist with an opportunity to make a final decision that is informed by actual group experience. In regard to particular interview measures and psychological tests, familiarity with the literature can allow clinicians to try out those that correspond to the specific characteristics of their groups.

DEMOGRAPHIC AND DIAGNOSTIC VARIABLES

Many of the 83 studies reported findings for demographic and diagnostic variables. The findings are summarized for each variable in terms of box-scores for the four types of dependent variables (attendance, remaining, process, outcome). Process refers to intratherapy events that are reported by the patient, therapist, or an external observer. Space limitations require a selective rather than complete listing of the studies for each variable. Complete listings are available from the author.

Age

Of the two studies that included attendance, one reported a direct relationship and the other a nonsignificant relationship. Of the 10 studies that included remaining, one reported a direct relationship, one an inverse relationship, and eight nonsignificant relationships. Of the two studies that included process variables, both reported nonsignificant relationships. Of the 16 studies that included outcome variables, two reported a direct relationship, four an inverse relationship, and 10 nonsignificant relationships. The two direct relationships involve general symptomatology (Myers, 1975; Pilkonis et al., 1984). The four inverse relationships all involve depression (Cabeen & Coleman, 1962; Mohr et al., 1990; Steinmetz et al., 1983; Youssef, 1990); the older the client the less the improvement. Thus, only in the outcome area is there evidence for the importance of age.

Sex

No studies included attendance, and of the six studies that include remaining, one reported a direct relationship for males and five reported nonsignificant relationships. Of the three studies that include process variables, none reported significant relationships. Of the nine studies that include outcome variables, one reported a direct relationship for males, two a direct relationship for females, and six nonsignificant relationships. Overall, there is little evidence for the importance of sex.

Marital Status

There were no studies that included attendance or process variables. Of the 11 studies that include remaining, two reported a direct relationship with being married, one a direct relationship with being single, and 8 nonsignificant relationships. Of the eight studies that include outcome variables, one reported a direct relationship with being single and seven nonsignificant relationships. Thus, there is little evidence for the importance of marital status.

Educational Status

The one study that includes attendance was nonsignificant. Of the seven studies that include remaining, two reported direct relationships with amount of education and five reported nonsignificant relationships. No studies include process variables. Of the nine studies that include outcome variables, two reported direct relationships and seven reported nonsignificant relationships. Thus, there is only minimal evidence for the importance of educational status.

Employment Status

There were no studies that include attendance or process variables. Of the six studies that include remaining, none reported significant findings. Of the four studies that include outcome variables, one reported a direct relationship and three reported nonsignificant relationships. There is little evidence for the importance of employment status.

Social Status

Ratings of social status are often based on one or more of the previous variables. No studies include attendance. Of the four studies that include remaining, two reported a direct relationship and two reported nonsignificant relationships. The one study that uses a process variable reported a nonsignificant relationship. Of the four studies that include outcome variables, one reported a direct relationship and three reported nonsignificant relationships. Thus, there is only minimal evidence for the importance of social status.

Formal Diagnosis

There were no studies that included attendance. Of the eight studies that include remaining, two reported direct relationships for diagnoses of anxiety and depression (Frank et al., 1957; Rabin, Kaslow, & Rehm, 1985), three reported inverse relationships for personality disorders (Connelly et al.,

1986), paranoid disorders (Holmes, 1983), and hysterical disorders (Sethna & Harrington, 1971), and three reported nonsignificant relationships. The only study including a process variable was nonsignificant (Holmes, 1983). Of the six studies that include outcome variables, two reported direct relationships for diagnoses of neurosis (Cabeen & Coleman, 1962), anxiety, and depression (Frank et al., 1957), and four reported nonsignificant relationships. Thus, there is some evidence for the importance of formal diagnosis in the areas of remaining and outcome.

For the set of demographic variables, there was little or no evidence for the importance of sex, marital status, educational status, employment status, or social status. Only age emerged as having an impact, favorable in the case of general symptomatology and unfavorable in the case of depression. Similarly, there was some evidence for the impact of formal diagnosis in the areas of remaining and outcome. Better results were associated with what have traditionally been regarded as the "neurotic" disorders that are characterized by anxiety and depression. This should come as no surprise to clinicians.

INTELLIGENCE AND EXPECTANCY VARIABLES

Intelligence

No studies include attendance. Of the two studies that included remaining, neither reported significant findings. Of the two process variable studies, one reported a direct relationship with social interaction (McFarland, Nelson, & Rossi, 1962) and one reported a nonsignificant relationship. None of the four studies that involved outcome variables reported a significant relationship. Overall, there is little evidence for the importance of intelligence.

Expectancy

There are several different kinds of expectancy variables in the psychotherapy literature. The client expectancy variables from the studies reviewed can be summarized under favorable expectancies of what therapy will be like (process) and favorable expectancies of what therapy will achieve (outcome). No studies include attendance, and of the three studies that include remaining, two reported direct relationships for favorable process expectancies (Connelly et al., 1986; Rabin et al., 1985) and the other, a nonsignificant relationship (McCallum et al., 1992). The one study including a process variable (positive responder) reported a direct relationship with what appears to be a combination of favorable process and outcome expectancies (Caine & Wijesinghe, 1976). Of the six studies including outcome variables, four reported a positive relationship with favorable outcome expectancies (Bloch, Bond, Qualls, Yalom, & Zimmerman, 1976; Hoberman et al., 1988; Pearson & Girling, 1990; Steinmetz et al., 1983), and two reported nonsignificant relationships (Brown & Lewinsohn, 1984; Sandahl & Ronnberg, 1990). Thus, of the available studies there does appear to be evidence for the importance of expectancy variables. Given their ease of measurement, the findings suggest that they should be used more frequently by both clinicians and researchers.

ADDITIONAL PERSONALITY VARIABLES

In addition to the personality variables that were included in the interaction effect studies, a number of others have been investigated as predictor variables. For example, psychological mindedness has been found to be directly related to remaining (McCallum & Piper, 1990; McCallum et al., 1992) and improvement (de Carufel & Piper, 1988). Confidence in the former study's findings was enhanced by utilization of a cross-validation procedure. Ego strength has also been found to be directly related to favorable outcome (Lazic & Bamburac, 1991; Sexton et al., 1990). Measures of approval dependency (Anchor, Vojtisek, & Berger, 1972), emotional lability (Bossert, Schmolz, Wiegand, Junker, & Krieg, 1992), and suggestibility (Frank et al., 1957) similarly were significantly related to important dependent variables.

Although client predictor variables have been studied much less frequently by behaviorally oriented therapists, some investigators have demonstrated significant relationships with such variables as perceived mastery and learned resourcefulness (Hoberman et al., 1988). In addition, a variety of personality dimensions from standard personality inventories have yielded significant findings. These include studies using the MMPI (Grosz & Wagoner, 1971), Edward's Personal Preference Schedule (Payne, Rasmussen, & Shinedling, 1970), the Maudsley Personality Inventory (Stern & Grosz, 1966), Cattell's 16 PF Questionnaire (Hoy, 1969), and the Jourard Self-Disclosure Questionnaire (Yalom et al., 1967). However, a number of the limitations characterizing the entire area of client variables as predictors curtail enthusiasm that might otherwise be derived from these studies. There is a lack of replication or cross-validation and an absence of more than one type of therapy group in each study. Additionally, for most of the studies that investigated a large number of variables (e.g., those using multiple personality factor inventories), only a few out of the many variables emerged as significant. Until such limitations are remedied, the results of each study stand as relatively isolated findings. Clinicians may wish to try out certain personality measures; however, it is clear that particular measures cannot as yet be recommended upon the basis of cumulative research evidence.

HISTORICAL AND INITIAL DISTURBANCE VARIABLES

Historical Variables

Historical information about clients is easily and commonly acquired. Two variables investigated as predictors in a number of the reviewed studies were previous treatment and chronicity of problems. Previous treatment was usually defined as a dichotomous variable (presence/absence), although the type and amount varied. Of the ten studies investigating the relationship between previous treatment and outcome variables, three reported inverse relationships and seven reported nonsignificant relationships. Of the six studies investigating the relationship between chronicity of problems and outcome variables, two reported inverse relationships and four reported nonsignificant relationships. Thus, for both previous treatment and chronicity of problems there is some, although no substantial, evidence for an inverse relationship with outcome. A variety of other types of historical variables (e.g., age of onset, developmental abuse) have been investigated, but because the number of studies for each is small, generalizations are not warranted.

Initial Disturbance Variables

Measures of initial (pretherapy) disturbance are perhaps the most popular of all predictor variables. Approximately 40% of the studies reviewed explicitly reported results for initial disturbance. In a number of cases, the investigators merely reported a significant relationship between the initial and post-therapy levels of various outcome variables. Such findings are common in studies of both group and individual therapy. Among the other studies reviewed, where the investigators used different measures for the predictor and outcome variables, a frequent pattern emerged. In most cases, there was evidence from each study for both inverse relationships (i.e., the greater the initial disturbance, the poorer the outcome) and nonsignificant relationships. Evidence for direct relationships was nearly nonexistent. Thus, when there was a significant relationship, greater initial disturbance predicted poorer outcome. Although the evidence is not that strong, the implication for clinicians is that they may wish to take care not to overload their groups with patients who have a history of previous treatments and chronic problems, or who are high in initial disturbance.

RESEARCH EVIDENCE AND PREVIOUS CONCLUSIONS

As indicated earlier, previous reviewers have formed a number of conclusions and have made a number of recommendations for research investigating the impact of client characteristics. The 83 studies of the present review and their findings can be viewed in light of those recommendations. The most promising body of research is that of the interaction studies. During the past 20 years, three times as many interaction studies have been conducted than in the past preceding 20 years and 83% of the studies have yielded significant findings.

By definition, an interaction study involves a client characteristic and at least one additional type of variable. Therefore, a multivariate model and the notion of interaction between the different types of variables are inherent. In most cases, the additional type of variable is the type of group therapy, which fulfills another recommendation of previous reviewers. In addition, interaction studies require a theoretical rationale that explains why the findings should differ for different levels of the variables. Some of the explanations offered by previous investigators were admittedly post hoc, but more studies are being carried out where the hypotheses concerning interactive effects are being formulated a priori upon the basis of a clear theoretical rationale.

Although progress in the area of interactive studies has definitely occurred, further progress can be made. The current review revealed that investigators typically consider only two-way interaction effects. Higher order interaction effects are known to occur and offer a better representation of the complexity of the clinical situation. Type of therapist and type of outcome variable are investigated as additional interactive dimensions only infrequently. Also infrequent is the use of multivariate statistical procedures, which can provide both an indication of the total amount of variance accounted for and the unique contribution of individual predictors. Another improvement involves a greater use of interpersonal variables as predictors in interaction studies. Of the 22 interaction studies reviewed, only four investigated interpersonal variables. After reviewing all of the studies (i.e., both interaction studies and noninteraction studies), it is clear that researchers rarely have considered the issue of base rates and infrequently have attempted to replicate and cross-validate findings. These two recommended objectives remain unfulfilled.

Aside from making recommendations about future research, previous reviewers have formed conclusions about the value of certain types of predictors. One theme of previous reviewers is to invest in interpersonal variables as predictors, but to eschew the dyadic interview as the source of such variables. The present review clearly supports the use of direct observation of group behavior as a source of interpersonal variables. There is mixed evidence about the value of the dyadic interview. On the one hand, the use of direct observation of dyadic behavior as a source of interpersonal variables appears to be nonproductive. On the other hand, the use of the dyadic interview to derive an historical assessment of interpersonal traits and problems has met with some success. It is likely premature to reject the dyadic interview as a source of useful predictors. Similarly, the use of psychological tests as a source of interpersonal variables has met with some success and should not be rejected entirely at this time. At the risk of making a tiring refrain, replication and cross-validation studies would go a long way toward resolving uncertainties about the value of these predictors.

Two other types of predictors that generally are viewed negatively by reviewers are demographic variables and formal diagnosis. The current review also revealed minimal evidence for the usefulness of demographic variables, with the possible exception of age. Some evidence for the importance of formal diagnosis was found in the areas of remaining and outcome. Some supportive evidence was also found for previous treatment, chronicity of problems, and initial level of disturbance. One of the more positive findings concerned expectancy variables, which are relatively easy to assess.

CLINICAL IMPLICATIONS

As pointed out in the introduction, a number of previous reviewers of the client variable literature have complained about the lack of specific guidelines for practitioners that have arisen from research studies. That state of affairs has not changed appreciably despite the increase of predictor studies in the past 20 years. Psychotherapy research tends to be characterized by a slow accumulation of information, not by dramatic breakthroughs. Although 83 studies may seem like a large number, when one focuses on particular combinations of patients, group techniques, and therapists, typically only a few studies are relevant.

From the findings of the available studies, certain generalizations can be made. Clinicians can be urged to devise group assessment procedures where direct observations of potential patients' behavior can be observed. They can be encouraged to take a careful client history that explores interpersonal traits and problems. Certain psychological tests that assess interpersonal variables may prove useful. Clinicians can be advised not to overstock their groups with patients with chronic problems, multiple previous treatments, and intense initial disturbance. They can be reminded that pessimistic expectations can be prophetic of later experience. While guidelines such as these seem to constitute reasonable advice from researchers, they may not satisfy clinicians' wishes for specific criteria to optimize outcomes in their specific clinical groups.

There is no doubt that the predominant issue for clinicians is patient selection. That typically involves decisions between group therapy or no therapy, group therapy or individual therapy, and between different types of group therapy. In recent years, more and more studies have been addressing such questions. The interaction studies are probably the best examples. Over time, as more complex and more methodologically sophisticated studies are conducted, the chances that the practitioner will have available a relevant body of knowledge to consult for his/her specific needs will increase. Even so, a nagging and potentially problematic question remains, "Will clinicians be attentive and allow the findings to influence their practice?" For that to occur, the gulf that often exists between "researchers" and "clinicians" will have to narrow. A good deal of responsibility will fall on researchers who must make their findings clear and clinically relevant.

As Yalom (1985) and others have noted, clinicians have traditionally paid more attention to exclusion rather that inclusion criteria. In Yalom's words, "Given a pool of patients, they determine that certain ones cannot possibly work in a therapy group and should be excluded, and then proceed to accept all the other patients" (p. 228). For example, in the case of intensive, interactional outpatient group psychotherapy, typical exclusion categories have been patients who are brain-damaged, paranoid, hypochondriacal, drug-dependent, psychotic, sociopathic, suicidal, deeply depressed, and in crisis. The common rationale is that such patients are likely to be viewed as deviants who do not share the objectives of the group and who are unable to participate in the required interpersonal processes of the group. While this position continues to be held, there is growing recognition among clinicians that there are few patients for whom some type of group is not appropriate. In Bond and Lieberman's words, "Deviant behavior, whether it be delinquency, alcoholism, or child abuse, has been successfully approached in a variety of situations" (p. 682). Groups with homogeneous composition in regard to a particular "deviant" population are frequently touted as the solution. Such an approach has its merits. However, it too, has its limits as those who have attempted to treat groups of borderline patients have found. Clinicians have frequently struggled with the irony that the patients most in need of group therapy seem to be those least able to benefit. They have not wanted to simply prove the aphorism that in regard to client characteristics and group therapy, "The rich get richer." A contribution that researchers could make would be to advise the clinician about what to do with excluded patients. An alternative may very well be a different type of therapy group.

There is a related factor that is relevant to the issue of exclusion and clinicians' willingness to use research findings. Clinicians may be unwilling to deny a "high risk" patient an opportunity to have a valuable experience in a therapy group. Risky clients sometimes surprise us. We may not want to deprive all risky patients of an opportunity to benefit even if we know that a number of such patients will not. In a 1972 article about dropouts, Martin Grotjahn made this point in regard to giving doubtful patients a chance in his own practice. In the same article, however, he expressed surprise and dismay at the high number of dropouts in his practice. A contribution that researchers can make is to clarify who represents high risk patients for specific types of groups and therapists, and then inform clinicians, who can make their own decisions about how much risk or how many risky patients to accept for their groups. Having one of two risky patients in a group is far different than having five or six.

In a 1975 review of the clinical literature, Mullan and Rosenbaum highlighted a number of contradictory positions involving such issues as the range of patients deemed suitable for group therapy and the degree of homogeneity among patients that is considered to be desirable. As an aside, they made an important point regarding the exclusion of patients for group therapy, "As the group therapist gains experience, he will become less selective." It is possible that the same point can be made for the entire group therapy field (i.e., as the field gains experience, it will become less selective). This already seems to have begun to happen.

In conclusion, there is an additional issue that researchers must face. A strong consensus exists among those who have carefully reviewed the literature about what is desirable in future research that investigates client characteristics. However, conducting sophisticated studies that both inform the researcher and clinician (e.g., multivariate research that explores interaction effects) will require considerable resources. It is reasonable to wonder whether institutions and granting bodies will be willing to allocate the necessary funds, staff, and time. Thus, it will be up to the researcher to convince administrators and granting bodies that tangible clinical benefits justify this complexity and the associated costs. Hopefully, clinicians will collaborate with researchers in making such requests and carrying out future projects.

REFERENCES

Note: The 83 research studies that met the inclusion criteria for the review are indicated by an asterisk.

*Abramowitz, C. V., Abramowitz, S. I., Roback, H. B., & Jackson, C. (1974). Differential effectiveness of directive and non-directive group therapies: A function of client internal-external control. *International Journal of Group Psychotherapy, 42*(6), 849–853.

*Abramowitz, S. I., & Abramowitz, C. V. (1974). Psychological-mindedness and benefit from insight-oriented group therapy. *Archives of General Psychiatry, 30*(5), 610–615.

*Anchor, K. N., Vojtisek, J. E., & Berger, S. E. (1972). Social desirability as a predictor of self-disclosure. *Psychotherapy: Theory, Research and Practice, 9*(3), 262–264.

*Anchor, K. N., Vojtisek, J. E., & Patterson, R. L. (1973). Trait anxiety, initial structuring and self-disclosure in groups of schizophrenic patients. *Psychotherapy: Theory, Research and Practice, 10*(2), 155–158.

*Annis, H. M., & Chan, D. (1983). The differential treatment model: Empirical evidence from a personality typology of adult offenders. *Criminal Justice and Behavior, 10*(2), 159–173.

*Aston, P. J. (1970). Predicting verbal participation in group therapy. *British Journal of Psychiatry, 116*, 45–50.

Barrett-Lennard, G. T. (1962). Dimensions of therapist response as causal factors in therapeutic change. *Psychological Monographs, 76,* (43, Whole No. 562).

Bednar, R. L., & Kaul, T. J. (1978). Experiential group research: Current perspectives. In S. L. Garfield & A. E. Bergin (Eds.), *Handbook of psychotherapy and behavior change* (2nd ed., pp. 769–815). New York: Wiley.

*Beutler, L. E., Engle, D., Mohr, D., Daldrup, R. J., Bergan, J., Meredith, K., & Merry, W. (1991). Predictors of differential response to cognitive, experiential, and self-directed psychotherapeutic procedures. *Journal of Consulting and Clinical Psychology, 59*(2), 333–340.

*Beutler, L. E., Jobe, A. M., & Elkins, D. (1974). Outcomes in group psychotherapy: Using persuasion theory to increase treatment efficiency. *Journal of Consulting and Clinical Psychology, 42*(4), 547–553.

*Bloch, S., Bond, G., Qualls, B., Yalom, I., & Zimmerman, E. (1976). Patients' expectations of therapeutic improvement and their outcomes. *American Journal of Psychiatry, 133*(12), 1457–1460.

Bond, G. R., & Lieberman, M. A. (1978). Selection criteria for group therapy. In C. Brady & K. Brodie (Eds.), *Controversy in psychiatry* (pp. 679–702). Philadelphia, PA: W.B. Saunders.

*Bossert, S., Schmolz, U., Wiegand, M., Junker, M., & Krieg, J. C. (1992). Case history and shorter communication: Predictors of short-term treatment outcome in bulimia nervosa inpatients. *Behavioral Research Therapy, 30*(2), 193–199.

*Brown, R. A., & Lewinsohn, P. M. (1984). A psychoeducational approach to the treatment of depression: Comparison of group, individual, and minimal contact procedures. *Journal of Consulting and Clinical Psychology, 52,* 774–783.

*Budman, S. H., Demby, A., & Randall, M. (1980). Short-term group psychotherapy: Who shall succeed and who shall fail? *Group, 4*(3), 3–16.

*Butler, T., & Fuhriman, A. (1983). Level of functioning and length of time in treatment variables influencing patients' therapeutic experience in group psychotherapy. *International Journal of Group Psychotherapy, 33*(4), 489–505.

*Cabeen, C. W., & Coleman, J. C. (1962). The selection of sex-offender patients for group psychotherapy. *International Journal of Group Psychotherapy, 12,* 326–334.

*Caine, T. N., & Wijesinghe, B. (1976). Personality, expectancies and group psychotherapy. *British Journal of Psychiatry, 129,* 384–387.

*Connelly, J. L., & Piper, W. E. (1989). An analysis of pretraining work behavior as a composition variable in group psychotherapy. *International Journal of Group Psychotherapy, 39*(2), 173–189.

*Connelly, J. L., Piper, W. E., de Carufel, F. L., & Debbane, E. G. (1986). Premature termination in group psychotherapy: Pre-therapy and early therapy predictors. *International Journal of Group Psychotherapy, 36*(1), 145–152.

*Cooney, N. L., Kadden, R. M., Litt, M. D., & Getter, H. (1991). Matching alcoholics to coping skills or interactional therapies: Two-year follow-up results. *Journal of Consulting and Clinical Psychology, 59*(4), 598–601.

*Covi, L., Lipman, R. S., Alarcon, R. D., & Smith, V. K. (1976). Drug and psychotherapy interactions in depression. *American Journal of Psychiatry, 133*(5), 502–508.

*de Carufel, F. L., & Piper, W. E. (1988). Group psychotherapy or individual psychotherapy: Patient characteristics as predictive factors. *International Journal of Group Psychotherapy, 38*(2), 169–188.

*Derr, J., & Silver, A. W. (1962). Predicting participation and behavior in group therapy from test protocols. *Journal of Clinical Psychology, 18,* 322–325.

*Dyck, R. J., & Azim, H. F. (1983). Patient satisfaction in a psychiatric walk-in clinic. *Canadian Journal of Psychiatry, 28*(1), 30–33.

Ellsworth, R. B. (1957). *The MACC behavioral adjustment scale.* Los Angeles, CA: Western Psychological Services.

*Finney, J. W., & Moos, R. H. (1979). Treatment and outcome for empirical subtypes of alcoholic patients. *Journal of Consulting and Clinical Psychology, 47*(1), 25–38.

*Follette, V. M., Alexander, P. C., & Follette, W. (1991). Individual predictors of outcome in group treatment for incest survivors. *Journal of Consulting and Clinical Psychology, 59*(1), 150–155.

*Frank, J. D., Gliedman, L. H., Imber, S. D., Nash, Jr., E. H., & Stone, A. R. (1957). Why patients leave psychotherapy. *Archives of Neurology and Psychiatry, 77,* 283–299.

*Gallagher, E. B., & Kanter, S. S. (1961). The duration of out-patient psychotherapy. *Psychiatric Quarterly Supplement, 35,* 312–331.

Garfield, S. L. (1986). Research on client variables in psychotherapy. In S. L. Garfield & A. E. Bergin (Eds.), *Handbook of psychotherapy and behavior change* (3rd ed., pp. 213–256). New York: Wiley.

*Giedt, F. H. (1961). Predicting suitability for group psychotherapy. *American Journal of Psychotherapy, 15,* 582–591.

*Gliedman, L. H., Stone, A. R., Frank, J. D., Nash, Jr., E., & Imber, S. D. (1957). Incentives for treatment related to remaining or improving in psychotherapy. *American Journal of Psychotherapy, 11,* 589–598.

*Grosz, H. J., & Wagoner, R. (1971). MMPI and EPPS profiles of high and low verbal interactors in therapy groups. *Psychological Reports, 28,* 951–955.

Grotjahn, M. (1972). Learning from dropout patients: A clinical view of patients who discontinued group psychotherapy. *International Journal of Group Psychotherapy, 22,* 306–319.

*Hargreaves, W. A., Showstack, J., Flohr, R., Brady, C., & Harris, S. (1974). Treatment acceptance following intake assignment to individual therapy, group therapy or contact group. *Archives of General Psychiatry, 31*(3), 343–349.

Harvey, O. J., Hunt, D. E., & Schroder, H. M. (1961). *Conceptual systems and personality organization.* New York: Wiley.

Hawkins, D. M., & White, E. M. (1978). Indications for group psychotherapy. In C. Brady & K. Brodie (Eds.), *Controversy in psychiatry* (pp. 703–720). Philadelphia, PA: Saunders.

*Heckel, R. V. (1972). Predicting role flexibility in group therapy by means of a screening scale. *Journal of Clinical Psychology, 28,* 570–573.

Hill, W. F. (1965). *HIM: Hill Interaction Matrix.* Los Angeles, CA: Youth Studies Center, University of Southern California.

*Hinshelwood, R. D. (1972). Patients who lapse from group psychotherapy. *British Journal of Psychiatry, 120*(558), 587–588.

*Hoberman, H. M., Lewinsohn, P. M., & Tilson, M. (1988). Group treatment of depression: Individual predictors of outcome. *Journal of Consulting and Clinical Psychology, 56*(3), 393–398.

Hollon, S. D. (1984). Clinical innovations in the treatment of depression: A commentary. *Advances in Behavioral Research and Therapy, 6,* 141–151.

*Holmes, P. (1983). "Dropping out" from an adolescent therapeutic group: A study of factors in the patients and their parents which may influence this process. *Journal of Adolescence, 6*(4), 333–346.

Honigfeld, G., & Klett, C. J. (1965). The nurses observation scale for inpatient evaluation. *Journal of Clinical Psychology, 21,* 65–71.

Horowitz, L. M., Rosenberg, S. E., Baer, B. A., Ureno, G., & Villasenor, V. A. (1988). Inventory of interpersonal problems: Psychometric properties and clinical applications. *Journal of Consulting and Clinical Psychology, 56,* 885–892.

*Hoy, R. M. (1969). The personality of inpatient alcoholics in relation to group psychotherapy, as measured by the 16-P.F. *Quarterly Journal of Studies on Alcohol, 30*(2), 401–407.

*Jacobs, M. A., Spilken, A. Z., Norman, M. M., Wohlberg, G. W., & Knapp, P. H. (1971). Interaction of personality and treatment conditions associated with success in a smoking control program. *Psychosomatic Medicine, 33*(6), 545–556.

*Kadden, R. M., Cooney, N. L., Getter, H., & Litt, M. D. (1989). Matching alcoholics to coping skills or interactional therapies: Posttreatment results. *Journal of Consulting and Clinical Psychology, 57*(6), 698–704.

*Kalb, M. (1987). The effects of biography on the divorce adjustment process. *Sexual and Marital Therapy, 2*(1), 53–64.

Kaul, T. J., & Bednar, R. L. (1986). Experiential group research: Results, questions, and suggestions. In S. L. Garfield & A. E. Bergin (Eds.), *Handbook of psychotherapy and behavior change* (3rd ed., pp. 671–714). New York: Wiley.

*Kilmann, P. R., Albert, B. M., & Sotile, W. M. (1975). Relationship between locus of control, structure of therapy, and outcome. *Journal of Consulting and Clinical Psychology, 43*(4), 588.

*Kilmann, P. R., & Howell, R. J. (1974). Effects of structure of marathon group therapy and locus of control of therapeutic outcome. *Journal of Consulting and Clinical Psychology, 42*(6), 912.

*Koran, L. M., & Costell, R. M. (1973). Early termination from group psychotherapy. *International Journal of Group Psychotherapy, 23*(3), 346–359.

*Kotkov, B. (1955). The effect of individual psychotherapy on group attendance: A research study. *International Journal of Group Psychotherapy, 5,* 280–285.

*Kotkov, B. (1958). Favorable clinical indications for group attendance. *International Journal of Group Psychotherapy, 8,* 419–427.

*Kotkov, B., & Meadow, A. (1952). Rorschach criteria for continuing group psychotherapy. *International Journal of Group Psychotherapy, 2,* 324–333.

*Lazic, N., & Bamburac, J. (1991). The functioning of personality and the success of group psychotherapy of alcoholics. *Acta Medica Iugoslavica, 45*(1), 77–86.

*Levine, D. G., Levin, D. B., Sloan, I. H., & Chappel, J. N. (1972). Personality correlates of success in a methadone maintenance program. *American Journal of Psychiatry, 129*(4), 456–460.

*MacKay, W., & Liddell, A. (1986). An investigation into the matching of specific agoraphobic anxiety response characteristics with specific types of treatment. *Behavior, Research & Therapy, 24*(3), 361–364.

*McCall, R. J. (1974). Group therapy with obese women of varying MMPI profiles. *Journal of Clinical Psychology, 30*(4), 466–470.

*McCallum, M., & Piper, W. E. (1990). A controlled study of effectiveness and patient suitability for short-term group psychotherapy. *International Journal of Group Psychotherapy, 40*(4), 431–452.

*McCallum, M., Piper, W. E., & Joyce, A. S. (1992). Dropping out from short-term group therapy. *Psychotherapy, 29,* 206–215.

*McFarland, R. L., Nelson, C. L., & Rossi, A. M. (1962). Prediction of participation in group psychotherapy from measures of intelligence and verbal behavior. *Psychological Reports, 11,* 291–298.

*McLachlan, J. F. (1972). Benefit from group therapy as a function of patient-therapist match on conceptual level. *Psychotherapy: Theory, Research and Practice, 9*(4), 317–323.

*McLachlan, J. F. (1974). Therapy strategies, personality orientation and recovery from alcoholism. *Canadian Psychiatric Association Journal, 19*(1), 25–30.

Megargee, E. I. (1972). *The California Psychological Inventory handbook.* San Francisco, CA: Jossey-Bass.

*Meichenbaum, D. H., Gilmore, J. B., & Fedoravicius, A. (1971). Group insight versus group desensitization in treating speech anxiety. *Journal of Consulting and Clinical Psychology, 36*(3), 410–421.

*Mintz, J., O'Brien, C. P., & Luborsky, L. (1976). Predicting the outcome of psychotherapy for schizophrenics: Relative contributions of patient, therapist and treatment characteristics. *Archives of General Psychiatry, 33*(10), 1183–1186.

*Mohr, D. C., Beutler, L. E., Engle, D., Shoham-Salomon, V., Bergan, J., Kaszniak, A. W., & Yost, E. B. (1990). Identification of patients at risk for nonresponse and negative outcome in psychotherapy. *Journal of Consulting and Clinical Psychology, 58*(5), 622–628.

*Moos, R. H., & Bromet, E. (1978). Relation of patient attributes to perceptions of the treatment environment. *Journal of Consulting and Clinical Psychology, 46*(2), 350–351.

Mullan, H., & Rosenbaum, M. (1975). The suitability for the group experience. In M. Rosenbaum & M. M. Berger (Eds.), *Group psychotherapy and group function* (pp. 415–426). New York: Basic.

*Myers, E. D. (1975). Age, persistence and improvement in an open out-patient group. *British Journal of Psychiatry, 127,* 157–159.

*Nash, E. H., Frank, J. D., Gliedman, L. H., Imber, S. D., & Stone, A. R. (1957). Some factors related to patients' remaining in group psychotherapy. *International Journal of Group Psychotherapy, 7,* 264–274.

*Neimeyer, R. A., & Weiss, M. E. (1990). Cognitive and symptomatic predictors of outcome of group therapies for depression. *Journal of Cognitive Psychotherapy, 4*(1), 23–32.

*Osborne, D., & Swenson, W. M. (1972). Counseling readiness and changes in self-evaluation during intensive group psychotherapy. *Psychological Reports, 31*(2), 646.

*Pattison, E. M., & Rhodes, R. J. (1974). Clinical prediction with the N-30 scale. *Journal of Clinical Psychology, 30,* 200–201.

*Payne, R., Rasmussen, D. M., & Shinedling, M. (1970). Characteristics of university females who lose weight. *Psychological Reports, 27*(2), 567–570.

*Pearson, M. J., & Girling, A. J. (1990). The value of the Claybury Selection Battery in predicting benefit from group psychotherapy. *British Journal of Psychiatry, 157,* 384–388.

*Pilkonis, P. A., Imber, S. D., Lewis, P., & Rubinsky, P. (1984). A comparative outcome study of individual, group, and conjoint psychotherapy. *Archives of General Psychiatry, 41*(5), 431–437.

Piper, W. E., Debbane, E. G., Bienvenu, J. P., & Garant, J. (1984). A comparative outcome study of four forms of psychotherapy. *Journal of Consulting and Clinical Psychology, 52,* 268–279.

*Piper, W. E., & Marrache, M. (1981). Selecting suitable patients: Pretraining for group therapy as a method of patient selection. *Small Group Behavior, 12*(4), 459–476.

Power, M. J. (1985). The selection of patients for group therapy. *International Journal of Social Psychiatry, 31*(4), 290–297.

*Puder, R. S. (1988). Age analysis of cognitive-behavioral group therapy for chronic pain outpatients. *Psychology and Aging, 3*(2), 204–207.

*Rabin, A. S., Kaslow, N. J., & Rehm, L. P. (1985). Factors influencing continuation in a behavioral therapy. *Behavior, Research and Therapy, 23*(6), 695–698.

Roback, H. B., & Smith, M. (1987). Patient attrition in dynamically oriented treatment groups. *American Journal of Psychiatry, 144*(4), 426–431.

*Rosenzweig, S. P., & Folman, R. (1974). Patient and therapist variables affecting premature termination in group psychotherapy. *Psychotherapy: Theory, Research and Practice, 11*(1), 76–79.

Rutan, J. S., & Stone, W. N. (1984). *Psychodynamic group psychotherapy.* Lexington, MA: D.C. Heath.

*Salzberg, H. C. (1969). Group psychotherapy screening scale: A validation study. *International Journal of Group Psychotherapy, 19,* 226–228.

*Sandahl, C., & Ronnberg, S. (1990). Brief group psychotherapy in relapse prevention for alcoholic dependent patients. *International Journal of Group Psychotherapy, 40*(4), 453–476.

Schutz, W. C. (1958). *FIRO: A three dimensional theory of interpersonal behavior.* New York: Holt, Rinehart and Winston.

*Sethna, E. R., & Harrington, J. A. (1971a). A study of patients who lapsed from group psychotherapy. *British Journal of Psychiatry, 119,* 59–69.

*Sethna, E. R., & Harrington, J. A. (1971b). Evaluation of group psychotherapy. *British Journal of Psychiatry, 118,* 641–658.

*Sexton, H., Fornes, G., Kruger, M. B., Grendahl, G., & Kolset, M. (1990). Handicraft or interactional groups: A comparative outcome study of neurotic inpatients. *Acta Psychiatrica Scandinavica, 82*(5), 339–343.

*Simons, A. D., Lustman, P. J., Wetzel, R. D., & Murphy, G. E. (1985). Predicting response to cognitive therapy of depression: The role of learned resourcefulness. *Cognitive Therapy and Research, 9,* 79–89.

Smith, M. H., Glass, G. V., & Miller, P. I. (1980). *The benefits of psychotherapy.* Baltimore, MD: Johns Hopkins University Press.

*Steinmetz, J. L., Lewinsohn, P. M., & Antonuccio, D. O. (1983). Prediction of individual outcome in a group intervention for depression. *Journal of Consulting and Clinical Psychology, 51*(3), 331–337.

*Stern, H., & Grosz, H. J. (1966). Personality correlates of patient interactions in group psychotherapy. *Psychological Reports, 18,* 411–414.

*Stone, W. R., & Rutan, J. S. (1984). Duration of treatment in group psychotherapy *International Journal of Group Psychotherapy, 34,* 93–109.

*Stoppard, J. M., & Henri, G. S. (1987). Conceptual level matching and effects of assertion training. *Journal of Counseling Psychology, 34*(1), 55–61.

*Truax, C. B. (1971). The initial status of the client and the predictability of psychotherapeutic change. *Comparative Group Studies, 2*(1), 3–16.

Woods, M., & Melnick, J. (1979). A review of group therapy selection criteria. *Small Group Behavior, 10*(2), 155–175.

*Yalom, I. D. (1966). A study of group therapy dropouts. *Archives of General Psychiatry, 14,* 393–414.

Yalom, I. D. (1985). *The theory and practice of group psychotherapy* (3rd ed.). New York: Basic.

*Yalom, I. D., Houts, P. S., Zimerberg, S. M., & Rand, K. H. (1967). Prediction of improvement in group therapy: An exploratory study. *Archives of General Psychiatry, 17,* 159–168.

*Youssef, F. A. (1990). The impact of group reminiscence on a depressed elderly population. *Nurse Practitioner, 15*(4), 32–38.

CHAPTER 4

Therapist Variables in Group Psychotherapy Research

ROBERT R. DIES

Group psychotherapy is widely regarded as a viable and vital treatment format. The empirical foundation for group treatments has been firmly established (Dies, 1993; in press-a), and considerable attention is now being devoted to the refinement of our understanding of the complex processes that contribute to client improvement through group participation. Many of the unique advantages of this modality are documented, but there is still much to be learned about how group psychotherapists can enhance the quality and effectiveness of their interventions during the treatment process. Generalizations about leadership based on the empirical literature have often been compromised by either the limited quantity or inferior quality of the research; nevertheless, it has been possible to offer recommendations that have direct implications for clinical practice (Dies, 1983b, 1993; Dies & Dies, 1993a).

This chapter provides an overview of recent research on the therapist's influence during group treatments including a comprehensive survey of research published since 1980. The conclusions from an extensive review of the literature on therapist variables during the 1970s (Dies, 1983b) are extended or modified through an evaluation of more recent empirical findings. This critique is not exhaustive; however, it reflects a detailed sampling of the articles appearing in more than 50 different professional journals. Of the thousands of empirical studies of group treatments that have emerged during the past 20 years, only those with direct evaluations of leadership are considered in this review. Rather than a listing of methodological problems and pitfalls, a pragmatic set of guidelines is offered that is consistent with the accumulated empirical results.

Two types of investigations are covered in this summary: those including various instruments that are used to assess the influence of the therapist on group process and/or outcome, and those that compare different forms of group intervention (e.g., interpersonal versus psychodynamic, or cognitive-behavioral versus supportive). Moreover, when group treatments are contrasted with other forms of intervention, it is seldom possible to identify what aspects of leadership account for the findings. Thus, numerous reviewers show that group and individual therapies are roughly comparable in their efficacy (e.g., Dies, in press-a; Orlinsky & Howard, 1986; Toseland & Siporin, 1986), but it is not clear whether "nonspecific factors" or particular therapist techniques produce the results. Consequently, in this review, group-versus-other-modality studies are not included unless instruments to assess leadership variables are also integrated.

There are other areas of investigation that have clear implications for therapists' interventions during the treatment process, but no attempt has been made to address these areas. The extensive bodies of literature on pre-group contracting and therapeutic factors are not reviewed (Dies, 1993), nor is the material on group treatments for children and adolescents (Dies & Riester, 1986).

THE NATURE OF THE GROUPS

The author's previous review of group leadership included 95 investigations of both treatment and personal growth groups designed to promote therapeutic change. The present survey adds another 135 studies to this body of evidence, although related articles and recent reviews of other aspects of group process and outcome are cited to provide a broader foundation for the conclusions. Tables 4.1 and 4.2 furnish an overview of the research published since the author's last synopsis.

The largest single category of "client" remains the nonpatient group (27% of the studies), which generally consists of students or trainees who are participating in an intensive encounter group experience, or mental health practitioners who are seeking refinement of their own intervention skills through involvement in a concentrated experiential group. This figure is substantially below that of ten years ago, when the percentage of nonpatients represented nearly two-thirds of the investigations (Dies, 1983b). Reviewers of the group treatment literature have commonly included the nonpatient groups in their surveys, based on the strong process and intervention parallels that exist between these groups and more treatment-oriented models. The significant advantage of these projects is the convenience of evaluating large numbers of groups in a brief period of time (e.g., the studies by Coché, Dies, & Goettelmann, 1991 and MacKenzie, Dies, Coché, Rutan, & Stone, 1987 both incorporate more than 40 groups). Moreover, it is possible with nonpatient samples to examine group processes that are difficult to control in more naturally occurring treatment contexts (e.g., variations in how interpersonal feedback is delivered) (Morran, Robison, & Stockton, 1985).

The three largest patient groups investigated include diagnostically mixed outpatient groups (16%), depressed (12%), and anxious clients (8%). Ten studies were conducted within inpatient settings (8%). Furthermore,

TABLE 4.1.   Diagnostic Composition of Groups in Leadership Research
(n = 135 Studies)

Sample	n	Group Composition	Percent
Abusive/Angry males	3	*Composition:*	
Alcohol/Substance abusing	5	Homogeneous	79%
Anxious/Unassertive	11	Heterogenous	21%
Depressed	16	Closed	94%
Eating disordered	6		
Geriatric	3	Open	6%
Inpatient:		*Selection:*	
Mixed	8		
Schizophrenic	2	Recruited	53%
Nonpatient	37	Routine	47%
Outpatient—Mixed	21		
Personality disordered	3		
Prisoners	3		
Sexually abused	3		
Special populations:			
Cancer patients	2		
Caregivers	1		
Chronic back pain	4		
Foster mothers	1		
Herpes sufferers	2		
Marital distress	2		
Mastectomy patients	1		
Physically disabled	1		
Smokers	2		
Type A personalities	3		

numerous special populations were evaluated, including cancer and chronic
back pain patients, smokers, and Type A personalities. In a majority of the
investigations (53%), patients were specifically recruited for the research
project and the groups were composed homogeneously (79%). To alleviate
any concern about biased sampling, most investigators established meaningful cut-offs to ensure that their syndrome-specific volunteers (e.g., anxious,
bulimic, or depressed) were genuinely symptomatic and distressed.

Table 4.2 reveals that two-thirds of the studies that provide such information contain fewer than seven groups (85 of 127) and that most of the investigations focus on short-term interventions; from the descriptions available,
71% of the projects (86 of 121) conduct no more than a dozen sessions. The
average number of groups is 6.8, with a mean number of sessions of 11.6.
Although about half the groups function with co-therapists and many of the
clinicians are rather inexperienced (65% of the 106 studies furnishing such
information), the impact of these variables is seldom researched. The issues
of co-leadership and the group psychotherapists' level of experience are addressed later in this chapter.

TABLE 4.2.   Leadership and Groups Examined in Research (n = 135 Studies)

Leaders	Percent	Groups	Percent
Studies with solo therapists	51	*Number of groups:*	
Studies with co-therapists	45	1 to 6 groups	63
Unknown	4	7 to 12	19
		13 or more	12
Experience level:		Unknown	6
Nondegree/Interns	30		
1 to 3 years	21	*Number of sessions:*	
More than 3 years	27	1 to 6 session	19
Unknown	22	7 to 12	44
		13 or more	26
		Unknown	10

*Average number of groups = 6.8 and sessions = 11.6.

RESEARCH EXPEDIENCY OR CLINICAL REALITY?

Some readers may question whether much confidence can be placed in research findings based on such time-limited group treatments conducted by relatively inexperienced therapists. However, the temptation to dismiss this body of research as unrepresentative should be resisted, at least until we have had the opportunity to examine the critical evidence of treatment effects and to explore whether the findings on leadership are commensurate with our own practical experiences as group psychotherapists.

There is little question that a considerable proportion of the research on therapist variables is driven by pragmatic issues and matters of expediency. It is much easier to entice less experienced practitioners to become involved in research than it is to cajole our more seasoned colleagues to devote the amount of time and effort that is necessary to implement a systematic research project. Many investigators have noted the reluctance of experienced clinicians to become involved in research (e.g., Bernard & Drob, 1989; Cappon, 1981; Dies, 1992a); however, it seems clear from recent evidence that this "resistance" is not related to beliefs that research is unimportant, or that it is incompatible with the goals of treatment. Rather it is more a matter of time management (Dies, 1992a, 1993). It is not that inexperienced clinicians are any less busy, but rather that they are willing to balance priorities, because involvement in group research facilitates their professional development (e.g., they are provided with additional supervision; it is part of their internship training; or the study is related to their dissertation research).

The apparent inexperience of the therapists who participate in group research is somewhat misleading, however, for several reasons. In many of the studies, the leaders are guided by detailed treatment manuals (manuals carefully developed by experts in the field) that furnish extensive directions on how to conduct the group sessions (see Table 4.3). Moreover, many of the

TABLE 4.3.   A Sampling of Treatment Manuals (n = 30 Studies)

Therapeutic Approach and Patient Samples	Investigators
Cognitive-behavioral	
Anxious/Unassertive	Eayrs, Rowan, & Harvey, 1984; Shaffer, Sank, Shapiro, & Donovan, 1982; Stoppard & Henri, 1987
Avoidant disorders	Alden, 1989
Depressed	Fine, Forth, Gilbert, & Haley, 1991; Neimeyer & Feixas, 1990; Nezu, 1986; Sanchez, Lewinsohn, & Larson, 1980; Steuer et al., 1984; Zettle & Rains, 1989
Herpes sufferers	Drob, Bernard, Lifshutz, & Nierenberg, 1986
Inpatient—Mixed	Coché, Cooper, & Petermann, 1984
Low back pain patients	Turner, Clancy, McQuade, & Cardenas, 1990; Turner & Clancy, 1988
Sexual assault victims	Resnick, Jordan, Girelli, Hutter, & Marhoefer-Dvorak, 1988
Social/Dating anxiety	Gormally, Varvil-Weld, Raphael, & Sipps, 1981; Neumann, Critelli, Tang, & Schneider, 1988
Type A personality	Thurman, 1985
Interpersonal-experiential	
Alcoholics	Getter, Litt, Kadden, & Cooney, 1992
Depressed	Fleming & Thornton, 1980
Nonpatients	Richardsen & Piper, 1986
Sexually abused women	Alexander, Neimeyer, & Follette, 1991
VA patients—Mixed	Monti, Curran, Corriveau, DeLancey, & Hagerman, 1980
Psychodynamic	
Depressed	Steuer et al., 1984
Herpes sufferers	Drob et al., 1986
Loss patients	McCallum & Piper, 1990
Psychoeducational/Social Skills	
Career counseling	Robbins & Tucker, 1986
Depressed	Brown, 1980; Hoberman, Lewinsohn, & Tilson, 1988; Lewinsohn, Steinmetz, Antonuccio, & Teri, 1985
Family caretakers	Abramowitz & Coursey, 1989
Schizophrenics	Jensen, 1982
VA patients—Mixed	Monti et al., 1980

studies highlight how the less experienced clinicians are monitored and supervised throughout the treatment process to ensure that the "experimental treatment" is implemented reliably. Indeed, many investigators devote considerable time to the preparation of their group leaders. Hoberman, Lewinsohn, and Tilson (1988), for example, indicate that their doctoral students completed a specialized three-month training program before their research project was inaugurated. Finally, many researchers argue that their treatments proved to be quite effective in spite of their therapists' relative inexperience and suggest that the findings might be even more robust with more experienced practitioners. It may be important to remind ourselves that relatively inexperienced therapists are not just involved in group research, but also represent a significant proportion of those professionals who conduct group treatments in our various mental health facilities (Dies, 1993).

It is common for researchers to recruit clients for homogeneously composed, closed, short-term group treatments. Recruitment of "special interest" groups (e.g., test-anxious students, depressed elderly, abuse victims, cancer patients) ensures an adequate sample size for appropriate assignment to alternative treatments. Moreover, the abbreviated and closed group format shields the investigator from the disruptive effects that dropouts have on group process. Once again, however, a critical question is whether these pragmatic constraints or concerns about expediency render these types of groups inappropriate for judgments about clinical practice. It is apparent from the literature that this is not the case, since such short-term, symptom-oriented groups are quite popular in a wide range of mental health contexts (Dies, 1992b). Indeed, pressure from third-party payers, legislators, and patient-consumers for more effective and cost-efficient treatments fuels this trend toward brief forms of psychosocial intervention that require the establishment of more modest goals, greater attention to task focus, prompt interventions, and more directive participation on the part of therapists (Dies & Dies, 1993a, 1993b).

Investigators have examined a variety of methods for augmenting the impact of their brief group treatments, including "booster sessions," the involvement of family members and "buddies" in the treatment process, homework assignments, the completion of research instruments between sessions, and concentrated efforts to foster generalization from treatment to outside settings. These efforts have direct parallels to the types of activities that are found in clinical practice (Dies & Dies, 1993a).

It would be ill-advised and premature to disqualify the empirical work as unrepresentative, especially if our review of the findings can identify central dimensions of leadership that have been consistently linked to beneficial outcomes over the past two decades.

THE ROLE OF STRUCTURE IN GROUP TREATMENTS

The increased emphasis on streamlining group treatments to meet the demands for less expensive and more effective psychosocial interventions appears to be related to a shift away from the nonspecific and personal aspects of leadership so frequently emphasized throughout the 1970s (e.g., genuineness, empathy, support, and self-disclosure) to a focus on the critical ingredients of treatment that foster therapeutic change. Whereas the author's earlier review began with personal and relationship factors (Dies, 1983b), it now seems more appropriate to first highlight variations in group structure and therapist technique.

In an effort to explore the broad implications of group structure, studies were classified according to the nature of the group comparisons that were evaluated by the investigators. Judgments about structure focused on the level of activity of the therapists within the alternative treatment formats, independent of the content of that structure. Seventy-eight studies were identified in which contrasts between two or more group treatments were examined. Fifty-one of these investigations were classified as varying the level of therapist directiveness. In the majority of these studies (69%), the researchers themselves provided the criteria for differentiating between the groups, using such concepts as "structured versus nonstructured," "directive versus nondirective," or "active/planned versus nonspecific and supportive." When these key words were not used, the investigators made it clear that their experimental groups were designed to be more structured; for example, the therapists assumed more responsibility in guiding the group sessions by following a focused treatment manual, by using various exercises or instruction in cognitive-behavioral skills, and/or incorporating specialized techniques (e.g., contracts, homework assignments). In the less structured groups, the leaders typically "did for the group only what the group was unable to do for itself" (Steuer et al., 1984, p. 183). In the remaining 27 studies, it was not possible to distinguish differences in level of therapist activity; the treatments were designed to vary the treatment focus (e.g., cognitive versus behavioral skills training), but not the degree of structure. Most of the investigators attempted to match their experimental groups along the activity dimension. Table 4.4 summarizes the outcome and process findings in relation to structural variations. Conclusions about differential treatment effectiveness were formulated by the original investigators.

There is a distinct pattern to the findings, with the more structured group treatments demonstrating their advantage in the vast majority of the studies. Thus, in the 51 projects exploring differential group structure, the more directive treatments were favored in 40 instances (78%). In seven studies, the authors concluded that results were comparable, while in four others, the less programmed alternatives proved to be more effective. Although outcome was assessed most commonly by self-report measures of symptomatic amelioration, behavioral criteria generally demonstrated parallel results.

TABLE 4.4. Structure and Outcome in Group Treatments

Outcomes	Equally Active Treatments	Structured versus Less Structured
Comparable outcomes	20	7
Differential outcomes	7	44*
Totals	27	51

*40 of these 44 (91%) comparisons favor the structured treatments. After removal of the four inconsistent studies, the chi-square on structure by outcome is 25.9, $p < .001$.

Twenty-seven other researchers compared two equally active group formats and found that in 20 instances (74%), differential main effects could not be established. A statistical analysis of the structure by outcome interaction in Table 4.4 proves to be quite significant (chi-square = 25.9, $p < .0001$).

Although this finding convincingly documents the value of active structuring within short-term group treatments, it does very little to clarify the components of that contribution (e.g., content, timing, focus). What is clear, however, is that structure provides more than a "nonspecific" therapeutic ingredient. When all forms of group therapy are compared with "no treatment" or "wait-list" controls, or with "routine institutional care," it is possible to demonstrate the value of group treatments. Yet this advantage might indeed be nonspecific. For example, there are 70 different comparisons between any form of group treatment and nonactive control groups in the present pool of 135 articles, and the group interventions are superior in 85% of these contrasts. But these results may only relate to increased attention, the opportunity to feel support from fellow sufferers, or some other nontechnical aspect of group treatment. The results from Table 4.4, however, provide evidence that structure has the potential to augment whatever nonspecific factors exist within group interventions.

Two questions that must be addressed are, "Why is more structure better than less?" and "Why do two equally active group treatments generally fail to differentiate?" To answer these questions, it is necessary to examine the variations in structure that have been explored during the past two decades of research. However, it is unrealistic to expect that we can pinpoint the exact structural components (or personal aspects of leader style) that foster more productive group processes and treatment benefits, since direct associations between process and outcome are virtually impossible to establish. Treatment is just too complex and individual differences too complicated to expect that level of precision. Nevertheless, it may be feasible to highlight contributions of therapeutic structure that relate quite consistently to treatment outcome. To do this, it is necessary to examine the types of studies that serve as the basic foundation for leadership research.

THE EMPIRICAL FOUNDATIONS FOR LEADERSHIP RESEARCH

Comparison of Outcomes by Model of Group Therapy

It was noted earlier (Table 4.4) that 78 different investigators compared two or more group treatments in their efforts to understand the role of structure in therapeutic outcome. The types of groups represented in these studies are summarized in Table 4.5. The classification of studies is based on the primary comparison made by the investigators, although this simple scheme

TABLE 4.5.   Structural Comparisons in Leadership Research (n = 78 Studies)

Alternative Treatment	Primary Treatment			
	Cognitive-Behavioral	Traditional	Psycho-educational	Structure A
Cognitive-Behavioral	30	0	0	0
Traditional	22	4	6	0
Psychoeducational	0	0	3	0
Structure B	0	0	0	13
Total	52	4	9	13
Percent	(67%)	(5%)	(11%)	(17%)

overlooks the fact that in many projects multiple treatment groups are evaluated. Thus, a study may contrast two different forms of cognitive-behavioral therapy and a less active "supportive" treatment. This type of study appears in Table 4.5 as a comparison between the cognitive-behavioral alternatives, since that was the investigator's main interest.

Cognitive-behavioral approaches cover a wide range of treatments including assertiveness training, stress management, progressive relaxation, operant techniques, behavioral practice, and cognitive restructuring. Two-thirds of the investigations are focused on these types of groups, and in most instances the comparisons are between two different cognitive-behavioral treatments (30 studies). Traditional group therapies, such as interpersonal, psychodynamic, and supportive group discussion, are often employed as contrast groups in the cognitive-behavioral research (22 of 52 studies), but rarely serve as the principal focus of investigation (4 studies). Psychoeducational programs (e.g., topic-centered, combined didactic-experiential) appear more frequently as the primary treatment (9), most commonly using traditional models as the alternative method (6). The structure A versus structure B comparisons represent 13 studies in which the level of therapist directiveness is systematically varied in some fashion, such as in the use of research measures or contracts.

There is a major concentration on structured group treatments that use a group comparison experimental design. This represents a shift away from the emphasis on correlational studies so popular during the 1970s (Dies, 1983b). Two issues become apparent when the comparisons in Table 4.5 are reviewed more carefully. The first derives from a comparison of cognitive-behavioral and traditional group therapies; 22 such contrasts are identified. The more conventional approaches represent three forms of therapy: supportive group discussion (13), psychodynamic/insight-oriented models (5), and interactive-interpersonal approaches (4). In the vast majority of cases, the supportive and psychodynamic approaches are less structured than the cognitive-behavioral alternatives (17 out of 18 comparisons), and prove to be less effective in most instances (82%). The four studies contrasting interactional and cognitive-behavioral models describe equally active treatment alternatives, and the results do not differentiate between the two approaches. Although the numbers may be too small to draw meaningful conclusions, it seems clear that when traditional methods fail to provide a coherent structure for therapeutic change in short-term group treatments, patients do not achieve substantial benefit. This conclusion becomes even more viable when the earlier findings from Table 4.4 are recalled, showing clear superiority of structured treatments; in a substantial proportion of the nonstructured treatments, the comparison group is described as "supportive."

The second issue derived from a review of Table 4.5 findings relates to the failure of equally active treatments to demonstrate differential outcomes. A review of the reasons offered by investigators to explain their nonsignificant findings is informative. Although the brevity of treatment, diagnostic heterogeneity, and shortcomings in the theoretical models of psychopathology are mentioned by several authors, four other problems appear with greater regularity. First, and by far the most frequent observation, the two treatments share *common nonspecific ingredients,* such as opportunities for interpersonal support, affective expression, and feedback; some treatment alternatives may even share specific treatment components, such as relaxation and assertiveness training. The second most frequently cited factor relates to *interaction effects,* whereby client variables and treatment type interact to cancel out the differential effects of intervention. For example, Coché, Cooper, and Petermann (1984) found that their gender balanced treatments were comparable, but that the males benefited more from the cognitive approach, whereas the females gained more from the affect-oriented model. A third observation is related to *instrument insensitivity.* Thus, research measures may either be too global to detect subtle symptomatic or behavioral improvements, or the battery of change measures may show conflicting results; certain instruments may favor one treatment mode, while others may prove to be more effective with others. Finally, investigators often mention the problem of *small sample sizes.* Deffenbacher, McNamara, Stark, and Sabadell (1990), for example, note that tests of statistical significance may lack power, given the limited number of subjects in group research.

Treatment Manuals

Another way to understand the structure provided by group psychotherapists is to examine the treatment manuals that guide their therapeutic interventions (Table 4.3). These directive treatment plans have become much more common in recent years as investigators have attempted to describe their treatment formats in greater detail. The use of manuals represents a substantial methodological improvement, since it allows researchers to demonstrate that different therapists conducting a particular treatment are reasonably comparable in their approach. Moreover, investigators can empirically corroborate differences across treatment types that are consistent with their experimental design. Getter, Litt, Kadden, and Cooney (1992), for example, used a Group Sessions Rating Scale to substantiate the planned differences between their coping skills and interactional groups for treating alcoholics in an aftercare program. Earlier these authors demonstrated interesting patient by treatment-type interactions that become even more meaningful when it is possible to systematically measure process differences between treatments (Kadden, Cooney, Getter, & Litt, 1989).

A careful analysis of the treatment manuals outlined in Table 4.3 reveals several common ingredients relevant to our consideration of structure, despite differences in models of treatment and therapeutic application. Generally, investigators attempt to furnish a coherent framework for therapeutic change. The basic rationale for treatment, ground rules for interaction (e.g., confidentiality, attendance), clarification of patient and therapist roles, and similar issues are reviewed early in treatment. Goal-setting and evaluation of expectations also occur early in therapy, and sessions are planned to ensure meaningful progress toward individually defined goals. Session-by-session plans for how to guide interaction (process) and what topics to address (content) are typically provided to guarantee continuity across sessions. Homework and other between-session activities are frequently introduced. Concerted effort is made to establish a supportive climate for interaction by highlighting strategies for promoting group cohesion and efforts to provide reinforcement for individual participants.

Although the manuals vary in the specific skills that are addressed (e.g., active listening, self-talk, behavior-targeting, self-reinforcement), most outline a sequence of learning involving general instruction, followed by problem identification, individual sharing and behavioral practice (often using role playing and modeling), and then interpersonal feedback (shaping and reinforcement); these steps are not limited to the cognitive-behavioral approaches, but include interpersonal and psychoeducational models as well. Although the psychodynamically oriented manuals focus less on the aforementioned sequence of individual learning, the system-level parameters are highlighted (i.e., coherent framework, supportive climate) as are the efforts to concertize treatment objectives.

Instruments to Evaluate the Influence of the Therapist

Since the author's review of research, (Dies, 1983b), a substantial reduction in the use of research measures to evaluate leadership has occurred. In the prior survey, extensive tables were provided to summarize three categories of instruments: self-report inventories completed by the therapists (29 different measures), ratings provided by group members (48 methods), and independent assessments supplied by trained observers (42 rating systems). Tables 4.6 and 4.7 list the measures applied in the publications reviewed for the present chapter. Only the client and observer ratings are furnished, since only four authors used therapist self-reports.

TABLE 4.6. Client Ratings of Leadership

Instrument (Number of Studies)	Dimensions and Investigations
Adjective Rating Scales (21)*	Evaluative scales such as warm-cold, involved-detached, skillful-unskillful (e.g., Hurley, 1986; MacKenzie, Dies, Coché, Rutan, & Stone, 1987)
Couples Therapy Alliance Scale (1)	Therapist-client bond, agreement on goals, and engagement in therapy tasks (Bourgeois, Sabourin, & Wright, 1990)
Critical Events (5)	List of most important session events (e.g., Coché, Dies, & Goettelmann, 1991; Drob et al., 1986)
Group Atmosphere Scale (1)	Multiple dimensions of group process but includes leader support (Braaten, 1989)
Group Attitude Scale (1)	Attraction to group and the leader (Evans, 1984)
Group Environment Scale (3)	Various dimensions of group process, including leadership (e.g., Beutler, Frank, Scheiber, Calvert, & Gaines, 1984).
Group Evaluation Form (2)	Six subscales, including perception of the leader (Kivlighan, Hageseth, Tipton, & McGovern, 1981; Robbins & Tucker, 1986)
Group Leader Behavior Instrument (2)	Personal and technical dimensions of leadership (e.g., Phipps & Zastowny, 1988)
Group Leadership Behavior Inventory (1)	Many facets of leadership are measured (Alexander, Neimeyer, & Follette, 1991)
Interviews (3)	To determine critical therapeutic events (e.g., Bernard & Drob, 1989)
Leadership Questionnaire (3)	Four major categories of intervention (e.g., Piper, Connelly, & Salvendy, 1984)
Leader Style Questionnaire (1)	Assesses six styles of leadership (Alexander, 1980)
Relationship Inventory (2)	Measures empathy, regard, congruence (e.g., Clarke, Kramer, Lipiec, & Klein, 1982)
Taxonomy of Interventions (2)	Eighteen clusters of leader behaviors (e.g., Kuriloff, Babad, & Kline, 1988)
Therapist Evaluation Questionnaire (2)	Interest, clarity of communication (e.g., Deffenbacher, McNamara, Stark, & Sabadell, 1990)

*Many different versions of the adjective checklists are available to assess both personal and technical dimensions of therapeutic interventions.

Several reasons can be offered to explain the decline of interest in research measures to evaluate leadership in short-term group treatments. The shift from correlational to experimental design probably accounts for most of this disinterest in instrumentation. The efforts to structure and monitor group process with carefully developed treatment manuals undoubtedly reduces the impact of individual differences across group leaders, since structure overrides personal styles to a large extent in short-term groups. Moreover, stylistic variables, such as genuineness, empathy, and warmth, are now so well-established that investigators train their therapists to ensure that these qualities are evident during treatment.

The fact that therapist self-reports are so unpopular in recent years undoubtedly relates to the finding that global personality variables seldom

TABLE 4.7. Observer Ratings of Leadership

Instrument (Number of Studies)	Dimensions and Investigators
Confrontation Ratings (1)	Assesses the client-centered form of confrontation (Roffers & Waldo, 1983)
Empathy Ratings (1)	Therapist's empathic understanding (Roffers & Waldo, 1983)
Flanders Interactional Analysis System (1)	Personal and technical qualities of leadership (Antonuccio, Davis, Lewinsohn, & Breckenridge, 1987)
Frequency of Self-Disclosures (1)	Therapist sharing of feelings or beliefs (Linehan & O'Toole, 1982)
Group Environment Scale (1)	Various dimensions of group process, including leadership (Beutler et al., 1984)
Group Session Rating Scale (1)	Personal style and specific behaviors (Getter et al., 1992)
Hill Interaction Matrix—Group	Classification of interpersonal communication style and content (Barlow, Hansen, Fuhriman, & Finley, 1982)
Interpretation Ratings (1)	Different types of interpretations (Flowers & Booraem, 1990)
Leader Interventions Rating System (1)	Seven different leadership categories (Richardsen & Piper, 1986)
McDaniel Observer Rating Scale (1)	Personal and technical aspects of behavior (Antonuccio et al., 1987)
Member-to-Leader Behavior (1)	Positive and negative exchanges with the leader (Burrows, 1981b)
Structure Rating Scale (1)	Measures degree of structuring (Stoppard & Henri, 1987)
SYMLOG (1)	Member to leader behaviors (Burrows, 1981a)
Therapy Rating Scale (1)	Cognitive vs. behavioral approach (Stoppard & Henri, 1987)

relate to treatment outcome; specific interactional styles and behaviors within treatment are more likely to be salient, but these are usually assessed by client and observer rating systems. Nevertheless, the "scripting" of treatment has contributed to a reduced interest in individual differences in therapists overall. This observation probably accounts for the less frequent use of client ratings as well. Table 4.6 lists 15 different approaches compared to 48 methods used ten years ago, in spite of the increased number of studies. The most popular approach to client ratings is the adjective checklist; it is versatile and quite easy to apply. For example, MacKenzie et al. (1987) administered a list of 40 leader adjectives in their large-scale study of intensive training groups. Factor analysis of this instrument identified personal and technical "clusters" of leadership (e.g., caring, charismatic, skillful, noncontrolling) that correlated meaningfully with group members' reports of learning. Many other investigations that evaluate open-ended or "nonmanualized" leadership styles continue to find such process-outcome correlations.

Client ratings of leadership remain much more common than observer-based rating systems (the ratio is about 4 to 1); the latter are much more time-consuming and expensive to implement. Consistent with findings in the previous review (Dies, 1983b), most investigators rely on only one perspective on leadership (85%); very few use two viewpoints (13%), and only one researcher used all three. Similarly, there are few standard rating scales in the field that are incorporated by many investigators. Nevertheless, the available findings contribute meaningfully to the body of literature on leadership in group psychotherapy; these results, integrated with information on variations in therapeutic structure, offer generalizations about therapist's interventions.

GENERALIZATIONS ABOUT LEADERSHIP

The vast majority of research on the therapist's contribution to group treatments examines general methods (e.g., assertiveness training versus supportive group discussion, or interactional versus psychodynamic models), rather than specific intervention strategies, such as particular forms of interpretation, dimensions of self-disclosure, or styles of confrontation. The treatment manuals (Table 4.3) outline broad dimensions of intervention, such as a here-and-now focus, directive inquiries, role plays and modeling, selective reinforcement, and interpersonal feedback. Consequently, it is virtually impossible to disentangle the specific factors that promote constructive group interaction and beneficial outcomes. Although the findings clearly indicate that structured treatments are typically more effective than less directive alternatives, the meaning of "structure" is highly variable across and very confounded within investigations. Nevertheless, certain dimensions emerge rather consistently.

Providing a Meaningful Framework for Therapeutic Change

The therapist is faced with the responsibility of helping clients accept assignment to a therapy group as an appropriate form of treatment. Although most clients acknowledge that group psychotherapy is probably just as effective as one-to-one treatment, most prefer to be seen individually (Dies, 1993). Budman et al. (1988), for example, noted that most of their patients did not wish to be placed in a group and that many dropped out of their study when this assignment was made. Despite the fact that their individual and group treatments were equally effective, patients in group therapy were less satisfied with their experience.

Patients have a variety of negative expectations regarding group interventions: fears of attack, embarrassment, emotional contagion or coercion, and actual harmful effects (Slocum, 1987; Subich & Coursol, 1985). Potential group members also have various misconceptions about how group treatments foster therapeutic growth, and initially have difficulty setting goals compatible with effective group interaction (Dies, in press-a; Dies & Dies,

1993a). Finally, the role of the therapist is less clear in group treatments. Brykczynska (1990) found that perceptions of the therapist are different in group therapy, and Bond (1984) discovered that norm regulation around leadership is more confusing.

Many group therapists address these issues during the pretreatment preparation of group members. During this "negotiation phase" (Dies & Dies, 1993b), clinicians attempt to reduce apprehensions about group treatment while instilling positive role and outcome expectations, and to inform patients about constructive interpersonal behaviors (e.g., self-disclosure, feedback, here-and-now interaction), group developmental issues, and helpful therapeutic factors. Researchers have explored the efficacy of various methods to introduce these concepts, including audiotape and videotape interventions, verbal instructions, printed materials, interviews, trial groups, and combinations of these procedures (see Chapter 5 in this volume). The literature suggests that multiple strategies yield better results than single methods (Kivlighan, Corazzini, & McGovern, 1985) and that more realistic interventions (e.g., videotapes and practice sessions as opposed to written handouts) are more productive (Tinsley, Bowman, & Ray, 1988). These pregroup interventions are designed to provide a coherent framework for understanding individual experiences and events within the group, and to minimize the likelihood of premature attrition and therapeutic casualties (Dies, 1993).

The Role of Structure in Relationship to Group Development

Many clinicians do not have the opportunity to spend much time in pretherapy preparation with group members. Instead, they actively structure their initial treatment sessions to integrate the type of material that is typically covered in the "contract." Thus, a majority of the treatment manuals (Table 4.3) address how the group leader should manage the first few sessions in order to provide a meaningful rationale for treatment, by highlighting procedural guidelines (e.g., time boundaries, attendance, confidentiality) and process norms (e.g., turntaking, avoiding a question-and-answer format), therapist and patient responsibilities, and the nature of group interactions.

Bednar, Melnick, and Kaul (1974) offered a developmental model for initiating group psychotherapy, proposing that "lack of structure in early sessions not only fails to facilitate early group development but actually feeds client distortions, interpersonal fears, and subjective distress, which interferes with group development and contributes to premature client dropouts" (p. 31). Recent research adds further confirmation to past generalizations (Dies, 1983b): When treatment goals are clear, appropriate client behaviors are identified, and the group process is structured to provide a framework for change, clients tend to engage in therapeutic work more quickly.

For example, interviews with dropouts reveal that the failure of the therapist to prepare patients effectively for group treatment, as well as the leader's inactivity in early sessions, are central factors in patients' decision to forgo treatment (Bernard & Drob, 1989; Budman, Demby, & Randall, 1980; Connelly, Piper, de Carufel, & Debbane, 1986; Roback & Smith, 1987). Earlier studies suggest that the value of structure depends on the nature of the intervention. Therapist activity and directiveness are only useful when patients feel that task-oriented or therapeutic events have occurred (Anderson, Harrow, Schwartz, & Kupfer, 1972; Schwartz, Harrow, Anderson, Feinstein, & Schwartz, 1970). More recent projects report similar findings. For example, Bourgeois, Sabourin, and Wright (1990) found that treatment outcome is improved when clients have the sense that there is agreement about goals and that there is engagement in tasks relevant to the process of therapy. Borgers (1980) documented the value of a specific treatment contract, whereas Brekke's (1989) use of brief orientation groups with "hard-to-reach clients" was successful in educating, building cohesion, and preparing members for further group treatment.

Caple and Cox (1989) demonstrated that groups with early structure are more cohesive, whereas McGuire, Taylor, Broome, Blau, and Abbott (1986) found increased levels of self-disclosure. Kivlighan and Jauquet (1990) studied agenda-setting activity to show that when participants formulate more realistic goals during early sessions, they see the group as engaged in more productive interactions. Moreover, when members set increasingly realistic, interpersonal, and here-and-now agendas over the life of the group, these changes are related to the perceptions of the group climate along important dimensions of interpersonal work. The issue of timing was also evaluated by Kivlighan, McGovern, and Corazzini (1984), who discovered that group therapy process and outcome are enhanced when therapists coordinate the content and timing of structuring interventions with group developmental issues around themes of anger and intimacy.

Fuehrer and Keys (1988) directly tested the Bednar, Melnick, and Kaul (1974) model of early group development by comparing high and low amounts of structure to explore the impact on group cohesion and the members' sense of "ownership" of group functioning. They concluded that "structuring by the group leaders can have both positive and negative effects and must be used judiciously. With too little structure, participants may not realize the importance of performing constructive group member behaviors and thus may impede the development of group cohesion. With too much structure, participants are less likely to feel ownership of group accomplishments" (Fuehrer & Keys, 1988, p. 339).

It has been suggested that the amount of structure should be sequenced to match the needs of clients within the evolving social microcosm of the group. Kinder and Kilmann (1976) indicated that groups were more productive when they began with a more structured format and then reduced the amount of therapist directiveness. Reviews of the literature provide support for this position (Bednar, et al., 1974; Dies, 1993; Stockton & Morran, 1982). One implication is that therapists should gradually reduce their level of activity and the focus of their structuring as group members improve in their understanding of the therapeutic task and their role in helping each other to accomplish individual goals (Dies, 1993).

Lichtenberg and Knox (1991) note that this activity-shift is consistent with Yalom's (1985) argument that as therapy groups evolve, they should become increasingly "leaderful," with group members assuming more of the responsibility for directing the sessions. However, Lichtenberg and Knox could not detect this progressive change from leader dominance to member or shared dominance in their detailed analysis of group process. It is likely that in many short-term structured groups this pattern will not unfold because of the directive nature of treatment.

Indeed, in a significant proportion of the current studies, therapists continue to maintain an active role in structuring their group treatments. Alden (1989) encouraged specific weekly social targets for his patients and then followed through on these during subsequent sessions; he later learned from his patients that these procedures were particularly helpful in changing their avoidant personality styles. Neimeyer and Feixas (1990) evaluated the value of regular homework assignments and found support for this method of maintaining task orientation during treatment. Graff, Whitehead, and LeCompte (1986) proposed that assigning specific homework projects might be a principal factor in accounting for the success of cognitive-behavioral approaches to group intervention. Many of the noted treatment manuals outlined in Table 4.3 offer guidelines for therapists in how to employ homework assignments to enhance the quality of treatment.

Other investigators incorporate research instruments into treatment in order to provide more effective structure. Caple and Cox (1989) had members discuss the results from a personality test, and Hisli (1987) requested his patients to periodically complete a group behavior self-evaluation form as a feedback mechanism to enhance treatment outcome. Elsewhere, a developmental model is proposed that outlines how to integrate research instruments into four stages of group treatment to improve the quality of service delivery (Dies & Dies, 1993b). The issue of structuring through research instruments continues to receive considerable attention (Dies, 1983a; 1987; 1992a).

The various investigations show that continuing to monitor and structure treatment in light of group developmental themes may play a vital role in facilitating constructive group process and in improving therapeutic gains. Corazzini, Heppner, and Young (1980) demonstrated that even during the termination phase of group treatment, clients appreciate the contribution of therapeutic structure; members in their experimental group who were prepared for termination through a detailed written handout felt more able to work through the ending process. Kivlighan and Jauquet (1990) also noted the importance of members setting the agenda for the latter phases of group work. The overall implication of the various research findings is that the type of therapist activity or structure that seems most beneficial in the group setting is that which gives meaning and significance to the group enterprise throughout the group's existence (Dies, 1983b; Dies & Teleska, 1985).

The classic study by Lieberman, Yalom, and Miles (1973) reveals, however, that it is necessary to define "structure" quite carefully. These authors found that guidance offered by leaders in terms of "meaning attribution" (providing concepts for how to understand individual experiences or group events) is highly conducive to positive group outcome. On the other hand, structure in terms of the "executive function" (setting limits, suggesting rules, managing time) has mixed effects: either too much or too little structure is counterproductive. Both inactive, laissez-faire leaders and overly active ones are far less effective than leaders who assume a more moderate stance. More recently, others have confirmed that nonactive therapists may contribute to disappointing or even deleterious effects for group members (Alexander, 1980; Kanas et al., 1980), as might those leaders who are more domineering or controlling in their styles (Beutler, Frank, Scheiber, Calvert, & Gaines, 1984; MacKenzie et al., 1987). On the other hand, therapists who provide effective levels of structure through "meaning attribution" are likely to provide a framework for change that will have both immediate and enduring consequences for group members (Coché et al., 1991; Piper, Connelly, & Salvendy, 1984). Richardsen and Piper (1986) found that leaders who are more consistent in their meaning-attributive interventions are most effective.

Structure in Relationship to Levels of Psychopathology

In a prior review of leadership research, it was noted that structure is especially important in groups with more psychologically impaired inpatient groups (Dies, 1983b). More recent research supports this generalization. Thus, on the basis of their discharge debriefing interviews with their inpatients, Leszcz, Yalom, and Norden (1985, p. 430) concluded that, "Almost every respondent commented on the necessity for group leaders to be active in structuring, integrating, and focusing, and how wasteful meetings were when the therapist seemed to be waiting for the group to 'activate itself.' Leaders' passivity and silence was unanimously criticized as harmful to group morale, either through failure to set limits to monopolistic, disturbing patients, or through permitting multiple tangential comments which fragmented the group."

Reviewers of the literature on group treatments with inpatient populations generally concur with these observations that therapists not only need to be more active, but also more focused in their efforts to provide a cognitive integration of therapeutic experiences (Erickson, 1982; Mosher & Keith, 1980; Leszcz, 1986). The hallmark of social skills training programs for schizophrenics, for example, is the emphasis on structured activities that provide concrete training through instruction, role play practice, and behavioral reinforcement (Halford & Hayes, 1991). Kanas (1986) reviewed 30 years of group therapy research with both inpatient and outpatient schizophrenics. He established that group therapy is often effective in producing constructive change for these patients, but this is only true for treatments classified as interaction-oriented rather than insight-oriented; the latter were found to be harmful for some schizophrenics.

The summary of diagnostic findings (Table 4.1) indicates that 10 inpatient studies were conducted. Several of these investigations fail to provide information on the value of group interventions with more disturbed populations, since they were not treatment-effects studies. Three research projects revealed the advantages of more structured methods. Monti, Curran, Corriveau, DeLancey, and Hagerman, (1980) and Spencer, Gillespie, and Ekisa (1983) showed that social skills training procedures are more beneficial than less structured group approaches. Fromme and Smallwood (1983) demonstrated the merits of reinforcement techniques in promoting behavioral change. Although these studies indicate that structured techniques are more effective, this finding is not unique to more impaired populations.

Kanas et al. (1980), however, discovered that certain forms of group psychotherapy might even prove to be harmful. Their results revealed that acutely psychotic inpatients in psychodynamic group psychotherapy actually did worse on both psychological and behavioral measures of change following treatment. Similarly, Beutler et al.(1984) found that their inpatients deteriorated as a result of participation in expressive-experiential group therapy. Although this group was highly structured, these leaders exerted more dominance and control, and the approach was confrontational (emphasizing emotional expression, the breaking down of defenses, and emotional release). Erickson's (1987) review found little evidence of casualties in inpatient group treatment programs, so the findings from the studies by Kanas et al. (1980) and Beutler et al. (1984) are unique.

Other investigators have detected interaction effects in their studies. Kadden, Cooney, Getter, and Litt (1989) found that neurologically impaired subjects did better in interactional therapy, whereas nonimpaired individuals fared better in the coping skills program. They surmised that "this may have occurred because our coping skills therapy, with its agenda of training a number of skills and reliance on homework assignments, overwhelmed the more impaired subjects, who felt supported in interactional therapy with its emphasis on interpersonal relationships and feelings" (p. 703). Similarly, Goldwasser, Auerbach, and Harkins (1987) were unable to produce changes in cognitive or behavioral measures with their more structured treatment for demented elderly patients.

Fine, Forth, Gilbert, and Haley (1991) failed to demonstrate the superiority of a more structured group format. In fact, their therapeutic support group proved to be more effective than social skills training with their depressed clients. They proposed that "individuals in the throes of a mood disturbance may require this supportive atmosphere before they can approach a more cognitive task like social skills" (p. 83). A review of those studies that failed to document the advantages of structured treatments over supportive methods (Table 4.5) uncovers a curious finding, which is too consistent to be dismissed as happenstance. In each instance, the treatment focused on the alleviation of depressive symptomatology (Fine et al., 1991; Fleming & Thornton, 1980; Hogg & Deffenbacher, 1988). The authors generally argue that for these patients, such nonspecific treatment factors as interpersonal acceptance and support may be very powerful components of treatment. The studies by Comas-Díaz (1981), Hodgson (1981), and Shaffer, Sank, Shapiro, and Donovan (1982) lend further credence to this observation. Finally, although Flowers and Booraem (1991) found more significant changes in their patients exposed to psychoeducational interventions, their depressed patients actually expressed more satisfaction with the less-structured experiential group.

Overall, the number of studies may be too limited, and the diagnostic classifications too unreliable, to offer specific recommendations for how to match treatments and patients with particular clinical syndromes. Nevertheless, the results suggest that therapists need to be sensitive to how their therapeutic structuring may interact with levels of distress and cognitive abilities such that they maximize the value of group interventions.

Specific Therapist Techniques for Structuring

As noted earlier, very little research exists regarding specific therapeutic techniques. The two areas that have received some attention, however, are interpretation and reinforcement/modeling.

The findings on therapeutic structuring suggest that group members benefit most from treatment when there is a coherent conceptual framework for change. The research on pretreatment contracting, structure in relationship to group development, and "meaning attribution" all suggest that cognitive input by the therapist clarifies the task for group members, thereby facilitating the learning process. In a prior review of 15 studies relevant to this issue of *cognitive input* (Dies, 1983b), it was noted that: (1) patients consistently value understanding and insight as mechanisms of therapeutic change, (2) interpretations that serve to integrate complex personal and group-related events encourage client investment in therapy, (3) interpretations that foster generalization from interactions within the group sessions to personal experiences outside the treatment context are more beneficial, and (4) patients often appreciate simple cognitive input such as advice, instruction, and feedback more than abstract analyses or "genetic insight."

Fourteen additional studies were identified for the present review. Seven of these investigations invited participants in intensive growth or training group experiences to evaluate the factors that contributed to their learning (Coché et al., 1991; Kuriloff, Babad, & Kline, 1988; Kuriloff et al., 1984; MacKenzie et al., 1987; Piper et al., 1984; Richardsen & Piper, 1986; Smith, 1987). The accumulated findings uniformly endorse the importance of the leader's ability to offer meaningful interpretations, to clarify understanding of complex group process, and to teach effective leadership strategies. Coché et al. (1991) found that the leader's capacity to demonstrate techniques, provide information, clarify process, stimulate discussion, and confront difficult process issues were critically important for the transfer of learning several months after the group experience; these leadership factors were even more influential than satisfaction with the group and the members' own work during the sessions. Several leadership dimensions differentiated between the most and the least successful groups in the large-scale study by MacKenzie and his colleagues (1987); these related primarily to the ability of the leaders to conduct their groups skillfully (the items in this factor included knowledgeable, perceptive, and nonvague).

It should be of little surprise that cognitive input by the leader in these intensive training experiences is judged to be critical to learning for the group participants. However, it is quite plausible that these conclusions are appropriate for psychotherapy groups as well. For example, Phipps and Zastowny (1988) studied a large sample of outpatient groups to evaluate the association between leadership variables, group climate, and outcome. They found that clarification, confrontation, and interpretations of the group dynamics are particularly effective interventions. Antonuccio, Davis, Lewinsohn, and Breckenridge (1987) found that clarity, on-task activity, and specificity of feedback are valued. Similarly, Maton (1988) reported that higher levels of order and organization within his groups were associated with greater treatment benefit.

Many of the treatment manuals (Table 4.3) stress the importance of instruction and interpretation by the group therapists, as well as efforts that guide the group interactions to ensure that members will acquire understanding of their dysfunctional thoughts, troubling feelings, or counterproductive interpersonal patterns. Alden (1989) summarized the factors that his socially avoidant clients reported as important to their improved outcome, "Overall, these elements can be seen as a cognitive reframing of the social avoidance and cognitive and behavioral exposure to fearful situations" (p. 763). One of the distinguishing factors that accounts for the psychological improvement in Drob, Bernard, Lifshutz, and Nierenberg's (1986) herpes patients was reported to be the specific information provided by the therapists. Indeed, many of the psychoeducational and cognitive-behavioral programs appearing in this body of leadership literature incorporate specific teaching by the therapist about relevant concepts (e.g., the identification of distorted thinking, stress management, concepts of disease or medical malfunctioning).

Two additional studies offer more direct evaluations of therapist cognitive input. Morran et al. (1985) studied feedback exchange in counseling groups and established differential leader-versus-member effects. These authors found that leader feedback is generally of higher quality than that of members, and more effective earlier in treatment. As time progressed, clients became increasingly able to deliver valuable feedback to their fellow members. Flowers and Booraem (1990) carefully studied four types of interpretations offered during group sessions: (1) the client's impact on his or her environment, (2) patterns of behavior, (3) motives for behavior, or

(4) historical causes of behavior. The interpretations producing the greatest client change were those that address interpersonal impact and behavioral patterns. These results are consistent with those from the earlier summary of research on cognitive input by the therapist (Dies, 1983b).

The second specific leadership variable that has received some attention is that of *reinforcement/modeling*. Integrated research indicates that token and natural reinforcers can be used to modify a variety of behaviors in group treatment settings, including rate of interaction, direction of verbalization, sequence of speakers, group cohesiveness, and hostility toward the leader (Dies, 1983b). Selective reinforcement by the therapist through attention, approval, and interest seems most effective when it is immediate, direct, and uncomplicated. The research suggests that as the group develops, "the group members take over from the therapist some of his influence in shaping behavior. While the therapist initially is important in establishing a group culture, later some of his influence is mediated by the group members themselves" (Liberman, 1970, p. 172). Moreover, the therapist may intervene to establish group members as effective role models within treatment sessions. The quality of the therapist-client relationship influences the effectiveness of reinforcement and modeling procedures.

The 17 studies contained in the prior review clearly document the intimate connection between reinforcement and modeling; this is confirmed once again by the detailed comments furnished in the various treatment manuals, which invariably link these two concepts (Table 4.3). A majority of these treatment programs offer specific recommendations for how therapists can first model or demonstrate effective interpersonal behaviors and then reinforce group members in their efforts to modify their own actions accordingly.

Most of the 11 new studies, however, provide only indirect support for the importance of reinforcement and modeling, since it is difficult to isolate the specific contributions of these therapeutic ingredients from the complex array of other factors influencing group process and outcome (Falloon, 1981; Hansen, St. Lawrence, & Christoff, 1985; Moon & Eisler, 1983; Oei & Jackson, 1982, 1984; Turner & Clancy, 1988). Nevertheless, these authors endorse the value of modeling and reinforcement to effect meaningful modifications in their group members' behaviors. Changes are effected through both verbal and model reinforcement, that is, through direct interactions with particular clients or indirectly as group members observe others receiving support and encouragement (vicarious learning).

The two investigations directed by Fromme are more focused in their examination of reinforcement and modeling. In the first, Fromme and Smallwood (1983) used operant techniques in a group setting to increase the frequency of here-and-now affect, feedback, and empathy statements. Their inpatient subjects were also able to demonstrate transfer of this learning to new social situations. Fromme, Dickey, and Schaefer (1983) used reinforcement methods with differing leader styles in an experimental analog study, and found an additive effect beyond that achieved with either modeling or direct elicitation of affective verbalizations.

Linehan and O'Toole (1982) systematically varied therapist self-disclosures to explore the influence of modeling, whereas two other studies examined modeling by analyzing therapist "sponsoring and maintaining" behaviors during group interactions (Barlow, Hansen, Fuhriman, & Finley, 1982; Kanas, Barr, & Dossick, 1985). Each of these investigations demonstrates that group members increase in those behaviors displayed by their therapists. Borgers (1983) has argued that modeling may be used to shape group norms or to effect behaviors of individual group members. The impact of modeling is mediated by timing, reinforcement or feedback, and the quality of relationship the therapist has established with group members.

Overall, the various results suggest that therapists should be aware of the potential effects of their own behavior on their clients' involvement in and benefit from treatment. Although many group therapists are uncomfortable with the suggestion that they can manipulate (facilitate) group process through modeling and selective reinforcement, there is no doubt that these subtle influences are present (Dies, 1985).

Providing a Positive Climate for Therapeutic Change

The role of structure is to reduce the ambiguity about the therapeutic task so that clients have a better understanding about how to involve themselves meaningfully in constructive interactions. But this task clarity will not produce increased levels of self-disclosure, risk-taking, and interpersonal feedback unless clients also believe that a secure and supportive group atmosphere exists. Thus, clients may *know* that self-disclosure is necessary, but unless they *feel* "safe" they will not discuss their problems openly. Fears of nonacceptance, criticism, humiliation, or attack from either the leader or other group members will preclude substantial commitment to the task.

The author's previous review summarized 34 studies on the quality of relationship established between the therapist and group members (Dies, 1983b). The consistent findings led to a number of generalizations: (1) that a positive relationship between the therapist and group members plays a significant role in the development of constructive group norms and in facilitating therapeutic change, (2) that a relationship with the leader which is experienced as warm, caring, and supportive is essential, but is not "sufficient" to promote therapeutic growth, especially with more seriously disturbed patients, and (3) that intermember bonding is often more important than the relationship between the therapist and group members.

The large body of literature on therapeutic factors (see Chapter 8 in this volume) suggests that although the therapist plays a vital role in fostering an open and supportive climate within the group, it is the interaction among group members that is the most direct mechanism of change in the therapeutic process. Reviews of the therapeutic factors literature show that five dimensions are regarded as central by most clients: (1) interpersonal feed-back, (2) catharsis, (3) self-understanding, (4) group cohesiveness, and (5) the development of socializing skills (Dies, 1993; in press-a). These factors highlight interpersonal processes unique to group treatments that do not necessarily involve direct client-therapist relationships. According to Yalom (1985, pp. 115–116), "to a large extent, *it is the group that is the agent of change*. Here lies a crucial difference in the basic roles of the individual therapist and the group therapist. In the individual format, the therapist functions as the solely designated direct agent of change; the group therapist, however, functions far more indirectly."

It is this *indirect* contribution that often leads to an underestimation of the leader's importance during group treatments. Certainly, the therapist's interventions to create a meaningful learning environment through pregroup contracting, early structuring, interpretation, reinforcement, and modeling are absolutely vital to the creation of the therapeutic potential of the group, but these activities will not have the *intensity* of emotional impact on individual members as will the mutual sharing of painful experiences, the courageous risk-taking, or the powerful interpersonal validation that members experience with each other.

However, it is important to note that the vast majority of research on therapeutic factors uses the 60-item measure developed by Yalom (1985). This instrument clearly favors the view that member-to-member interactions are pivotal to the clients' experience of therapy. Only *four* items are directly focused on the leader's contributions to treatment! Two of these items are rated by clients as quite unimportant; an item relating to transference (therapist compared to parent) and another regarding "admiring and behaving like" the therapist. The other two items call for direct comparisons between clients and therapists. According to Yalom's (1985) findings, clients report more benefit in expressing negative or positive feelings toward other members than toward their leader, but the therapist's advice or suggestions are *much more* valuable than those from other group members. Moreover, it should be recognized that many other items in Yalom's questionnaire fail to isolate the source of the benefit (therapist versus members), although most reviewers assign credit to the members. The therapist could be just as influential as the other clients, however, in the types of items Yalom (p. 75) reports as among the 10 most helpful, for example, "learning how to express my feelings," "the group's teaching me about the type of impression I make on others," and "learning how I come across to others" (the therapist is part of the group, and as we noted above, may give higher quality feedback than the members).

The salience of member-to-member interactions for therapeutic change should not be minimized, but neither should the fundamental importance of the quality of therapist-client relationships be overlooked. Recent research demonstrates that even in highly structured cognitive-behavioral or psychoeducational interventions, a positive view of the therapist is associated with client improvement (Drob et al., 1986; Falloon, 1981). Twenty-six additional studies published since 1980 support the general conclusions offered in the earlier review (Dies, 1983b).

For example, 12 investigations using encounter groups or training groups examined associations between outcome and the participants' perception of the group leader. In each instance, group members who changed more substantially on personality measures or who reported more significant learning, had more favorable views of their group leader (Alexander, 1980; Barlow et al., 1982; Braaten, 1989; Coché et al., 1991; Evans, 1984; Hurley, 1986; Kuriloff et al., 1984; MacKenzie et al. 1987; Piper et al., 1984; Richardsen & Piper, 1986; Roffers & Waldo, 1983; Smith, 1980). These findings are not limited to groups with nonpatients and have been obtained with various patient samples as well (e.g., Antonuccio et al., 1987; Bourgeois et al., 1990; Clarke, Kramer, Lipiec, & Klein, 1982; Phipps & Zastowny, 1988). Correlations between constructive group processes, such as cohesiveness, self-disclosure, and quality of feedback, and favorable impressions of the group leader, are typically quite substantial. Which is "cause" and which is "effect" is virtually impossible to establish, but it does seem clear that a positive relationship with the therapist is essential for constructive change to occur. The contributions of the leader to therapeutic structure may be even more important than these "relationship" issues, especially with more disturbed patients, but a foundation of care, concern, and support from the therapist is vital.

The highlighted treatment manuals (Table 4.3) usually contain recommendations regarding how therapists can intervene to provide a supportive atmosphere for interpersonal learning. The manuals furnish directions for how to create opportunities for members to share personal strengths, rather than simply to highlight their maladaptive patterns, and how to reward behaviors that are conducive to effective therapeutic work (e.g., mutual sharing, honest communication, reciprocity of risk-taking). Methods for building group cohesion, establishing trust, and promoting supportive exchanges are also frequently highlighted.

Studies of patients who prematurely terminate from group psychotherapy typically find that these dropouts fail to develop a favorable view of their therapist or their fellow members (Bernard & Drob, 1989; Budman et al., 1980; Connelly et al., 1986; Falloon, 1981); these findings are underscored in reviews of this body of literature (Bostwick, 1987; Roback & Smith, 1987), as well as in surveys of those who are regarded as treatment casualties (Dies & Teleska, 1985).

Ironically, when individual clients view group treatments as successful, they typically cite the helpfulness of client-to-client interactions, but when treatments fail, therapists are generally implicated, either for their negligence in protecting members from hostile or counterproductive interactions with other clients, or for their own position of negative dominance within the treatment setting (Dies, 1983b). In the absence of a positive therapist-client relationship, confrontations by the leader are likely to be experienced as threatening and intrusive (Dies, 1985). Barlow et al. (1982) and Bonney, Randall, and Cleveland (1986) report clients feeling defensive in the face of confrontation by the therapists. MacKenzie and his colleagues (1987) found that leaders of less successful training groups were experienced as inhibiting and controlling. Beutler et al. (1984) showed that therapists who were actively confronting, but negatively focused, actually produced therapeutic deterioration among their inpatients in expressive-experiential group treatment. Neimeyer, Harter, and Alexander (1991) found that the tendency to perceive group leaders in extremely negative terms was associated with poorer outcome, whether it occurred at early or late stages of therapy; moreover, this pejorative view of the therapist was predictive of outcome even six months after treatment.

On the other hand, numerous investigators show that *clients value confrontation by the group psychotherapist when the orientation is more positive.* Alexander (1980) linked "warm-energizing" and "positive confronting" leadership styles to constructive group norms and favorable group outcomes. Other investigators have established similar connections between positive qualities, along with active confrontation by the leader: "warmth" and "dominance" (Hurley, 1986); "reassurance-approval" and "clarification-confrontation" (Phipps & Zastowny, 1988); "empathy" and "confrontation" (Roffers & Waldo, 1983); "support" and "confrontation" (Smith, 1980). Finally, Coché et al. (1991) found that members regarded leader support and capacity to confront difficult issues as two of the most helpful items from a list of 29 process variables.

From their critique of the individual psychotherapy literature, Beutler, Crago, and Arizmendi (1986) asserted that more effective therapists tend to confront and interpret patient affect more often than do their less helpful counterparts. Furthermore, clinicians who do not shy away from demonstrations of anger promote "more realistic and goal-directed expressions of affect on the part of their clients. Indeed, evidence from many sources suggests that rousing patient affect and motivating them to confront their fears enhances both cognitive and behavioral changes" (p. 294). Because group members may be reluctant to confront potentially volatile feelings and are disinclined to deliver negative feedback (Kivlighan, 1985), it appears that the group psychotherapist is uniquely qualified to shoulder this therapeutic responsibility (Dies, 1993).

It seems quite apparent that the conclusion offered more than 10 years ago continues to receive empirical corroboration, "that group members favor and seem to benefit more from a positive style of intervention, and that as leaders become more actively negative, they increase the probability that participants will not only be dissatisfied but also potentially harmed by the group experience" (Dies, 1983b, p. 39). Yet, therapists who are active in providing structure and willing to confront difficult individual and group-level problems, within the framework of a supportive and caring therapeutic stance, are more likely to promote constructive engagement in the group process and meaningful clinical progress (Dies & Dies, 1993a).

Therapist Self-Disclosure

One aspect of the therapist-patient relationship receiving some attention is that of the therapist's willingness to share personal feelings and experiences during the treatment sessions. Although 13 studies were examined in the previous review, many dimensions of self-disclosure (valence, focus, depth, breadth, frequency) and numerous qualifiers of content (such as credibility, perceived intent, timing, and context) were simply overlooked in the empirical work (Dies, 1983b).

The available findings suggest that therapists who are willing to be open with their group members, especially in terms of here-and-now feelings and their rationale for therapeutic interventions, are more likely to facilitate the development of openness among group members, but there is no consistent link with treatment outcome (Dies, 1993). Therapist transparency can encourage corresponding behaviors among group members, but there are alternative interventions that may be even more productive in stimulating open dialogue among group members (e.g., reinforcement of sharing by other group members, invitations for candid disclosure). Fromme, Dickey, and Schaefer (1983), for example, found that although self-disclosure by the therapist contributes to more openness among members, as well as to positive intermember feelings, direct elicitation techniques are even more effective. Linehan and O'Toole (1982) found that therapist self-disclosure produces more revelations by group members, but the association is often not direct.

Three other studies evaluated variations in self-disclosures by therapists and found differential results, but it was not possible to isolate the impact of the leader's openness from other components of their interventions, such as, reinforcement (Oei & Jackson, 1982; 1984; Robbins & Tucker, 1986). Coché et al. (1991) found that leaders' level of self-disclosure was regarded as one of the least important intervention strategies, and ranked far below other tactics, such as support of members, confrontation of difficult issues, demonstration of techniques, and clarification of group process.

We investigated self-disclosure by co-therapists to test the modeling hypothesis regarding co-leadership (McNary & Dies, 1993). Three dimensions of therapist transparency were explored: positive or negative *valence,* low or high *risk,* and the *target* of the disclosure, that is, the individual members, the group as a whole, the therapist her/himself, or the co-leader. Although the overall level of therapist self-disclosure was quite low, results were consistent with expectations showing that most of the personal comments were positive, low risk, and rarely directed to the co-therapist.

Co-Therapy

One of the principal arguments in behalf of co-leadership in group treatments is the opportunity for the leaders to use their own relationship to model effective interpersonal behaviors. The self-disclosure study by McNary and Dies (1993), however, failed to support this position, since the co-therapists rarely interacted with each other during the treatment sessions. In a survey of experienced group psychotherapists, these practitioners ranked both group-oriented and member-focused disclosures as much more common in their own groups than either self or co-leader oriented remarks of a personal nature (Dies, 1990).

Although a substantial proportion of treatment groups are conducted by two therapists, research on co-therapy is rare: only five studies were identified in the previous review (Dies, 1983b). There is no evidence that the presence of two therapists enhances the quality or efficacy of therapeutic outcome, but the limited findings suggest that co-leadership may complicate group process unless the leaders manage their relationship effectively within the sessions. "Compatibility despite dissimilarity appears to be the key consideration in establishing co-therapist teams, and the capacity to model an open and positive relationship within the sessions seems to be the critical dimension in maintaining an effective team" (Dies, 1983b, p. 59).

Although nearly half (45%, see Table 4.2) of the studies compiled for the present chapter were co-led, only a few investigators examined the implications of this arrangement. Hajek, Belcher, and Stapleton (1985) note that the presence of co-therapists had no significant effect on outcome; Falloon (1981) failed to find many effects when he examined the differential attraction to the co-leaders. This was also the case in the study by McNary and Dies (1993) who found that members did not differentiate much between their leaders. Other investigators, however, have established differences in perceptions of co-therapists that have important treatment implications.

Burrows (1981b) linked early childhood memories with client-leader interaction patterns and found support for the concept of transference, that is, early experiences within the primary family were related to the group members' styles of interacting with co-leaders in terms of therapist gender. Greene, Morrison, and Tischler (1980; 1981) also found gender-based differences: Group members tended to attribute greater power to leaders of their own sex. In two other reports, Greene, Rosenkrantz, and Muth (1985; 1986) examined perceptions of co-leaders by borderline patients and demonstrate evidence of splitting mechanisms, as well as some support for the concept of countertransference; their co-therapists tended to diverge in their clinical judgments of group members in relationship to their patients' polarization of co-leadership.

We need more research on the topic of co-therapy. The findings imply that the presence of two leaders may indeed introduce more complexity into the treatment situation. The critical issue, however, is how well these complications are managed by the co-therapists. Effective working through of issues precipitated by the presence of two group therapists may offer unique opportunities for client growth, but the failure to understand and confront these difficulties might hamper effective treatment (Dies, 1983b).

CONCLUSIONS

Several prominent reviews of the psychotherapy research literature demonstrate that therapist experience and competence play an instrumental role in treatment outcome (Beutler et al., 1986; Lambert, Shapiro, & Bergin, 1986; Orlinsky & Howard, 1986). Although this topic has not been centrally highlighted in the group literature, it would not be unreasonable to assume that therapist experience and competence affect treatment outcome in the group setting as well, especially in light of the widespread belief that group interventions are inherently more complicated and difficult to master (Dies, 1993).

Many investigators provide extensive guidelines for the therapists in the form of detailed treatment manuals, often furnish specialized training before the research is launched, and then supervise the group leaders throughout the study. These precautions may serve to compensate for the relative inexperience of the therapists, but the question remains whether these adjustments are sufficient.

Kivlighan and Quigley (1991) found differences between novice and expert group therapists in their conceptualizations of group process, and Dies (1980), in a survey of experienced supervisors, reported a variety of problems with their supervisees (e.g., insensitivity to group process, difficulties in moderating level of activity, ill-timed interventions). Dies (in press-b) noted that beginners are likely to ask too many closed-ended questions and focus too long on less productive group issues or problematic clients; furthermore, they are not able to anticipate the impact of their comments or to sequence their interventions very skillfully, and often miss important opportunities to pick up on "feeling words" or subtle nuances of group process. Frequently, potentially fruitful issues are prematurely diverted by "problem-solving" efforts or interpretations that discourage further elaboration.

Several researchers express concern that the limited training of the group leaders may have compromised the effectiveness of the treatments (e.g., Beutler et al., 1984; Moon & Eisler, 1983), while others provide more direct evaluation of this issue. Azim and Joyce (1986) used feedback from patients to improve their outpatient group treatment program; while numerous aspects of their program were modified, patients expressed satisfaction specifically related to their view of increased skill and knowledge on the part of the therapists. MacKenzie et al. (1987) compared successful and less successful training groups on various process and outcome criteria and found that skillful leadership was one of the main differentiating variables.

Four studies have examined the issue of leader expertise with participants in support groups and psychoeducational programs. Thompson, Gallagher, Nies, and Epstein (1983) failed to detect differences between professional and nonprofessional leaders (32 different instructors) in their "Coping with Depression Course," but their leaders participated in 24 hours of training, and subsequently implemented a highly structured treatment program (e.g., Lewinsohn, Steinmetz, Antonuccio, & Teri, 1985). The remaining three studies allowed for greater flexibility on the part of the group leaders, and in each case there were clear differences related to level of expertise (Lieberman & Bliwise, 1985; Maton, 1988; Toseland, Rossiter, Peak, & Hill, 1990). The latter authors noted that even with careful training and supervision, the leaders often did not follow the explicit model called for in the group protocol.

These findings suggest that experience and competence make a difference, but are most likely to be manifest in less tightly structured treatment programs. Waltman and Zimpfer (1988) conducted a meta-analytic review of the literature on group composition in relationship to group structure and treatment duration. They conclude that "highly structured groups may suppress composition effects and that there is a minimum exposure time necessary if composition is to be a significant factor in determining outcome" (pp. 178–179). This generalization may also hold true for the effects of leadership in many of the investigations appearing in the literature. A significant proportion of the studies evaluate structured short-term interventions that are sufficiently powerful to produce meaningful changes in the types of clients and on the measures used by the investigators. Since the researchers did not have the option of using more experienced group leaders, the question is seldom raised whether this factor may have made a difference.

However, it is common for researchers to express concern about the brevity of their treatments. Fifteen different investigators in this review argue that their results may have been compromised by the short-term nature of their interventions. A majority of these authors worked with patients experiencing more pervasive or chronic problems, for example, avoidant personality disorders (Alden, 1989), women sexually abused as children (Alexander, Neimeyer, Follette, Moore, & Harter, 1989), generalized anxiety disorders (Eayrs, Rowan, & Harvey, 1984), obsessive-compulsive disorders (Enright, 1991), and bulimics (Kirkley, Schneider, Agras, & Bachman, 1985). Similarly, an examination of those projects that failed to detect differences between some form of group intervention and no treatment controls shows that many of these patients were more seriously impaired, for example, inpatients (Beutler et al., 1984), prisoners (Annis & Chan, 1983; Leak, 1980), and demented elderly (Goldwasser et al., 1987).

Despite the popularity of short-term interventions, there is concern that brief forms of therapy may furnish only transitory or circumscribed relief for many individuals whose conflicts are long-standing and deeply ingrained. Many of these unfortunate individuals may become "group recidivists," seeking a new short-term group experience with each exacerbation of their interpersonal problems, or find a more appropriate long-term psychotherapy experience (Dies, 1992b). When the duration of group treatment is extended, the focus is less likely to be on simple symptomatic relief, peer

TABLE 4.8.   Variables Linked to Outcome in Group Research

Category	Pre-Treatment	Treatment
Individual		
Client	Demographics	Defenses/Resources
	Diagnosis	Level of psychopathology
	Expectations	Specific vulnerabilities
	Medical condition	Stress level
	Motivation	
	Personality variables	
	Prior experience	
Therapist	Demographics	Cotherapist relationship
	Expectations	Focus of intervention
	Orientation	Personal style (many)
	Personality	Skill/Expertise
		Techniques (many)
		Treatment manuals
Client × Therapist	Contract (nature)	Quality of relationship
	Match (alliance)	Restructuring of goals
	Preparation	Transference
System		
Composition	Homogeneity	Attendance patterns
	Open vs. closed	Attrition/Dropouts
	Short vs. long-term	Boundary issues (many)
		Cohesion
		Group size
		Massed vs. spaced session
		Norms
		Stage phenomena
		Therapeutic factors
Group × Client	Group availability	Activity/Involvement
	Selection factors	Dominance patterns
	Voluntary/Mandated assignment	Role (system "fit")
		Subgrouping
Context		
Confounds	In/Outpatient	Concomitant treatments
	Referral source	Presence of observers
		Ward/Social climate
Life Events	Convenience/Travel	Family involvement
	Social network	Life changes/Stress
	Stressful events	
Research	Instruments used	Contract for research
	Therapists' role	Integration of measures
		Timing of assessments

and self-acceptance, or training in basic social skills and immediate problem-solving strategies. Long-term group interventions focus more on maladaptive behavioral patterns that are rigidly entrenched, conflicts that are less accessible to conscious awareness, or a greater understanding of the pathogenic developmental experiences that predispose patients to personal suffering and interpersonal strife (Dies, in press-a). The extended time in treatment gives patients more opportunities to *work through* their chronic dysfunctional patterns of relating to others (Tschuschke & Dies, in press).

Long-term groups are also more typically open-ended, with greater membership turnover than the abbreviated, closed, and homogeneous groups that characterize most of the research found in the literature. The increased demands to manage system-level stresses (e.g., attrition, phase transitions, termination of individual patients) and to address more pervasive interpersonal problems undoubtedly require more experience on the part of the clinician. The challenges to maintain a meaningful structure and positive climate for intensive interpersonal work, and to use technical skills competently (e.g., interpretation, confrontation), also demand more expertise of the therapist.

The contributions of the clinician to effective group treatment are important, but outcome is also influenced by a host of other considerations. Table 4.8, for example, provides a list of variables found to relate to treatment outcome in various empirical studies. Many of the items represent broad categories that could be further refined (e.g., therapeutic factors), and the table does not list post-treatment factors that may contribute to an understanding of outcome (e.g., how improvement is assessed); however, it shows the enormous complexity of attempting to comprehend the critical ingredients that foster therapeutic gain. Realistically, we will never develop the regression equation that neatly summarizes the complex weightings assigned to each of the variables that contribute to treatment outcome. Nevertheless, we have made some progress in our understanding of the therapist's contribution to treatment; clearly there is still much to be learned.

REFERENCES

Abramowitz, I. A., & Coursey, R. D. (1989). Impact of an educational support group on family participants who take care of their schizophrenic relatives. *Journal of Consulting and Clinical Psychology, 57,* 232–236.

Alden, L. (1989). Short-term structured treatment for avoidant personality disorder. *Journal of Consulting and Clinical Psychology, 57,* 756–764.

Alexander, C. (1980). Leader confrontation and member change in encounter groups. *Journal of Humanistic Psychology, 20,* 41–55.

Alexander, P. C., Neimeyer, R. A., & Follette, V. M. (1991). Group therapy for women sexually abused as children: A controlled study and investigation of individual differences. *Journal of Interpersonal Violence, 6,* 218–231.

Alexander, P. C., Neimeyer, R. A., Follette, V. M., Moore, M. K., & Harter, S. (1989). A comparison of group treatments of women sexually abused as children. *Journal of Consulting and Clinical Psychology, 57,* 479–483.

Anderson, C. M., Harrow, M., Schwartz, A. H., & Kupfer, D. J. (1972). Impact of therapist on patient satisfaction in group psychotherapy. *Comprehensive Psychiatry, 13,* 33–40.

Annis, H. M., & Chan, D. (1983). The differential treatment model: Empirical evidence from a personality typology of adult offenders. *Criminal Justice and Behavior, 10,* 159–173.

Antonuccio, D. O., Davis, C., Lewinsohn, P. M., & Breckenridge, J. S. (1987). Therapist variables related to cohesiveness in a group treatment for depression. *Small Group Behavior, 18,* 557–564.

Azim, H. F. A., & Joyce, A. S. (1986). The impact of data-based program modifications on the satisfaction of outpatients in group psychotherapy. *Canadian Journal of Psychiatry, 31,* 119–122.

Barlow, S., Hansen, W. D., Fuhriman, A. J., & Finley, R. (1982). Leader communication style: Effects of members of small groups. *Small Group Behavior, 13,* 518–531.

Bednar, R. L., Melnick, J., & Kaul, T. J. (1974). Risk, responsibility, and structure: A conceptual framework for initiating group counseling and psychotherapy. *Journal of Counseling Psychology, 21,* 31–37.

Bernard, H. S., & Drob, S. L. (1989). Premature termination: A clinical study. *Group, 13,* 11–22.

Beutler, L. E., Frank, M., Scheiber, S. C., Calvert, S., & Gaines, J. (1984). Comparative effects of group psychotherapies in a short-term inpatient setting: An experience with deterioration effects. *Psychiatry, 47,* 66–76.

Beutler, L. E., Crago, M., & Arizmendi, T. G. (1986). Research on therapist variables in psychotherapy. In S. L. Garfield & A. E. Bergin (Eds.), *Handbook of psychotherapy and behavioral change* (3rd ed., pp. 257–310). New York: Wiley.

Bond, G. R. (1984). Positive and negative norm regulation and their relationship to therapy size. *Group, 8,* 35–44.

Bonney, W. C., Randall, D. A., & Cleveland, J. D. (1986). An analysis of client-perceived curative factors in therapy group of former incest victims. *Small Group Behavior, 17,* 303–321.

Borgers, S. B. (1980). An examination of the use of contracts in groups. *Journal for Specialists in Group Work, 5,* 68–72.

Borgers, S. B. (1983). Uses and effects of modeling by the therapist in group therapy. *Journal for Specialists in Group Work, 8,* 133–139.

Bostwick, G. J. (1987). "Where's Mary?" A review of the group treatment dropout literature. *Social Work with Groups, 10,* 117–132.

Bourgeois, L., Sabourin, S., & Wright, J. (1990). Predictive validity of therapeutic alliance in group marital therapy. *Journal of Consulting and Clinical Psychology, 58,* 608–613.

Braaten, L. J. (1989). Predicting positive goal attainment and symptom reduction from early group climate dimensions. *International Journal of Group Psychotherapy, 39,* 377–387.

Brekke, J. S. (1989). The use of orientation groups to engage hard-to-reach clients: Model, method and evaluation. *Social Work with Groups, 12,* 75–88.

Brown, S. D. (1980). Coping skills training: An evaluation of a psychoeducational program in a community mental health setting. *Journal of Counseling Psychology, 27,* 340–345.

Brykczynska, C. (1990). Changes in the patient's perception of his therapist in the process of group and individual psychotherapy. *Psychotherapy & Psychosomatics, 53,* 179–184.

Budman, S., Demby, A., & Randall, M. (1980). Short-term group psychotherapy: Who succeeds, who fails? *Group, 4,* 3–16.

Budman, S. H., Demby, A., Redondo, J. P., Hannan, M., Feldstein, M., Ring, J., & Springer, T. (1988). Comparative outcome in time-limited individual and group psychotherapy. *International Journal of Group Psychotherapy, 38,* 63–86.

Burrows, P. B. (1981a). Parent orientation and member-leader behavior: A measure of transference in groups. *International Journal of Group Psychotherapy, 31,* 175–191.

Burrows, P. B. (1981b). The family-group connection: Early memories as a measure of transference in a group. *International Journal of Group Psychotherapy, 31,* 3–23.

Caple, R. B., & Cox, P. L. (1989). Relationships among group structure, member expectations, attraction to group, and satisfaction with the group experience. *Journal for Specialists in Group Work, 14,* 16–24.

Cappon, J. (1981). Reality in analytic group psychotherapy: Beyond transference and countertransference. *Group, 5,* 41–53.

Clarke, D. L., Kramer, E., Lipiec, K., & Klein, S. (1982). Group psychotherapy with mastectomy patients. *Psychotherapy: Theory, Research and Practice, 19,* 331–334.

Coché, E., Cooper, J. B., & Petermann, K. J. (1984). Differential outcomes of cognitive and interactional group therapies. *Small Group Behavior, 15,* 497–509.

Coché, E., Dies, R. R., & Goettelmann, K. (1991). Process variables mediating change in intensive group therapy training. *International Journal of Group Psychotherapy, 41,* 379–397.

Comas-Díaz, L. (1981). Effects of cognitive and behavioral group treatment on the depressive symptomatology of Puerto Rican women. *Journal of Consulting and Clinical Psychology, 49,* 627–632.

Connelly, J. L., Piper, W. E., de Carufel, F. L., & Debbane, E. G. (1986). Premature termination in group psychotherapy: Pretherapy and early therapy predictors. *International Journal of Group Psychotherapy, 36,* 145–152.

Corazzini, J. G., Heppner, P. P., & Young, M. D. (1980). The effects of cognitive information on termination from group counseling. *Journal of College Student Personnel, 21,* 553–557.

Deffenbacher, J. L., McNamara, K., Stark, R. S., & Sabadell, P. M. (1990). A comparison of cognitive-behavioral and process-oriented group counseling for general anger reduction. *Journal of Counseling & Development, 69,* 167–172.

Dies, R. R. (1980). Group psychotherapy: Training and supervision. In A. K. Hess (Ed.), *Psychotherapy supervision: Theory, research and practice* (pp. 337–366). New York: Wiley.

Dies, R. R. (1983a). Bridging the gap between research and practice in group psychotherapy. In R. R. Dies & K. R. MacKenzie (Eds.), *Advances in group psychotherapy: Integrating research and practice* (pp. 1–26). New York: International Universities Press.

Dies, R. R. (1983b). Clinical implications of research on leadership in short-term group psychotherapy. In R. R. Dies & K. R. MacKenzie (Eds.), *Advances in group psychotherapy: Integrating research and practice* (pp. 27–78). New York: International Universities Press.

Dies, R. R. (1985). Leadership in short-term group therapy: Manipulation or facilitation? *International Journal of Group Psychotherapy, 35,* 435–455.

Dies, R. R. (1987). Clinical application of research instruments: Editor's introduction. *International Journal of Group Psychotherapy, 37,* 31–37.

Dies, R. R. (1990, Feb.). *The cotherapy relationship: Establishing a good marriage.* Paper presented at the meeting of the American Group Psychotherapy Association, Boston, MA.

Dies, R. R. (1992a). Clinician and researcher: Mutual growth through dialogue. In S. Tuttman (Ed.), *Expanding domains of psychodynamic group therapy* (pp. 379–408). Madison, CT: International Universities Press.

Dies, R. R. (1992b). The future of group therapy. *Psychotherapy, 29,* 58–64.

Dies, R. R. (1993). Research on group psychotherapy: Overview and clinical applications. In A. Alonso & H. I. Swiller (Eds.), *Group therapy in clinical practice* (pp. 473–518). Washington, DC: American Psychiatric Press.

Dies, R. R. (in press-a). Group psychotherapies. In A. S. Gurman & S. B. Messer (Eds.), *Modern psychotherapies: Theory and practice.* New York: Guilford Publications.

Dies, R. R. (in press-b). The therapist's role in group treatments. In H. Bernard & K. R. MacKenzie (Eds.), *Manual of group psychotherapy.* New York: Guilford Publications.

Dies, R. R., & Dies, K. R. (1993a). Directive facilitation: A model for short-term group treatments. *Independent Practitioner, 13,* 103–109.

Dies, R. R., & Dies, K. R. (1993b). The role of evaluation in clinical practice: Overview and group treatment illustration. *International Journal of Group Psychotherapy, 43,* 77–105.

Dies, R. R., & Riester, A. E. (1986). Research on child group therapy: Present status and future directions. In A. E. Riester & I. A. Kraft (Eds.), *Child group psychotherapy: Future tense* (pp. 173–220). New York: International Universities Press.

Dies, R. R., & Teleska, P. A. (1985). Negative outcome in group psychotherapy. In D. T. Mays & C. M. Franks (Eds.), *Negative outcome in psychotherapy and what to do about it* (pp. 118–141). New York: Springer.

Drob, S., Bernard, H., Lifshutz, H., & Nierenberg, A. (1986). Brief group psychotherapy for herpes patients: A preliminary study. *Behavior Therapy, 17,* 229–238.

Eayrs, C. B., Rowan, D., & Harvey, P. G. (1984). Behavioral group training for anxiety management. *Behavioral Psychotherapy, 12*(2), 117–129.

Enright, S. J. (1991). Group treatment for obsessive-compulsive disorder: An evaluation. *Behavioral Psychotherapy, 19,* 183–192.

Erickson, R. C. (1982). Inpatient small group psychotherapy: A survey. *Clinical Psychology Review, 2,* 137–151.

Erickson, R. C. (1987). The question of casualties in inpatient small group psychotherapy. *Small Group Behavior, 18,* 443–458.

Evans, N. J. (1984). The relationship of interpersonal attraction and attraction to group in a growth group setting. *Journal for Specialists in Group Work, 9,* 172–178.

Falloon, R. H. (1981). Interpersonal variables in behavioral group therapy. *British Journal of Medical Psychology, 54,* 133–141.

Fine, S., Forth, A., Gilbert, M., & Haley, G. (1991). Group therapy for adolescent depressive disorder: A comparison of social skills and therapeutic support. *Journal of the American Academy of Child and Adolescent Psychiatry, 30,* 79–85.

Fleming, B. M., & Thornton, D. W. (1980). Coping skills training as a component in the short-term treatment for depression. *Journal of Consulting and Clinical Psychology, 48,* 652–654.

Flowers, J. V., & Booraem, C. D. (1990). The frequency and effect on outcome of different types of interpretation in psychodynamic and cognitive-behavioral group psychotherapy. *International Journal of Group Psychotherapy, 40,* 203–214.

Flowers, J. V., & Booraem, C. D. (1991). A psychoeducational group for clients with heterogeneous problems: Process and outcome. *Small Group Research, 22,* 258–273.

Fromme, D. K., Dickey, G. V., & Schaefer, J. P. (1983). Group modification of affective verbalizations: Reinforcement and therapist style effects. *Journal of Clinical Psychology, 39,* 893–900.

Fromme, D. K., & Smallwood, R. E. (1983). Group modification of affective verbalizations in a psychiatric population. *British Journal of Clinical Psychology, 22,* 251–256.

Fuehrer, A., & Keys, C. (1988). Group development in self-help groups for college students. *Small Group Behavior, 19,* 325–341.

Getter, H., Litt, M. D., Kadden, R. M., & Cooney, N. L. (1992). Measuring treatment process in coping skills and interactional group therapies for alcoholism. *International Journal of Group Psychotherapy, 42,* 419–430.

Goldwasser, A. N., Auerbach, S. M., & Harkins, S. W. (1987). Cognitive, affective, and behavioral effects of reminiscence group therapy on demented elderly. *International Journal of Aging and Human Development, 25,* 209–222.

Gormally, J., Varvil-Weld, D., Raphael, R., & Sipps, G. (1981). Treatment of socially anxious college men using cognitive counseling and skills training. *Journal of Counseling Psychology, 28,* 147–157.

Graff, R. W., Whitehead, G. I., & LeCompte, M. (1986). Group treatment with divorced women using cognitive-behavioral and supportive-insight methods. *Journal of Counseling Psychology, 33,* 276–281.

Greene, L. R., Morrison, T. L., & Tischler, N. G. (1980). Aspects of identification in the large group. *Journal of Social Psychology, 111,* 91–97.

Greene, L. R., Morrison, T. L., & Tischler, N. G. (1981). Gender and authority: Effects on perceptions of small group co-leaders. *Small Group Behavior, 12,* 401–413.

Greene, L. R., Rosenkrantz, J., & Muth, D. Y. (1985). Splitting dynamics, self-representations and boundary phenomena in the group psychotherapy of borderline personality disorders. *Psychiatry, 48,* 234–245.

Greene, L. R., Rosenkrantz, J., & Muth, D. Y. (1986). Borderline defenses and countertransference: Research findings and implications. *Psychiatry, 49,* 253–264.

Hajek, P., Belcher, M., & Stapleton, J. (1985). Enhancing the impact of groups: An evaluation of two group formats for smokers. *British Journal of Clinical Psychology, 24,* 289–294.

Halford, W. K., & Hayes, R. (1991). Psychological rehabilitation of chronic schizophrenic patients: Recent findings on social skills training and family psychoeducation. *Clinical Psychology Review, 11,* 23–44.

Hansen, D. J., St. Lawrence, J. S., & Christoff, K. A. (1985). Effects of interpersonal problem-solving training with chronic aftercare patients on problem-solving component skills and effectiveness solutions. *Journal of Consulting and Clinical Psychology, 53,* 167–174.

Hisli, N. (1987). Effect of patients' evaluation of group behavior on therapy outcome. *International Journal of Group Psychotherapy, 37,* 119–124.

Hoberman, H. M., Lewinsohn, P. M., & Tilson, M. (1988). Group treatment of depression: Individual predictors of outcome. *Journal of Consulting and Clinical Psychology, 56,* 393–398.

Hodgson, J. W. (1981). Cognitive versus behavioral-interpersonal approaches to the group treatment of depressed college students. *Journal of Counseling Psychology, 28,* 243–249.

Hogg, J. A., & Deffenbacher, J. L. (1988). A comparison of cognitive and interpersonal-process group therapies in the treatment of depression among college students. *Journal of Counseling Psychology, 35,* 304–310.

Hurley, J. R. (1986). Leaders' behavior and group members' interpersonal gains. *Group, 10,* 161–176.

Jensen, J. L. (1982). The relationship of leadership technique and anxiety level in group therapy with chronic schizophrenics. *Psychotherapy: Theory, Research and Practice, 19,* 237–248.

Kadden, R. M., Cooney, N. L., Getter, H., & Litt, M. D. (1989). Matching alcoholics to coping skills or interactional therapies: Post-treatment results. *Journal of Consulting and Clinical Psychology, 57,* 698–704.

Kanas, N. (1986). Group therapy with schizophrenics: A review of controlled studies. *International Journal of Group Psychotherapy, 36,* 339–351.

Kanas, N., Barr, M. A., & Dossick, S. (1985). The homogeneous schizophrenic inpatient group: An evaluation using the Hill Interaction Matrix. *Small Group Behavior, 16,* 397–409.

Kanas, N., Rogers, M., Kreth, E., Patterson, L., & Campbell, R. (1980). The effectiveness of group psychotherapy during the first three weeks of hospitalization: A controlled study. *Journal of Nervous and Mental Disease, 168,* 487–492.

Kinder, B. N., & Kilmann, P. R. (1976). The impact of differential shifts in leader structure on the outcome of internal and external group participants. *Journal of Clinical Psychology, 32,* 857–863.

Kirkley, B. G., Schneider, J. A., Agras, W. S., & Bachman, J. A. (1985). Comparison of two group treatments for bulimia. *Journal of Consulting and Clinical Psychology, 53,* 43–48.

Kivlighan, D. M. (1985). Feedback in group psychotherapy. Review and implications. *Small Group Behavior, 16,* 373–385.

Kivlighan, D. M., Corazzini, J. G., & McGovern, T. V. (1985). Pregroup training. *Small Group Behavior, 16,* 500–514.

Kivlighan, D. M., Hageseth, J. A., Tipton, R. M., & McGovern, T. V. (1981). Effects of matching treatment approaches and personality types in group vocational counseling. *Journal of Counseling Psychology, 28,* 315–320.

Kivlighan, D. M., & Jauquet, C. (1990). Quality of group member agendas and group session climate. *Small Group Research, 21,* 205–219.

Kivlighan, D. M., McGovern, T. V., & Corazzini, J. G. (1984). Effects of content and timing of structuring interventions on group therapy process and outcome. *Journal of Counseling Psychology, 31,* 363–370.

Kivlighan, D. M., & Quigley, S. T. (1991). Dimensions used by experienced and novice group therapists to conceptualize group process. *Journal of Counseling Psychology, 38,* 415–423.

Kuriloff, P. J., Babad, E. Y., & Kline, M. (1988). Mechanisms that contribute to learning in experiential small groups. *Small Group Behavior, 19,* 207–226.

Kuriloff, P. J., Babad, E. Y., Samuels-Singer, M., & Sutton-Smith, K. (1984). Teaching and learning in small groups: An analysis of trainer interventions. *Small Group Behavior, 15,* 187–203.

Lambert, M. J., Shapiro, D. A., & Bergin, A. E. (1986). The effectiveness of psychotherapy. In S. L. Garfield & A. E. Bergin (Eds.), *Handbook of psychotherapy and behavior change* (3rd ed., pp. 157–211). New York: Wiley.

Leak, G. K. (1980). Effects of highly structured versus nondirective group counseling approaches on personality and behavioral measures of adjustment in incarcerated felons. *Journal of Counseling Psychology, 27,* 520–523.

Leszcz, M. (1986). Inpatient groups. In A. J. Frances & R. E. Hales (Eds.), *American psychiatric association annual review, Vol. 5.* (pp. 729–743). Washington, DC: American Psychiatric Press.

Leszcz, M., Yalom, I. D., & Norden, M. (1985). The value of inpatient group psychotherapy: Patients' perceptions. *International Journal of Group Psychotherapy, 35,* 411–433.

Lewinsohn, P. M., Steinmetz, J. L., Antonuccio, D., & Teri, L. (1985). Group therapy for depression: The Coping with Depression Course. *International Journal of Mental Health, 13,* 8–33.

Liberman, R. (1970). A behavioral approach to group dynamics: I. Reinforcement and prompting of cohesiveness in group therapy. *Behavior Therapy, 1,* 141–175.

Lichtenberg, J. W., & Knox, P. L. (1991). Order out of chaos: A structural analysis of group therapy. *Journal of Counseling Psychology, 38,* 279–288.

Lieberman, M. A., & Bliwise, N. G. (1985). Comparisons among peer and professionally directed groups for the elderly: Implications for the development of self-help groups. *International Journal of Group Psychotherapy, 35,* 155–175.

Lieberman, M. A., Yalom, I. D., & Miles, M. B. (1973). *Encounter groups: First facts*. New York: Basic Books.

Linehan, E., & O'Toole, J. (1982). Effect of subliminal stimulation of symbiotic fantasies on college student self-disclosure in group counseling. *Journal of Counseling Psychology, 29,* 151–157.

MacKenzie, K. R., Dies, R. R., Coché, E., Rutan, J. S., & Stone, W. N. (1987). An analysis of AGPA institute groups. *International Journal of Group Psychotherapy, 37,* 55–74.

Maton, K. I. (1988). Social support, organizational characteristics, psychological well-being, and group appraisal in three self-help group populations. *American Journal of Community Psychology, 16,* 53–77.

McCallum, M., & Piper, W. E. (1990). The psychological mindedness assessment procedure. *Psychological Assessment, 2,* 412–418.

McGuire, J. M., Taylor, D. R., Broome, D. H., Blau, B. I., & Abbott, D. W. (1986). Group structuring techniques and their influence on process involvement in a group counseling training program. *Journal of Counseling Psychology, 33,* 270–275.

McNary, S. W., & Dies, R. R. (1993). Co-therapist modeling in group psychotherapy: Fact or fantasy? *Group, 17,* 131–142.

Monti, P. M., Curran, J. P., Corriveau, D. P., DeLancey, A. L., & Hagerman, S. M. (1980). Effects of social skills training groups and sensitivity training groups with psychiatric patients. *Journal of Consulting and Clinical Psychology, 48,* 241–248.

Moon, J. R., & Eisler, R. M. (1983). Anger control: An experimental comparison of three behavioral treatments. *Behavior Therapy, 14,* 493–505.

Morran, D. K., Robison, F. F., & Stockton, R. (1985). Feedback exchange in counseling groups: An analysis of message content and receiver acceptance as a function of leader versus member delivery, session, and valence. *Journal of Counseling Psychology, 32,* 57–67.

Mosher, L. R., & Keith, S. J. (1980). Psychosocial treatment: Individual, group, family, and community support approaches. *Schizophrenia Bulletin, 6,* 10–41.

Neimeyer, R. A., & Feixas, G. (1990). The role of homework and skill acquisition in the outcome of group cognitive therapy for depression. *Behavioral Therapy, 21,* 281–292.

Neimeyer, R. A., Harter, S., & Alexander, P. C. (1991). Group perceptions as predictors of outcome in the treatment of incest survivors. *Psychotherapy Research, 1,* 148–158.

Neumann, K. F., Critelli, J. W., Tang, C. S. K., & Schneider, L. J. (1988). *Journal of Behavior Therapy and Experimental Psychiatry, 19,* 135–141.

Nezu, A. M. (1986). Efficacy of a social problem-solving therapy approach for unipolar depression. *Journal of Consulting and Clinical Psychology, 54,* 196–202.

Oei, T. P. S., & Jackson, P. R. (1982). Social skills and cognitive behavioral approaches to the treatment of problem drinking. *Journal of Studies on Alcohol, 43,* 532–547.

Oei, T. P. S., & Jackson, P. R. (1984). Some effective therapeutic factors in group cognitive-behavioral therapy with problem drinkers. *Journal of Studies on Alcohol, 45,* 119–123.

Orlinsky, D. E., & Howard, K. I. (1986). Process and outcome in psychotherapy. In S. L. Garfield & A. E. Bergin (Eds.), *Handbook of psychotherapy and behavior change* (3rd ed., pp. 311–381). New York: Wiley.

Phipps, L. B., & Zastowny, T. R. (1988). Leadership behavior, group climate and outcome in group psychotherapy: A study of outpatient psychotherapy groups. *Group, 12,* 157–171.

Piper, W. E., Connelly, J. L., & Salvendy, J. T. (1984). Variables related to reported learning in brief experiential groups held at professional meetings. *Group, 8,* 43–51.

Resnick, P. A., Jordan, C. G., Girelli, S. A., Hutter, C. K., & Marhoefer-Dvorak, S. (1988). A comparative outcome study of behavioral group therapy for sexual assault victims. *Behavior Therapy, 19,* 385–401.

Richardsen, A. M., & Piper, W. E. (1986). Leader style, leader consistency, and participant personality effects on learning in small groups. *Human Relations, 39,* 817–836.

Roback, H. B., & Smith, M. (1987). Patient attrition in dynamically oriented treatment groups. *American Journal of Psychiatry, 144,* 426–431.

Robbins, S. B., & Tucker, K. R. (1986). Relation of goal instability to self-directed and interactional career counseling workshops. *Journal of Counseling Psychology, 33,* 418–424.

Roffers, T., & Waldo, M. (1983). Empathy and confrontation related to group counseling outcome. *Journal for Specialists in Group Work, 8,* 106–113.

Sanchez, V. G., Lewinsohn, P. M., & Larson, D. W. (1980). Assertion training: Effectiveness in the treatment of depression. *Journal of Clinical Psychology, 36,* 526–529.

Schwartz, A. H., Harrow, M., Anderson, C., Feinstein, A. E., & Schwartz, C. C. (1970). Influence of therapeutic task orientation on patient and therapist satisfaction in group psychotherapy. *International Journal of Group Psychotherapy, 20,* 460–469.

Shaffer, C. S., Sank, L. I., Shapiro, J., & Donovan, D. C. (1982). Cognitive behavior therapy follow-up: Maintenance of treatment effects at six months. *Journal of Group Psychotherapy, Psychodrama, and Sociometry, 35,* 57–64.

Slocum, Y. S. (1987). A survey of expectations about group therapy among clinical and nonclinical populations. *International Journal of Group Psychotherapy, 37,* 39–54.

Smith, P. B. (1980). The T-group trainer: Group facilitator or prisoner of circumstance? *Journal of Applied Behavioral Science, 16,* 63–68.

Smith, P. B. (1987). Laboratory design and group process as determinants of the outcome of sensitivity training. *Small Group Behavior, 18,* 291–308.

Spencer, P. G., Gillespie, C. R., & Ekisa, E. G. (1983). A controlled comparison of the effects of social skills training and remedial drama on the conversational skills of chronic schizophrenic inpatients. *British Journal of Psychiatry, 143,* 165–172.

Steuer, J. L., Mintz, J., Hammen, C. L., Hill, M. A., Jarvik, L. F., McCarley, T., Motoike, P., & Rosen, R. (1984). Cognitive-behavioral and psychodynamic group psychotherapy in treatment of geriatric depression. *Journal of Consulting and Clinical Psychology, 52,* 180–189.

Stockton, R., & Morran, D. K. (1982). Review and perspective of critical dimensions in therapeutic small group research. In G. M. Gazda (Ed.), *Basic approaches to group psychotherapy* (pp. 37–85). Springfield, IL: Thomas.

Stoppard, J. M., & Henri, G. S. (1987). Conceptual level matching and effects of assertion training. *Journal of Counseling Psychology, 34,* 55–61.

Subich, L. M., & Coursol, D. H. (1985). Counseling expectations of clients and nonclients for group and individual treatment modes. *Journal of Counseling Psychology, 32,* 245–251.

Thompson, L. W., Gallagher, D., Nies, G., & Epstein, D. (1983). Evaluation of the effectiveness of professionals and nonprofessionals as instructors of "Coping with Depression" classes for elders. *Gerontologist, 23,* 390–396.

Thurman, C. W. (1985). Effectiveness of cognitive-behavioral treatments in reducing Type A behavior among university faculty. *Journal of Counseling Psychology, 32,* 74–83.

Tinsley, H. E. A., Bowman, S. L., & Ray, S. B. (1988). Manipulation of expectancies about counseling and psychotherapy: Review and analysis of expectancy manipulation strategies and results. *Journal of Counseling Psychology, 35,* 171–201.

Toseland, R. W., Rossiter, C. M., Peak, T., & Hill, P. (1990). Therapeutic processes in peer led and professionally led support groups for caregivers. *International Journal of Group Psychotherapy, 40,* 279–303.

Toseland, R. W., & Siporin, M. (1986). When to recommend group treatment: A review of the clinical and the research literature. *International Journal of Group Psychotherapy, 36*(2), 171–201.

Tschuschke, V., & Dies, R. R. (in press). Intensive analysis of therapeutic factors and outcome in long-term inpatient groups. *International Journal of Group Psychotherapy.*

Turner, J. A., & Clancy, S. (1988). Comparison of operant behavioral and cognitive-behavioral group treatment for chronic low back pain. *Journal of Counseling Psychology, 56,* 261–266.

Turner, J. A., Ciancy, S., McQuade, K. J., & Cardenas, D. D. (1990). Effectiveness of behavioral therapy for chronic low back pain: A component analysis. *Journal of Consulting and Clinical Psychology, 58,* 573–579.

Waltman, D. E., & Zimpfer, D. G. (1988). Composition, structure, and duration of treatment: Interacting variables in counseling groups. *Small Group Behavior, 19,* 171–184.

Yalom, I. D. (1985). *The theory and practice of group psychotherapy.* New York: Basic Books.

Zettle, R. D., & Rains, J. C. (1989). Group cognitive and contextual therapies in treatment of depression. *Journal of Clinical Psychology, 45,* 436–445.

CHAPTER 5

Pretraining and Structure:
Parallel Lines Yet to Meet

THEODORE J. KAUL and RICHARD L. BEDNAR

Entering group therapy is like riding in an open-cockpit airplane, especially if you have never done it before. You might feel exhilaration or apprehension, or both. The exhilaration might come from the nearly perfect novelty of the experience, but that might arouse dread, too. It would be fun to just sit back and be taken through the sky, but unless you are an experienced pilot, the feeling that your safety depends upon someone else's skill could be disconcerting.

Analogies always break down if you push them too far, so we won't push our luck with this one. We only wanted to highlight a fact that experienced group leaders seem often to ignore. Just because you have participated in dozens, or hundreds, of groups, and you know what probably will happen in this one, and you know how to perceive, think, and act in most group situations, it doesn't mean that your perceptions, thoughts, and actions are appropriate to the group's purposes or needs. It doesn't necessarily mean that they are consistent with *your* purposes or needs.

Even more, your expert perception, intimate knowledge, and facile skill do not necessarily translate into any useful understanding on the part of your group members. To walk into the woods with a botanist does not mean that you will know more about trees and plants and how they live together. The botanist must teach you in a way that makes contact with your knowledge and expectations. To watch a trial with an attorney does not mean that you will understand the unique epistemology of the law, or its procedures and rituals. You need guidance; how much depends on what you already know (including how much you know that is false), what you want to know, and how well you learn, among other considerations.

The overarching question in this volume is, "How can we be more effective in our treatments?" More specifically, we want to focus on questions of pregroup training and group structure. The usual point of origin is to define what we mean by these concepts and to place them in a useful context. We

155

will then review some of the better research pertinent to the goal of enhancing treatment through training and structure, and propose conclusions and suggest guidelines for practice that we have drawn from the research. We will nominate what we find to be interesting, creative, and clever, and suggest ways in which future research can add even more to practice. Proceeding from the literature review and critique, we will review some pretheory and a model for considering pretraining and structure. We will present some of the literature relevant to the model and conclude with general recommendations about practice and research.

STRUCTURE, PRETRAINING, AND THE THERAPEUTIC ROLE OF AMBIGUITY

The strategic use of ambiguity in systems of psychological help-giving has occupied a particularly important historical role. Its highly favorable conceptual and applied status usually is traced to the classical psychoanalytic model of psychotherapy. As Fenichel (1945) observed, the therapist remains as ambiguous as possible to provide a neutral background against which the patient's irrational thoughts and feelings can more readily be displayed. To this end, the therapist (a) sits behind, where his or her reactions cannot be observed by the analysand, (b) seldom speaks, and (c) provides little direction as to the course the client should pursue.

According to Bordin (1955), these techniques are in the service of a number of vital therapeutic operations that cannot be accomplished in a more structured atmosphere. For example, in classical psychoanalysis, ambiguity is essential for the therapeutic use of free association, a form of projection that contains the seeds for understanding the client's pathology. Ambiguity, which is the inevitable consequence of therapist "objectivity," also is a prerequisite for the development of transference, a phenomenon that is at the very core of successful treatment.

Neo-analytic therapies have modified some of these presuppositions about the salutary role of therapist ambiguity. For instance, they may substitute the notion of "technical neutrality" (a neutrality to the patient's material, but not to the patient's person) for the objectivity notion (cf. Slipp, 1982). While this would almost certainly reduce ambiguity in the client, it would with equal certainly not eliminate it.

The therapeutic use of ambiguity is not limited to psychoanalysis or, for that matter, individual forms of psychological treatment. It is a central component in person-centered therapies, for example, and small group treatments as well. In the person-centered approach, nondirectiveness is assumed to help foster a permissive and accepting atmosphere that encourages clients to explore the meaning and significance of their inner feelings more fully and completely (Rogers, 1951; Rosenbaum & Berger, 1963) and to reduce the salience of conditions of worth. In some encounter and

T-group approaches, ambiguity about role expectations and goals is intentionally preserved to create situations stressful to the client that can elicit typical coping strategies. These coping strategies then provide experiential materials that group members can use to learn about their own adaptive and maladaptive modes of behavior. The group leader's diagnostic certainty supposedly is enhanced as well by this opportunity to observe the client deal with an emotionally charged ambiguous situation.

In brief, some of the most important elements of psychological helpgiving are based on the working assumption that externally imposed structure actively interferes with clients' capacity to become more aware and responsive to the workings of their internal mental and emotional life. It is this assumption that has established the conceptual and applied preeminence of ambiguity in systems of interpersonal influence. This influence seems to have had a remarkable effect on shaping both individual and group forms of psychological treatment. In the individual therapies, it is one of the guiding influences of such critical treatment operations as facilitating access to learned conditions of worth, encouraging client self exploration and self direction, and transference. In group treatments, it is assumed to encourage the style and pace of group development so that they are in harmony with the unique needs of each group. It is believed to enhance the clarity with which problem behaviors are displayed as well as lead to meaningful self exploration and behavior change.

Clearly then, ambiguity has been awarded a position of great moment and grave consequence in some therapeutic constructions. But it is not an award by acclamation. Other notions of psychotherapy seem as adamant in their conclusion that ambiguity in the client, while probably inevitable, is a potential source of serious mischief in individual or group therapy. Adherents of these alternative approaches believe that a characteristic of an expert therapist is sensitivity to nascent ambiguity and the skillful administration of antidotes to it. The issue has waxed and waned for over 50 years. Why have we not resolved it? What is a reasonable stance for the contemporary practitioner or researcher?

Conceptions and Misconceptions

In discussions of therapy, ambiguity usually is thought of as one endpoint on a single continuum. Its opposite generally is structure. So we have come to think of treatments as structured or ambiguous. Therapies supposedly could be arrayed along this line, ranging from the most structured, to those moderately so, through those that are neither structured nor ambiguous, and so on out to those that are highly ambiguous. This intuitively appealing conceptualization has gradually evolved to the point where the structure—ambiguity continuum is a major dimension often used to describe and compare different forms of treatment. One of the major implications of this conception is obvious enough; it suggests that structure and ambiguity seemingly are incompatible. As one increases, the other must of necessity decrease. You cannot have both.

Even though this view has been historically popular and inviting, it may be misleading. We think that it is seriously flawed, both conceptually and semantically, specifically in the context of group psychotherapy. We suggest that it is quite possible to have psychological treatment systems that are simultaneously highly structured and ambiguous.

In discussions of group treatment, structure refers to events or ideas that are made up of interdependent elements having a definite organization or pattern. It is an "organized" entity or an "organization" of interrelated events. The literal meaning of structure emphasizes organization and order. Whether you can separate them in quantum mechanics or chaos theory, we don't know. But we are unable to conceive of structure without organization in the consideration of group psychotherapy. Structure *is* organization in some meaningful sense of the word.

Where we part company with the conventional view is with the opposite of structure. We argue that the opposite of structure is not ambiguity; it is the presence of disorganization or, more precisely, the absence of organization and order. It is a lack of conceptual orderliness and clarity! Given this assumption, it does not seem practical to array theories of psychological help-giving on a continuum of structure-versus-ambiguity. As a matter of fact, with the possible exceptions of a few perhaps chemically induced speculations, it does not even make much sense to array them on the organization-versus-disorganization dimension. *All* approaches to psychological treatment that are worth discussing are highly structured (or organized), at least conceptually. Virtually all such approaches that warrant the title of theory, and many that don't, have rather well-organized assumptions and expectations of how clients and therapists are to behave if the treatment is to be successful.

If systems of psychotherapy do not vary on levels of structure, at least not in a fundamentally useful way, where does ambiguity enter into the equation? We think that systems vary on the clarity or vagueness with which they impose their structure, and the clarity of the attendant expectations and demands on client behavior. This point of view was recently summarized by Bednar, Wells, and Peterson (1989). They said:

> [I]t is clear with even a modest understanding of classical psychoanalytic theory that client insight is a staple element in the cure, and client introspection and self exploration are essential ingredients in the process. The treatment process is also highly structured, so that clients are encouraged to respond to internal cues and stimuli as a means of enhancing insight, introspection, and self exploration. During treatment sessions, the therapist maintains a neutral posture because neutrality is assumed to be the optimal condition for encouraging material to come bubbling up from the client's unconscious for review. Note that all of these conditions are structured for the client. Actually, this treatment orientation is highly structured, with the

appropriate behavior of the client and therapists well defined. It is misleading and unfortunate that this treatment has mistakenly been referred to as
"unstructured," and by implication, a treatment with low demand characteristics for client behavior. Its demand characteristics are high, as is its
level of imposed structure. (p. 251)

These authors went on to suggest that the same analysis also applies
to client-centered and group approaches as well. The essence of their view
was that all systems of psychological treatment are highly structured events,
but some of them are structured in a way designed to obscure what is expected, and perhaps even required, of clients if they are to improve. Others
simply convey these role expectations more openly and clearly. To para-
phrase Watzlawick, Beavin, and Jackson (1967), one cannot not structure.

The implications that flow from this observation are indeed significant.
The idea that person-centered or psychoanalytic treatments, for example,
are less structured with fewer demand characteristics imposed on clients is
not a particularly accurate or relevant description of these approaches. Demand characteristics are not eliminated or, for that matter, even minimized
because they remain vague. In any event, they are anything but vague to the
therapist! They are just more difficult for the client to respond to, or even
recognize. So the very idea of structure and ambiguity as major elements of
different types of psychological treatment seems misleading. Perhaps it is
more accurate and useful to shift the emphasis away from the influence of
structure and ambiguity and towards the influence of intentional vagueness
or clarity about our expectations of clients during the therapy process.

With this idea in mind, we can now shift the central question of concern
in the historical debate about the value of therapeutic structure and ambiguity. Now we can ask why, and under what circumstances, does intentional
vagueness about client roles and therapeutic demand characteristics benefit
client learning in any system of psychotherapy? And equally important
why, and under what conditions, are clear and obvious role expectations and
demand characteristics beneficial to client learning in any system of psychotherapy? At the most fundamental level, these questions ask us carefully
to consider such obvious therapeutic operations as determining if it is helpful or harmful to start sessions by asking clients to start talking about what
is most important to them instead of saying nothing and waiting to see how
the client fills the void created by the therapist's silence. Or we might determine the therapeutic efficacy of specific exercises designed to enhance
feelings of universality compared to exercises designed to teach effective
listening skills. Or, more broadly still, we could investigate the superiority
of individual sessions with a therapist versus videotaped instruction in fostering skills for shifting appropriately from helper to helpee roles. The list
could be expanded infinitely, of course. Questions of this type can readily
be approached with the empirical tools already at hand. And in spite of the
range of penetrating questions that can be formulated from this premise,

our generic concern is always the same. We want to know when, and under what conditions clients benefit from having their role in the therapeutic process remain vague and implicit, and when and how we should openly and expeditiously clarify it regardless of the orientating theory. This question is also the central concern in the group literature regarding the role of structure and pregroup preparation for new group members.

PRETRAINING AND STRUCTURE

We have argued elsewhere that many of the concepts in group treatment suffer from inadequate specification (cf. Bednar & Kaul, 1994; Kaul & Bednar, 1986). This vehicle will not enable us to remove pretraining and group structure from the gossamer list, but we need to move toward ad hoc explications that will serve our purposes. Part of the problem lies in the fact that if you drew a Venn diagram of the two concepts, the circles would show substantial overlap. They seem to share common elements. They seem inextricable to a large degree.

Pretraining

In general, pregroup training involves preparing individuals for their client/member roles. The preparation has included an impressive variety of variables, some with generality across groups and clients, others highly specialized to a setting, treatment, or client concern. The more general ones can be summarized as concerning group members' expectations, perceptions, or actions.

At least since Rosenthal and Frank (1956), practitioners have had reason to concern themselves with client expectations for treatment. Though Rosenthal and Frank's work dealt with individual therapy, group workers have become acutely aware of the power of member expectations as well. The novice member often has many expectations about what happens in groups, most of them far-fetched, and some almost beyond science fiction. Reasoning correctly from these incorrect premises, novices commonly translate their expectations into an array of possible emotional consequences. Indeed, why should group therapy be anything but ambiguous to the uninitiated? It is in many respects unlike anything that most of us have experienced elsewhere in our lives. But the likely readers of this narrative are exquisitely aware of the uniquity of group treatment and don't need to hear it repeated by us. Suffice it to say that pregroup training can involve educating potential members about what is likely to happen, and not happen, in their group. It can help create appropriate expectations, neither too high nor too low, that are believed to enable or enhance treatment.

Closely associated with creating appropriate member expectations is educating them about what is important in a group and how to perceive it. Two examples clarify this point. Feedback from other members is commonly accepted as a critical therapeutic factor in group treatment. This is so widely held that we would be embarrassed to mention it to an audience of group leaders. But novice members often cannot recognize feedback's importance. Indeed, many find it impossible to recognize feedback at all. It has been confused with criticism, personal attack, story telling, and just about anything other than information intended to benefit the recipient. A second example is cohesion. Again, this is widely held to be necessary for effective group functioning and among the most therapeutic elements found in the group setting. But sometimes in cohesive groups "it may be difficult to confront negative aspects of the group's experience . . . and may create a sense of the group's uniqueness that can limit the member's ability to transfer learning . . ." (Stockton & Morran, 1982, p. 54). There is little wonder, then, that group workers often feel compelled to present pregroup training in the perception of important therapeutic elements.

Finally, it may be appropriate to train participants in the skills of group membership. If giving feedback is as important as we all believe it to be, it seems egregious to leave acquisition of the skills involved in effective feedback to chance. Similarly, learning how most beneficially to obtain feedback may involve the teaching of certain behaviors. The same is true of assuming the reciprocal roles of giver and receiver in the group, reinforcing desired responses, creating a healthy interpersonal confrontation, and many other instances where specific behaviors are presumed to be critical to effective group treatment. Here again, pregroup training has responded.

Any classification system can be found wanting, and there doubtlessly are occasions when dividing the variables of pretraining among expectations, perceptions, and behaviors is flawed. They are not independent events. Still, for the purposes at hand, expectations, perceptions, and behaviors seem to cover just about all of what has been called pregroup training.

Structure

As suggested earlier, structure most often seems to represent a deliberate attempt by the group leader to create specific therapeutic circumstances for the group. Sometimes the goal is to avoid the consequences of the unavoidable ambiguity involved in becoming a group member. Other times, the objective seems more to create opportunities for the ordered experiencing of phenomena believed to be important, including the managed introduction of aversive events, while controlling their negative consequences. Structure also is employed to manipulate the degree of interpersonal risk taken or accepted by group members. In any event, a common element of group structure is that, while it may be carefully planned for by the group leader, it is observed in the ongoing group. Its purpose is to create specific opportunities in the group, opportunities that almost necessarily must include influences on members' perceptions, expectations, or behavior. So the Venn diagrams overlap and concepts may become confused. The confounding does not necessitate confusion, however, at least not the kind of confusion that makes impossible normal conversation about the two constructs by experienced group workers.

No group is unstructured. Even the most casual, insouciant, wing-it group leader must have some structure in mind in order to think about the group. But there are vast differences in the awareness of the structure among leaders and among members. No matter what, it seems, some want to demolish the structure, others want to change it, and some want to pretend that it is not there. And there are vast differences in the depth of organization of thought about structure on the part of different leaders or members. Some have only the faintest comprehension of the structure of the treatment, some choose to ignore its details, and still others have a thorough understanding about how things fit within the group.

Even so, differences in the comprehension of structure among leaders tells us nothing about the innate structure of the treatment, or, especially, the structure of the theory underlying the treatment. Because one does not understand or is overpowered by quantum mechanics does not mean that quantum mechanics is unstructured. Structure may facilitate understanding, but it does not entail it.

Pretraining and Structure

At least part of the ineluctable confounding of pretraining and structure lies in their mutual necessity. One cannot conceive of pregroup training worthy of the name that did not involve substantial elements of structure. Training demands thoughtful organization.

When you consider pretraining as being a part of the treatment itself (often the most sensible way to view it), the relationship becomes even tighter. For example, teaching neophyte group members how to recognize and emit assertive sentences, give and receive feedback, or assume the role of therapist or client, may be carried on before the group treatment is begun. Each of these activities or roles is presumed to be potentially therapeutic in group treatments, but also may be therapeutic in its own right. When the target of the training is potentially beneficial to the client, it may be reasonable to consider the pregroup training as a part of the treatment. Or it may not. The issue is almost never an important one in practice, but it is in research. There, theoretical and methodological considerations would determine the most salubrious decision.

THE RESEARCH LITERATURE

Over the years, there has been a consistent empirical and applied interest in the value of pregroup preparation for group members. The underlying rationale driving this research has remained essentially unchanged. The small group situation is inherently difficult and awkward for many inexperienced group members, at least initially. They do not know what to expect from the group, the group leader, other group members, or themselves. Additionally, the expectation that group treatment can be helpful almost always exists, if only as a faint hope, but group members generally have little understanding of what they are to do during this process. As importantly, when members have an idea of what to do in the group, they seldom know how and almost never know why. When they do have an understanding, it often bears no discernable relation to the understandings and expectations of the leader or other members of the group. The very nature of early group meetings seems to generate anxiety and discomfort for many group members, probably because of the uncertainty of what is about to happen and how it will happen. Pregroup training is a way of preparing clients to respond to these difficulties more realistically and constructively.

Pregroup preparations historically have included a variety of activities including: (1) teaching clients vital interpersonal skills such as self-disclosure or the purpose and value of feedback, (2) clarification of expectations about problems in early group development that most groups will have to face and resolve, (3) watching role models in videotaped segments perform vital behaviors during critical incidents in group development, and (4) receiving instructions in a variety of formats on how to recognize and respond to personal feelings of resistance, anger, affection, anxiety, or fear in a small group setting. It is generally assumed that these orientating activities help clients respond more easily as well as therapeutically to the difficulties of early group sessions. Fortunately, some of these assumptions have been put to empirical test under controlled conditions. Before we look at the accumulated literature, however, we will review a few studies in some detail to illustrate the types of questions asked, samples drawn, methods employed, and conclusions offered.

Examples

The outcome question is, not surprisingly, a primary question of interest to those studying pregroup training. Piper, Debbane, Garant, and Bienvenu (1979) wondered if learning the objectives and procedures of group psychotherapy prior to entering a group would improve attendance rates and reduce dropouts. Their ongoing program of long-term outpatient group therapy was demanding of patients in the early sessions, and about one in five was dropping out. They decided to train their clients in "here-and-now events, interpersonal processes, group processes, and member-leader relations in a safe, structured situation" (p. 1253) independent of the presenting problem.

Cognitive material and related structured group exercises were developed for each of the four concepts. Four hours of pretraining, one hour for each concept, were given in a group setting to screened clients. Five groups were constituted, three given the cognitive-experiential training and two serving as no-training controls. Clients were matched according to age, sex, and screening data and randomly assigned to treatment or control conditions. Each group was led by a trained leader or co-leaders. Attendance and dropout rates were taken for the first four months of therapy.

The three pretrained groups produced one dropout (4.3% rate), compared to five (31.3% rate). They found significantly fewer missed sessions for the pretrained members, too, but were able to ascribe almost all of the difference to the difference in dropout rate.

With the appropriate caveats, Piper et al. (1979) were cautiously encouraged by the results. They speculated about the causes of the observed differences, wondering if they were due to informational enhancement of the group members, or if they were the result of "positive interpersonal bonds" (p. 1255) that strengthened members' ability to persist in the treatment. That would await follow-up investigations.

The Piper et al. (1979) study is thoughtfully derived from practice and carefully anchored in the research literature. They asked an important, and basic, question. They involved actual clients and leaders, and apparently did not modify the treatment to make it fit an experimental protocol. The extra four hours of contact given to the experimental groups probably was attenuated by the four-month duration of treatment. They treated their data and their readers with respect. It is a good (not perfect) example of how to study the outcomes of pregroup training.

The Piper et al. study tells us about whether pregroup training has an effect on actual clients in real-life treatment. The authors properly acknowledge that this particular study does not tell us how the effect occurs (it could be a Hawthorne effect), but that was not their purpose.

A second, and probably more representative, example of pregroup training was reported by Muller and Scott (1984). They wondered whether there were important differences between pretraining media, and if there were, how they affected group process.

Four treatment methods were created and were randomly assigned to college student volunteers (N = 67) for personal growth groups. The experimental treatments were: (1) film presentation (participants observed a 17-minute film about group process), (2) written material (participants read "material equivalent to the film" [p. 123] that took about 20 minutes to read), (3) film-plus-written-material (participants received both interventions mentioned), (4) minimum-treatment (participants read "general material about groups" [p. 123]), and (5) there were no-treatment control participants. Subjects from each of these five conditions were randomly placed in personal growth groups. Each group was led by the same facilitator and met three times.

Data were drawn pretraining, after the first group session, and after the third group meeting. The pregroup Experience Checklist (Cartwright,

1976), Reaction to Group Situation Test (Thelen, 1974), and Personal Orientation Inventory (Shostrom, 1963), each with subscales, combined for 18 dependent variables, for which 7 significant main effects were obtained by pre-post analyses of covariance.

Muller and Scott (1984) concluded that the "benefits of previous training for participants in short-term group counseling were supported once again" (p. 124). Some members responded positively to the film, others to the written material, and these treatments separately "produced more positive results than those from the treatment combining these two methods" (p. 124). The results appear to suggest to Muller and Scott that the effects of the pregroup training were noticeable in the group process.

As with Piper et al. (1979), Muller and Scott (1984) investigated an important question. The questions differed in that Muller and Scott were more concerned about the effects of pretraining on group processes, rather than outcome. Differences in the methods are apparent, even from the abbreviated reports given here. An important similarity is that both seem driven by practical concerns. Neither seemed deeply committed to theory development or to deeper understanding of basic processes. Each wanted to uncover what worked.

A final example of the pretraining and structure research should suffice to illustrate the general style and substance of this type of work. The pretheoretical ideas of Bednar, Melnick, and Kaul (1974) suggested that pregroup preparation could reduce the psychological risk, and therefore anxiety, associated with small group participation. This rationale led Evensen and Bednar (1978) to test the relationship between different types of pregroup preparation with clients who differed in their initial risk-taking disposition. These investigators employed a randomized design with a 2 × 4 factorial arrangement of treatments. The first factor was two levels of client risk-taking disposition (high and low). The second factor was four types of pregroup preparation (cognitive, behavioral, a combination of cognitive and behavioral, and minimal preparation). After receiving one of these four types of pregroup preparation, the participants from each treatment condition were asked to "form a group and get better acquainted using the information and skills they had learned" (p. 69).

The dependent measures in this study were of three types, which included: (1) group behavior, which was rated from audiotapes using the Hill Interaction Matrix (Hill, 1965), (2) self-disclosure and feedback, which were assessed through a self-report instrument developed for the study, and (3) group cohesion, which was measured by the Gross Cohesion Scale (Gross, 1957).

The results of the Evensen and Bednar (1978) study suggested that a high risk-taking disposition was related to higher levels of interpersonal communication, group cohesion, and high levels of self-disclosure and feedback. The implication of this finding was that the psychological risk-taking inherent in early group development was more easily accommodated by those with a higher risk-taking disposition. Evensen and Bednar suggested that, since most therapy clients probably are of the low risk-taking vintage, it is important for group leaders to be cognizant of, and appropriately manage, the levels of risk taking involved in early group development.

More importantly to Evensen and Bednar, however, were the findings that revealed a consistent pattern of risk-taking × treatment interaction effects on all dependent measures. These results indicated that pregroup behavioral practice was most interpersonally productive with the high risk-taking participants. These participants also showed the highest levels of communication, cohesion, and perceived self disclosure. The low risk-takers showed the opposite patterns on these variables. It seemed to the investigators that to be most effective even the type of pregroup training that is provided must take into account the personality attributes of the participants.

Evensen and Bednar's pattern of results suggested that the explicitness of the training provided high risk-taking participants with both a willingness and skill to engage in more meaningful interactions that subsequently enhanced the quality of their small group experience. These participants had the highest ratings of group cohesion and intimate interactions, and more favorable evaluations of the group experience. These results were also consistent with the general idea that clear role expectations and the development of skills related to early group development enhanced the group experience for some group members.

The Evensen and Bednar (1978) study differed from those of Piper et al. (1979) and Muller and Scott (1984) in several ways. Most importantly to this current discussion, however, is its grounding in theory (pretheory, actually, but the consequence is the same). The questions, independent variables, and dependent variables largely were determined by the model developed earlier by Bednar, Melnick, and Kaul (1974). We will return to this later, but given three examples of the research conducted in the pretraining and group structure arena, it is time to shift perspectives and examine more generally the body of research.

Research Scope

There is an abundance of research on pregroup preparation and how it seems to affect both group processes and client outcomes. The collective body of research in this fertile field of study is sophisticated and somewhat informative and contains some distinct as well as significant trends that we will identify and discuss. We will summarize and comment on some important elements of it.

We selected some of the most significant research in this area over the last 25 years or so to summarize the state of the art in pregroup training and group structure. To be included, they had to involve at least a quasi-experimental design and independent or dependent variables that seemed relevant to the topic. From that set, we chose what we consider among the most useful. Our choices are not representative of the entire literature, nor are they intended to be. They do represent the subset of literature that contributes to the understanding of pretraining and structure. These studies have been abstracted with regard to (1) experimental conditions, (2) sample characteristics, (3) dependent measures, and (4) major results. The summary is displayed in Table 5.1.

Table 5.1 contains 21 pregroup training and structure studies. Almost all of these studies have been included in our earlier reviews of the experiential group research (Bednar & Kaul, 1978, 1994; Bednar & Lawlis, 1971; Kaul & Bednar, 1986). This was not by desire; we had hoped to summarize new, exciting contributions to our understanding. Additional reports have been published; however, some are not included because they essentially replicate studies already chosen, others because of serious design limitations (many involve pre-experimental designs), while others have been omitted because they did not appear to contribute significantly to our specific understanding of therapeutic groups.

On the whole, the body of research represented in Table 5.1 is rather impressive. It includes studies with some of the following characteristics: (a) actual clinical samples, and not just undergraduate students recruited for the study, (b) experienced professional as opposed to student therapists, (c) advanced design, analysis, and measurement procedures, (d) long-term follow-up procedures, and (e) conceptual considerations that are more relevant to group theory and practice than is often the case. Individually and collectively, these studies contribute to our understanding of the components and consequences of pregroup training and group structure.

Inspection of Table 5.1 reveals the following noteworthy trends:

1. The breadth and diversity of psychological variables included in attempts to prepare clients for group participation or provide more explicit structure to group events is impressive. They include such salient personality characteristics as risk-taking disposition, levels of anxiety, self-esteem, and internal-external locus of control. There are others that demand empirical explication, but that does not mitigate the importance of the variables selected for investigation in these studies.

2. Pretraining activities varied substantially in the type of training offered and the way it was presented. For example, expectations about group roles were clarified with role induction films, interviews, audiotapes, and written materials. Similarly, specific group skills were clarified or taught with role-playing exercises, cognitive instructions, audiotaped instructions, and written materials. Generally speaking, pregroup preparation activities in our sample of better studies seem to vary with respect to their emphasis on: (a) various forms of behavioral practice or modeling, (b) cognitive clarification, and (c) self-involving experiential learning.

TABLE 5.1. Pretraining and Structure Studies

Author	Purpose	Experimental Comparison	Dependent Variable	Participants/Leaders	Results
PRETRAINING STUDIES					
Wogan et al. (1977)	To see if cognitive-experiential pretraining in a clinical situation would affect process variables.	Taped pretraining using cognitive-experiential instruction (3 groups). Structured T-group experience in pretraining (2 groups). No pretraining control. Placebo control.	Patient-identified problem. Group interaction.	P: Undergraduate students referred by marital health clinic for group therapy. L: Three Ph.D. psychologists. Three M.S.W.O. Two Clinical Psychology graduate students. Two graduate Social Work Students. One graduate student in Ed. Psychology.	No significant effects of pretreatments on group interactions or outcomes. However, groups in tape pretreatment had highest overall outcome ratings and placebo condition had lowest; significant affects appear due to therapist and group composition differences.
Garrison (1978)	Compare the impact of a verbal preparation and attention placebo for group therapy.	Preparatory interview. Written introduction. Attention placebo interview.	Patient expectations toward group. Patient behavior. Dropout rate.	P: Applicants for services at an outpatient clinic. L: Master's level Social Work students. Experienced clinical social worker.	Prepared patients had better attendance records and were judged as manifesting better patient role behavior. No difference between the two treatment groups.
Piper et al. (1979)	Implement a pretraining procedure combining cognitive and experiential approaches to pretraining.	Three pretraining groups. Two control groups.	Attendance and dropout.	P: Patients referred for group therapy. L: Co-therapist teams composed of a psychiatric resident and a nonmedical professional (psychologists, social worker, or nurse).	Fewer dropouts and higher attendance with a cognitive-experiential pretraining program.
Piper & Marrache (1981)	Investigate the potential of using pretraining group behavior to predict therapy group behavior.	Pretraining group behavior.	Therapy group behavior.	P: Patients referred for group therapy. L: Co-therapist teams composed of psychiatrist resident and a nonmedical professional (psychologists, social worker, or nurse).	Significant, positive relationships between a number of pretraining behaviors and therapy behavior. However, psychiatric interview variables were poor predictors of pretherapy and therapy behavior variables.

Piper et al. (1982)	To determine the relative importance of material highly relevant versus minimally relevant to the orientation of therapy groups in a pretraining procedure.	Primary pretraining-emphasizing here-and-now, interpersonal processes, group processes, leader's role. Secondary pretraining-emphasizing individual patient, past history control condition—no pretraining.	Attendance and remaining in therapy (HIM content and work categories) and outcome (interpersonal functioning and general psychiatric symptoms).	P: Patients referred for group therapy. L: Co-therapist teams composed of a psychiatric resident and a nonmedical professional (psychologist, social worker, or nurse).	No significant differences among treatments on outcome measures or work levels, although content (percentage of personal and relationship statements) was influenced: 0:1, primary; 3.5.1, secondary; 2:1, control.
Hilkey et al. (1982)	To measure the effects of videotape pretraining on selected process and outcome variables.	Videotape presentation and guided performance experience prior to group. Control group.	Anxiety prior to group, self-report of readiness for group, group interaction, movement toward behavioral goals.	P: Inmates at a medium-security penitentiary L: Counseling psychology, doctoral students, and Ph.D.s.	Pretraining clients had expectations of group treatment, demonstrated more desirable behaviors in the early stages of therapy, and made more progress toward individual goals.

STRUCTURE STUDIES

Whalen (1969)	Investigate the affects of pregroup instructions and modeling on early group interactions.	Factorial arrangement of treatments (2 × 2) including: 1. Film model and detailed instructions 2. Detailed instructions only. 3. Film model and minimal instructions.	College students.	Ratings of observable behavior.	Film model and detailed instructions associated with more interpersonal openness.
Warren & Rice (1972)	Investigate the effects of outside therapy structuring on group participation style and attrition.	1. Therapy and out of group structuring and stabilization. 2. Therapy and out of group stabilization interviews. 3. Therapy only.	Low prognosis college center clientele.	Group process analysis. Therapist-rated changes. Q-sort. Group sessions attended.	Out of therapy structure and stabilization interview associated with lower attrition, improved group participation, and more perceived personal change.
Anchor, Vojtisek, & Patterson (1973)	Investigate the effects of initial group structure on the group behavior of high- and low-anxiety subjects.	1. Specific cognitive instructions to self. 2. Placebo control. 3. High- and low-anxiety group participants.	Hospitalized patients.	Group process ratings.	High-anxiety subjects talked more in both treatment conditions.

TABLE 5.1. (*Continued*)

Author	Purpose	Experimental Comparison	Dependent Variable	Participants/ Leaders	Results
Strupp & Bloxom (1973)	Investigate the effects of pregroup role induction procedures on lower-class patients.	Group introduced to group treatment by: 1. Role induction film. 2. Role induction interview. 3. Control film.	Lower-class patients.	Rating of improvement. Satisfaction with treatment. Symptom discomfort. Role expectancies. Motivation for treatment in therapy behavior.	The two role induction procedures were associated with more favorable therapy experience, and on several measures the role induction film was superior to the control film.
Abramowitz, Abramowitz, Roback, & Jackson (1974)	Investigate the effects of direction and nondirective group therapy on internal-external locus of control subjects.	1. Relatively directive group. 2. Relatively nondirective group. 3. Internal-external locus of control group participants.	College outpatients.	Expectations for successful life. Social alienation scale. Feelings of guilt and shame. State-trait anxiety inventory. Client self-report.	Subjects in group more closely matched for their locus of control orientation, generally showed a more favorable response to group treatment. This was particularly true for internally oriented clients.
D'Augelli & Chinsky (1974)	Investigate the effects of interpersonal skills and pregroup training on meaningful group participation.	Cognitive instruction. Cognitive instruction and behavioral practice. Placebo control.	College students.	Group process ratings.	Subjects receiving any type of meaningful pretraining engaged in high levels of interpersonal communications. Cognitive pretraining was associated with the highest levels of pretraining; this was particularly true of interpersonally skilled subjects.
Zarle & Willis (1975)	Investigate the effects of pregroup stress management techniques on client deterioration from encounter groups.	Induced-affect training. Induced-affect training and encounter group. Induced-affect training only.	College students.	Eysenck Personality Inventory.	Group participants not receiving induced affect training showed significant increase on Neuroticism scales whereas group members receiving such training demonstrated significant increases on the Extraversion scale.

Study	Purpose	Design	Sample/Measures		Results
Bednar & Battersby (1976)	Investigate effects of pregroup cognitive structure in early group development.	Factorial arrangement of treatments (2 × 2 × 2) including: 1. Behavioral instructions. 2. Goal instructions. 3. Persuasive explanation.	College students.	Behavior ratings. Group cohesion. Attitudes toward groups.	Specific behavioral instruction associated with more productive group behavior, more favorable attitudes, and higher levels of group cohesion.
Crews & Melnick (1976)	Investigate effects of initial and delayed structure and social avoidance on short- and long-term outcomes.	Factorial arrangement of treatments (2 × 3) including: 1. Early group structure. 2. Delayed group structure. 3. No structure. 4. Social anxiety and avoidance.	College students.	Group behavior. Group cohesion. Attitudes toward group situational anxiety.	Early group structure associated with increased self-disclosure as well as higher levels of anxiety. The effects of structure dissipated over time.
Lee & Bednar (1977)	Investigate affects of group structure, risk-taking, disposition, and sex on early group development.	Factorial arrangement of treatments (3 × 2 × 3 × 2) including: 1. Group structure. 2. Risk-taking disposition. 3. Sex. 4. Behavioral tasks.	College students.	Group behavior. Attitudes toward group. Group cohesion.	Risk × structure interaction with high structure most beneficial for low risk-taking subjects. Experimental conditions associated with highest levels of interpersonal communications generally had lowest levels of group cohesion.
Lundgren (1977)	Analyze developmental trends in sensitivity training groups by exploring the sequence of interpersonal issues of problem areas emerging at different points in the group life span.	A record of communication patterns and content themes occurring in five T-groups.	Categorization of content themes.	P: MTL participants. L: MTL leaders.	Average trends for the five groups suggest a temporal sequence of concerns with involvement, control, openness, conflict, and solidarity problems, respectively.
Ware & Barr (1977)	The effects of leader structure on self-concept and self-actualization.	Structured experience. Unstructured experience. Control.	Self-concept, self-actualization, social desirability, and locus of control.	P: Undergraduate student volunteers. L: Not specified.	Both experimental groups scored higher on self-actualization and self-worth than controls. Subjects in structured groups showed more openness, less defensiveness, a higher

TABLE 5.1. (Continued)

Author	Purpose	Experimental Comparison	Dependent Variable	Participants/ Leaders	Results
Ware & Barr (continued)					degree of social desirability, and reported higher feelings of personal worth than the other two conditions.
Roach (1977)	Compare the effects of cognitive vs. behavioral presentation of structure, high vs. low level of specificity, and interpersonal vs. intrapersonal content on early group development.	Eight separate treatments reflecting the two levels of the three dimensions of structure compared ($2 \times 2 \times 2$).	Change in attitudes concerning interpersonal feedback and honesty, group discussion of feelings: the group, awareness of feelings, openness, self-exploration, subject anxiety level, group interaction and cohesion, member satisfaction and level of discomfort.	P: Undergraduate student volunteers. L: Not specified.	Superiority of behavioral structure over cognitive. The effects of varied content or specificity of structure differed according to the method of presentation.
Evensen & Bednar (1978)	Investigate the effects of specific pregroup cognitive and behavioral structure and risk-taking disposition on early group development.	Factorial arrangements of treatments (2×4) including: 1. Cognitive structure. 2. Behavioral structure. 3. Cognitive and behavioral structure. 4. Minimal structure. 5. Risk-taking disposition.	College students.	Group behavior. Self-reports. Group cohesion.	Risk × structure interaction variables with the high risk-behavioral structure conditions associated with highest levels of group performance on all variables and low risk-behavioral structure lowest performance on most variables.
DeJulio, Bentley, & Cockayne (1979)	Investigate the effects of high and low initial structure on short- and long-term group development.	1. Audiotaped instructions and examples of desired behaviors at first group meeting. 2. Comparable groups without audiotape instruction.	College students.	Observational group behavior. Self-closure questionnaire. Self-esteem scale. Personal orientation inventory.	The high structure started at higher levels of group interaction, but moved toward less productive interaction over time. Low-structure groups began at lower levels of interactions but moved to high levels of group functioning over time.

It is encouraging to see that many of the core elements of pregroup preparation have been studied in conjunction with equally important personality characteristics; a procedure that is required to clarify the vital treatment × personality interaction effects that are so central in any attempt to understand the power and limitations of psychological treatments.

3. The breadth and diversity of measures employed to assess the effects of group structure and pregroup training activities are equally broad. It should be noted that the effects of structure and pregroup preparation have been assessed in terms of both group processes and client improvement, both crucial for improved scientific understanding and professional practice. Variables studied include such considerations as symptom improvement, dropout rates, group interaction patterns, cohesion, client self-evaluations, attitudes toward the group experience, changes in self concept, and reductions in anxiety.

   Regrettably, the technical psychometric qualities of many of these measures are less than we might desire or should be willing to continue to accept. This problem is not one the group disciplines are likely to escape in the near future because of the limited availability measurement instruments that are designed to capture the most relevant effects of group activities (Bednar & Kaul, 1994).

4. The breadth and diversity of populations studied and group leaders employed is equally apparent. Clients were rather diverse, ranging from college undergraduates, to NTL participants, to incarcerated prisoners, to outpatients. The lack of racial or ethnic diversity in the group members is a concern, and the effects of these demands further investigation. That lack does not obviate the diversity on other dimensions. Group leaders ranged from students in training, to NTL leaders, and included MSWs, MDs, and PhDs. More racial and ethnic variability might be desirable here, too.

5. The results of these reports are equally diverse, a fact that should not be too surprising given the variability of treatment conditions, leaders, outcome measures, and populations studied. But there is one observation about this collective body of research that may be more significant than the results of any individual or combination of individual studies.

Over the years, it has become more and more apparent that psychotherapy researchers have consistently reported favorable results for virtually all types and forms of psychological treatments (e.g., Garfield & Bergin, 1986; Smith & Glass, 1977; Whitehouse, 1966). What makes this finding interesting is not the consistency with which we can generate evidence that psychotherapy can be effective, but that we have precious little reliable evidence to suggest that any one type of treatment is superior to any others.

While some claim there is sufficient evidence to assert the superiority of some approaches with specific diagnostic categories, most others remain unconvinced that such a conclusion is warranted by the research. There seems to be an abundance of evidence that all treatments can be effective, but nothing seems consistently and generally to work better than anything else—a curious and puzzling finding. But if our research methods and procedures are sensitive enough to demonstrate treatment effectiveness, it certainly seems reasonable to assume that they could also detect differential treatment effectiveness, if it existed. Failing that, we could expect our methods to enable the data to hint broadly, at least. But it seems that differential treatment effectiveness just doesn't present itself as yet! The implication is that therapeutic success may be mediated by the common underlying elements of all treatments (or all treaters, or all clients, both of which seem unlikely given the evidence) much more than the specific and obvious techniques of each treatment.

The same pattern may be emerging in the pregroup training literature. Almost all the cognitive, behavioral, and experiential components of pregroup preparation have been demonstrated to produce favorable effects, but none of them seems to be consistently superior to any other variables. We can't be sure if this early trend is reliable or robust, but it is certainly suggestive. Consider, for example, that more desirable patterns of group communication and interaction, as well as actual client improvement have been shown to be favorably affected by such diverse considerations as: (a) behavioral instructions (Bednar & Battersby, 1976), (b) cognitive instructions (D'Augelli & Chinsky, 1974), (c) high levels of initial group structure (DeJulio, Bentley, & Cockayne, 1976), (d) high risk-taking disposition coupled with behavioral preparation (Evensen & Bednar, 1978), (e) high initial group structure coupled with low risk-taking disposition (Lee & Bednar, 1977), (f) filmed models coupled with detailed instructions (Whalen, 1969), (g) verbal and written preparation (Garrison, 1978), (h) videotaped pretraining activities (Hilkey, Wilhelm, & Horne, 1982), (i) leader imposed structure (Ware & Barr, 1977), (j) directive or nondirective group activities that were matched to participants' locus of control (Abramowitz, Abramowitz, Roback, & Jackson, 1974), and (k) role induction films and interviews (Strupp & Bloxom, 1973).

As can be seen, a wide variety of variables has been successfully related to improved group processes and, in some cases, client improvement. How or why these variables seem to work, however, remains something of a mystery. In some cases, these variables have failed to produce their desired effects; and more importantly, there are relatively few attempts to explain their success or failure in relevant theoretical terms.

Even though this collective body of research is not as secure and specific as we might choose, we do not conclude that it is practically sterile. We find clinical implications that are far from inconsequential. If compelled to place a significant wager now, we would bet that preparing clients for group therapy through role inductions, cognitive instructions, or exposure to models would prove to be one of the most important elements in effective group treatment.

This raises an intriguing dilemma for consideration. Have group researchers successfully identified such potent pretreatment considerations that subjects cannot resist their powerful and pervasive influence? Or, is something like the Hawthorne effect alive and well in the group literature? How are we to interpret and explain this body of literature collectively and what implications does it have for the group practitioner and researcher?

These are not easy questions to answer. It is obvious to us (in the practical sense) that pregroup preparation specifically, and group structuring generally, shows considerable promise for influencing group development and client outcomes. But we must attempt to interpret these data in ways that will help us understand their core ingredients so we can understand (in the scientific sense) how they operate, rather than just duplicate the techniques that create them. As scientists, we do not want to replicate these group activities nearly as much as we want to understand their most potent ingredients and how they may work.

HOW CAN WE FIND OUT WHY AND HOW THEY WORK?

About 20 years ago, we published a model of how we thought structure affected the development of growth and therapeutic groups (Bednar, Melnick, & Kaul, 1974). Our model primarily was based on observations and experience—our own and those of some scientist-practitioners whose perceptions struck us as acute and astute—and a few empirical inquiries.

Twenty years ago, there was a controversy among group theorists and practitioners over the preferability of ambiguity or structure in initiating group therapy. This is not to say that there was any difference of opinion about the therapist's ambiguity. There was near-unanimity. Everyone agreed that, while there always is some uncertainty about unique clients in unique groups, it is always preferable for group leaders to have some integrated plan of action. Everyone agreed that it is always preferable for group leaders to understand what they are doing. The debate about the benefits of ambiguity was limited to the client's ambiguity, not the leader's.

To summarize what was mentioned earlier, some argued that ambiguity enhanced development of the transference relationship, encouraged more thorough client self-direction and genuineness, and facilitated the leader's diagnostic activities. These gains supposedly were worth any incidental costs that clients might incur while trying to deal with the demands of a novel and undefined circumstance—among which one of the most salient was unearthing just what the demands were.

On the other hand, others were not so sanguine about the benefits of ambiguity in initiating groups. Bednar, Melnick, and Kaul (1974), for example, held that "lack of structure in early sessions not only fails to facilitate early group development, but actually feeds client distortions, interpersonal fears, and subjective distress that interfere with group development and contribute to premature client dropouts" (p. 31). Clients are better off with knowledge and understanding of what is happening and what is being demanded in the group, and worse off without them. We argued that the subjective state of certainty that often accompanies structure often facilitates client cooperation and growth.

Briefly, the early model posited in part that ambiguity brought out the worst in clients, and that the "predictable consequence of placing anxious and socially inept clients in an ambiguous group environment is enhanced anxiety and the manifestation of inappropriate behavior patterns" (Bednar, Melnick, & Kaul, 1974, p. 32). People just don't seem concerned about their housekeeping habits when there is the smell of smoke in the house. In short, the ambiguity (to the client) of a supposedly unstructured (to the client) introduction to something potentially threatening and risky (to the client) would be more likely to bring out the worst in the client.

We postulated that if group leaders thoughtfully structured at least the early group sessions, clients would be able to take greater interpersonal risks and engage in less stereotyped, exaggerated, and ineffective behavior—the types of behavior that often persuade them to join a group in the first place. The reason for the increased interpersonal risk-taking, we claimed, was the reduction in personal responsibility that clients would have to assume for actions taken in a leader-structured environment. Giving feedback in a helpful way to relative strangers who would evaluate the feedback openly, and perhaps reciprocate, might be an example of a high-risk situation developed in a leader initiated activity. If the emitted behavior proved ineffectual or inept or "wrong," at least clients did not have to attribute the attempt and the "failure" to their own volition. It would be the leader's responsibility, or that of the activity, but not that of the participating members. While denying responsibility, however, they would be acting in ways supposedly different from those that made them clients in the first place. If those different ways of acting included appropriate self-disclosure, the giving and receiving of therapeutic feedback, and increasingly mature participation in processing the activities and progress of the group as a whole, the group would become increasingly more cohesive and potentially more therapeutic.

The general model, then, was that leader-initiated structure reduced ambiguity, which reduced anxiety or other subjective distress, which then reduced ineffective client responding. Structure instead encouraged the consideration of new and more adaptive behaviors. Because clients were behaving differently at the behest of the group leader, any inefficiencies, inadequacies, or failures could be attributed to the leader's demands and not to personal shortcomings of the client. But as long as the leader's requirements were in the direction of more effective ways of perceiving, processing, and behaving, the group was likely to be more cohesive and the client was at risk of positive change.

The model attracted some attention, whether more or less than it deserved we leave to others to decide. Sometimes it has been operationalized in ways that range from highly imaginative to far-fetched, but seldom has it been operationalized similarly in any two investigations. Sometimes it was cited as undergirding a specific study, but no part of the model seems realistically to have been put at risk of rejection. A few times, the model has been discussed in ways that are nearly alien to us. (This is not meant to blame the researchers. We take responsibility for acting as though such variables as interpersonal risk and personal responsibility were anything but ineffable.) In general, the model seems to have been corroborated, but candor requires the acknowledgment that many of the studies are wanting in rigor, less carefully structured than might be hoped, and often have resulted in more ambiguity about ambiguity.

In the decade following its publication, the risk, responsibility, and structure model stimulated a series of investigations by Bednar and his colleagues. Most were analogue studies, designed to explicate the relationships among risk, responsibility, structure, and cohesion. One (Evensen & Bednar, 1978) has been presented in some detail earlier. A few others will be briefly summarized now.

Roach (1976) crossed method of presentation of material (behavioral or cognitive), level of specificity (high or low latitude for interpretation of the material), and content (intrapersonal or interpersonal) in a 2 × 2 × 2 design. Undergraduates were given one-half hour of structure. Roach concluded that "results of this investigation clearly indicate the superiority of behavioral structure" (p. 915-B). In general, specificity and content interacted with method of presentation (e.g., little latitude for interpretation [high specificity] facilitated interaction in behavioral groups).

Client risk-taking disposition was probed in another analogue study by Lee and Bednar (1977). They crossed risk-taking disposition (high versus low), sex, group structure (high, intermediate, low), and group tasks (self-disclosure, interpersonal feedback, group confrontation) in a factorial arrangement. Undergraduate students were assigned to same-sex groups. High risk-takers in high structure groups produced the more therapeutically relevant behavior than any other combination. Low risk-taking disposition members performed best under conditions of high structure. This study began to unravel one of the components of the risk, responsibility, and structure model. Evensen and Bednar (1978), presented earlier, continued analysis of the interaction between risk and structure.

Finally, Robison and Hardt (1992) employed behavioral and cognitive structure, crossed with high or low risk-taking disposition and with a discussion of anticipated undesirable reactions to their feedback expected by the members. Undergraduate students met for four hours in groups homogeneous for risk-taking disposition. Like Evansen and Bednar, they found that low risk-takers in the behavioral structure condition showed lower attraction to the group and lower cohesion. Unlike them, however, Robison and

Hardt reported that both high and low risk-takers produced more feedback under the combined cognitive-behavioral structure condition.

In none of these reports was structure conceptually defined. Nor was risk. Nor was responsibility. They were operationally defined, of course. Each was operationalized in ways that made sense given the state of conceptual development at the time. Each was put to experimental challenge under relatively stringent conditions. Individually and collectively, they suggest how risk, responsibility, and structure interact in early group development. Insofar as they achieve relevance, they offer guides to practice of varying specificity. That desirable contribution should not blind us to what these studies fail to tell us, however. Alone and in combination, they allow us no inferential wattage with regard to the elements of the model, or of the model itself.

Uniquely, however, Fuehrer and Keys (1988) reported a rather direct and relatively unambiguous attempt at testing the risk-responsibility-structure model as a model. They adapted the model to what they called "mutual-aid groups" and replaced the variable of risk with one they called "the importance of constructive group member behaviors" (p. 327). College students interested in insight about their feelings of isolation or alienation were recruited and randomly placed in a high- or low-structured group. The structured group received "instructions concerning constructive group member behaviors . . . and an opportunity to practice self-disclosure and giving feedback" (p. 323). The low-structured group received no specific instruction on constructive behavior, but instead was left to develop its own preferred ways of progressing. Three dependent variables included measures of member ownership of group functioning (what we had called responsibility), the importance of performing constructive group behaviors (what we had called risk), and an adaptation of Lieberman, Yalom, and Miles's (1973) feelings-about-the-group questionnaire as an indicator of group cohesion. Observations were taken at the second (Time 1) and fourth (Time 2) sessions.

Among the several analyses of the data was a path analysis. Their data "provided considerable support for the initial processes of development posited by the model" but that "at Time 2 the relations . . . were evident but to a somewhat lesser degree" (Fuehrer & Keys, 1988, pp. 334–336). They discussed how their data might reconcile inconsistencies in previous research and how the original risk-responsibility-structure model might be modified. Perhaps the conclusions of Fuehrer and Keys are unduly charitable (they seem so to us). Their work is almost singular in that it attempted to test not just the components of a model, but the model itself.

The purpose of this reminiscence is not to suggest that we were prescient in 1974. Nor is it to suggest that we were mistaken in our model-positing. It is to confess that we really don't know, and there seem to be no encouraging omens and portents in the group research that we could know. Between 1974 (the model) and 1988 (Fuehrer & Keys), and indeed up to the end of

1992, our research has told us practically nothing about psychological risk, personal responsibility, or group structure, beyond what we knew in 1974.

Those who have read our previous commentaries on the group literature (Bednar & Kaul, 1994; Kaul & Bednar, 1986) may recall our repeated, and perhaps repetitious, lamentations about the lack of cumulativity in the group literature. We will not cover that ground again, except to reiterate: Years of effort that result in a mass of research that, *as a whole,* may have putative practical implications, but has little more conceptual relevancy than a table of random numbers, is a tragic waste of time and talent.

This time, we are going to do more than lament. We instead will explicate an approach that takes no more time or talent than the current group research, and in some respects may take less of each. It sacrifices whim and poetry for potential cumulativity and understanding. We think that the cost-benefit ratio is favorable. This line is meant to augment, not replace, research such as that reviewed above.

An Additional Line of Research

We propose briefly to summarize research done in other areas that may inform group practitioners and researchers. To keep from gratuitously stepping on toes, we will use the risk-responsibility-structure model as a specimen. The purpose is to show how important a parallel line of research might be to those of us in the field. It is not to say that "Does this work?" is bad research, but to say instead that "What is this that may or may not work?" is worth our time, too.

Risk

In 1974, we defined risk as the "possibility of loss or injury" (p. 34). That literary definition, almost empty of meaning, is among the deeper definitions to be culled from the group literature. Most often, risk is given no conceptual definition. The operationalization of risk through most of 1992 usually has involved administration of the Social Risk-Taking subscale of Jackson, Hourany, and Vidmar's (1971) four-dimensional assessment of risk-taking. The specific subscale is composed of 30 true-false questions. You would think that, if the dimension of risk and the disposition to take risks is important to the provision of group therapy, we might have achieved more progress in the conceptual or operational definitions.

There is an entire body of scholarship dedicated to the analysis of risk, complete with its own associations and journals. For example, Slovic, Fischoff, and Lichtenstein (1985) studied the perception of risk. They wanted "to discover what people mean when they say that something is risky; to develop a psychological taxonomy of risk that can be used to understand people's perceptions . . ." (p. 91). Samples of students, community members, activists, and risk assessment experts rated the relative risk of 30 activities (e.g., bicycling, construction work, smoking) and technologies (e.g., nuclear weapons, home appliances, chlorinated water, DNA technology) on nine characteristics. Among their many interesting findings were several that may have relevance to group leaders.

Experts' judgments about risk differed from those of nonexpert citizens and students. First, experts discriminated much more widely among the various risks. Second, experts were substantially more homogeneous in their assessment of risk than were other groups. Third, unlike the nonexperts, the experts' estimates of risk were to a large degree independent of the subjective characteristics of risk, but instead were "closely related (r = .92) to technical estimates of the average annual fatalities from each activity" (p. 102).

But experts and nonexperts were not completely unlike one another. They showed some interesting similarities, as well. For instance, as experts and nonexperts perceived more risk in an activity, they expressed greater desire to reduce that risk. Furthermore, two factors accounted for most of the variance in perceptions of risk across all groups. The first factor was called Unknown Risk. Toward one end were cases with novel, unknown, and involuntary risks, such as food coloring and pesticides. At the opposite extreme of Unknown Risk were familiar and involuntary risks such as mountain climbing and fire fighting. They named the second factor Dread Risk. At one extreme were phenomena with dire consequences for large numbers of persons, such as nuclear war, nerve gas accidents, and coal mining accidents. Toward the other extreme were circumstances that cause nonfatal harm to one person at a time, such as caffeine, aspirin, and power mowers.

No, group therapy is not like food coloring or nuclear war. Nor is it like fire fighting or mountain climbing, except in the most metaphorical ways. We don't know if novice clients view joining a group along Unknown and Dread dimensions. And we don't know if group leaders view group risks more like risk assessment specialists or more like citizens and students. That is the point—we don't know much about the perception of risk in group treatment.

Would we profit by looking separately at the perception of risk when members are asked to choose from among several risky alternatives ("risk-risk" situations), as compared with situations in which they are to decide how much of other activities they will sacrifice for increased safety ("how safe" situations)(Lave, 1987). Maybe.

Is the perception of threat a function of primary appraisal (the amount of threat present) and secondary appraisal (one's resources for dealing with the threat)? Are the severity of the threat, its imminence, and its likelihood, "all necessary and together sufficient" to produce threat or be perceived as risky by group clients (Paterson & Neufeld, 1987)? Perhaps.

Is there an analogue to "signal accidents" (Freudenberg, 1988; Slovic, 1987) in the group setting? That is, might things happen at one time or to one person that alert the rest of the group that there is reason for concern. If so, the capacity to control signal accidents and their interpretation might be a reason to structure.

If, as Freudenberg (1988) says, we can be sanguine about discrepancies between real risk and perceived risk when "the stakes are low, consensus is high, experience is vast, and decisions do not impose burdens on one group for the benefit of another" (p. 48) should we as group leaders relax our vigilance? Or, is the group situation more characterized by a high guesswork to knowledge ratio, one that would call for more careful scrutiny? You probably would respond differently from the group leader's perspective than you would from the member's.

Ambiguity

Since there was no ambiguity about ambiguity in our minds in 1974, we didn't bother to define it. Kahn and Sarin (1988) used the term to "distinguish the class of risky decisions for which the odds of an uncertain event are not precisely known . . . there is 'uncertainty about the uncertainty'" (p. 265). That certainly seems to cover some of the phenomenology of group participants. But does their model of decision-making under ambiguity apply to group therapy? Kahn and Sarin concluded that, contrary to some predictions of subjective expected utility theory, people do consider ambiguity when making decisions under uncertainty, and that they will tolerate more or less of it depending upon the context. They reported individual differences in ambiguity approach or avoidance. In one sample of students, for example, nearly half preferred to avoid it, about one-third were indifferent to it, and about one-fifth indicated a preference for ambiguity. In another experiment, there was an indication that people would back up their ambiguity preferences with action, and perhaps money. They concluded that "if ambiguity is present in consumer decisions, the overall attitude toward risk may be accentuated" (p. 271).

Kahn and Sarin were interested in consumer decisions. How much aversion one might feel to applying their model to group treatment may be accounted for by their model. We cannot help but wonder if this model may account for some of the discrepancies in the risk-responsibility-structure literature. It could not help but refine our view of members' decisions in groups.

Curley, Yates, and Abrams (1986) defined ambiguity much like Kahn and Sarin did. After summarizing evidence that people respond to ambiguity, and do not just ignore it (similar to the Kahn and Sarin model above), they wondered what leads people to avoid it. Five competing explanations were found in the literature: (1) hostile nature—when you don't have control, the situation is biased against you, (2) uncertainty avoidance—you avoid ambiguity because it is a subset of uncertainty and you don't like uncertainty, (3) forced-choice—you avoid ambiguity only when all other considerations are equal, (4) self-evaluation—later on, when you get more information, you will regret your decisions made under ambiguity, and (5) other evaluation—you fear that others will evaluate your decision later.

Employing a series of five rather ingenious experiments, they reported results that seem almost directly applicable to group research and practice. First, they determined that responses to risk and ambiguity were independent of one another. Second, like Kahn and Sarin, they found that some subjects would pay to avoid ambiguity. And third, only the other evaluation explanation for ambiguity avoidance was corroborated! In these studies, evaluation was implicit, not explicit. Participants showed a stronger reaction against ambiguity when their choices were made publicly than when they were made privately. Apparently, they tried to avoid the evaluation of their public choices by others by choosing the course of action supposedly most acceptable to others. They seemed to choose the most "justifiable" course of action under ambiguous circumstances.

Two final points deserve mention. One is that ambiguity avoidance may not be irrational. To the degree that others evaluate our behavior, it is not necessarily irrational to try to avoid uncertainty. There cannot be much doubt that members evaluate the behavior of other members early in the group. And if the leader is using ambiguity to assess a member's style, pathology, and personality, it may not be irrational for the member to squirm a bit. The second point is that Curley, Yates, and Abrams (1986) speculated that people believe that avoiding ambiguity is more justifiable "because they evaluate decisions on the basis of decision outcomes, and not on the basis of the decision process" (p. 253). That probably is a more succinct and testable statement that was our notion of responsibility 20 years ago.

Responsibility

We defined responsibility as "accountability for actions . . . clear acknowledgement of ownership of one's thoughts and feelings, relative candor in self-expression, and mature processing of feedback . . ." (p. 34). We knew what that meant then, and we still have a reasonable idea of what we meant. But that doesn't dim its glaring inadequacy as a conceptual definition, and near impossibility of operationalization. Even this vapidity has not seemed to challenge group workers and researchers, however. The field has gone no further.

Social psychologists have. There is an immense and fascinating body of literature on attributions, for example. Quite a bit is known about proclivities for assigning responsibility to self or others, for instance. The effects of schemas, memories, learning, and experience have been probed. Context effects and biases (in both senses of the word) have been dragged into the open where we can look at them, describe them, and deal with them.

The sheer enormity of material precludes any attempt to summarize this literature. Interested practitioners or researchers can narrow their search and begin with any of a number of valuable summaries (cf. Weary, Stanley, & Harvey, 1989). Even so, a few potentially relevant questions arise.

Does the manipulation of responsibility early in the group obviate *causal* attributions of ability and effort (internal attributions) in favor of attributions of task difficulty or luck (external attributions)? Or are the attributions of group members better considered as attributions of *responsibility?* If the latter, then they may be a function of the member's " (a) . . . apparent causal contribution to the outcome, (b) knowledge of the consequences of the action taken, (c) intention to produce the outcome, and (d) degree of volition versus coercion . . ." (Weary, Stanley, & Harvey, 1989, p. 10). Each of these functions suggests methodological and practical considerations.

If the assertion that emotional arousal makes more likely the emission of strongly habitual responses is correct, and there is reason to believe so, does the manipulation of structure (and, therefore, responsibility) change the quality of the feedback given group members? Suppose we assume that "interpersonal accountability provides the archetype for social regulation" (Schlenker & Weigold, 1992, p. 137) and that group members have a need for acceptance and approbation. Is that need enough incentive to divert attention from the inferential information in feedback (information about the structure of the task) to the evaluation information (about how well you are doing)? Hogarth, Gibbs, McKenzie, and Marquis (1991) present a model and data that suggest that it does.

CONCLUSION

What does all of this literature mean to practitioners and researchers in the area of group therapy? We have presented a body of research on pregroup training and structure, research that suggests that these can be important adjuncts to group treatment. Though there may be little warrant for choosing one pregroup training medium over another, there is reasonable consistency across a methodologically diverse body of research. So, too, with structure. Introduced in a variety of ways, it seems capable of influencing group process indicators, and perhaps through them, outcomes as well.

We think that practice would be improved with the judicious application of pregroup training. It is unreasonable for the leader to expect participants to possess high, or perhaps even adequate, levels of all important skills as the group begins. Furthermore, the research suggests quite strongly that naive members seem to profit from vicarious or personal exposure to the skills and understandings putatively important to success in group treatment. And we can find little justification for insisting that they be acquired in the heat of battle.

This is not to say that member skills should go untested in the group; we think they should be tested. Indeed, two of the major conclusions drawn by the National Research Council's Committee on the Enhancement of Human Performance (Bjork & Druckman, 1991) are relevant here. First, their report suggested that increasing the variability of conditions under which skills are practiced will increase transfer of training. And, second, reducing external feedback during practice may enhance resistance to extinction.

In addition, we think that group leaders should deliberately structure their groups in the service of their overall therapeutic goals. The research suggests to us that some of the specific effects of overt structure probably will interact with person and situation variables. But that should not be handicapping, since just about all specific treatment effects also seem to interact with person and situation variables. The overall advantage of structure probably lies in the increased capacity of the group leader to control the learning environment. Better control would permit more efficient acquisition and more effective transfer of training functions.

If we understand Einstein correctly, under some conditions parallel lines eventually will meet. That seems a desirable goal in research on groups. For group researchers, it seems to us that cumulativity of inference probably is enhanced when the research is theory-driven. That state may elicit more programmatic research efforts. We examined some research that, with a little charity, can be described as model-driven, and we saw budding additive inferential power. But the real potential of theory- or model-driven research in groups is lost if researchers limit their concerns to whether the intervention "works."

But model- or theory-driven research alone does not seem enough. Parallel research is necessary to consider simultaneously other important questions such as, "What does my independent variable mean?" and "What does my dependent variable mean?" That is, we need constantly to refine our understanding of what our terms and concepts mean or represent. If requisitioning research from cognate areas helps in that refinement, all the better. But we cannot blindly apply requisitioned ideas to our field without testing them.

When (if) the two lines of research merge, understanding could accelerate. As the meaning of terms becomes more clear, the models of relations among those terms should become more tractable. Research in one line can improve research in the other. Improved research can lead to knowledge. If we judiciously meld that knowledge with our experience, we may improve our practice.

REFERENCES

Abramowitz, C., Abramowitz, S., Roback, H., & Jackson, C. (1974). Differential effectiveness of directive and nondirective group therapies as a function of client internal-external control. *Journal of Consulting and Clinical Psychology,* 42, 849–853.

Anchor, K., Vojtisek, J., & Patterson, R. (1973). Trait anxiety, initial structuring and self-disclosure in groups of schizophrenic patients. *Psychotherapy: Theory, Research and Practice, 10,* 151–158.

Bednar, R., & Battersby, C. (1976). The effects of specific cognitive structure on early group development. *Journal of Applied Behavioral Science, 12,* 513–522.

Bednar, R., & Kaul, T. (1978). Experiential group research: Current perspectives. In S. Garfield & A. Bergin (Eds.), *Handbook of psychotherapy and behavior change: An empirical analysis* (2nd ed.). New York: Wiley.

Bednar, R., & Kaul, T. (1994). Experiential group research: Can the canon fire? In A. Bergin & S. Garfield (Eds.), *Handbook for psychotherapy and behavior change* (4th ed.). New York: Wiley.

Bednar, R., & Lawlis, F. (1971). Empirical research in group psychotherapy. In A. Bergin & S. Garfield (Eds.), *Handbook for psychotherapy and behavior change.* New York: Wiley.

Bednar, R., Melnick, J., & Kaul, T. (1974). Risk, responsibility, and structure: A conceptual framework for initiating group counseling and psychotherapy. *Journal of Counseling Psychology, 21,* 31–37.

Bednar, R., Wells, M., & Peterson, S. (1989). *Self-esteem: Paradoxes and innovations in clinical theory and practice.* Washington, DC: American Psychological Association.

Bjork, R., & Druckman, D. (1991). How do you improve human performance? *APS Observer, 4,* 13–15.

Bordin, E. (1955). The implications of client expectations for the counseling process. *Journal of Consulting Psychology, 2,* 17–21.

Budman, S., Demby, A., Feldstein, M., & Gold, M. (1984). The effects of time-limited group psychotherapy: A controlled study. *International Journal of Group Psychotherapy, 34,* 587–603.

Cartwright, M. (1976). A preparatory method for group counseling. *Journal of Counseling Psychology, 23,* 75–77.

Crews, C., & Melnick, J. (1976). The use of initial and delayed structure in facilitating group development. *Journal of Counseling Psychology, 23,* 92–97.

Curley, S., Yates, J., & Abrams, R. (1986). Psychological sources of ambiguity avoidance. *Organizational Behavior and Human Decision Processes, 38,* 230–256.

D'Augelli, A., & Chinsky, J. (1974). Interpersonal skills and pretraining. *Journal of Counseling and Clinical Psychology, 42,* 65–72.

DeJulio, S., Bentley, J., & Cockayne, T. (1976). Pregroup norm setting: Effects on encounter group interaction. *Small Group Behavior, 10,* 368–388.

Evensen, E., & Bednar, R., (1978). Effects of specific cognitive and behavioral structure on early group behavior and atmosphere. *Journal of Counseling Psychology, 25,* 66–75.

Fenichel, O. (1945). Neurotic acting-out. *Psychoanalytic Review, 32,* 197–206.

Freudenberg, W. (1988). Perceived risk, real risk: Social science and the art of probabilistic risk assessment. *Science, 242,* 44–49.

Fuehrer, A., & Keys, C. (1988). Group development in self-help groups for college students. *Small Group Behavior, 19,* 325–341.

Garfield, S., & Bergin, A. (Eds.). (1986). Introduction and historical overview. *Handbook of psychotherapy and behavior change: An empirical analysis* (3rd ed.). New York: Wiley.

Garrison, J. (1978). Written vs. verbal preparation of patients for group psychotherapy. *Psychotherapy: Theory, Research and Practice, 15,* 130–134.

Geen, R. (1991). Social motivation. *Annual Review of Psychology, 42,* 377–399.

Gross, E. (1957). *An empirical study of the concepts of cohesiveness and compatibility.* Unpublished honor's thesis, Harvard University, Department of Social Relations.

Hilkey, J., Wilhelm, C., & Horne, A. (1982). Comparative effectiveness of videotape pretraining versus no pretraining on selected process and outcome variables in group therapy. *Psychological Reports, 50,* 1151–1159.

Hill, W. (1965). *HIM: Hill Interaction Matrix.* Los Angeles, CA: University of Southern California, Youth Study Center.

Hogarth, R., Gibbs, B., McKenzie, C., & Marquis, M. (1991). Learning from feedback: Exactingness and incentives. *Journal of Experimental Psychology: Learning, Memory, and Cognition, 17,* 734–752.

Jackson, D., Hourany, L., & Vidmar, N. (1971). *A four-dimensional interpretation of risk taking* (Research Bulletin No. 185). London, Canada: University of Western Ontario.

Kahn, B., & Sarin, R. (1988). Modeling ambiguity in decisions under uncertainty. *Journal of Consumer Research, 15,* 265–272.

Kaul, T., & Bednar, R. (1986). Experiential group research: Results, questions, and suggestions. In S. Garfield & A. Bergin (Eds.), *Handbook of psychotherapy and behavior change: An empirical analysis* (pp. 671–714). New York: Wiley.

LaTorre, R. (1977). Pretherapy role induction procedures. *Canadian Psychological Review, 18,* 308–321.

Lave, L. (1987). Health and safety risk analyses: Information for better decisions. *Science, 236,* 291–295.

Lee, F., & Bednar, R. (1977). Effects of group structure and risk-taking disposition on group behavior, attitudes, and atmosphere. *Journal of Counseling Psychology, 24,* 191–199.

Lieberman, M. A., Yalom, I. D., & Miles, M. B. (1973). *Encounter groups: First facts.* New York: Basic Books.

Lundgren, D. (1977). Developmental trends in the emergence of interpersonal issues in T groups. *Small Group Behavior, 8,* 179–200.

Muller, E., & Scott, T. (1984). A comparison of film and written presentations used for pregroup training experiences. *Journal for Specialists in Group Work, 9,* 122–126.

Paterson, R., & Neufeld, R. (1987). Clear danger: Situational determinants of the appraisal of threat. *Psychological Bulletin, 101,* 404–416.

Piper, W., Debbane, E., Bienvenu, J., & Garant, J. (1982). A study of group pretraining for group psychotherapy. *International Journal of Group Psychotherapy, 32,* 309–325.

Piper, W., Debbane, E., Garant, J., & Bienvenu, J. (1979). Pretraining for group psychotherapy. *Archives of General Psychiatry, 36,* 1250–1256.

Piper, W., & Marrache, M. (1981). Selecting suitable patients: Pretraining for group therapy as a method of patient selection. *Small Group Behavior, 12*, 459–475.

Roach, A. (1976/1977). The comparative effects of behavioral vs. cognitive presentation, high vs. low levels of specificity, and interpersonal vs. intrapersonal content of structure on early group development. *Dissertation Abstracts International, 38*, 914B–915B.

Robison, F. F., & Hardt, D. A. (1992). Effects of cognitive and behavioral structure and discussion of corrective feedback outcomes on counseling group development. *Journal of Counseling Psychology, 39*(4), 473–481.

Rogers, C. R. (1951). *Client-centered therapy, its current practice, implications, and theory*. Boston, MA: Houghton Mifflin.

Rosenbaum, M., & Berger, M. (Eds.). (1963). *Group psychotherapy and group treatment*. New York: Basic Books.

Rosenthal, D., & Frank, J. (1956). Psychotherapy and the placebo effect. *Psychological Bulletin, 53*, 294–302.

Schlenker, B., & Weigold, M. (1992). Interpersonal processes involving impression regulation and management. *Annual Review of Psychology, 43*, 133–168.

Shostrom, E. (1963). *The personal orientation inventory*. San Diego, CA: Educational and Industrial Testing Service.

Slipp, S. (Ed.). (1982). *Curative factors in dynamic psychotherapy*. New York: McGraw-Hill.

Slovic, P. (1987). Perception of risk. *Science, 236*, 280–285.

Slovic, P., Fischoff, B., & Lichtenstein, S. (1985). Characterizing perceived risk. In R. Kates, C. Hohenemser, & J. Kasperson (Eds.), *Perilous progress: Managing the hazards of technology*. Boulder, CO: Westview.

Smith, M., & Glass, G. (1977). Meta-analysis of psychotherapy outcome studies. *American Psychologist, 32*, 752–760.

Steuer, J., Mintz, J., Hammen, C., Hill, M., Jarvik, L., McCarley, T., Motoike, P., & Rosen, R. (1984). Cognitive-behavioral and psychodynamic group psychotherapy in treatment of geriatric depression. *Journal of Consulting and Clinical Psychology, 52*, 180–189.

Stockton, R., & Morran, D. (1982). Review and perspective of critical dimensions in therapeutic small group research. In G. Gazda (Ed.), *Basic approaches to group psychotherapy and group counseling* (3rd ed.). Springfield, IL: Thomas.

Strupp, H., & Bloxom, A. (1973). Preparing lower class patients for group psychotherapy: Development and evaluation of a role induction film. *Journal of Consulting and Clinical Psychology, 41*, 373–384.

Thelen, H. (1974). Reactions to Group Situations Test. In J. Pfeiffer & J. Jones (Eds.), *Annual handbook for group facilitators*. LaJolla, CA: University Associates.

Ware, J., & Barr, J. (1977). Effects of a nine-week structured and unstructured group experience on measures of self-concept and self-actualization. *Small Group Behavior, 8*, 93–99.

Warren, N., & Rice, L. (1972). Structure and stabilizing of psychotherapy for low-prognosis clients. *Journal of Consulting and Clinical Psychology, 39*, 173–181.

Watzlawick, P., Beavin, J., & Jackson, D. (1967). *Pragmatics of human communication: A study of interaction patterns, pathologies and paradoxes.* New York: Norton.

Weary, G., Stanley, M., & Harvey, J. (1989). *Attribution.* New York: Springer-Verlag.

Whalen, C. (1969). Effects of a model and instructions on group verbal behaviors. *Journal of Consulting and Clinical Psychology, 33,* 509–521.

Whitehouse, F. (1966). *The concept of therapy: A review of some essentials.* Paper presented at the Annual Convention of the American Psychological Association, New York City.

Wilson, R., & Crouch, E. (1987). Risk assessment and comparisons: An introduction. *Science, 236,* 267–270.

Wogan, M., Getter, H., Amdur, M., Nichols, M., & Okman, G. (1977). Influencing interaction and outcomes in group psychotherapy. *Small Group Behavior, 8,* 25–45.

Zarle, T., & Willis, S. (1975). A pregroup training technique for encounter group stress. *Journal of Counseling Psychology, 22,* 49–53.

PART THREE

Therapeutic Components of the Group Ecosystem

CHAPTER 6

Interaction Analysis:
Instrumentation and Issues

ADDIE FUHRIMAN and SALLY H. BARLOW

Acknowledgment of the complexity of the group psychotherapeutic process is clearly documented in the literature, and calls for conceptual clarity in process analyses are replete in the multiple reviews available on the subject (Bednar & Kaul, 1978; Kaul & Bednar, 1986). In recent years, the group research literature has witnessed increased attention on the analyses of group process via the spoken word as the viable portion of the interactional behavior of group participants. In part, this focus exists as a response to the persistent request to unravel the contextual complexity posed by multiple players and purposes, by bifurcated and convoluted influences, and by dynamic and interactive relationships (Fuhriman, Drescher, & Burlingame, 1984). It is becoming increasingly apparent that recognizing the *presence* of therapeutic or change mechanisms is a necessary, but far from sufficient, condition. More importantly, it is critical to understand the interactive *responsiveness* of these mechanisms to one another, their interactive *influence* on the participants involved, and the relevant *context* within which these occur.

A number of reviews addressing the interactive nature of group process have emerged in the past decade, each attending to specific issues and concerns related to the analysis of interaction (Fuhriman & Packard, 1986; Overlaet, 1991; Trujillo, 1986). All acknowledge the trend to focus more specifically on the verbal interaction and, for the most part, to do so by means of observational techniques. Issues regarding the adequacy of the conceptual underpinnings and operational procedures of interaction analysis are illustrated in the sole use of observational techniques, singular focus on verbal and rational behavior, lack of synthesized research findings across studies, and the use of minimally standardized and replicated instruments.

The analysis of interaction as a means to describe and understand "process" is not without precedent. Although articulated as social interaction, evidence can be found in the related fields of social psychology and communications to justify the analysis of verbal behavior in defining and explaining the interpersonal and group processes. Investigators of individual therapy process, certainly closer relatives to group research, likewise lend voice to the benefits of describing "in-situation" performance (Greenberg, 1986), attending to different levels of interaction (Greenberg & Pinsof, 1986), examining groups of episodes (Rice & Greenberg, 1984), and delineating multifactor, dynamic properties (Luborsky, Barber, & Crits-Christoff, 1990), most of which escape us by our neglect of moment-by-moment analyses.

Interaction analysis attempts to unravel and understand the dialogue of the participants through observational techniques. Basically, the rating systems function as coding schemes, assigning behaviors to predetermined categories deemed important by the clinician or researcher. Distinguished from (although often confused with) content analysis, interactional analysis unitizes behavioral events and codes to a categorical framework. Fisher (1980) observes that the "event-nature" of the data is retained and "time-oriented" analyses (i.e., sequentiality, redundant patterning) can be applied. It is true that moving from the measurement of a global to a more specific phenomenon lends precision to the description of the group by identifying intricate parts of the system and concomitantly their relationship to one another. If the "message is the medium," then the act of analyzing the actual, verbal behavior increases the likelihood of understanding and addressing the current problems and issues within the group.

The verity of interaction analysis systems lies within the adopted coding scheme, the worth of which is highly dependent on the conceptual and empirical value of the category classes. The conceptual underpinnings have not gone unnoticed; in fact, much concern remains regarding the adequacy of  classes based only on verbal and rational behavior and grounded on the communication "sender-receiver" model (Overlaet, 1991). From Overlaet's point of view, these category classes lack reference to the context of the communicative behavior and to the occurrence of time. Additionally, the observational ratings fail to measure the internal processes surrounding the verbal behavior and thus cannot account for the "creation of meaning" (Overlaet, 1991). In a similar vein, Scheflen (1974) cautions against attributing meaning to any single act or behavior for "meaning is not a property of the behavior itself" (p. 179). Without these various and contextual dimensions of information, the probability of success in identifying and measuring change processes occurring within individuals and groups via their verbal interaction is attenuated.

Nevertheless, the precision of interaction analysis ultimately affords the capability of viewing micro and macro processes more effectively than the cumulative average of one time period. More specifically, overall *patterns* can be recognized either within a single session, or over the entire length of the group. Such patterns lend contextual meaning that speaks, in part, to Overlaet's concern. They are also more likely to capture the dynamic properties of the process. Interactional analysis in this sense is not a single or isolated unit or behavior. . . . "You must not be satisfied to isolate bits of behavior and merely measure or count them. It is in the *relations* of the elements or events, the configuration, the pattern we are after" (Scheflen, 1969, p. 210). Thus, interaction analysis facilitates the discovery of patterns: "We should be studying patterns" (Rice & Greenberg, 1984); "observing patterns . . . can help reveal the dynamics of social interaction" (Bakeman & Dabbs, 1976).

Interactional analysis likewise affords an additional capability, that of dealing with complexity by "sorting out the sundry elements" (Stein & Kibel, 1984), facilitating "multidimensional thinking," thereby not confusing the levels of abstraction (Agazarian, 1983). The combination of pattern discovery and complexity unentanglement could well be the distinctive contribution of interaction analysis. In a sense, interactional analysis facilitates the creation of meaning from micro to macro, from singular to cumulative, and from individual to group perspectives through its moment-by-moment data collection and analysis.

INSTRUMENTATION

During the past 40 years, numerous measures have been developed for the purpose of analyzing the ongoing verbal and communicative behavior of members in small group settings. A review of available instruments (Fuhriman & Packard, 1986) revealed some 26 measures of varying capability and popularity. Utilizing predetermined criteria, all measures were rated according to their value (high, moderate, and low), resulting in only six instruments being given the high value in assessing the verbal interaction occurring within small groups. High value instruments generally were theory-driven, provided sufficient information for implementation, had available standardization data, and were the most frequently used measures. Four of the six were intended for therapy and counseling groups; all were appropriate for therapy groups. Since that time, 13 additional measures have emerged, accompanied by studies reporting findings from their various applications.

All the instruments purport to measure constructs and components applicable to the various purposes for which groups are organized. Some are most appropriate for task, work, or discussion groups (Bales, 1950; Benne & Sheats, 1948; Borgotta, 1963; Chapple, 1940, 1949; Ellis, 1976; Fisher, 1976; Isaacson, 1977; Just, 1968; Mills, 1964; Ruback, Dabbs, & Hopper, 1984). Others are more suited to tap the processes occurring within training and personal growth groups (Anchor, 1973; Bales, 1950; Beck, Dugo, Eng, & Lewis, 1986; Borgotta, 1963; Chapple, 1949; Cooper, 1977; Fisher, 1976; Gibbard & Hartman, 1973; Hill, 1965; Mann, 1967; Reisel, 1959; Watson, 1970). Several measures, including a number more recently developed, are applicable to counseling and psychotherapy groups (Anchor, 1973; Bales, 1950; Beck et al., 1986; Cooney, Kadden, Litt, & Getter, 1991; Cox, 1973; Ellis, 1976; Fisher, 1976; Friedlander & Heatherington, 1989; Gottschalk

THE GROUP EMOTIONALITY RATING SYSTEM:

& Gleser, 1969; Hahlweg et al., 1989; Halliday & Hasan, 1976; Heckel, Holmes, & Rosecrans, 1971; Hill, 1965; Karterud & Foss, 1989; Klein, Mathieu, Gendlin, & Kiesler, 1969; Mann, 1967; Mills, 1964; Nichols & Taylor, 1975; Noble, Ohlsen, & Proff, 1961; Ohlsen & Pearson, 1965; Piper & McCallum, 1992; Vogel, 1977; Watson, 1970). A more limited number of instruments claim application to all group formats (Bales, 1950; Gazda & Mobley, 1980; Stone, Dunphy, Smith, & Ogilvie, 1966).

Included in this review and analysis are 29 instruments that meet the 1986 high and moderate criteria (Table 6.1). Measures deemed of low value in the 1986 review and those receiving little or no further attention in the literature were excluded. It is of note that only one "low-value" measure is represented in a published study during the past decade. The foci of the selected instruments span a wide range of interactional, interpersonal, and therapeutic constructs. Most often, the constructs are observed in the member or client action; in a few cases, the instruments are specifically earmarked for the therapist, and in some, ownership of the action is irrelevant. Numerous instruments focus on constructs describing interpersonal interaction and member relationships, and either classify the content (supportive, negative, etc.) or identify the object of the interaction, such that sociometric linkages can be observed. Typical discussion skills (giving information, asking questions, encouraging comments, etc.) and problem-solving behaviors are indicated in a number of measures. Processes relating to the climate existing within the group (cohesion, member roles, here-and-now focus) are dimensions of some measures. While most of the measures respond to interpersonal functioning, some focus entirely on the individual member (self-exploration, level of experiencing, fight, flight, dependency, and affective involvement and expression). Interpretations, modes of engagement, and general involvement are constructs underlying some of the measurement of therapist interaction. Phase boundaries that define the group's development are the target of interest in Beck's et al. (1986) measures. They suggest using all three measures in tandem such that process characteristics across multiple levels of functioning—intrapersonal, interpersonal, and group as a whole—can be described.

The selected constructs of these instruments provide some insight into the conceptual values of the designers. Far and away, the interpersonal dimension (roles, relationships, influence) is a core interest. The climate or atmosphere that exists or is developed and the personal dynamics (particularly as they relate to personal involvement and relationship to others) also appear to be central concerns. In a statement, the designers are saying: The core of small group functioning is the interpersonal context of small groups, the atmosphere that exists within the group, and the individual member's engagement with self and others.

These instruments vary not only in the constructs they measure, but also in their formating of the data, sampling procedures, and validity and reliability evidence. The systems are capable of rating the entire dialogue occurring within sessions of any length, although individual studies vary with regard to the quantity of the interaction being analyzed. Ratings are generally made from live action, audio or video recordings, or transcripts of the interaction. In some cases, data contained on audio recordings are fed directly into a computer (Chapple, 1949), thus facilitating data analysis. A notable strength of the instruments is their capability to measure the moment-by-moment process; nevertheless, the labor intensive and costly procedures of recording, transcribing, and so on, are probably a major reason for their disuse.

Many of the instruments define the unit of measurement to be used in the analyses, while some leave that in the hands of the individual researcher. It is not a requirement, and perhaps not even desirable, that similar units be unitized by all instruments. But it does become problematic when one tries to compare or relate constructs and themes across the measures, further impeding progress in untangling a complex process. Although all utterances are included in a rating, the unit to which some categorical value is placed varies across instruments. A unit may be an uninterrupted utterance, a single sentence, the subject and predicate of a sentence, a series of sentences receiving the same value, a thought, a singular act (perhaps a word or an entire monologue), or a time unit (e.g., every 5 seconds). While the designated unit may be conceptually tied to the focal construct (e.g., member utterance), in some cases it merely seems to ensure a uniform, segmented measurement (e.g., a rating every 5 seconds). A conceptual base to the unit of measure would make a stronger case for the specific use.

While most measures report reasonable to excellent reliability data, few document any validation efforts. For the most part, the user must rely on the "word" of the author that the instrument is valid, usually in terms of face validity and construct validity (relating to the theoretical basis of the instrument). Some of the more recent measures go beyond this normative practice and report the instrument's success when compared with another instrument (e.g., RCCC), with subjects' perceptions (e.g., RCCC), and with treatment (e.g., GSRS, PWORS), making some claim not only to construct validity, but to predictive and criterion validity as well. *Groups Sessions*

A re-analysis of the available interaction measures provides some conclusions regarding their utility for understanding the complexity of a group's interaction. Many of the instruments simply have gone without use; many have not been employed by anyone other than the original authors; and some relate to or were intended for broad communicational analyses of small groups in general. On the other hand, the recently developed measures are more oriented toward therapy groups and the relational dynamics of the group. Additionally, they are conceptually tied to a theoretical orientation (i.e., psychodynamic), a specific purpose (i.e., familial communication), or presumed therapeutic factors (i.e., cohesion, self-exploration) and dynamics (i.e., development) of the group. To date, little has transpired to alleviate the cost and labor-intensive nature of moment-by-moment analysis.

Although the appearance of additional measures is encouraging, nonetheless we are still in a relative state of poverty when it comes to having a pool

TABLE 6.1. Group Process Instrument*

Instrument	Description	Data Format	Reliability
Interaction Process Analysis (IPA) (Bales, 1950)	Measures task and social emotional behavior using 12 categories; emphasizes problem-solving behavior.	Two types of profiles are constructed: one summarizes the number of behavioral acts; the other analyzes responses in the 12 categories and subcategories.	Inter-rater reliabilities for highly trained observers range between .75 and .95 depending on the scoring category.
System for Multiple Level Observations of Groups (SYMLOG) (Bales, Cohen, & Williams, 1979)	An observational system designed to measure interpersonal behavior and values. Measures behavior as dominant (U) vs. submissive (D), friendly (P) vs. unfriendly (N), task oriented (F) vs. emotional (B).	Incorporates an act-by-act scoring method as well as a retrospective behavioral rating method. Dimensions are collapsed into three, measured in three-dimensional space and yielding a total of 26 vectors. Clients rate self and others respectively along these dimensions. Act-by-act live scoring method is also conducted by expert raters through 1-way mirror using same dimensions.	In one study, positive vs. negative dimension reliability was .60; all other dimensions ranged from .87 to .95. Variables more reliable by rating method than by the observational scoring method.
The Experiencing Scales (Beck, Dugo, Eng, & Lewis, 1986)	Measures aspects of a patient's involvement in self-exploration and level of experiencing, the manner in which this is done (therapist), and the therapist's means of exploration.	Client scale has seven stages; the content and the manner in which the speaker is using feelings are taken into account in forming a judgment about level of experiencing, and in assigning a rating to a sample segment. Therapist experiencing scale has seven stages; the Therapist Manner Scale rates the mode in which the therapist engages in the exploratory therapy process.	Inter-rater reliability was assessed with both cross tabulation and Pearson Correlation methods. For the cross-tabulation, percentages of complete agreement (Item-by-Item EXP rating) were .67, .63, and .66. Pearson average rating per page was .80, .74, and .60.
Hostility/Support Scale (Beck, Dugo, Eng, & Lewis, 1986)	A three-category measure that makes a gross assessment of the basic supportiveness or negativity of the speaker in relation to the person being addressed.	Three ratings are given: 1 is given when the statement expresses acceptance, agreement, or neutrality toward the person addressed; 2 is given when a statement expresses disagreement, mild, or veiled negativity or criticism; and 3 is given when a statement expresses openly negative, angry, or aggressive feelings toward the person addressed.	A cross-tabulation assessed the percentage of complete agreement between the two raters, followed by Pearson correlation on the average rating per page of transcript. Cross tabulation % agreement was 74.32, 71.85, and 75.78. Pearson correlations were .83, .66, and .61.
Behavior Scores System (Borgatta, 1963)	Focuses on definitions that maximize content areas corresponding to peer assignments. Similar to Bales' and Chapple's systems.	Behavior is scored in six categories; two prominent factors are assertiveness and sociability. Five additional scales describe the nature of the behavior (e.g., laughter, tension)	Not indicated.

Instrument	Description	Scoring/Analysis	Reliability
Group Session Rating Scale (Cooney, Kadden, Litt, & Getter, 1991)	Rates communication in categories: education (skill training), problem solving, role playing, identifying high risk situations, interpersonal learning, expression of feeling, and here and now focus.	Raters indicate the occurrence of any of the seven categories during each one-minute period.	Inter-rater reliabilities, in one study, using Cronbach's alpha-coefficient ranged from .83 to .97. Coping skills items were moderately correlated with one another, and negatively correlated with those items characteristic of interactional therapy; exception was "identifying high-risk situations," which was not highly correlated with any of the other rated behaviors.
Group Rating Schedule (Cooper, 1977)	Focuses on five factors (21 scales): process orientation, social atmosphere, trainer involvement, trainer-client involvement, and emotional cohesiveness.	Scales are rated via Likert procedures; provides measure of the group on five basic factors. Percentage of time in each category is then calculated.	Inter-rater reliabilities reported to range from .75 to .81.
Group Therapy Interaction Chronogram (Cox, 1973)	Represents interactions and relationships between group members; similar to a sociogram but more complex. Derived from Chapple's Interaction Chronograph.	Each member is represented as a circle divided into specific time phases; relationships between group members are recorded by arrows including an affective component as well as strong vs. ambivalent feelings.	Not indicated.
Relational Communication Control System (RCCCS) (Friedlander & Heatherington, 1989)	Classifies verbal messages among two or more people and subsequently maps the relational control sequences in the flow of talk. Is an extension to the Family Relational Communication Control Coding System. Major change from the RCCCS is the identification of "triadic" moves (speaking turns in which there are two or more targets).	Control codes are assigned to elements of speech flow. They are: up (messages used to assert control), down (messages that attempt to give up control), across (messages that are neutral with respect to control), direct and indirect targets, intercepts (a speaker's intrusion), disconfirmations, simple moves (two targets in which at least one is across), complex moves (messages with multiple control implications), and levels of analysis (indices which can be used depending on the objectives of the investigation).	Inter-rater reliability ranged from .52–.97 with a mean of .82. Kappas for unitization, determination of participants, and format were high; reliability for response modes was lower (adequate to good range).
The Time by Event by Member Pattern Observation (TEMPO) (Futoran, Kelly, & McGrath, 1989)	Divides categories into two sets: production (propose & evaluate content and process), nonproduction (member support and group well-being).	One task performance period of a group is a single protocol. A protocol consists of an event string, each event of which is referenced with respect to three facets: the member who originated the act, the type of act, and its temporal address (the second at which it began). Intended to perform some analyses on the matrix resulting from a single protocol. In	Authors' report only.

TABLE 6.1. (*Continued*)

Instrument	Description	Data Format	Reliability
The Time by Event (*continued*)		its extended three-dimensional form, usually only one entry is in each one-sec layer on the time address axis. Collapsing the matrix accumulates more than one act in the cells of the other dimensions (member by type).	
Individual Differences Scaling (INDSCAL) (Carroll & Chang, 1970)	Provides a means for analyzing intrapersonal issues and gestalt issues; based upon what group members believe to be important; is a multidimensional scaling program.	Members rate each possible combination of dyads, leader, and each of the other members to each other, from 1 (very similar) to 9 (very dissimilar). The computer algorithm processes the ratings and prints the results in two dimensional maps. Using correlational techniques, a comparison of the various trends is produced by the INDSCAL computer. With the geometric expression in front of them (via. computer), group members are asked to name the dimensions. Also occasional weights offer an assessment of the individual within the system.	Not indicated.
Anxiety and Hostility Verbal Content Analysis Scales (Gottschalk-Gleser, 1969)	Measures verbal content; provides objective categories of anxiety and hostility states; based on psychoanalytic concept: overt affective statement and projected, negated, displaced, and weakened affect cures are scored.	Raw scores on each scale are summed for all members and therapists for each session and then are transformed using the score formula to yield a single score. O-factor analysis can also be done to determine which sessions have the same mix of content scales. This helps determine the interactional climate of the sessions.	Average inter-rater reliability in one study was .80.
Category System for Partners Interaction (KPI) (Hahlweg, Doane, Goldstein, Nuechterlein, Magana, Mintz, Miklowitz, & Snyder, 1989)	Assesses speaker and listener skills that form the basis of behaviorally-oriented communication and problem-solving treatments; includes both verbal and nonverbal components.	Twelve verbal categories are: self-disclosure, positive solutions, acceptance of the other, agreement, problem description, meta-communication, personal criticism, specific criticism, negative solution, justification, and disagreement. Content categories receive a nonverbal rating as well. In an hierarchical order, the facial cues of the speaker or listener are evaluated first as positive, negative, or neutral; if unable to code the utterance as positive or	Reports reliability kappas over .80. In one study, inter-rater agreement between pairs of the six coders ranged between .71 to 95.3%. Kappa values were .83 (verbal) and .84 (nonverbal) codes. A 91% agreement rate was found between the two sets of codes, indicating minimal rater drift.

Category System (continued)		Method	Reliability
	negative, the voice tone cues are scanned. If unable to code the utterance as positive or negative, the body cues are scanned until an appropriate rating can be applied.		
Sematic Cohesion Analysis (Halliday & Hasan, 1976, adapted by Friedlander, et al., 1985)	Measures spoken discourse-semantic cohesion; is nonreactive and a theoretical indicator of conversational involvement.	All adjacent turns are coded for number, location, and type of cohesive tie. Cohesive ties are analyzed both for the group members and the therapists.	Interjudge reliability 93%, 88%, and .75 on Cohen's Kappa.
Hill Interaction Matrix (HIM) (Hill, 1965)	Classifies content and style of interaction. Sixteen cells are in hierarchial value of therapeutic quality.	Sixteen cell matrix of categories for content (topic, group, person, relationship) and style (conversational, assertive, speculative, & confrontive) of interaction.	Mean reliability indices for three judges rating three groups were 70% agreement, .76 product-moment correlation, and .90 rank order correlation.
Group Emotionality Rating System (GERS) (Karterud & Foss, 1989)	Simplifies and revises Thelen's system (which was based on concepts of Bion); classifies individual statements of group participants.	Every verbal statement (per minute) is rated as fight, flight, dependency, pairing, group reaction, very short statements, very long statements, mixed emotionality, psychotic statements, and revision of the data protocol.	A reliability study (act-by-act scrutiny of 4,343 verbal statements) revealed an overall agreement of .77. The range for the emotionality sub-categories was from .57 to .67. Mean correlation coefficient for emotionally charged statements was .80.
A Method For Classifying Group Interaction (Ohlsen & Pearson, 1965)	Classifies roles used by principal actors and the reaction of group members to these roles.	Actors are rated on 28 categories which focus on the intent of the communication; rated on four categories of moving toward, away, or against the principal actor or passive attendance.	Inter-rater reliabilities for principal actors range from .73 to .93, and the same for response roles are from .76 to .87.
Psychodynamic Work and Object Rating Systems (PWORS) (Piper & McCallum, 1992)	Assesses two basic constructs in group therapy: presence and complexity of psychodynamic work, and reference to objects (one or more types or persons). Precursor was the Therapist Interventions Rating System.	Five components are in the system: four dynamic (wishes, reactive anxiety, defensive process, and one nondynamic dynamic expressions) and one nondynamic (objects). To be scored as dynamic, the expression must be presented as being in conflict with, causing, giving rise to, or impacting on another expression. This second expression (resultant) must be stated and the connection between the dynamic and resultant expressions must be clear in the rater's mind. Objects refer to people internal or external to the group: two	The average percentages of perfect category agreement for categories 1 through 4 (inter-rater reliability) were: .87, .83, .67, and .66 respectively. The average Kappa coefficient after removing chance-expected agreement was .69. The mean Kappa coefficient for four raters over twelve sessions on the work-nonwork distinction was .75.

TABLE 6.1. (Continued)

Instrument	Description	Data Format	Reliability
Psychodynamic Work and Object Rating Systems (continued)		aspects of objects are monitored: object focus and object linking. There are two nonwork categories: externalizing statements and descriptive statements; two work categories: single dynamic component and two or more dynamic components.	Article reports inter-rater reliability was "adequate."
Analysis with Individual and Group Vocal Parameters (AIGVP) (Ruback, Dabbs, & Hopper, 1984)	Vocal behavior recorded uses a data acquisition system built around an Apple II computer; sound and silence define more meaningful units.	Functions like an expanded version of the Automatic Vocal Transaction Analyzer (AVTA) used by Jaffe and Feldstein to study dyads. Scans the microphones of each individual continuously and identifies signals from solitary speakers as well as from several persons speaking at once. The computer records the on-off state of each voice every quarter second; also records signals from push-button switches held by the two coders. Whenever a coder identifies a new idea from the group, a switch button is pressed, time recorded, idea, and who said it. Vocalizations and button presses representing ideas were recorded by the computer on the same quarter-second time base; data transmitted via telephone line to a Univac mainframe computer.	
Social Information Processing Analysis (SIPA) (Fisher, 1976)	Based on systems theory; defines four dimensions: source of information, time orientation, information assembly rules, and equivocality reduction.	The unit of information coded into the analytical system is the "act" (each uninterrupted verbal comment emitted by a single individual). Each act is coded on each of the four dimensions.	Reliabilities among coders was computed using Guetzkow's formula. Among three pairs of raters correlation coefficients ranged between .70 and .80 on the four rating dimensions.
Process Analysis Scoring System (Gibbard & Hartman, 1973)	Extends Mann's system for analyzing member-leader relationships; includes element of member-member interchanges.	General categories (similar to Mann's format) are revised to include hostility, affection, power relations, and ego states. Eighteen specific content categories define the four general areas.	Not indicated.
Factor Analysis of Process Variables (Heckel, Holmes & Rosecrans, 1971)	A factor analysis of 11 rating categories derived six factors; early and later factors were distinct from one another.	All responses were coded into either environmental, personal, or group responses. Responses scored on categories described as negative responses, initiating activity, seeking information, giving information, seeking opinion, giving opinion, elaborating, and group building roles.	Inter-rater reliability on pilot study of .86 was reported.

Instrument	Description	Procedure	Reliability
Program for Conservation Analysis (Just, 1968)	Analyzes conversation into word counts, act counts, and act duration for each speaker.	Specified in formal computer program.	Not indicated.
Experiencing Scale (Klein, Mathieu, Gendlin, & Kiesler, 1969)	Seven stage scale co-assesses the degree to which one is affectively involved and trying to understand communications.	Rating of each unit on a seven stage continuum from high to low.	Pearson r = .73.
Member-to-Leader Scoring System (Mann, 1967)	Analyzes member-leader relationships; primary emphasis on how members relate to group leaders.	Rater uses a multiple category system to classify the type of interaction occurring. Four areas (hostility, affection, anxiety, and depression) are rated in 16 specific content categories (e.g., resisting, expressing self esteem).	73% average agreement between scorers reported for content categories.
Sign Process Analysis (SPA) (Mills, 1964)	Measures the course of interaction by determining the nature of input from two perspectives: the nature of the object and its corresponding value standard.	An 11×12 object matrix is used with a positive, negative, and neutral breakdown in each cell (396 possible classifications). For each statement, general categories include: internal, external, principal, and secondary objects.	Percentage of rater agreement equalled 80% across several trials.
Group Therapist Interventions Scale (Nicols & Taylor, 1975)	Classifies type, degree of confrontation, and direct object of statements made by group leader.	Three general categories include: type of intervention, confrontation scale, and object of intervention. Additional subcategories under each of the three general areas.	73%, 88%, and 93% agreement between trained raters on three rating scales. Pearson R of .66 between raters on confrontation scale.
A Method for Quantifying Interaction in Counseling Groups (Nobel, Ohlsen, & Proff, 1961)	Based on Bales' system but directed to counseling groups. Specifies three categories of observation: client statements, counselor statements, and nonverbal behavior.	Client and counselor categories each contain 12 coding possibilities; the nonverbal category includes six possibilities. Each coding is listed by frequency of occurrence after which a percentage of each subcategory is calculated.	Rank order correlations between observer teams ranged from .92 for client observations to .78 for counselor observations to .60 for nonverbal observations.
The General Inquirer (Stone, Dunphy, Smith, & Ogilvie, 1966)	Analyzes content of psychological protocols or other textual materials; has three main aspects: dictionary lookup, question format, syntax identification.	Procedures include: preparation of text, composition of dictionary, checking of dictionary format, sorting and listing of entry words, tag tally, composition of questions, tagging of text words, and inquiry of text and tags.	Not indicated.

*Revised updated table (Fuhriman & Packard, 1986)

of varied instruments or instruments capable of measuring multiple issues. Few of the instruments have been applied in more than one type of group (e.g., population, purpose, theortical orientation), leaving us in the dark regarding the constancy of therapeutic themes and issues evident across groups. It is also unfortunate that the existing measures do not accompany one another in specific studies, further impeding our ability to determine conceptual overlap or to relate relevant processes to one another. The apparent singularity of interest and intent, and the lack of cooperative interplay among designers and investigators also restrict our ability to understand process in a comprehensive fashion.

STUDY CHARACTERISTICS AND FINDINGS

Pragmatics reign in psychological research, as in most heuristic endeavors. Thus, while some instruments clearly possess superior construction, they may not be utilized as often as others, given their accompanying complexities, such as investment in time to ensure rater reliability, level of intrusiveness, coding of data, the ease with which data yield to statistical procedures, and the constraints of the research design, just to name a few.

Table 6.2 reports the interactional instruments most utilized during the past decade, the kinds of studies and populations involved, and the significant results. In some cases, instruments per se are only peripherally related to such results. That is, the instrument may be designed for distinguishing family patterns (e.g., Hahlweg), but have little to do with obtaining those findings. There is a wide range in the relationship between the stated purpose of an instrument, its capacity to measure those processes, and its actual ability to do so. Nevertheless, it is of interest to note how each process measure plays a part in the construction of meaning in group process research.

In the past decade, the instruments that appear to be utilized in studies most frequently are Bale's Interaction Process Analysis (IPA) and System for the Multiple Level Observations of Groups (SYMLOG) (12 studies), followed by the Hill Interaction Matrix (HIM SS) developed by William Hill (five studies). The Individual Differences Scaling instrument (INDSCAL) developed by Carroll and Chang (1970) is visible in three studies, while the remaining instruments are seen only once or twice in the past decade. Over the past 40 years, the Bales and Hill instruments have attracted the largest proportion of research interest involving an interactional analysis perspective. Of the two, the HIM captures the greater clinical interest (therapy and personal growth populations).

Types of Groups

Table 6.2 also reveals that the groups studied represent an interesting spectrum of populations and types, from long-term therapy groups to 15-minute analogue groups. Specifically, these include three case studies (though only one labeled itself as such), 12 leaderless analogue studies of under-graduates (half of whom were in a course) being rated on a variety of behaviors, specialized treatment groups (aged, bereaved, convicted DUI vi-olators, families of recently diagnosed schizophrenics), and a garden-variety of outpatient and inpatient therapy groups. All groups were made up of adults ranging in age from 18 to "retired"; only two studies specified demographics regarding distribution of race and ethnicity. With the excep-tion of two studies involving married couples and families, the group popu-lations were ahistorical, people who came together having had no prior experience with each other.

It is also of interest to note which instruments are typically used with which kinds of groups. For example, in the 12 studies using the IPA or SYMLOG (Jarboe, 1991; Jurma & Wright, 1990; Kelly & McGrath, 1985; Keyton & Springston, 1990; Kressel, 1987; Mabry, 1985; Mabry, 1989; Mabry & Attridge, 1990; McDermott, 1988; Polley, 1987; Polley, 1992; Seibert & Gruenfeld, 1992), all but one are analogue studies. The utilization of groups organized specifically for the purpose of study appears to come from the social psychology literature, which traditionally measures vari-ables in task groups. This is certainly understandable given the relatively easy format and the availability of subjects. Still, this practice raises some concern regarding the applicability to different settings. The SYMLOG and IPA were both developed originally from the writings of Bales (1950), and although applicable to therapeutic settings, the theory and resulting studies are based mainly on task groups.

The IPA is a fairly straightforward categorization of 12 thought units of discourse based on the four underlying clusters of interactive messages: task responses, task questions, positive affect, and negative affect. The SYMLOG includes these categories, somewhat reorganized to yield three-dimensional scores or positions along 26 vectors. This extension of the IPA system was influenced by the first factor-analytic study of interpersonal behavior conducted by Arthur Couch (1960). Bales based his dimensions of up/down, friendly/unfriendly, and forward/backward on the thousands of data points collected from Couch's exhaustive study (Bales, Cohen, & Williams, 1979).

As the SYMLOG studies suggest, this group process measure is appro-priate for organizational behavior groups with an applied communication focus in a work setting as well as for small groups with a therapeutic focus. Still it does not appear to be utilized equally by both kinds of groups. The five studies using the Hill Interaction Matrix statement-by-statement rating system, in contrast, deal almost exclusively with some kind of treatment group. The number of studies incorporating Hill's interactive model would be somewhat larger if studies involving the questionnaire variations of the HIM (i.e., HIM-B, HIM-G) and unpublished dissertations were included. It is also interesting to note the context of the HIM beginnings in contrast to SYMLOG's. William Hill developed his conceptual framework while work-ing countless hours with psychiatric inpatients at a state hospital. Though it

P. 204
P. 209

TABLE 6.2. Group Process Instrumentation: Study Results

Instrument	Population	Type of Group	Results
Interaction Process Analysis (Bales, 1950)			
Jarboe (1991)	160 male and female undergraduates	40, 4-member 30-minute discussion groups leaderless 10 sessions	While particular outcomes were of interest to the researchers, the main focus of the study was a comparison of log-linear vs. MANOVA statistical analysis. Both analyses yielded procedure as a main effect. However, different results were tapped by each analysis.
Jurma & Wright (1990)	120 male and female undergraduates	4, 30-minute analogue task groups leaderless 1 session	Inconclusive findings regarding how male and female leaders affected member contributions in power maintenance and power-loss situations.
Mabry & Attridge (1990)	176 male and female undergraduates	44, 3–5 member analogue task groups leaderless	Unstructured outcome indicated significant associations between four sets of enacted messages and task products. No significance for structured outcome.
Mabry (1989)	45 male and female undergraduates	4, 70-minute "t groups" facilitators weekly sessions for a term	Attempted to test sex-role differentiation theory against role-status expectation and contextual role adaptation theories; yielded role-status theory as more explanatory framework for results which included differentiation on task vs. social-emotional dimensions for males and females.
McDermott (1988)	Adults in a "partial hospital" program	3, 60-minute groups (1 task, 1 verbal, 1 activity) facilitators	Task group formats had more positive social-emotional communications, more interaction between members. Verbal and activity-based verbal groups had more discussion of feelings and more leader involvement.
Mabry (1985)	168 male and female undergraduates	44, 3–5 member analogue task groups leaderless 20-minute sessions	Influence of gender composition (male and female) and task (high structure vs. low) on group communication behaviors provided weak support for both variables significantly affecting group interaction.
Kelly & McGrath (1985)	344 male and female undergraduates	86, 4-member analogue task groups leaderless 2 trials (10 and 20 minutes)	Groups with a 20-minute first trial produced products higher in quality and quantity, and engaged in more interpersonal activity which persisted in subsequent 10-minute trials. Specific processes leading to social entrainment yet to be found.

[handwritten annotations: "Anderson", "Umpoli", "TASK GROUPS", "I"]

Systems for Multiple Level
Observations of Groups
(Bales, Cohen, & Williams, 1979)

HIM—SEE P.204 AS WELL

THERAPY GROUPS

Study	Sample	Method/Design	Findings
Seibert & Gruenfeld (1992)	85 male and female undergraduates	4 "in class" discussion groups (observational ratings collected on subsample of 34) 16 weeks	Masculinity was positively associated with dominant behavior while the predicted positive relationship between femininity and friendly interpersonal behavior was found only with retrospective ratings, not when using an observational method.
Polley (1991)		Statistical analysis comparing level of agreement between theoretical and item to scale correlations on SYMLOG and GFD (Group Field Dynamics form).	Polley's GFD appears to be a more robust instrument given its refinement of SYMLOG and its ability to identifying subgroups, polarizations, and scapegoats. Both are ideally suited to case-study approach as they provide detailed information concerning individual behavior, interpersonal perception, and group dynamics which can be utilized with management, market research, and therapy groups.
Keyton & Springston (1990)	248 male and female undergraduates	47, 3–7 member "in class" analogue task groups 13 weeks	Measures of cohesiveness (polarization, unification, group attitude, and solidarity) measured group cohesiveness, as operationalized by one another. But predicting group effectiveness from cohesiveness constructs may be premature.
Polley (1987)	800 male and female adults	Item-to-scale correlations based on 6,432 sets of original ratings of 800 students and office workers in a variety of settings. The average subject rated self, 5 other group members, and hypothetical most/least effective member.	SYMLOG's pattern of poor or reversed correlations appears not to be random and thus represents a problem with the dimensions themselves rather than poor wording. In the revised version, all 54 correlations were in the right direction. The most notable improvement was in the measurement of the F-B dimension which heretofore has undergone serious criticism.
Kressel (1987)		Position paper	SYMLOG, a "new social psychological system" is useful in both individual and group behavior therapy and can serve as a way to bring psychoanalytic and humanistic techniques to behavior therapy.

Hill Interaction Matrix
(Hill, 1965)

Study	Sample	Method/Design	Findings
Toseland, Rossiter, Peak, & Hill (1990)	"Older" adult males and females	4 therapy groups 2 peer, 2 professionally led 8, 2-hour sessions	The opportunity to vent feelings, affirm coping abilities, mutual sharing, and support variables accounted for outcome regardless if group was peer or professionally led.

TABLE 6.2. (*Continued*)

Instrument	Population	Type of Group	Results
Barlow (1988)	102 male and female adults	10 therapy outpatient groups 4 expert, 4 natural helper leaders, 2 wait list controls 2-hour sessions	Nonspecific affects of warmth and empathy (as measured by client perception of therapeutic relationships) were necessary but not sufficient conditions for client improvement. The specific effect of skill or expertise accounted for initial client deterioration and subsequent improvement at post and six-month follow-up.
Hammonds & Worthington (1985)	16 males and females, married	Assessment-only control group (10) & marriage enrichment group (6) facilitators 3, 2½-hour sessions	Couples in enrichment group were more dissatisfied with their marriages and reported poorer communication than assessment-only group at the beginning. At post treatment, enrichment group improved mental satisfaction and communication skills equal to assessment-only group. Researchers noted HIM was easier to use than HCS (Heckel Classification System) but provided less information.
Barlow, Hansen, Finley, & Fuhriman (1982)	48 male and female undergraduates	6, 30-hour personal growth groups leaders trained to use either speculative, confrontive, or unspecified (controls) verbal style	Regardless of condition, members perceived leaders as caring. Confrontive leaders were seen as more charismatic, speculative, and more peer-oriented. In all conditions, group members followed leader verbal style up to three lags. Experimental variable of leader talk (spec. vs. conf.) was confirmed.
Peterson & Pollio (1982)	8 male and female adults	1, 8-member outpatient therapy group co-leaders 17, 1½-hour sessions	Majority of humorous remarks, categorized according to target (self, others in group, generalized other) were directed at a specific target and were negative. Humorous remarks directed towards others in group tended to decrease therapeutic effectiveness. Remarks targeted outside the group increased therapeutic effectiveness.
The Experiencing Scales and Hostility/Support Scale (Beck et. al., 1986)			
Beck, Dugo, Eng, & Lewis (1986)	Male and female adults	3 outpatient groups co-leaders 15–20 weekly sessions	Rating hostility and support allowed researchers to track a major shift in group behavior. Nevertheless, the most relevant variable in the identification from phase 2 (group concerns) to 3 (personal concerns) was based on statements made to scapegoat leader by group members.

Individual Differences Scaling (Carroll & Chang, 1970)			
Pace (1990)	141 male and female undergraduates	32, 4–5 member analogue task groups weekly sessions for the semester	High consensus groups had significantly higher differentiation scores on personalized-positive, depersonalized-negative and depersonalized-positive conflicts than did low consensus groups. Also, a thorough differentiation of cooperative attitudes does not ensure cohesion. A prolonged differentiation of competitive conflict is counterproductive.
Gazda & Mobley (1980)	9 adult males and females	1 organizational/staff group consultant/leader	Through use of a case study, authors present usefulness of INDSCAL as a measure of individual perceptions of each possible dyad and overall group gestalt by applying a computer algorithm.
Sprouse & Brush (1980)	10 adult males (3 Black, 7 White)	1 "quasi-therapy" DUI group facilitator 8, 2½-hour sessions	Results of similarity ratings indicated three major dimensions across group time: (1) self-disclosure about alcoholism, (2) talking as opposed to silence, and (3) racial perception which diminished in salience over time. Also, members were shown their configurations which allowed them to see themselves as others saw them.
Anxiety and Hostility Verbal Content Analysis Scales (Gottschalk & Gleser, 1969)			
Tschuschke & MacKenzie (1989)	18 male and female adults	2 outpatient therapy groups leaders 150, 1½-hour sessions	Using scores from Gottschalk and Glaser procedure to demonstrate sequential interactional climate, Group 1 demonstrated better outcome. This was likely based on sequential periods of interactional stability.
Tschuschke (1986)	Adult males and females	1 outpatient therapy group leader 57, 1½-hour sessions	Verbal statements were correlated with EKGs and breathing rate, indicating that members who reacted psychophysiologically to affects, acknowledged afterwards an increased emotional involvement. Therapist and members reacted in similar fashion.
Category System for Partners Interaction (Hahlweg, Doane, Goldstein, Nuechterlein, Magana, Mintz, Miklowitz, & Snyder, 1989)	107 male and female adults (43 family "units")	Recently diagnosed schizophrenics (43) meeting in 2, 10-minute problem-solving tasks with family members	Family interaction patterns of expressed emotion (EE) indicated that high EE critical relatives were more negative in direct interactions and showed extreme negative escalation patterns. Inability of the KPI to distinguish family patterns may have to do with way in which data are summarized.

TABLE 6.2. *(Continued)*

Instrument	Population	Type of Group	Results
Psychodynamic Work and Object Rating Systems (Piper & McCallum, 1992)	58 male and female adults	16 psychodynamic outpatient bereavement groups 12 sessions	The PWORS was evaluated as a reliable instrument able to differentiate between therapists' theoretical orientations. Pre-group measures of psychological mindedness correlated with self-based work but not with group participation or group-based work.
Relational Communication (Ellis, 1976) and Interaction Analysis System (Fisher, 1976)	84 male and female undergraduates	19, 4–6 member analogue task groups leaderless	RELCOM and IAS findings indicated that both relational and content levels of communication were significantly different for high vs. low consensus groups in the final stages of task performance. High consensus groups engaged in interpretation in response to clarification.
DeStephen (1983)	Inpatient substance abuse	Coping skills vs. interactional therapy groups 26 sessions	Education and skill training correlated with fewer group members reporting drinking-related problems.
Group Session Rating Scale (Cooney, Kadden, Litt, & Getter, 1991)	Counseling center clients Neurotic/personality disorder and defensive style	Interactional psychotherapy groups Leadership styles: self-disclosing vs. facilitating 8 sessions	Client cohesive ties more associated with nondisclosing therapists. Therapists' cohesive ties more associated with nondisclosing therapists. Nondisclosing style may be most critical in early life of group.
Sematic Cohesion Analysis (Friedlander, Thibodeau, Nichols, Tucker, & Snyder, 1985)	Undergraduate psychology students	Task (brainstorming) analogue groups 1, 20-minute session	Examined content free patterns. Ideas appear most rapidly at beginning of session and often come "in clusters." Leaders talk more than other members.
Analysis with Individual and Group Vocal Parameters (Ruback, Dabbs, & Hopper, 1984)			

is difficult to determine if the context for development determines usability in that same context, it is interesting to note the differences in development and later usage between the SYMLOG/IPA and HIM.

The remaining instruments representing studies during the past decade (Table 6.2) have a similar development history, having originated primarily from one setting (i.e., INDSCAL-task) or another (i.e., PWORS-therapy). Thus far, it appears that certain process instruments are not what they say they are, are not utilized equally across therapy and analogue settings, and rely heavily on expert observer/raters to determine presence or absence of the phenomenon being observed in members.

Sampling Procedures

While incidental on first inspection, how researchers sample the communication process to be rated has an important effect on significance. These studies represent the variety of sampling procedures extant in group research, sampling chunks of communication data ranging from mere seconds to entire sessions. They also illustrate different purposes for sampling (i.e., ensuring calibrated tallies, tracking developmental phenomenon). For instance, in the Kelly and McGrath study (1985), the observers record a code for each group member comment that occurred on the 10th second of each 10-second interval. Several HIM studies select beginning, middle, and end segments or 10- to 15-minute segments from each group (Barlow, Hansen, Fuhriman, & Finley, 1982; Peterson & Pollio, 1982; Toseland, Rossiter, Peak, & Hill, 1990), while one HIM study (Barlow, 1988) rates three group sessions in their entirety. Several other therapy studies also use entire sessions as their time sample (Beck, 1986; McCallum & Piper, 1990; Peterson & Pollio, 1982; Tschuschke, 1986; Tschuschke & MacKenzie, 1989). Keyton and Springston (1990) sought predetermined segments from each session based on the rationale that certain phenomena would occur in specified stages. One study hypothesized that the variable of interest to the researchers occurs in the final session, and thus only coded those end segments (Jurma & Wright, 1990). In the main, therapy studies sample larger session segments than do analogue and task group studies. Unfortunately, until the validity of the sampling procedure is ensured, those relying on the results are in an untenable position.

In addition to the length and timing of samples, it is interesting to note what behaviors are actually rated. The majority of studies regarded verbalizations as the most important process variable, defined as everything from an utterance to a complete thought (i.e., grammatical clause; Tschuschke, 1986). Very few studies rated nonverbal movements within the group, unless indirectly inferred by the category descriptions. For instance, the dimensions on the SYMLOG (i.e., friendly versus unfriendly) and the Hostility/Support Scale suggest that expert raters employ act-by-act, behavioral scoring methods that may involve nonverbal behaviors as well. Only the KPI actually includes a distinct category for nonverbal ratings. Also, the majority of studies used transcripts made from audiotapes, suggesting that, for the most part, visuals were not available to be rated or were deemed irrelevant. The exceptions include the live-ratings obtained in the Seibert and Gruenfeld (1992) SYMLOG study and three IPA studies (Kelly & Mc-Grath, 1985; Mabry, 1989; McDermott, 1988).

Variables Manipulated and Measured

When one surveys the results across all Table 6.2 studies, it is also clear that a variety of variables are manipulated: group composition (i.e., proportion of males/females in problem solving groups), kinds of tasks, length of time, type of leader, power-maintenance or power-loss situations, structured tasks, unstructured tasks). An equal number of dependent variables are measured: frequency and type of verbal statements, task products, member satisfaction, leader involvement, friendly interpersonal behavior, number of humorous remarks, therapeutic effectiveness, types of conflict, physiological indicators (breathing, heart rate), levels of consensus, levels of cohesiveness, reduction of symptoms, acquisition of new skills, and more.

Study Results

An enlightening array of results was also found by these various researchers represented in Table 6.2, from correlational connections between process consensus and outcome consensus (DeStephen, 1983) to in-group indicators of physiological arousal with member acknowledgement of increased emotional involvement afterwards (Tschuschke & MacKenzie, 1989). Again, study results appear to be influenced by sampling procedures, statistical analysis, and so on. Such variability across these influences hampers a subsequent comparison of findings across studies. Nevertheless, imbedded within the plethora of results are possible prescriptions and proscriptions for clinicians: prolonged competitive conflict could be counterproductive (Pace, 1990); groups enjoy a sense of satisfaction if there are sufficient, sustained levels of interactional stability (Tschuschke & MacKenzie, 1989); members and leaders are likely to have similar states of physiological arousal (Tschuschke, 1986); opportunity to vent and confirm abilities with like-minded retired persons may be more important than if the group is led by an expert or paraprofessional (Toseland et al., 1990); members are able to attend less to the variable of race and more to a variable of commonly shared feelings when they disclose distress about alcoholism (Sprouse & Brush, 1980); role status theory is a more useful framework when explaining the task/emotional differences between males and females (Mabry, 1989); positive interpersonal traits of leaders are a necessary but not sufficient condition for member change to occur in therapy groups—leaders must also demonstrate specific skills (Barlow, 1988); humor may mask actual group member hostility (Peterson & Pollio, 1982); therapists should be careful when attempting marital change with couples in enrichment groups as couple communication may deteriorate rather than improve! (Hammonds & Worthington, 1985); and finally, clinicians might attend to their verbal styles more, as members are apt to follow them into those styles (Barlow et al., 1982).

These process measures may also point the way towards potential problem resolution. For instance, the IPA could alert therapists to the percent of talk time being driven by task rather than emotion. The HIM could help leaders be aware of the proportion of time spent on various topics, as well as the effect of the communication style engaged in during conflicts. The SYM LOG, with its view from the inside (member self-report) as well as the outside (expert rater), could add a dimension which more clearly illuminates how different positions may influence the phenomena being perceived, illustrating the age-old axiom that beauty (in this case, meaning attribution) is in the eye of the beholder.

The studies' findings contain caveats for researchers as well. While the variables under scrutiny are interesting, and many of the outcomes enlightening, the prominent relationship between heretofore suspected group process variables and their supposed relationship to other process and outcome variables is not always clear. This may have to do with a variety of problems, all of which could be subsumed under construct validity and reliability. For instance, many of the measures did not perform as expected. The KPI (Category System for Partners Interaction) used in the Hahlweg et al. 1989 study was unable to distinguish family patterns, yet it was designed specifically to determine patterns among family members; in this case, expressed emotion proved to be a better predictor. The IPA (Interaction Process Analysis) has as its foremost variable Dominant (Up)-Submissive (Down); yet in a study designed to measure power-maintenance and power-loss of group leaders, it failed to differentiate between male and female leaders. In addition, the studies in Table 6.2 suggest the appropriateness of some, rather than other, design and analyses procedures: log linear analysis could yield different findings than MANOVA (Jarboe, 1991); retrospective member ratings may be different than on-site expert observers (Seibert & Gruenfeld, 1992); some instruments may be easier to use (HIM), but may provide less information than others (HCS) (Hammonds & Worthington, 1985).

Identifying sets or combinations of process variables that are capable of influencing treatment outcome no longer involves a simple linear relationship between single factors and outcome. The reality of this conclusion is made clear through moment-by-moment analyses. Rather, we will need to construct a complex interactive model capable of defining an explanatory framework that has the capacity to embrace the rich interconnecting processes inherent in small groups. Meaningful data cannot be obtained from simply matching treatment to group member, or even by determining which member requires which factors and to what degree. Tracking the array of possibilities requires multiple instruments capable of measuring many dimensions at various levels via a moment-by-moment record. Such efforts could assist researchers not only in describing *content, context* (including

rpersonal, and group relationships), and *time,* but also in ac-
e *responsiveness* and *influence* of these variables. Such efforts
ʲᵒˡᵈ a complex model of immense proportion and innumerable detail,
which hopefully could explain how and why groups work. *or how +*
why risk behavior
groups work
successful change

Interaction Analysis: In Search of a Structure

Interwoven throughout the analysis of these interactional instruments and
issues is the scientist/practitioners' wish for a group heuristic. As these authors and instruments define and articulate moment-by-moment process
within a group, it becomes apparent that the driving force behind such efforts is the discovery of a structure that underlies, and perhaps governs, the
dynamic and interpersonal nature of the group as a whole. It is such a structure that may give meaning to the concept of the group as a whole, as an
entity much greater than the sum of its parts, with just possibly a replicable
life of its own, capable of influencing individual change.

Perhaps somewhere between Darwin and deconstructionism a paradigm
for complex interacting systems already exists. The comparison might have
been drawn earlier had the social sciences not been so bent on their own
separate and independent system, choosing to place men and women "outside nature . . . It was the easiest thing in the world to float the social
sciences off their scientific foundations" (Darrington, 1961, pp. 70–71).
About the time the first process measures were being developed in group
research, Watson and Crick made the discovery of the double helix, or as
Crick modestly wrote, "DNA made the discovery of Watson and Crick"
(Crick, 1988). Watson and Crick's discovery, which was a follow-up on the
work of Avery, Wilkins, and Franklin (Talaro & Talaro, 1993), allowed scientists to apply the laws of chemistry to biology, opening up an entirely new
vista of cell life subject to predictable patterns. That simple nucleic acids
were the basic building blocks of life surprised everyone. But that they
mixed, divided, and matched to create the genetic code inspired nothing
less than awe from scientists who were struck by the elegance of the structure of this living, interacting system. A therapy group is just such a living,
interacting system that might benefit from such a biological model. With
apologies to microbiologists, we wish to borrow the double helix as an analogy, its constituents as well as dynamic process, for the purpose of elucidat-
ing the complexity of the small group and the need for a structural model.

The following are the essential elements forming the structure of DNA:
The external rails (phosphates and sugars) are always present and spiraling.
Nitrogenous bases make up the steps between these stable rails and are of
four basic chemical compounds that always pair with their complementary
partner. Nevertheless, the arrangement of pairs can be quite varied, and it is
this permutation of sequences that allows for an infinite variety of outcomes. The double helix is not entirely symmetrical; depending on the order
of the bases, one rail can be slightly larger than the other, and depending
upon how tightly the strands are twisted, can be condensed or expanded.

Finally, at the midpoint of each step, hydrogen bonds (the least stable of the three forms of molecular bonding) connect the various pairs. These unstable bonds facilitate the "unzipping" that begins the dynamic process of replication. Thus, through this transfer of complex messages contained within basic constituents, the renewal of life occurs.

If we had a structure such as this, which could designate the predictable sine qua non of a small, interpersonal therapy group, and subsequently were able to add the permutations of possibilities within that structure, we might know much more clearly the essential processes to be measured. In other words, if our pursuant investigations rested on conceptualizing an organizing "structure," we would be in a better position to grasp the complexity and nonlinearity of the dynamic group process. We know, for instance, from 40 years of research that the essential definition of group includes a certain number of persons with a particular purpose, otherwise it is not a "small group," but rather any one of a variety of biological or social phenomena from a gaggle of geese to a gathering of third graders. We also know from 40 years of research that a therapy group has not only a certain number of persons, but a more focused purpose surrounding social/emotional issues, and most usually includes a designated professional, therapist, or leader(s) at its helm. Even research from leaderless self-help groups or task/analogue groups suggests that leaders quickly emerge, given the demands of the situation. Perhaps then, the structuring (always present, always moving) rails of group process are people (i.e., patients, therapists, specific group composition) who share a common purpose.

What basic group constituents in certain pairings of infinite sequences might make up the steps between the two permanent structuring rails? Here our 40 years is more sparse regarding what phenomena exist or pair together to create change. Table 6.2 suggests that a variety of phenomena could compete for a place on the steps: words, interaction sequences, emotions, behaviors, tasks, demographics, time, and so on. The research has yet to offer indisputable proof that two specific factors must be paired with and only with each other, as cytosine must always pair with guanine and thymine with adenine in the double helix. Nevertheless, some good guesses appear that could be defined under the rubric of therapeutic factors. For instance, it is just possible that catharsis and insight must always be paired to effect long-lasting change (that is, involve a genuine transfer of learning). Another possible pairing might be identification and universality. Humans appear to respond to nomothetic as well as idiographic influences. They wish to be unique and yet long for a common bond with all of humanity. In the therapy group, our testing of individual need fulfillment with the needs of the group as a whole may well be just such a permanent pairing that leads to change of behavior. Our neglect in using multiple interactional analyses in a single study precludes understanding such presumed structural pairs.

And what might be the connecting (hydrogen bond) elements that exist to link these two pairs? In our illustration, that bond is most likely cohesion, here-and-now interactions which manifest a sense of "groupness," or a willingness to be influenced by one another. The dimension of time (spiraling, expanding, moving) can also be added to the structure by observing the effects of length of time in group (short-term and long-term groups). Just as the helix condenses or expands its basic components by twisting tightly (i.e., 30-hour intensive group) or loosely (i.e., long-term, once-a-week group), so too could the influence of time be tracked and understood within the structure of the group process. Moment-by-moment measurement may well be the methodological means by which to observe the presence of time, the occurring patterns, and the structural framework. These then may represent a structure: basic parts of differing sizes within certain parameters, which can be condensed or expanded, then divided and replicated—that constitute the group therapeutic process.

This analogy highlights some critical points in interaction analysis and group process research as well. It focuses us on slightly different concerns than those we have pursued. What is always there? What aspects are always present together? What connects these parts, yet facilitates movement? The instruments and accompanying studies address, in part, the first question.

But few of the extant instruments actually encompass all of the potential elements of such a structure: Group process is an organized whole played out within a context over the passage of time. All of the instruments together do not encompass all the elements. Perhaps the most evident absence is an instrument which would help us understand the individual characteristics of group members and the way they respond to one another. The impact of composition is both intrapersonal and interpersonal. Our proposed external rail of people includes these intrapersonal and interpersonal styles (dyads, larger subgroups, the group-as-a-whole) that shift and change over time yet are always present as part of the small group experience. While some of the instruments attend to an inferred intrapsychic process (PWORS, Experiencing Scale, Hostility/Support Scale, Process Affective Scoring System, [Gibbard & Hartman, 1973], and others attend to interpersonal aspects (HIM, SYMLOG, etc.), no group process scale includes intra- and interpersonal dimensions. There is such a scale, the Structural Analysis of Social Behavior (SASB) (Benjamin, 1993), which includes the complex planes of interpersonal (other and self) and intrapsychic functioning. To date, it has had limited exposure to group therapy. The second external rail, agreed-upon purpose, is uniquely social/emotional in therapy groups. For whatever reason—alienation in society, lack of skill building, and so on—the recent surge of self-help groups and the steady subscription to therapy groups attests to this emotional need. The group process instruments that clearly measure emotional components become essential. Some of the instruments attempt this (KPI, GSRS), but affect is not a predominant construct to be rated by many others.

It is not possible here to do justice to the elegance of the double helix; group process research lacks such elemental precision. The purpose is merely to illustrate the importance of a unifying structure in a dynamic entity—in this case, an intimately varied therapeutic process of interpersonal interaction in which humans come to learn and grow and change.

Concluding Comments

While interaction analysis holds promise for measuring complex, dynamical properties of the group, this review makes clear the persistent and remaining problems that plague its use. Such analysis demands great effort in time and resources, more so than other methodological approaches; many of us lack the means and commitment required to engage in continuous recording, transcribing, and coding. An examination of the existing instruments indicates a few viable measurement options covering limited areas of focus. The good news is that most of the recently developed measures are focused and oriented toward therapeutic populations, which ought to encourage clinicians in their attempts to understand the intra- and interpersonal processes occurring within their groups. The lack of instrument replication across varying populations, structures, and purposes creates large holes in our understanding of what is most effective and with whom; thus, we are left knowing less about the usefulness of the specific instrument. Many of the study findings relate to other dependent measures and fail to relate to the interactional instrument. Use of a process measure in conjunction with *multiple* variables would increase the probability of linking process with outcome, as well as discovering probable pairing variables (e.g., Beck et al., 1986). Additionally, this type of information could lend greater credence to the meaning and influence of the group as a whole.

All extant measures are category dependent so that even when capturing the dynamic properties of interpersonal responsiveness the significance is limited to the categorical definition. Overlaet's (1991) concern, the failure to capture the contextual meaning, is well taken. Missing here are the various perspectives on the same moment, event, or response. Most measures identify behaviors; few describe emotions, and none catalog the cognitive processes. The dynamic interplay of these three most likely overlies the dynamic interpersonal qualities of the group members. The lack of detail in various dimensions and across varying levels of functioning surely calls for increased interactional instrumentation capable of such measurement.

It is clear that the problems plaguing interaction analysis do not rest solely on the shoulders of the instruments themselves. Some problems relate to the design, some to the aggregation of data, some to ill-designed or poorly conceptualized constructs, some to inappropriate statistical strategies. It may be that at the point of design articulation we need to ask different questions such that the available methodology and techniques can be utilized, or alternatively, seek a different way to ask the questions of concern.

Still there are many reasons to be encouraged about the possibilities of utilizing interactional analysis to further our understanding of group process. Analysis stands positioned to measure the dynamic properties—those transitions, linkages, and bifurcations that may well contain the interpersonal mechanisms of change. The moving and transitional parts of the group can only be represented by a moment-by-moment analysis (i.e., that which accounts for time); hence the importance of having multiple measures capable of identifying a wide range of therapeutic themes.

At issue here is the construct of the group as a whole, an entity capable of changing and developing, capable of influencing individual members. Interactional analysis as a methodological tool can facilitate a greater understanding of the influential properties governing the group. It is by measuring the moment-by-moment process *over time* that group patterns become visible and reveal the workings of the entire group. This begs us to consider measuring not only representative segments of interpersonal functioning or therapeutic segments, but also the group in its entirety (See MacKenzie, Chapter 7). Although the available instruments are capable of such measurement, most studies rely on the analyses of relatively small periods of time. This then reduces their ability to make a statement regarding the viability of the group as a whole, or to determine which influential properties are driven by individuals (members or therapist), which by subgroups, or which by the total group. Without a moment-by-moment analysis, it is also difficult to determine if an influence results from cumulative, progressive, or singular actions. Finally, without a time-related measurement, it is nigh impossible to distinguish an organizing structure.

The complexity of the therapy group is marked by multiple and diverse players (individual biospheres accompanied by individual contexts), multiple levels of interaction (intrapersonal, dyadic, subgroup, group as a whole), multiple dimensions of responsiveness (cognitive, affective, behavioral) and, no less, manifold interests, concerns, and abilities. Add to this complexity the fact that the therapeutic process is interpersonal, interactive, and nonlinear, and that it is a living entity wherein changes in one part of the group (itself a biosphere) ultimately affect the whole (Wallace, 1987); it then becomes apparent that our attempts to define and eventually affect therapeutic processes must be attended by multidimensional instrumentation capable of assessing micro and macro and static and dynamic influences over time.

REFERENCES

Agazarian, Y. (1983). Some advantages of applying multidimensional thinking to the teaching, practice, and outcomes of group psychotherapy. *International Journal of Group Psychotherapy, 33*(2), 243–247.

Anchor, K. N. (1973). *Interaction processes in experimental massed and spaced group experiences.* Paper presented at Midwestern Psychological Association, Chicago, Illinois.

Bakeman, R., & Dabbs, J. M. (1976). Social interaction observed: Some approaches to the analysis of behavior streams. *Personality and Social Psychology Bulletin, 2*, 335–345.

Bales, R. F. (1950). *Interaction process analysis: A method for the study of small groups.* Cambridge, MA: Addison-Wesley.

Bales, R. F., Cohen, S. P., & Williams, S. A. (1979). *SYMLOG: A system for the multiple level observation of groups.* New York: Free Press.

Barlow, S. (1988). *Interaction analysis of leader/member communication styles in time-limited group psychotherapy.* Presented at the American Psychological Association, Atlanta, Georgia.

Barlow, S., Hansen, W., Fuhriman, A., & Finley, R. (1982). Effects of leader communication style on members of small groups. *Journal of Small Group Behavior, 13*(4), 518–531.

Beck, A. P. (1974). Phases in the development of structure in therapy and encounter groups. In D. A. Wexler & L. N. Rice (Eds.), *Innovations in client-centered therapy.* New York: Wiley.

Beck, A. P. (1983). A process analysis of group development. *Group, 7*(1), 19–26.

Beck, A. P. (1986). Developmental characteristics of the system-forming process. *Living groups: Group psychotherapy and general system theory.* New York: Brunner/Mazel, Inc.

Beck, A. P., Dugo, J. M., Eng, A. M., & Lewis, C. M. (1986). The search for phases in group development: Designing process analysis measures of group interaction. In L. S. Greenberg & W. M. Pinsof (Eds.), *The psychotherapeutic process: A research handbook.* New York: Guilford Press.

Beck, A. P., Dugo, J. M., Eng, A. M., Lewis, C. M., & Peters, L. N. (1983). The participation of leaders in the structural development of therapy groups. In R. R. Dies & K. R. MacKenzie (Eds.), *Advances in group psychotherapy: Integrating research and practice.* New York: International Universities Press.

Bednar, R. L., & Kaul, T. J. (1978). Experiential group research: Current perspective. In S. L. Garfield & A. E. Bergin (Eds.), *Handbook of psychotherapy and behavior change* (2nd ed.). New York: Wiley.

Bednar, R. L, & Lawlis, G. F. (1971). Empirical research in group psychotherapy. In S. L. Garfield & A. E. Bergin (Eds.), *Handbook of psychotherapy and behavior change.* New York: Wiley.

Benjamin, L. S. (1993). Interpersonal diagnosis and treatment of personality disorders. New York: Guilford Press.

Benne, K., & Sheats, P. (1948). Functional roles of group members. *Journal of Social Issues, 4*, 41–59.

Borgatta, E. F. (1963). A new systematic interaction observation system: Behavior scores system. *Journal of Psychological Studies, 14*, 24–44.

Carroll, J. D., & Chang, J. J. (1970). Analysis of individual differences in multidimensional scaling via an N-way generalization of Eckart-Young decomposition. *Psychometrika, 35*, 238–319.

Chapple, E. D. (1940). Measuring human relations: An introduction to the study of interaction of individuals. *Genetic Psychology Monographs, 22*, 3–147.

Chapple, E. D. (1949). The interaction chronograph: Its evolution and present application. *Personnel, 25,* 295–307.

Cooney, N. L., Kadden, R. M., Litt, M. D., & Getter, H. (1991). Matching alcoholics to coping skills or interactional therapies: Two-year follow-up results. *Journal of Consulting and Clinical Psychology, 59,* 598–601.

Cooper, C. (1977). Adverse and growthful effects of experimental learning groups: The role of the trainer, participant, and group characteristics. *Human Relationships, 30,* 1103–1129.

Cox, M. (1973). The group therapy interaction chronogram. *British Journal of Social Work, 3,* 243–256.

Crick, F. (1988). *What mad pursuit: A personal view of scientific discovery.* New York: Basic Books.

Couch, A. (1960). *Psychological determinants of interpersonal behavior.* Unpublished doctoral dissertation, Harvard University, Cambridge, MA.

Darrington, C. D. (1961) *Darwin's place in history.* New York: Macmillan.

DeStephen, R. S. (1983). High and low consensus groups: A content and relational interaction analysis. *Small Group Behavior, 14*(2), 143–162.

Dugo, J. M., & Beck, A. P. (1983). Tracking a group's focus on normative organizational or personal exploration issues. *Group, 7*(4), 17–26.

Dugo, J. M., & Beck, A. P (1984). A therapist's guide to issues of intimacy and hostility viewed as group-level phenomena. *International Journal of Psychotherapy, 34*(1), 25–45.

Ellis, D. G. (1976). *An analysis of relations communication in ongoing group systems.* Unpublished doctoral dissertation, University of Utah, Salt Lake City, Utah.

Fisher, B. A. (1976). *Social information processing analysis (SIPA).* Paper presented at International Communication Association, Portland, Oregon.

Fisher, B. A. (1980). *RELCOM research: Rationale and results.* Unpublished manuscript.

Friedlander, M. L., & Heatherington, L. (1989). Analyzing relational control in family therapy interviews. *Journal of Counseling Psychology, 36*(2), 139–148.

Friedlander, M. L., Thibodeau, J. R., Nichols, M. P., Tucker, C., & Snyder, J. (1985). Introducing semantic cohesion analysis: A study of group talk. *Small Group Behavior, 16*(3), 285–302.

Fuhriman, A., & Burlingame, G. M. (1989). *Hill Interaction Matrix: Therapy through dialogue.* Unpublished manuscript.

Fuhriman, A., Drescher, S., & Burlingame, G. M. (1984). Conceptualizing small group process. *Small Group Behavior, 15,* 427–440.

Fuhriman, A., & Packard, T. (1986). Group process instruments: Therapeutic themes and issues. *International Journal of Group Psychotherapy, 36*(3), 399–425.

Futoran, G. C., Kelly, J. R., & McGrath, J. E. (1989). TEMPO: A time-based system for analysis of group interaction process. *Basic and Applied Social Psychology, 10*(3), 211–232.

Gazda, G. M., & Mobley, J. A. (1980). INDSCAL multidimensional scaling: A technological breakthrough for group work. *Group Psychotherapy, Psychodrama, and Sociometry, 54,* 54–73.

Getter, H., Litt, M. D., Kadden, R. M., & Cooney, N. D. (1991). Measuring treatment process in coping skills and interactional group therapies for alcoholism. *International Journal of Group Psychotherapy, 42*(3), 419–430.

Gibbard, G. S., & Hartman, J. J. (1973). The oedipal paradigm in group development: A clinical and empirical study. *Small Group Behavior, 4,* 305–354.

Gottschalk, L. A., & Gleser, G. C. (1969). *The measurement of psychological states through the content analysis of verbal behavior.* Los Angeles, CA: University of California Press.

Greenberg, L. S. (1986). Research strategies. In L. S. Greenberg & W. M. Pinsof (Eds.), *The psychotherapeutic process: A research handbook* (pp. 707–734). New York: Guilford Press.

Greenberg, L. S., & Pinsof, W. M. (1986). Process research: Current trends and future perspectives. In L. S. Greenberg & W. M. Pinsof (Eds.), *The psychotherapeutic process: A research handbook* (pp. 3–20). New York: Guilford Press.

Greenway, J. D., & Greenway, P. (1985). Dimensions of interaction in psychotherapeutic groups: Sensitivity to rejection and dependency. *Small Group Behavior, 16*(2), 245–264.

Guttman, M. A. J. (1987). Verbal interactions of peer led group counseling. *Canadian Journal of Counseling, 21*(1), 49–58.

Hahlweg, K., Doane, J. A., Goldstein, M. J., Nuechterlein, K. H., Magana, A. B., Mintz, J., Miklowitz, D. J., & Snyder, K. S. (1989). Expressed emotion and patient-relative interaction in families of recent onset schizophrenics. *Journal of Consulting and Clinical Psychology, 57*(1), 11–18.

Halliday, M. A. K., & Hasan, R. (1976). *Cohesion in English.* London: Longman.

Hammonds, T. M., & Worthington, Jr., E. L. (1985). The effect of facilitator utterances on participant responses in a brief acme-type marriage enrichment group. *The American Journal of Family Therapy, 13*(2), 30–49.

Heatherington, L., & Allen, G. J. (1984). Sex and relational communication patterns in counseling. *Journal of Counseling Psychology, 3*(31), 287–294.

Heckel, R. V., Holmes, G. R., & Rosecrans, C. J. (1971). A factor analytic study of process variables in group therapy. *Journal of Clinical Psychology, 27,* 146–150.

Hill, W. F. (1965). *Hill Interaction Matrix.* Los Angeles, CA: University of Southern California.

Isaacson, R. M. (1977/1976). Development of the interpersonal skills interaction analysis: An interaction analysis technique to measure interpersonal communication skills in small group settings. *Dissertation Abstracts International, 37,* 570A.

Jarboe, S. (1991). Two multivariate methods for analyzing small group interaction: A data base comparison. *Small Group Research, 22*(4), 515–547.

Jurma, W. E., & Wright, B. C. (1990). Follower reactions to male and female leaders who maintain or lose reward power. *Small Group Research, 21*(1), 97–112.

Just, R. (1968). IBM 7040 program for content analysis. *Behavioral Science, 13,* 427.

Kanas, N., & Smith, A. J. (1990). Schizophrenic group process: A comparison and replication using the HIM-G. *Group, 14,* 246–252.

Karterud, S., & Foss, T. (1989). The group emotionality rating system: A modification of Thelen's method of assessing emotionality in groups. *Small Group Behavior, 20*(2), 131–150.

Kaul, T. J., & Bednar, R. D. (1986). Research on group and related therapies. In S. L. Garfield & A. E. Bergin (Eds.), *Handbook of psychotherapy and behavior change* (pp. 671–714). New York: Wiley.

Kelly, J. R., & McGrath, J. E. (1985). Effects of time limits and task types on task performance and interaction of four-person groups. *Journal of Personality and Social Psychology, 49*(2), 395–407.

Keyton, J., & Springston, J. (1990). Redefining cohesiveness in groups. *Small Group Research, 21*(2), 234–254.

Klein, M. H., Mathieu, P. L., Gendlin, E. T., & Kiesler, D. J. (1969). *The experiencing scale: A research and training manual.* Madison: Wisconsin Psychiatric Institute.

Kressel, N. J. (1987). SYMLOG and behavior therapy: Pathway to expanding horizons. *Small Group Behavior, 18*(3), 420–436.

Luborsky, L., Barber, J. P., & Crits-Christoph, P. (1990). Theory-based research for understanding the process of dynamic psychotherapy. *Journal of Consulting and Clinical Psychology, 58*(3), 281–287.

Lustig, M. W. (1987). Bale's interpersonal rating forms: Reliability and dimensionality. *Small Group Behavior, 18*(1), 99–107.

Mabry, E. A. (1985). The effects of gender composition and task structure on small group interaction. *Small Group Behavior, 16*(1), 75–96.

Mabry, E. A. (1989). Some theoretical implications of female and male interaction in unstructured small groups. *Small Group Behavior, 20*(4), 536–550.

Mabry, E. A., & Attridge, M. D. (1990). Small group interaction and outcome correlates for structured and unstructured tasks. *Small Group Research, 21*(3), 315–332.

Mann, R. D. (1967). *Interpersonal styles and group development.* New York: Wiley.

McCallum, M., & Piper, W. E. (1990). A controlled study of effectiveness and patient suitability for short-term group psychotherapy. *International Journal of Group Psychotherapy, 40*(4), 431–452.

McDermott, A. A. (1988). The effect of three group formats on group interaction patterns. *Occupational therapy in mental health* (pp. 69–89). Haworth Press.

Mills, T. (1964). *Group transformation.* Englewood Cliffs, NJ: Prentice-Hall.

Nichols, M. P., & Taylor, T. Y. (1975). Impact of therapist interventions on early sessions of group therapy. *Journal of Clinical Psychology, 31,* 726–729.

Noble, F., Ohlsen, M., & Proff, F. (1961). A method for the qualification of psychotherapeutic interaction in counseling groups. *Journal of Counseling Psychology, 8,* 54–61.

Ohlsen, M., & Pearson, R. (1965). A method for the classification of group interaction and its use to explore the influence of individual and role factors in group counseling. *Journal of Clinical Psychology, 21,* 436–441.

Overlaet, B. (1991). Interaction analysis: Meaningless in the face of relevance. *International Journal of Group Psychotherapy, 41*(3), 347–364.

Pace, R. C. (1990). Personalized and depersonalized conflict in small group discussions: An examination of differentiation. *Small Group Research, 21*(1), 79–96.

Page, R. C., Davis, K. C., Berkow, D. N., & O'Leary, E. (1989). Analysis of group process in marathon group therapy with users of illicit drugs. *Small Group Behavior, 20*(2), 220–227.

Page, R. C., & Wills, J. (1983). Marathon group counseling with illicit drug users: Analysis of content. *Journal for Specialists in Group Work, 15*(4), 67–75.

Peterson, J. P., & Pollio, H. R. (1982). Therapeutic effectiveness of differentially targeted humorous remarks in group psychotherapy. *Group, 6*(4), 39–50.

Piper, W. E., Debbane, E. G., de Carufel, F. L., & Beinvenu, J. P. (1987). A system for differentiating therapist interpretations for other interventions. *Bulletin of the Menninger Clinic, 51*(6), 532–550.

Piper, W. E., & McCallum, M. (1992). *Psychodynamic work and object rating system.* Unpublished manuscript, University of Alberta, Canada.

Piper, W. E., McCallum, M., & Azim, H. F. A. (1992). *Adaptation to loss through short-term group psychotherapy.* New York: Guilford Press.

Polley, R. B. (1987). The dimensions of social interaction: A method for improving rating scales. *Social Psychology Quarterly, 50*(1), 72–82.

Polley, R. B. (1991). Group process as diagnostic: An introduction. *Small Group Research, 22*(1), 92–98.

Reisel, J. (1959). *A search for behavior patterns.* Unpublished doctoral dissertation, University of California at Los Angeles, CA.

Rice, L. N., & Greenberg, L. S. (1984). *Patterns of change.* New York: Guilford Press.

Rorer, B., & Tucker, C. M. (1988). Long-term nurse-patient interactions: Factors in patient compliance or noncompliance to the dietary regimen. *Health Psychology, 7*(1), 35–46.

Ruback, R. B., Dabbs, J. M., Jr., & Hopper, C. H. (1984). The process of brainstorming: An analysis with individual and group vocal parameter. *Journal of Personality and Social Psychology, 47*(3), 558–567.

Rugel, R. P., & Meyer, D. J. (1984). The tavistock group: Empirical findings and implications for group therapy. *Small Group Behavior, 15*(3), 361–374.

Scheflen, A. (1969). Templates, blueprints and programs on human behavior. In W. Gray, F. J. Duhl, & N. D. Rizzo (Eds.), *General systems theory and psychiatry.* Boston, MA: Little, Brown.

Scheflen, A. (1974). *How behavior means.* Garden City, NY: Anchor Press.

Seibert, S., & Gruenfeld, L. (1992). Masculinity, femininity, and behavior in groups. *Small Group Research, 23,* 95–112.

Sprouse, C. L., & Brush, D. H. (1980). Assessment of interpersonal perception: Assessing a quasi-therapy group by individual differences multidimensional scaling. *Small Group Behavior, 11*(1), 35–49.

Stein, A., & Kibel, H. D. (1984). A group dynamic-peer interaction approach to group psychotherapy. *International Journal of Group Psychotherapy, 34*(3), 315–333.

Stockton, R., Robison, F. F., & Morran, D. K. (1983). A comparison of the HIM-B with the Hill Interaction Matrix model of group interaction styles: A factor analytic study. *Journal of Group Psychotherapy, Psychodrama, and Sociometry, 36*(3), 102–113.

Stone, P. J., Dunphy, D., Smith, M.S., & Ogilvie, D. M. (1966). *The general inquirer: A computer approach to content analysis.* Cambridge, MA: MIT Press.

Talaro, K., & Talaro, A. (1993). *Foundations in Microbiology.* Dubuque, IA: Brown.

Toseland, R. W., Rossiter, C. M., Peak, T., & Hill, P. (1990). Therapeutic processes in peer led and professionally led support groups for caregivers. *International Journal of Group Psychotherapy, 40*(3), 279–303.

Tracey, T. J., & Guinee, J. P. (1990). Generalizability of interpersonal communications rating scale ratings across presentation modes. *Journal of Counseling Psychology, 37*(3), 330–336.

Trujillo, N. (1986). Toward a taxonomy of small group interaction-coding systems. *Small Group Behavior, 17*(4), 371–394.

Tschuschke, V. (1986). Relationships between psychological and psychophysiological variables in group therapeutic setting. *International Journal of Group Psychotherapy, 36*(2), 305–312.

Tschuschke, V., & MacKenzie, K. R. (1989). Empirical analysis of group development: A methodological report. *Small Group Behavior, 20*(4), 419–427.

Vogel, P. A. (1977). The development of a social integration measure (SIM) based on peer ratings for the study of small group process. *Dissertation Abstracts International, 37,* 5384B–5385B.

Wallace, D. R. (1987). *Life in balance.* San Diego, CA: Harcourt Brace Jovanovich.

Watson, P. J. (1970). A repertory grid method of studying groups. *British Journal of Psychiatry, 117,* 309–318.

CHAPTER 7

Group Development

K. ROY MACKENZIE

The concept of time pervades and perhaps drives the discussion herein of group development. The idea of development implies change over time, while arrested development suggests a discontinuity between actual and expected temporal change. Historically, time has been discounted in psychotherapy and psychotherapy research. Treatment continues until change occurs, often even in the absence of change. Only recently has there been an increased emphasis on the value of time-limited group psychotherapy, a conscious effort to manipulate the time variable as a method for promoting therapeutic work (MacKenzie, 1990). A thoughtful discussion of the philosophy of time and its implications for psychotherapy research is provided by McGrath and Kelly (1986). To quote from their introduction:

> Questions about the relations among time, motion, and change are both ancient and basic. Long ago, Heraclitus proffered the radical view that flux and motion and change are fundamental, whereas matter and structure and stability are illusion. That view was rejected by Democritus and other early Greeks in favor of a view in which matter and structure and stability were fundamental and fixed, whereas change was ephemeral and/or illusory. The latter view was favored by Aristotle, who was the channel for the major influence of Greek philosophy on the West. (p. 20)

Group development will be reviewed from three perspectives. First, major trends in the group development literature up to the mid-1960s will be detailed, emphasizing social psychology's underlying concepts with passing reference to specific studies. The intention behind this approach is to outline the major organizing theories that have guided research strategies. Without such higher order conceptualizations, the results of individual studies lack explanatory power. The findings of any given study must be placed in the context of a complex set of inter-related phenomena. For example, group process measures must be seen in the light of group composition, leadership style, goals of the experience, and outcome criteria. The actual formal research data base during this early period is relatively small. As might be expected in the early stages of a field of enquiry, many reports are based on informal observational impressions, with a greater reliance on theoretical concepts than on empirical data. Next follows a review of the decade through to the mid-1970s, during which time there was a major focus on process oriented studies largely based on self-analytic training groups. This material views groups as complex systems in which the designated leader and group members fulfilling role functions influence the development of the group. The theoretical background to this work is more abstract and draws heavily on psychoanalytic concepts. Third, a diverse set of research strategies are discussed, all having some relationship to how the development of a group might be conceptualized. This provides an overview of major themes and techniques that need to be considered in understanding the complexity of the small group. A final summary attempts to put this material into an integrated conceptual map of critical group processes.

ORIGINAL THEORIES OF GROUP DEVELOPMENT 1900–1965

Ideas about the way groups develop emerged as one component of the social psychology literature concerning small group dynamics. While interest in these topics goes back to the turn of the century (Cooley, 1909; Freud, 1921; LeBon, 1896; McDougall, 1920; Simmel, 1902), the first major formal studies stemmed from the work of Kurt Lewin. A second wave of original ideas came from Gordon Allport, Henry A. Murray, and Robert F. Bales who trained several generations of social scientists. The ideas of the British psychoanalyst Wilfred Bion were the basis for a major contribution from the University of Chicago under the direction of Herbert Thelen. Bennis and Shepard provided an early view of group development in psychoanalytically oriented groups. Tuckman's review (1965) pulls together much of this work and is used here as a marker of the end of the first wave of conceptualization concerning group development.

What Is a Group and What Is Group Development?

There is an intuitive appeal to the notion of the group. An appreciation of the social environment is part of our mammalian heritage and most of the basic dimensions reported in this chapter can be found in studies of higher primates as well (MacKenzie & Kennedy, 1991; Smuts, Cheney, Seyfarth, Wrangham, & Struhsaker, 1987). Participants in social groups as well as psychotherapy groups are willing to describe how they change over time without perhaps recognizing that the idea of "group" involves a conceptual shift to a higher order of structure.

For Cooley (1909/1968), the primary group "is characterized by intimate face-to-face association and cooperation. They (groups) are primary in several senses, but chiefly in that they are fundamental in forming the social nature and ideas of the individual. The result of intimate association, psychologically, is a certain fusion of individualities in a common whole, so that one's very self, for many purposes at least, is the common life and purpose of the group. Perhaps the simplest way of describing this wholeness is by saying that it is a "we" . . . One lives in the feeling of the whole and finds the chief aims of his will in that feeling" (p. 89). Cartwright and Zander (1960) state, "A group is a collection of individuals sharing a common goal who have relationships to one another that make them interdependent to some significant degree" (p. 46). Broom and Selznik (1968) consider a group to be "any collection of persons who are *bound together* by a distinctive set of social relations" (p. 30).

The idea of group development is intertwined with the nature of the history of the group and the passage of time. Krayer and Fiechtner (1984) describe the mature group as one that is able to function independently of its leader, is active and organized, brings an extended time perspective to its activities, and has an established working history. One recent review (Mennecke, Hoffer, & Wynne, 1992) describes group development in terms of "the degree of maturity and cohesion that a group achieves over time as members interact, learn about one another, and structure relationships and roles within the group." This definition provides some indication of the difficulty in capturing the nature of group development. What is a "mature" group? Can groups develop in the absence of "cohesion"? What is "cohesion"? Does "learning about each other" necessarily lead to a developed group?

A central definitional issue concerns the way in which one understands the purpose of the group. The laboratory approach to studying small groups tends to measure group development in terms of how well the assigned task of the group is addressed. For example, a group may need to solve a puzzle or design a solution to a complex situation. The measure of success is how well the objective is achieved, perhaps by elapsed time or by the complexity of the conclusions. That is, the group is judged in a global manner by its external output. In clinical studies, it is more common to judge a group by the outcome changes of each member. The sum of these then becomes a measure of how effective the group has been, for example, 6 of the 8 members are asymptomatic at the first follow-up visit. These two approaches are based on quite different assumptions about success: the group system versus the state of each member. The most specific question regarding a therapy group would be: Does a group that develops properly produce more change in its members than one that fails to develop?

This question of judging by output or by internal characteristics is particularly pertinent to the study of psychotherapy or training groups. The "output" from these types of groups is often defined in terms of the quality of the process of the group itself. The task of the group is stated to be a study of the group itself, or of one's behavior in the group. Indeed, it would be fair to say that historically psychotherapy research has been hampered by a disinclination to utilize objective measures of outcome. Therapists have tended to note impressionistic evaluations of subtle changes in interactional process. The assumption is made that these are then automatically translated into parallel changes in external adaptation. This question has direct relevance to the idea of group development. There is an implicit expectation that effective group development will allow the group to address its task more successfully. If that task is difficult to define, then one is left with no criteria by which to judge effective development. It presumably can be accepted that not all groups develop in a satisfactory manner. Outcome criteria seem essential for identifying enhancing versus retarding group developmental features.

Early Contributors

Kurt Lewin

Kurt Lewin, a German psychologist, moved to America in the early 1930s and eventually settled at the University of Michigan where he formed the Research Center for Group Dynamics. He and his graduate students had a profound effect on the field of social psychology (Lewin, 1947). He was also instrumental in the development of the National Training Laboratories in Bethel, Maine, where the concept of the T-group originated. The idea behind these training experiences was to provide a social field where individuals could explore their definition of self, not by a restatement of old roles, but in the reality of their current interaction. He drew upon Moreno's idea of the importance of the "moment" as well as the use of sociometric measures (Moreno, 1931). Lewin developed a "field theory" of small group functioning that is a precursor to general systems theory, an orientation that is further developed later in this chapter. Because Lewin's ideas are so seminal, he is quoted at some length here:

> A basic tool for the analysis of group life is the representation of the group and its setting as a "social field." This means that the social happening is viewed as occurring in, and being the result of, a totality of coexisting social entities, such as groups, subgroups, members, barriers, channels of communication, etc. One of the fundamental characteristics of this field is the relative position of the entities, which are parts of the field. This relative position represents the structure of the group and its ecological setting. It expresses also the basic possibilities of locomotion within the field.
>
> What happens within such a field depends upon the distribution of forces throughout the field. A prediction presupposes the ability to determine for the various points of the field the strength and directions of the resultant forces.
>
> According to general field theory the solution of a problem of group life has always to be finally based on an analytical procedure of this type. Only by considering the groups in question in their actual setting, can we be sure

that none of the essential possible conduct has been overlooked. (Lewin, 1947, p. 14)

Some of Lewin's most enduring work was concerned with the effect of group leadership on the social atmosphere of the group (Lewin, Lippitt, & White, 1939). He found, for example, that autocratic leadership resulted in either higher or lower levels of aggression in the group, depending upon the degree of control exerted by the leader. This resulted in either an atmosphere of aggressive autocracy or of apathetic autocracy, both characterized by low levels of "we-feeling" amongst the members. He found that the nature of dominating behavior would change for the same individual depending upon whether he was in low or high autocratic group environment. Within these studies, the role of the "scapegoat" was described as an interaction of both social environmental and personal characteristics of the individual. Lewin did not study group development per se, but inherent in his work is an appreciation of how the context of the group, the role of the leader, and the characteristics of the individual member must be considered as interacting variables in a complex interactive field of influences.

Robert F. Bales

Robert F. Bales is another important early influence in the field of group studies. Much of his work was based on the detailed analysis of groups run as problem solving laboratory exercises in the Department of Social Relations at Harvard University. Bales (1950) developed a system, Interactional Process Analysis, for analyzing interaction that consisted of 12 categories organized into four areas shown in Table 7.1. The four categories can be further consolidated into Task Functions (Attempted Answers and Questions) and Socioemotional Functions (Positive and Negative Reactions). Other terms describing the same phenomena are "Instrumental" and "Expressive" functions.

TABLE 7.1. Interaction Process Analysis (IPA) (Bales, 1950)

A. Positive reactions	1. Shows solidarity
	2. Shows tension release
	3. Agrees
B. Attempted answers	4. Gives suggestion
	5. Gives opinion
	6. Gives orientation
C. Questions	7. Asks for orientation
	8. Asks for opinion
	9. Asks for suggestion
D. Negative reactions	10. Disagrees
	11. Shows tension
	12. Shows antagonism

A series of publications (Bales, 1950; 1953; 1970; Bales, Cohen, & Williamson, 1980; Bales & Slater, 1955) has documented a recurring cyclical pattern in small groups. Instrumental functions apply to activities that are oriented toward the assigned task. Expressive functions deal with the management of emotional tension. These two functions tend to alternate over time. As a group works on its task, intermember process tensions build up. These begin to interfere with the task focus unless they are dispelled by socioemotional activity. Following this, the group can return again to its task focus. Bales also identified the importance of group members who functioned as leaders in promoting these two functions, called respectively the task leaders and the socioemotional leaders. The way a group achieves a resolution to this "equilibrium problem," the balance between task and socioemotional functions, is a critical characteristic of any group system. The oscillation between the two will occur in all group settings but with varying ratios.

Bales was working primarily with groups that had a clear task focus. Socioemotional activity was seen as a necessary process to clear the air for this task purpose. In itself, this body of work does not describe group development. The equilibrium balance is a micro pattern that would be expected to be found in all stages of group development.

Bales and Strodbeck (1951) also demonstrated that in single sessions there tends to be consistent patterns of group development (Figure 7.1). Using his 12 category system to code interaction acts, he found that Acts of Information Giving are highest at the beginning and steadily fall during the session. Acts of Suggestion Giving steadily rise throughout the session. Both

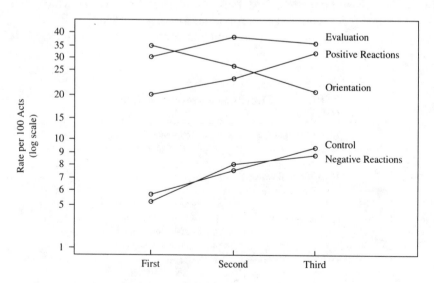

Figure 7.1. Three phases of group development (Bales & Strodbeck, 1951).

Positive and Negative reactions rise throughout the session. Acts of Opinion Giving are highest during the middle of the session. The rates of Negative reactions tend to be higher in response to Suggestion Giving. Groups reach a "decision point" when the problems of the task are resolved. Following this, the group devotes more time to socioemotional issues. These phenomena are summarized as demonstrating a progression through three phases: an initial phase primarily concerned with *orientation* of the members through Information Giving, followed by a phase of *evaluation* of the information, and concluding with a phase of decision making that involves more *control* processes with support for the opinions of some members and rejection of others.

Heinicke and Bales (1953) also studied, with the same methodology, groups meeting for a series of four sessions. The amount of time spent in task-related behavior gradually diminishes over the four sessions. Positive socioemotional behavior involving solidarity and tension release increases, especially in the last two sessions. At the same time, Showing Agreement decreases over the sessions. Negative socioemotional behavior is markedly higher in the second session in association with a status struggle to establish a dominance hierarchy among the members. Following that event, the interaction shows higher levels of group solidarity and emotionality, but without the need for agreement. These patterns are more strongly revealed in groups that have a high level of consensus about status issues. In those groups where there is ongoing disagreement about the status levels of the participants, more time has to be spent on resolving socioemotional tension, so that there is lower efficiency and lower satisfaction from the experience.

These findings of Bales and his colleagues are described in some detail because they serve as a starting point for most studies of small groups and the basic patterns emerge in many different types of groups. The sequence of *orientation* where there is a need to get information, followed by *evaluation* of this information with the expression of different opinions, and then a pressure for a decision in which there is a struggle for *control* of that process is fundamental to an evaluation of group development. Bales' recognition of the importance of the group roles of task and socioemotional leadership links group development to the characteristics of the members. It deepens the understanding of the relationship between the individual and the group that was first identified by Lewin. The two theoretical approaches of group development and group roles have formed the principal axes for understanding group level process. For the laboratory groups being studied by Bales, the task is clearly defined. In psychotherapy and training groups the task is internal to the group and its members. In some ways, socioemotional activity *is* the task. For task groups, socioemotional activities are a necessary adjunctive process to help address the task. In therapy groups, where the task is less clearly defined, the time spent on socioemotional problems is necessarily higher and at the same time more directly relevant to the purpose of the group.

Wilfred Bion

Wilfred Bion, a British psychoanalyst, stimulated a major theoretical shift in group understanding through a series of articles written between 1943 and 1952 which were eventually published as a book, "Experiences in Groups" (1961). His work is associated with the term "group-as-a-whole" school. Bion considered a group to be in either a "working" state or one of a variety of 'basic assumption' states. A working group has a clear idea of its tasks and is able to test rationally whether or not it is accomplishing these. The structure of the group is designed to facilitate cooperative task accomplishment and various members become active in fulfilling helpful leadership tasks. This "work group" atmosphere may be interrupted by "basic assumption" states in which primitive drives and reactions prevent the group from maintaining its task relevant activities.

The phrase "basic assumption" describes a collective reaction of the members; it appears 'as if' the members had arrived at some implicit understanding regarding the group's major problem at a given point in time. Bion describes three "basic assumption" states which he considers to be evidence that the group members are avoiding individual responsibility for therapeutic progress. An analogy may be drawn between "basic assumption" phenomena in the group and resistance in individual therapy.

Basic Assumption Dependency: The group acts as though it can only function effectively if a superior and wise person can be found who will lead it. Not surprisingly, the designated leader is often seen as the appropriate source of such leadership. Group members in this state behave "as if" they were helpless to direct their activities and instead address their problems from a position of passivity.

Basic Assumption Fight/Flight: Here the group clusters together "as if" threatened by a dangerous force. The language of the group centers around themes of threat and the need to defend itself or escape. There may be accusations about outside forces which are the locus of difficulty. Alternatively, individual members may be identified as the source of the group's problems. Such groups may experience rapid alterations between themes of fear and themes of revenge. The group may turn on the group leader for his failure to resolve issues and provide answers. A strong and absolute leader is sought.

Basic Assumption Pairing: This is the most obtuse of Bion's descriptions. The group is preoccupied with issues concerning two of its members and acts 'as if' a resolution of the problems presented by this pair would be of therapeutic value to the entire group. This may have a voyeuristic quality with sexual overtones. As in the other two "basic assumption" states, the responsibility for direction is displaced from the individual member to another source.

Bion attempts to apply a psychoanalytic point of view in which the group is regarded as a quasi-individual with its own "group mentality." This mentality consists of disavowed dependent, hostile, or shameful parts that the individual members project into the collective space of the group; each member resonates to this central theme according to personal predisposition. There will be varying degrees of "valency" in the eagerness of members to respond to a given "basic assumption" state. The group will seek out and pressure those members most in harmony with the theme to serve as leaders. Thus a member with a tendency to use projective defenses might be seen as a potential leader during "basic assumption Fight/Flight" states.

The descriptions of the "basic assumption" states vividly portray common group experiences. They are useful as a signal that a group is moving away from productive work into a resistant or regressed position. They do not provide an adequate general theory of group functioning. The assumption that all members of the group are preoccupied with the same defensive posture seems unrealistic. Nonetheless, Bion's descriptions draw attention to the power of the group to influence the emotional responses of the members, particularly under adverse circumstances. This idea of the group as an amplifier of emotion is a useful core conceptualization.

Bion himself did not accept that his 'basic assumption' states referred to developmental phenomena in a group. He saw an oscillation between work and basic assumption states as occurring in relationship to individual predispositions manifested in the group when the members are at a given point in time aligned around similar themes. The tension between work and basic assumption activity was clearly seen by Bion as a struggle that is never ending. The issues always require the need to be identified and addressed. In some ways, this is a slightly larger version of Bales' oscillation between task and socioemotional activities.

Herbert Thelen

Thelen and his colleagues at the University of Chicago (Martin & Hill, 1957; Stock & Thelen, 1958; Thelen, 1954; Whitaker & Lieberman, 1964; Whitman & Stock, 1958) developed a set of observational categories that had some elements drawn from Bales and others from Bion. They maintained Bales' division between instrumental and expressive functions and added categories related to "work" and "basic assumption" states. Rather than rating individual acts, they rated "natural units" of group interaction that were 3 to 18 minutes in length. Each unit was rated on both instrumental and expressive dimensions (Table 7.2).

The descriptions of Dependency, Fight/Flight, and Pairing appear to be parallel to group developmental stage descriptions of Engagement, Conflict, and Intimacy. However, Thelen and his coworkers were not able to detect systematically recurring sequences that would fit a developmental model. They raised the question rather that as each type of "group culture" arose over time, it might be managed by the group with increasing levels of maturity. They considered the group always to be showing a combination of work and basic assumption characteristics, with the balance between them moving more toward work with the passage of time. For example, a group in

TABLE 7.2.   Adaptation of Bion's Category System (Stock & Thelen, 1958)

A. The quality of work expressed; every statement receives one of four work ratings:

   1. Level of work is personally need-oriented and unrelated to group work.

   2. Level of work is maintaining or routine in character. It may involve attempting to define a task, searching for methodology, clarifying already established plans, and the like.

   3. Level of work is group-focused work that introduces some new ingredient; active problem solving.

   4. Level of work is highly creative, insightful, and integrative. It often interprets what has been going on in the group and brings together in a meaningful way a series of experiences.

B. The character of emotionality expressed: a statement may contain no detectable affect. If it does, the affect is placed in one of the following emotional categories:

   Fight (F): expressions of hostility and aggression.

   Flight (Fl): expressions of avoidance of the problem or withdrawal from participation.

   Pairing (P): expressions of warmth, intimacy, and supportiveness.

   Dependency (D): expressions of reliance on some person or thing external to the membership.

   E: This category is reserved for the relatively few statements in which some affect is clearly present but is too confused or diffuse to be placed in any one or any combination of the above categories.

a dependency culture may, at an early point in the group, be quite distracted from its task for some time. At a later time, dependency issues might be integrated with the work task. This idea of deepening levels anticipates the discussion in the third section of this chapter concerning personal construct changes. The work of the Chicago group incorporated role and sociometric considerations. They saw the manner in which the individual connected to a given group culture to be an expression of internal patterns of needs and associated conflicts. Thus, each type of group culture would elicit a predictable response from each of the group members. Members would express a sociometric preference for other group members with the same predisposition, that is, would feel "closer" to them. Some would find themselves drawn into the role of leader within a given particular culture while others would not be highly polarized on it. This provided an operational definition of what Bion had termed "valency" or predisposition to activation on a particular dynamic theme. Stock and Thelen (1958) used the triangle of conflict as a way of conceptualizing subgroups polarized around a common theme.

Bennis and Shepard

Bennis and Shepard (1956) presented the first detailed account of group development in longer term psychodynamically oriented training groups lasting about 17 sessions. Like Thelen, these investigators incorporated concepts drawn from the psychoanalytic tradition (Bion, 1961; Freud, 1921; Schein & Bennis, 1965). Their conceptualization of development centered around how the group addressed the problems of dependence and interdependence; power and love; authority and intimacy. From the standpoint of the group members, this involves working out how they would relate to authority in the person of the group leader, and how they would relate to their peers in the form of the other group members. The unstructured nature of human relations training groups allowed these issues to be played out without the usual constraints of social expectations and prescribed behaviors.

From a study of thematic developments in these groups, a developmental model evolved based on two phases, each with three subphases. Phase 1 deals with Dependence and Power Relations, with the subphases of Dependence-Submission, Counterdependence, and Resolution. Phase 2 shifts to issues of Interdependence and Personal Relations, with subphases of Enchantment, Disenchantment, and finally Consensual Validation. The transition from Phase 1 to 2 also is reflected in a shift from seeing other members in stereotypic role terms to understanding them as individual personalities, and a shift from focusing on group-related issues to individual-related concerns.

Bennis and Shepard (1956) speak of the group becoming split into polarized subgroups around these themes; some members for example, cling to their need to depend on the leader while others are pushing for independence and autonomy. This connects their work to that of Thelen who captured a similar dynamic through the idea of the triangle of conflict. Bennis and Shepard's stages can be aligned with a general model of group development, but their emphasis on a recurring cycle of polarization sets them somewhat apart. These authors are primarily theoreticians with considerable clinical experience, but have limited empirical data to support their model of development.

Other early contributions are found in the work of Schutz and Tuckman. W. C. Schutz (1958) developed his approach to group development by extrapolating ideas from the individual literature concerning basic human needs. He defined these as the needs for inclusion, control, and affection. He saw the early group being concerned with problems of how to become included, with individual members ranged along a continuum from wanting to be the center of attention to wanting to be quite isolated. The thematic focus then shifts to issues of wanting to be in control of others, or of wanting to be controlled by them. Having mastered these problems, the group then moves on to issues of how to deal with affection for others and a desire to be liked. Schutz suggests that groups may recycle through these three stages but will always do so in the same order. Finally, and in this he departs from all other theorists, the cycle is reversed at the end of the group so that the final three stages are dealing first with affection in the context of terminating relationships with other members, followed by releasing control/dependence bonds and finally relinquishing the sense of inclusion in the group. His three areas of interpersonal need reflect a psychoanalytic orientation. Schutz' ideas are reflected in much of the group developmental literature, although he himself did not present empirical findings to support his model.

Other authors have described group development in psychoanalytically derived terms purposefully selected as parallels to individual development (Kaplan & Roman, 1963; Saravay, 1978). Implicit in this approach is the idea that the individual members will relate to particular stages of group development in accordance with their own level of psychosexual development. The sequence is generally parallel to Erikson's progression from trust to autonomy to initiative. This work, while based on clinical observation of groups, is not grounded in empirical measures.

Tuckman (1965) provided a major review of the literature citing over 50 articles concerning group development drawn from a variety of types of groups: therapy groups, training groups, and natural or laboratory groups. He derived a common set of stages that recurred within these studies and then tested each study against this standard list. There was a generally good fit, although the exact terminology varied. The studies in the therapy and training categories most relevant for our purposes were, with few exceptions, based on observations made by clinicians and did not employ formalized measurement techniques. The only papers that stemmed from a consistent empirical study program were found in the laboratory group category.

Tuckman's classification perpetuated Bales' division of task and socioemotional functions although he acknowledges that in therapy and training groups there is a 'fuzzy' distinction between them. In his stage descriptions, he attempts to differentiate the members' "reactions to others as elements of the group task versus the reaction to others as social entities" (p. 386) (Table 7.3). In a later publication, Tuckman and Jensen (1977) added a final stage of adjournment. Garland, Jones, and Kolodny (1965), writing about the same time, outlined a schema for group development directly parallel to that presented by Tuckman, using the terms: pre-affiliation, power/control, intimacy, differentiation, and termination/separation.

Tuckman's paper can be seen as an important summary of a rather scattered field of enquiry. He raised questions regarding the effects on group development of group composition, time duration, and the nature of the task. However his data base did not permit any informed comment on such issues. Tuckman's paper can be seen as a summary of an existing belief system more than an empirically supported scientific tradition.

TABLE 7.3.   Stages of Group Development (Tuckman, 1965)

Stage	Task Activity	Group Structure
Stage 1: Forming	Orientation and testing	Testing and dependence
Stage 2: Storming	Emotional response to task demands	Intragroup conflict
Stage 3: Norming	Discussing oneself and other group members	Development of group cohesion
Stage 4: Performing	Emergence of insight	Functional role-relatedness

A number of important issues have been introduced by these various theorists, most of which will re-emerge in various forms in the more recent literature. These include, in addition to the idea of group development, the concept of recurring cyclic phenomena, role specialists who are characterologically well adapted for their roles, and the influence of the designated leader in shaping group norms and group climate. The power of the group to mould attitudes, including the sense of losing part of one's self in the group, the concept of group cohesion, and members learning about the nature of their group relationships have also been noted. Finally, a certain common shape has been detected in how groups move during the course of an hour and over the course of several meetings.

Much of the empirical literature concerning group development reviewed above is drawn from studies of artificially created small groups. Many of these groups are of quite short duration, often only 1 or 2 hours, and many are structured around specific group task challenges such as solving a puzzle. While some general ideas and principles might be derived from this work, the application to psychotherapy groups is somewhat problematic. Thus, the continuing overview of the small group literature concentrates in more detail on studies involving psychotherapy and experiential training groups that are more representative of clinical work.

Psychodynamic Group Psychology

In the mid 1960s, a series of studies were undertaken by a network of social psychologists who had trained under Bales (Dunphy, 1972; Gibbard & Hartman, 1973; Mann, Gibbard, & Hartman, 1967; Mills, 1964; 1978). These investigations were conducted primarily on student 'self-analytic' groups originally developed by Bales for the Harvard Social Relations 120 Course and replicated at the University of Michigan. These were large groups of 20–30 students that met from 1 to 3 times a week for a minimum of 40 sessions to a maximum of an entire academic year. The sessions were recorded for later text analysis. The atmosphere in these groups was somewhat like that of a T-group or sensitivity group. Indeed, many of these authors had connections with the National Training Laboratories. The role of the leader in these groups was relatively inactive and thus deprived the group of clear direction. The task of the group was to understand its own process, the format being much closer to the environment of a psychotherapy group than most of the group formats earlier reported. This group of investigators focused on translating psychodynamic principles into measurable dimensions.

Gibbard, Hartman, and Mann (1974), in summarizing a decade of work regarding the processes of self-analytic groups, provides a most provocative addition to the established literature of the time: the focus on boundary functioning. They built upon Slater's (1966) idea that the central issue driving group process is the individual member's continuing concern about how to resolve the dilemma of wanting to merge with the group versus wanting to retain an autonomous individuality. For Bales (1950), the equilibrium tension was polarized around a rational attention to the task versus the necessity of dealing with rising interpersonal emotional tension. To Gibbard and colleagues, the issues reflected a tension between powerful immature reactions to the desire/fear of merging with the group and the assigned task of understanding the process. To investigate these hypotheses, two scoring systems were utilized, each of which was able to achieve modest inter-rater reliability despite the abstract nature of the dimensions. Mills (1964) developed Sign Process Analysis which rated positive, negative, and neutral references to internal and external objects. This provided a content free measure of boundary maintenance. Mann (1966; with Gibbard & Hartman, 1973) created the Member-Leader Scoring System (Table 7.4) to describe the relationship between the leader and the members and between the members themselves. This system is based on Klein's (1948) distinction between the paranoid and depressive positions and Bibring's (1954) understanding of ego-states. The three ego state "expressing" measures, when plotted over time, showed peaks of distress characterized by one or more of the ego states.

Hartman and Gibbard (1974) describe a four stage model of group development. The first phase is centered around the leader who is endowed with both good and bad qualities. This culminates in a revolt against the leader, a process accompanied by rising evidence of distress. This phase is followed by "a process of assimilation, and inclusion, with boundaries becoming

TABLE 7.4. Process Analysis Scoring System (Gibbard & Hartman, 1973) (Based on Mann, 1966)

Category	Subarea	Area
1. Moving against	Hostility	Impulse
2. Disagreeing		
3. Withdrawing		
4. Guilt-inducing		
5. Making reparation	Affection	
6. Identifying		
7. Agreeing		
8. Moving toward		
9. Showing submission		Power relations
10. Showing equality		
11. Showing dominance		
12. Expressing anxiety	Anxiety	Ego state
13. Denying anxiety		
14. Expressing depression	Depression	
15. Denying depression		
16. Expressing guilt	Guilt	
17. Denying guilt		
18. Expressing self-esteem	Self-esteem	

relatively permeable to assimilate all members and ideas which are endowed with goodness in the creation of this utopia" (p. 173). Again distress levels rise as the group begins to address the third phase which is characterized by competition and sexual rivalry. Here there is again a focus on internal distinctions, exclusions, and boundary transformations. The final phase deals with the dissolution of group boundaries also associated with evidence of distress. The underlying group processes were seen to be a progression that begins with the group's efforts to establish indigenous norms through a sequence of giving up external norms, going through a period of relative normlessness, until an internally derived set of new norms was in place.

These phase developments are largely in keeping with Tuckman's sequence. The principal difference lies in the first phase. The Gibbard data did not reveal an initial bland phase characterized by attempts to establish commonalities, although there is a suggestion that this process might be found in a subtheme of the idealized "good group." These authors are more concerned with the recurring issues of self (differentiation, autonomy) versus group (we-ness, groupness). They suggest that group structure is determined by mechanisms that are reminiscent of early object relations processes of introjection and projection that are used to bind negative affects. Ego state distress is likely to emerge at those times when the equilibrium between inclusive and exclusive processes is breaking down. They thus serve as "marker variables" that mobilize efforts to find a group solution. The evolving group structure may therefore be conceptualized as a combination of primitive pre-Oedipal mechanisms involving the group-as-a-whole, combined with Oedipal competitive struggles centered around the person of the therapist.

These same authors offer a detailed consideration of the importance of group roles. The concept of group roles places them at the boundary between the needs of the group for a particular style of leadership, and the capacities of the individual members for performing that function. The result of this tension is the emergence of particular individuals who come to represent for the group the source of that type of group input. It is suggested that roles emerge more quickly and forcefully when the group is left without strong direction from the designated leader. This might be seen as one response to the fear of becoming overwhelmed by the group without the safety provided by a leader who is in clear control.

The ideas of this group of investigators have been discussed at length because they set new standards in applying psychodynamic concepts to understand group development. Their measures are complex but workable. Nonetheless, the body of their work, while stimulating, must be seen as preliminary in terms of empirical evidence. Their focus on the boundary issues of fusion and differentiation between the individual and the group must be accounted for in any comprehensive model of group functioning.

Martin and Hill (1957) describe a six stage group development system. A study of two groups composed of delinquent boys (Hill & Gruner, 1973) utilized the Hill Interactional Matrix (HIM) (Hill, 1965, 1977) to code sessions (Table 7.5). The interactional characteristics fit the hypothesized developmental sequence. The groups began with behavior primarily from Quadrant 1 concerned with socializing functions that entailed little risk. They then moved to a combination of Quadrants 2 and 3; Quadrant 2 dealing with individual differences and hostility, and Quadrant 3 with group level issues of responsibility. Following this, the groups shifted to Quadrant 4 behaviors concerned with more detail about each member and their relationships in the group. While only two groups were studied, the approach represents a sophisticated model for studying group development.

Hall and Williams (1966) compared brief ad hoc groups to established groups in terms of decision-making performance. They found that under high-conflict conditions, the ad hoc groups were more likely to use compromise strategies to short-circuit disagreement. This decreased the effectiveness of their problem-solving efforts. Established groups were more likely to attempt constructive resolution of differences. They also noted that the presence of conflict seemed to stimulate the group's problem-solving potential. While this study does not address group development specifically, it is pertinent to the issue of how groups address the intragroup tension associated with Tuckman's second stage of development. Braaten (1974/1975) provides a further review of developmental stages in groups.

Lundgren (1971) and Lundgren and Knight (1978) report on a large study of National Training Laboratory sensitivity groups using transcript analysis based on the ideas of Bales and Mills. They found a consistent three stage sequence consisting of initial encounter, interpersonal confrontation, and mutual acceptance. During the prolonged second stage of confrontation there was a decrease in the number of group references and in intermember directiveness. They noted that leader challenge was not high despite the confrontational atmosphere. They speculate that previous reports emphasizing the focus on leader attack might be an artifact of a student/teacher environment. Over time, the groups showed increasing self-disclosure, positive

TABLE 7.5.   Hill Interaction Matrix (Hill, 1965, 1977)

	Content Style Categories			
	Non-Member Centered		Member Centered	
	Topic	Group	Personal	Relationship
Work Style Categories				
Pre-work				
Responsive	Quadrant 1		Quadrant 2	
Conventional				
Assertive				
Work				
Speculative	Quadrant 3		Quadrant 4	
Confrontive				

openness, and identification with the group, as well as decreasing directiveness. These results appear to describe a combination of stage phenomena and progressive behavioral continuums.

A more complex stage development model (Beck, 1974) was developed through the detailed examination of transcripts from a series of client-centered psychotherapy groups at the University of Chicago during the 1960s. Beck's schema extends the number of stages to a total of nine (Table 7.6). The first four stages, perhaps the fifth, and the final stage are congruent with the literature outlined above. Stages six through eight of Beck's model extend the idea of group development to incorporate a growing independence of the group from the designated leader, requiring the designated leader to "gracefully acknowledge the group's emergent responsibilities" (p. 450). The leader must become more self-disclosing and behave as a more equal member of the group, thus allowing a deeper process of self-confrontation and transfer of learning to the outside world.

Beck integrates a number of group system characteristics into her approach. This includes identifying shifting norm standards (Beck, 1983; Dugo & Beck, 1983), the limits and criteria for membership and group level organizational issues (Beck, 1981; Lewis & Beck, 1983) and the group-level identity (Dugo & Beck, 1984). She has focused in particular on a detailed model of the contribution that different group roles play in the process of resolving the challenges of each stage of group development (Beck, Eng, & Brusa 1989; Peters & Beck, 1982). A sociometric instrument for completion by group members has been developed to test for role designation. This involves a four-role model: Designated Leader (Task Leader); Emotional Leader (Socioemotional Leader); Scapegoat; and Defiant Member (The Outsider). For example, in the first stage, the Designated Leader and the Emotional Leader offer complementary contributions that assist the group in forming. In the second stage, the role of the Scapegoat in polarizing issues is a necessary ingredient.

This set of four role types is a realistic minimum. The roles of task leader and socioemotional leader seem particularly important early in the group when there is the greatest ambiguity regarding the task and how to achieve it. The scapegoat serves as a repository of the group's projected anger. The

TABLE 7.6.   Phases of Group Development (Beck, 1974)

Phase 1: Making a contract: The agreement to work on becoming a functional group
Phase 2: Establishment of a group identity and direction
Phase 3: The exploration of individuals in the group
Phase 4: The establishment of intimacy
Phase 5: The exploration of mutuality
Phase 6: The achievement of autonomy through reorganization of the group's structure
Phase 7: Self-confrontation and the achievement of interdependence
Phase 8: Independence, the transfer of learning
Phase 9: Termination of group and separation from significant persons

fourth role is that of the distant member who rejects the group's control most vigorously. Varied lists of other roles are reported but with limited empirical support and often capturing personality dimensions that have only indirect relevance to group needs.

There is a general impression in the literature that role functions are seen most clearly earlier in the group's life. As the group members become more comfortable with their identification with the group there is less need for stereotypic and forceful role behaviors. This notion of 'distributed leadership' sits on the boundary between group needs and personal characteristics of the individual and would appear to be an important area for further research endeavors. It goes beyond the usual conceptualization of leadership to include people who may not be popular but have important functions for the group.

The Beck team has presented detailed descriptive work very much in the tradition of Gibbard and his colleagues, and has elaborated a comprehensive theory based on viewing the group as a system. A particularly important dimension to this work is the emphasis on understanding the nature of the transition process between stages (Beck, Dugo, Eng, & Lewis, 1986), so critical to the question of time segmenting. MacKenzie and Livesley (1983) augmented this approach by identifying tasks for both the group and the individual members in each stage.

Hare (1973, 1976) provides a variant on a life-cycle model of group development that contains the essence of Tuckman's stages (Table 7.7). He considers the final stage to be a recapitulation of the first L stage. This system incorporates the idea of four major dimensions of interpersonal behavior. Similar dimensions are also described by Bales and Couch (Table 7.7). Other important contributions to this notion of a small number of basic interactional dimensions is found in Leary (1957), Wiggins and Pincus (1989), and Schroeder, Wormworth, and Livesley (1992). A description of the "Big Five" personality dimensions, the most recent development in this field, is found in Costa and McCrae (1990). These consist of Neuroticism (emotional reactivity), Introversion/Extraversion, Openness, Agreeableness, and Conscientiousness. The value of this personality literature to

TABLE 7.7.   Four Dimensions of Interpersonal Behavior

Hare (1976)	Couch (1960)	Bales, Cohen, & Williamson (1980) SYMLOG
L = Pattern maintenance and tension management	Conforming vs. nonconforming	Forward-backward (task-oriented and conforming versus deviant)
A = Adaptation	Serious (task) vs. expressive	
I = Integration	Positive vs. negative	Positive-negative
G = Goal attainment	Dominant vs. submissive	Upward-downward (dominance vs. submission)

the investigation of group development lies in the identification of a small number of dimensions that might reasonably be tracked over time to demonstrate phasic shifts in the development of the group.

Caple (1978), in a review article, cites findings that suggest groups will spiral through thematic areas that will create tension and conflict. Such recurrences should not be seen in themselves as evidence of regression. Rather the investigator should look at how effectively the particular theme is addressed. The process of conflict resolution, not the thematic content per se, thus reveals group development. Cissna (1984) reviewed the literature for studies purporting to show no evidence of group development. Of the 13 studies he found, 5 were quite unacceptable because of inadequate data or extremely poor research design. Of the remaining 8 studies, none of them with very satisfactory design, at least half actually contain suggestive evidence of developmental phenomena.

EMERGING THEMES AND ISSUES IN GROUP DEVELOPMENT

This section reviews a number of themes from the more recent literature. Some of these have not been utilized specifically to track group development. However, all focus on important dimensions of group process that deal with changing phenomena over time.

Entrainment

Groups are often studied in isolation, without considering the context in which they are occurring. Considering context, McGrath and Kelly (1986) discuss the concept of entrainment, a term taken from the biological sciences meaning that an endogenous body rhythm has been 'captured' and modified by an external cycle. For example, the circadian rhythms that govern many bodily functions are influenced by the external day-night cycle, as any international traveller will attest. These authors argue that a similar process of temporal entrainment of social and organizational behavior also occurs. For example, such external forces as work schedules, assigned time limits, workdays and weekends, exert major effects on complex social behavior. Therefore, the state of boundary-regulation mechanisms cannot be properly understood by measuring at a single point in time, but only by following such phenomena over time, that is, by detecting dynamic patterning of behavior. Kelly and McGrath (1985) found that variations in time for completing a task resulted in enduring change in work patterns, as if the individuals had incorporated a new "frame of reference" for their performance. They argue that social behavior is replete with such "entrainment" phenomena and that only by taking them into account can group behavior be more fully understood:

People in interaction entrain one another; and their mutually entrained patterns of task performance and interaction in turn become entrained to external temporal markers and cycles. (p. 103)

Moreland and Levine (1988) and McGrath (1991) regard the group process from two perspectives: critical functions that must be resolved, and the stages in which they are addressed, producing a more complex map of group process (Table 7.8). The functions incorporate Bales' (1950) ideas of task and socioemotional needs, but in a manner that addresses the hierarchical nature of a systems model: the context of the group within an external environment, the group itself as an organism, and the individual member. The four modes identified by McGrath have a parallel to the life stage model. He suggests that a group may be at any point in time addressing the various functions with different mode levels. For example, a group may be dealing with task issues at one level, but be stuck at an earlier level in terms of socioemotional issues. This approach represents a fusion of the recurring cycle and the life cycle models of group process. It is an ambitious conceptualization likely to run into application difficulties when applied to psychotherapy groups. Conflict resolution, for example, could be understood both as a "production" goal and as a "member support" issue. The schema does highlight the complexity of understanding the group.

Early Group Structure

Bednar, Melnick, and Kaul (1974) suggest that increased early structure orchestrated by the group leader will free the group members to be more self-disclosing and to provide more interpersonal feedback. The structure provides less need for individual responsibility and therefore encourages greater levels of risk taking. This, in turn, promotes higher levels of cohesion. A series of studies have shown support for this hypothesis (Bednar & Battersbey, 1976; Crews & Melnick, 1976; Kirshner, Dies, & Brown, 1978; Levin & Kurtz, 1974; Rose & Bednar, 1980). Other studies have suggested that this is not entirely a benign process. Lee and Bednar (1977) found that while interpersonal behaviors were promoted by structure, this

TABLE 7.8. Group Development Model (McGrath, 1991)
(Adapted from Mennecke, Hoffer, & Wynne, 1992)

	Mode I Inception (Goal Choices)	Mode II Problem Solving (Means Choices)	Mode III Conflict Resolution (Political Choices)	Mode IV Execution (Goal Attainment)
Production	Production demand/ Opportunity	Technical problem solving	Policy conflict resolution	Execution
Well-being	Interaction demand/ Opportunity	Role network definition	Power and payoff distribution	Interaction
Member Support	Inclusion demand/ Opportunity	Position and status attainments	Contribution and payoff relationships	Participation

was associated with negative responses and some drop in group cohesion. Evensen and Bednar (1978) found variable results of structure on group cohesion.

MacKenzie, Dies, Coché, Rutan, and Stone (1987), in a study of 53 two-day experiential training groups compared those groups organized around a topic focus, and therefore containing more structure, with general psychodynamic process groups. The topic groups were rated by the participants as being significantly less defended than the general psychodynamic groups, an opinion echoed by group observers. On the other hand, the general process groups were rated as significantly more cohesive than the topic groups. These observations are in support of Bednar's hypothesis and also congruent with Fuehrer and Keys' (1988) findings concerning the effect of structure on cohesion.

Fuehrer and Keys (1988) studied 101 undergraduate students in four weekly "self-help" groups dealing with loneliness and alienation. Eight groups were given a high level of structure by a student facilitator and nine, a low structure. Self-report measures of group cohesion, ownership of group functioning, and constructive group behaviors were obtained. Bednar, Melnick, and Kaul's (1974) hypothesis was generally supported. Group structure promoted constructive group behaviors which, in turn, encouraged group cohesion. On the other hand, group structure was negatively correlated with early group cohesion and with ownership of personal responsibility in the group. Early group cohesion, early constructive behaviors, and early ownership of group responsibility were all strong predictors of final group cohesion. This study was based on group member self-report for most of its findings and no outcome measures were available. However, the findings are based on a relatively large sample size. They offer both support and caution regarding the effects of early group structuring. The impact on constructive behaviors is positive but the dampening of cohesion and self responsibility is less welcome.

Waltman and Zimpfer (1988) reviewed 23 studies of groups that focused on personal development and change in which group structure (high or low) was correlated with composition characteristics, length of treatment, and outcome. In 18 of these studies, the results were congruent with the following hypothesis: composition of membership has a relatively unimportant effect on outcome for brief (less than 12 hours) group experiences where there is a high degree of structure provided by the leader. Conversely, for longer term groups with less structure more care is warranted in choosing the group members. This review dealt with studies of greatly varying research sophistication so that the results must be interpreted with some caution. However, the number of studies with the same direction of results lends some support to the conclusions.

Stockton, Rohde, and Haughey (1992) describe the effects of group structuring exercises on group climate. The subject sample consisted of students seeking counselling at a campus-community counseling center. Eight groups met for six weekly 2-hour sessions. Four of the groups had a 15- to 20-minute structured exercise at the beginning of each session. These exercises were developed to facilitate the accomplishment of a particular task relevant to stage of group dynamics as described by MacKenzie and Livesley (1983). The Group Climate Questionnaire—GCQ-S (MacKenzie, 1983), the Attraction scale and the Reflective Questionnaire, both developed by Rohde (1988), were used to measure aspects of the group climate. Engaged and Avoiding (-) showed a linear trend over time. The experimental groups showed a quadratic pattern for Cohesion and Conflict consistent with a period of tension during the middle phase of the groups. The control groups showed less consistency. The importance of the study by itself is limited because of the low number of subjects and the brief duration of the groups. The results are compatible with an Engagement-Differentiation-Working stages model and with the helpful effect of structure in promoting these patterns.

The literature quoted above is largely supportive of the beneficial effects of early structure in promoting more active group involvement with higher levels of self-disclosure and interpersonal feedback, leading to associated positive feelings about the group itself. Most of these studies have been conducted on quite brief groups, most of them of a laboratory nature. Some of the studies had inconsistent findings. This idea of early structure is at odds with much of the psychotherapy literature which would hold that such early control might set a bad precedent for the group to rely on the leader for direction. Empirical evidence is clearly required to settle this issue.

Size and Gender Effects

The effect of group size on process has been well documented. As group size increases, cohesion and intimacy decrease, members report less satisfaction, and group participation becomes more skewed as some members dominate the interaction and others remain quiet (Bales & Strodbeck, 1951; Hare, 1976; Hare, Borgatta, & Bales, 1955; Kelley & Thibault, 1954). Gibb (1951) noted that larger groups inhibit creativity because of interpersonal threat. Efficiency also decreases (Gist, Locke, & Taylor, 1987).

Two separate studies were conducted on a group relations conference, one comparing groups composed of only men or women (Verdi & Wheelan, 1992) and the other comparing large and small group formats (Wheelan & McKeage, 1993). These authors employed a new category system based on the original conceptualizations of Bion and bearing resemblance to the measure used by Thelen (1954) and Stock and Thelen (1958). The seven categories in this system are as follows: Dependency, Counter-Dependency, Fight, Flight, Pairing, Counter-Pairing, and Work statements.

The authors rated each "thought unit" from a transcript of the sessions. A total of 11,528 units were coded, with only 3.13% of the units unscorable. Inter-rater reliability between two raters was 0.93. No difference was found between groups composed for homogeneity for gender. Flight and

Dependency were higher in earlier sessions, followed by an increase in Counter-Dependency and Fight, after which Pairing and Work increased. These results are compatible with the sequential stage hypothesis. In the second study, the larger group format was associated with significantly more Fight statements and fewer Pairing and Work statements. The authors suggest that the lower Work scores in the larger group reflected the initial higher Fight and lower Pairing scores and the later increase in Flight scores.

These two reports are of interest primarily for the methodology used. They achieved satisfactory inter-rater reliability on scales based on dynamic theme contents. Their analysis was based on the proportional dominance of a category relative to other categories, both within a time period, and as compared to other periods in the group's life. This is a more appropriate way of comparing periods than simple raw scores. Their findings also support the importance of considering group size as a variable in determining thematic development. The study is flawed because all of the groups were occurring within a single group relations conference and it would appear likely that behavior in one segment of the program, for example the small group or the gender-specific group, might have repercussions on other components such as the large mixed gender group. A similar measure of thematic content analysis has been developed by Karterud and Foss (1989) that uses only the categories of Fight, Flight, Dependency, and Pairing. This instrument also has reasonable inter-rater reliability figures.

Interpersonal Construct Change

Kelly (1955) described the process of construing interpersonal relationships as the mediating process in determining behavior. He used the Repertory Grid technology by which an individual is asked to rate a series of significant others using personalized construct terms. Factor analysis of the resulting Grid permits an analysis of major thematic dimensions used by the individual, as well as the way these are applied to each significant other. Kelly regarded "sociality" as the ability to construe the construction process of the other, a convoluted definition of empathy. This technique has been used to measure the manner in which an individual thinks about others over the course of therapy.

Duck (1973), following in this tradition, considered the changes in constructs that occur as relationships become more established. He found that construct changes moved from concrete and physical constructs such as neat/sloppy or outspoken/silent to more abstract and psychological constructs such as romantic/pragmatic or considerate/self-centered as therapy progressed. Neimeyer, Banikiotes, and Fami (1979) found empirical support for this concept of interpersonal development. Leichty (1989) reported that measures of construct differentiation and abstraction were associated with higher levels of intimacy between friends. Applegate, Kline, and Delia (1991) and Kline, Pelias, and Delia (1991) found that Crockett's (1965) measure of construct complexity was correlated with more "person-centered" communicative strategies. Catina, Gitzinger, and Hoeckh (1992) identified positive correlations between scores on Repertory Grid measures and a questionnaire concerning defense categories.

This area of empirical study as applied to small groups is reviewed in Neimeyer and Merluzzi (1982). The interactional group process is considered to provide in a systematic manner an opportunity for information exchange. With this increasing information base, the individuals become more psychologically knowledgeable about each other, making it possible to validate assumptions and initial impressions and to make finer discriminations in understanding. Therefore social relations increase in intensity leading to greater cohesion. It would appear that these investigational strategies would provide important information regarding the development of inter-member bonds in psychotherapy groups.

A group of investigators from The Netherlands also report a series of studies on 13 groups taking part in a 9-day residential training conference that featured 15 small group sessions of 1–2 hours duration (Kuypers, Davies, & Glaser, 1986; Kuypers, Davies, & Hazelwinkel, 1986; Kuypers, Davies, & van der Vegt, 1987). The ideas people use to describe themselves and others may be sorted into categories (Table 7.9). This investigation looked at how the use of such categories changed for the individual over time. In addition, the same category system was used to characterize how a group as a whole was functioning over time. This investigative model is built on the ideas of Bennis and Shepard (1956) and Harvey, Hunt, and Schroder (1961) who describe the group as moving into positions of dialectical tension regarding specific themes that split the membership. To this theoretical framework, these investigators have added the methodology of personal construct theory as a method for identifying construal patterns. Each succeeding phase is seen as a way of resolving the dilemma of the preceding phase.

The Repertory Grid constructs for each member were sorted into categories before therapy and at follow-up. A group observer recorded the thematic aspects of the group process using the same categories. The group members of different groups did not differ in their pretherapy Repertory

TABLE 7.9. Developmental Patterns in Self-Analytic Groups
(Kuypers, Davies, & Hazelwinkel, 1986)

Dilemma	Option	Constructs	Phase
Inclusion	External demands vs. own needs	External	Dependency
Authority	Law-and-order vs. anarchy	Moral	Counter-dependency
Intimacy	Symbiosis vs. self sufficiency	Psychological	Enchantment Disenchantment
		Expressive	Consensual validation
Separation	Retrospection vs. prospection	Interactional	Termination

Grid patterns. However there was sharp divergence in patterns of different groups at follow-up. Some of the groups became stuck at particular stages of development as indicated by their persistent use of the same construct style. The members of each group were found to be using a pattern of constructs that matched those of the phase at which the group was stuck. In short, the hypothesized relationships in Table 7.9 were confirmed. In addition, the authors found that feedback was taken in a defensive manner until the group had reached the stage of consensual validation, at which point it could be used to contribute to self-understanding. Cohesion increased over the duration of each group and was not directly related to the stage achieved by any particular group.

Group members were seen to act as role leaders in various stages, in part by the manner in which their interpersonal constructs matched the issues of the phase. The oppositional tension in the therapeutic milieu of each phase acts to "unfreeze" the internal state of the individual by invalidating constructs (Schein & Bennis, 1965). By definition, this system views the advanced group as showing positive member interdependence in which new roles and constructs can be validated. The authors suggest that these changes must be viewed as more than simply the effects of conformity to group norms because they remain in force when the individual describes his personal relationships at a follow-up testing several months later. Indeed, they found some indirect support for the idea that six months or more are required before the new patterns again become reconsolidated.

This work is based on a relatively brief training group experience, but with a group environment that approximates that of a psychotherapy group. The methodology is a sophisticated approach to matching developmental phenomena with outcome change. The study attempts to deal directly with the question of how far a group develops. The conclusions of the study are striking and call for validation. They suggest that the individual member benefits from the group only so far as the group itself develops.

Tschuschke and MacKenzie (1989) studied two long-term psychotherapy groups using the Gottschalk and Gleser (1969) verbal content analysis scales. The complete transcript of every fourth session was analyzed using six anxiety and four hostility scales. These scales are based on psychoanalytic concepts. Not only overt affective statements (states) are coded but also projected, negated, displaced, and weakened affect cues are scored. An average inter-rater reliability greater than 0.80 was achieved. One group had a successful outcome using general clinical assessments. The other group had a major loss of members and was ended prematurely because of the impending termination of several others. Thus is was reasonable to compare the process patterns in the two groups as representing a better and worse outcome for the members.

The verbal content analysis approach yields an independent view of the group climate. It stands in contrast to the more common method of measuring group climate through member self-report instruments. The transcript data base was analyzed using factor analysis. The usual P-factor approach identified thematic dimensions that occurred together; O-factor analysis identified group sessions that had similar interactional characteristics. The more successful group showed a pattern of prolonged periods spent in various states. These indicated a state of painful self-disclosure followed by a state of greater hostility directed towards others. These two states were then repeated and eventually followed by a final state of lowered affect. These patterns are compatible with the pendular swings described by Gibbard, Hartman, and Mann (1974), or alternatively with the idea that the group attempts to address the differentiation/conflict stage at first unsuccessfully, but on second approach is able to master it. While the study has weak outcome measures and would require replication with greater attention to change measurements, nevertheless, it is one of the few studies of long-term psychoanalytic group psychotherapy available in the literature. The process measures show robust evidence of enduring climate states in the successful group and no such evidence in the less successful group. The use of O-factor analysis appears to be a useful although not widely used tool for identifying stage shifts. It factors the data base in the opposite direction to P-factor analysis in which the scale results are factored over time. In O-factoring, the sessions are factored over time. The combination allows one to plot thematic scores for specific periods, all based on the same data base.

Interpersonal Intimacy

Another method for tracking change over time utilizes intimacy measures. Group participants commonly state that they feel much closer to each other as the group progresses. Sequential group development theories assume the deepening of intimacy as an underlying feature (Mills, 1978). Most of the literature concerning intimacy relates to dyadic relations and tends to emphasize positive characteristics such as familiarity, caring, and attraction. This ignores the fact that most intimate relationships also have significant negative interactions as well. When applied to groups, most authors cite the presence of interdependence with one another, where, for example, topics are pursued because of the value to the group, not necessarily to each individual (Berscheid & Walster, 1978; Cooley, 1909; Parsons & Shils, 1951; Walster, Walster, & Berscheid, 1978). A second feature is that intimacy is based on an extensive knowledge of each other (Chelune, Robison, & Kommor, 1984; Clark & Reiss, 1988). This might be manifested by an interest in personal issues as opposed to specific factual problems. Another feature of intimacy is self-disclosure regarding the effect each has on the other, what Perlmutter and Hatfield (1980) term "intentional metacommunication." Overall levels of emotionality, both positive and negative, tend to increase with greater intimacy (Dunphy, 1972). Using similar measures, Altman, Vinsel, and Brown (1981) take an alternate approach reminiscent of the earlier discussion of task and socioemotional recurring cycles. They suggest that social behavior is influenced by fundamental underlying dialectical processes of intimacy/privacy and stability/change that oscillate over time.

Barker (1991) develops these concepts into a preliminary measure of interpersonal intimacy. The progression from casual familiarity to intimacy would appear to be an essential component to the developing group environment. This concept is closely related to the earlier discussion concerning interpersonal constructs shifting from viewing others in superficial generalizations related to role stereotypes to understanding others in specific personal terms.

Group Climate

Another focus to measuring change over time in group process is to ask group members to describe the group as a whole on a climate measure. This is analogous to ascertaining the personal construct patterns of the individual. Both assume that the participant's perception of the situation is the operational link that determines response. Several instruments are available for this purpose: two longer questionnaires, the Group Environment Scale (GES) (Moos, 1974) and the Group Atmosphere Scale (GAS) (Silbergeld, Koenig, Manderscheid, Meeker, & Horning, 1975); and one short one, the Group Climate Questionnaire (GCQ-S) (MacKenzie, 1983).

MacKenzie, Dies, Coché, Rutan, and Stone (1987) studied 53 14-hour experiential training groups. Measures of group climate using the GCQ-S were compatible with stage phenomena. The groups with members who expressed a strongly positive evaluation of the experience demonstrated high levels of positive work and gradually decreasing levels of conflict. The groups with members who expressed less satisfaction with the experience began with lower levels of positive work that never approached the levels of the more positive groups. They began with similar levels of conflict, but these levels did not decrease over time, suggesting that the more successful groups mastered intra-group tension and could progress, while the less successful remained stuck in a more conflictual process. Interestingly, the factor structure of the group climate questions shifted in the final sessions of more successful groups to a pattern focusing on deeper psychological exploration. This suggests a change in construal patterns within the more successful groups, in keeping with the more complex use of interpersonal constructs. While this is a large study, the outcome measure is quite weak and measured only at the end of the final session when a halo effect would be most pronounced; nevertheless, the patterns do support the idea that group development is correlated with a more positive group experience.

Kivlighan and Jauquet (1990) studied six student personal growth groups that met for 26 sessions over a 13-week period. Every fourth session, the participants completed a problem agenda card that had the instructions: "What would you like to get accomplished in today's group?" Up to three items could be specified. This technique has generally been applied more to structured cognitive or behaviorally oriented groups than to process groups (Flowers & Schwartz, 1980; McGuire, Taylor, Broome, Blau, & Abbott, 1986). There was no requirement that the agenda items needed to be revealed in the group session itself. At the end of the session, the Group Climate Questionnaire (MacKenzie, 1983) was completed. Group climate patterns were similar in all six groups. The Engaged score rose steadily across time, while the Avoiding score decreased across time; the Conflict score was highest in the middle sessions. The agenda items were rated using the Goal Dimension Rating Manual (O'Farrell, 1986) on three dimensions: realistic versus abstract, here-and-now versus there-and-then, interpersonal regarding group relationships versus intrapersonal. Satisfactory inter-rater reliability was achieved among three judges. All groups showed a consistent progression over time for realistic, here-and-now, and interpersonal goals. The final analysis correlated the climate and cognitive style measures. In early sessions, realistic goals were significantly correlated with high Engaged scores. In middle sessions, a here-and-now focus was correlated with all three GCQ dimensions, and an interpersonal focus with Engaged and Avoiding (-). In later sessions, here-and-now and interpersonal focus were correlated with Engaged and Avoiding (-).

These results are congruent with a linear developmental process regarding 5 of the 6 measures, only conflict showed a quadratic effect. The climate-goal correlations also are understandable from a developmental perspective. Realistic goals are an early necessity, followed by intense submersion in group process that is accompanied by conflict, and then progression to a here-and-now and interpersonal focus with Engaged. These patterns fit an Engagement-Differentiation-Working stage model.

Critical Incidents

Another approach for tracking group development is through the analysis of group members' responses on critical incident forms. These approaches characteristically ask members to describe the most personally important experience within a particular session. These reports may then be scored using a therapeutic factor category system (Bloch, Reibstein, Crouch, Holroyd, & Themen, 1979). Alternatively, some studies use a therapeutic factor questionnaire or Q-sort in which the members are asked to rate a variety of types of experience directly (Butler & Fuhriman, 1983). Butler (1981) found that over time, members of psychotherapy groups tended to show higher levels of cohesion, self-understanding, and interpersonal learning. In general, this study demonstrated a deepening of interactional qualities that are compatible with a continuum concept of group involvement, not specifically stages per se.

MacKenzie (1987) studied four time-limited outpatient psychotherapy groups meeting for more than 20 sessions, in which members completed a critical incident form following each session. Modest inter-rater reliability was achieved in categorizing these incidents using Bloch et al.'s manual (1979). The results clustered into three broad dimensions: psychological work (self-understanding, learning from interpersonal actions, and vicarious learning), self-revelation (self-disclosure and catharsis), and morale (acceptance, instillation of hope, and universality). The morale cluster gradually dropped over time. Self-revelation dropped from initial levels during the middle time period (sessions 6–10), but then rose to its highest levels in the final sessions. Psychological work, the most frequently endorsed dimension, rose rapidly through the first quarter, was maintained during the second quarter, and then dropped slightly toward the end. These overall patterns also are compatible with a stage development process. The relatively nonspecific items in the morale cluster gradually became less important, while self-disclosure reflected a phasic pattern. The measures did not elicit material that would detect a negative atmosphere, but the phasic nature of self-disclosure is compatible with changing levels of safety within the group.

Kivlighan and Mullison (1988) studied 3 counseling groups of 11 sessions each. Critical incident scoring was found to contain three main dimensions: cognitive work (self-understanding, vicarious learning, guidance, universality), behavioral actions (self-disclosure, altruism, interpersonal actions), or affective experience (acceptance, hope, catharsis). Early sessions showed higher levels of cognitive learning, especially universality, while later sessions had more interpersonal learning and more behavioral application. Group members who were more affiliative in nature tended to rate cognitive experience as more helpful. Members who were less affiliative rated behavioral incidents as more helpful. This suggests that members rated experiences that were less characteristic of them as being more helpful, suggesting the operation of change-inducing tendencies. However, these were quite brief groups and were studied only using a split half analysis design that might have obscured a more sensitive tracking of climate shifts.

Inertial Forces

Not all authors support the idea of group development as an inevitable progressive force. Gersick (1988) suggests an alternate model of process change. She studied eight work group teams, meeting over varying lengths of time from 7 days to 6 months. The full text of all meetings was analyzed without preconceived theoretical dimensions. These groups tended to be controlled by inertial forces in the group and to maintain a "habitual routine," unless something happened to force a change. This phenomenon is termed the "Einstellung" effect: a tendency for individuals to persist with the same problem-solving approach regardless of the success of that approach. Gersick named this a pattern of "punctuated equilibrium," a term also currently being used concerning evolutionary theory. Change triggering events may include such things as an externally set time deadline, experiencing failure, structural changes in the group, leader changes, or receiving an intervention. A change in state is seen as a revolutionary process, not a natural progression.

In a second project, Gersick (1989) studied eight student groups as they worked over time on creative projects. All of the groups showed a similar pattern. An interactional style was established in the first meeting and maintained with little change until the midpoint, even though the nature of that initial climate varied considerably between the groups. The midpoint might be anywhere from a few days to a few months depending on the length of the assignment. At the midpoint, each group went through a transition process in which the goals and methods were reviewed. This new state was then maintained until the end, culminating in a flurry of activity in the final session.

The findings of these two studies were interpreted to mean that the context in which the group was meeting, particularly the time context, was an important factor in shaping the change process of the groups. This general effect was far more powerful than the exact nature of the environment established in each group at any point in time. While the groups studied were far removed from psychotherapy groups, the findings are provocative, particularly given the increasing use of time-limited formats in therapy where a clear emphasis on the passage of time is regularly maintained.

Putman (1979) suggested that the personality style of the group members may be a critical ingredient in triggering a change process. He identified a style dimension entitled 'preference for procedural order'. High procedural order persons strive for planned, sequential patterns for organizing task activities. They are concerned about time management and prefer regular, predictable procedures. These qualities appear to lie along the "compulsivity" or "conscientiousness" dimension. Mennecke, Hoffer, and Wynne (1992) have suggested that such individuals may supply the stimulus for the group to address developmental tasks, and that, in their absence, inertial forces rule. The presence of such characteristics among group members may provide a mechanism for promoting group climate change, particularly in relation to task accomplishment.

A DISCUSSION AND CONCEPTUALIZATION

This review of group development raises more questions than answers. There is substantial empirical evidence for the development of an initial group climate characterized by increasing cohesion and self-disclosure, followed by the emergence of a period of intragroup tension and conflict. These two stages can be reasonably tracked with group level measures that focus on positive and negative emotional tone. Beyond that point, the nature of the group interaction becomes more complex and measures that capture specific interpersonal dimensions or individual cognitive styles appear to be more relevant than global group level approaches. This makes the research task as well as the clinical implementation more challenging.

Few authors have taken a broad structural view of the group. This seems essential if a comprehensive understanding is to be achieved. It is apparent in the preceding review that many factors can influence group development. Some of the major dimensions might include: the context in which the group is taking place, the task of the group, time restraints, size of group, closed or open membership, personal characteristics of the members, style of leadership, degree of homogeneity on specific dimensions, and the interactional capacity of the members. All of these factors could reasonably be considered to influence the rate at which the group interaction deepens over time. A comprehensive framework is helpful in checking for possible influences, even if only a few dimensions are actually being measured. It is impossible to control for all possible variables, nevertheless, a healthy vigilance for likely influences is warranted.

A Systems Approach

A systems approach provides a model for the study of phenomena at various levels of group organization. A possible format is laid out in Figure 7.2. This schema identifies important boundary structures within the group. The term 'boundary' is used in a double sense. Boundaries can be conceptualized in physical terms; for example, closing the door of the group room reinforces the physical external boundary of the group; the individual participants in the room are separate entities. Of just as much interest, is the idea of a boundary being created from an awareness about differences on either side of that boundary. For example, the mechanism of universalization, one of the basic therapeutic factors (Yalom, 1985), can be understood as stemming from the experience of finding others with similar experiences in a way that has not been experienced in the outside world. Thus, the milieu inside the group begins to be seen as a different sort of environment and so establishes an information based external boundary. As the group develops, the nature of the therapist-membership boundary undergoes significant changes, generally described as moving from dependence, to confrontation, to collaboration. Group therapists must continually decide, knowingly or spontaneously, whether to make an intervention that addresses the group in its broader context, the group as a whole, the interaction between certain members, or issues pertinent to the internal world of a single member.

This systems schematic map offers one method of conceptualizing group events and encourages consideration of a variety of possibilities for understanding the meaning of a given situation. The studies reviewed in this chapter can be superimposed upon this map of the group. At a minimum, four levels of an organizational hierarchy are immediately evident: external factors, group level phenomena, interactional events, and intrapsychic processes.

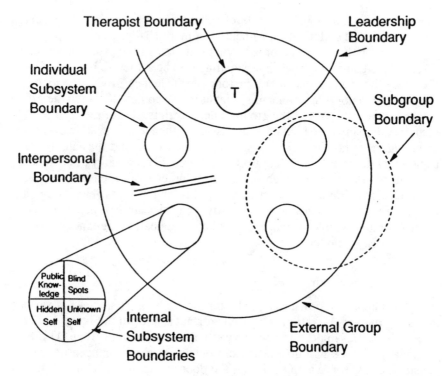

Figure 7.2. A structural diagram of the group system (MacKenzie, 1990).

The external boundary of the group differentiates the intragroup environment from that without. This is an important focus that deals with the effects of the context in which the group exists. For example, selection and composition decisions will significantly influence the type of group interaction that will emerge. Groups held in a prison setting spend an inordinately long time with early group issues centering around trust and confidentiality. An external decision regarding the amount of time the group is to meet will have profound effects on the process. The process of small groups operating within the context of a larger milieu such as an inpatient unit or a day treatment program are likely to be influenced by that milieu and to show parallel processes to those in the larger setting. For example, the clinical literature describes the emergence in ward groups of the sorts of tensions occurring within the staff system.

There is a major divide in the empirical literature between groups that have specific external group goals to accomplish and groups that depend on the process of the group for a therapeutic or learning effect on the individual members. Considerable caution needs to be exerted when applying findings from task groups to process groups. The context of these two types of groups are quite different and will exert major influence on the process.

While similar patterns may be found, it remains to be demonstrated that they have the same significance in each type of group. When considering outcome, a general group task can be assumed to be the result of group processes, for example, speed in resolving a task or the complexity of the result. However, individual change scores present a more complex problem. Should one simply calculate a mean outcome score based on all members? Would it be better to look at the number of members who achieve a particular target level in terms of symptoms or performance? Do members with particular characteristics respond selectively to certain types of group environments? Is outcome best understood as a team effort or as the efforts of individuals?

A different set of issues emerge when considering the organizational level of the whole group. From a technical point of view, the study of group development has the collectivity of the group as the focus of interest. For meaningful results, therefore, a statistically satisfactory number of groups must be studied, obviously a heretofore major short-coming in the literature. It is for this reason that so much of this review has had to report findings that are 'compatible' with a developmental stage hypothesis. Only with adequate numbers of groups can statistically meaningful answers be given to the question: Do groups that develop satisfactorily produce better results for the members?

Few studies deal with characteristics of the group-as-a-whole. Simple measures of group climate have been applied as well as attempts to track dynamic themes thought to be characteristic of the entire group. Such approaches present methodological problems in terms of how to represent the entire group organism. Is a simple summing of behaviors adequate? Is a global rating of the entire group really meaningful? Is the silent member to be assumed to be in agreement with the majority? What is the influence of group role on the individual's perception of the group? Should endorsement by a certain percentage of members be required to establish a feature such as a group norm?

There is an older established literature concerning group norms which has been largely neglected in recent studies. The effects of normative pressures in regard to attraction to the group, attitude change, conformity, and social facilitation seem worthy of further investigation. Do normative influences increase over time, or does the individual become more autonomous through the process of therapy? Similarly, little attention has been paid to dominance rank in groups, despite it being a fundamental characteristic of both human and primate small groups (Kennedy & MacKenzie, 1986).

Much of the group literature has focused on interactional events. Lewin's early work focused on leader behavioral variables and the resulting group climate, effects revealed across the leader-member interface. While the leadership boundary highlights the role of the leader, many laboratory groups function without a designated leader, allowing internal leadership functions to emerge spontaneously. However, psychotherapy groups do have a leader and the professional role status lends that role a particularly high profile. Relatively few studies have examined these features across time.

Most studies concentrate on intermember behaviors. In general, these behaviors are summed to describe the group. Relatively few studies examine the data in a more detailed way in an attempt to identify individual patterns and their effect on the group. Does this do justice to the group, or does it in fact blur important individual differences? Little use is made of interpersonal behaviors developed in current personality studies. Others take a more integrative view by examining group level changes and the roles of specific members in shaping these. The use of group role dimensions is, indeed, at an early stage of development.

The use of internal, or intrapsychic, concepts has taken two forms. Most outcome studies of group psychotherapy utilize some measurement of internal change for how individuals see themselves or their significant relationships. Such change is often assumed to be related to group experiences, but there is little data to connect in-group events with outcome changes. Personal construct researchers take the position that the perception of the group by the member is the most real and important aspect to study. This orientation suggests that actual measurement of behavior misses the most important point. The reactions of the individual members are based primarily upon what each "sees" happening in the group. Personal construct technology offers one way of systematically tapping this source of information but is used sparingly in group studies. In therapeutic factor studies, members report that a considerable part of their learning occurs through the vicarious learning opportunities provided by observing others in the group. The question of the effects of the interactional capacity of group members on group development has not been addressed, for example with a psychometrically sound measure of quality of relationships.

The Question of Time

The manner in which time is segmented for analysis purposes continues to pose major problems in the literature. Pre-set time periods are commonly used; however, it seems clear that group development is likely to evolve in accordance with the characteristics of the group and its context. Time segmentation therefore must be based on criteria within the group process. Several of the reviewed models incorporate time. Beck, Eng, and Brusa (1989) identify the process details around a phase-shift point, particularly role behaviors, in order to understand the change processes at work. From a statistical view, Brower (1986) uses the Pearson phi coefficient correlational matrix to compare all sessions with each other. This reveals patterns of commonality within the flow of sessions. Similarly, Tschuschke and MacKenzie (1989) achieve the same result with O-factor analysis, a method that lends itself to analysis of the grid of ratings spread over time. Markovian sequential analysis has also been utilized. The issue of time segmenting offers an opportunity for creative use of time analysis procedures (Francis, Fletcher, Stuebing, Davidson, & Thompson, 1991; Graham, Collins, Wugalter, Chung, & Hansen, 1991; Jensen, 1990).

Poole (1983) and Poole and Roth (1989) developed a strategy of sampling group events over a short duration of time. They argue that many studies use excessively long predetermined segments and are, in fact, picking up artifacts related to time duration. Poole found that only 25% of his groups followed a progressive developmental pattern. He identified three types of breakpoints that may interrupt group development: normal breakpoints reflecting topic shifts, breakpoints related to adaption or reflection on new contingencies that cause a reworking of earlier tasks, and disruptive breakpoints related to major conflict of other systemic failure. Poole's concept of "breakpoints" is reminiscent of Gibbard's documentation of tension points at the transition between stages. It is also the other side of the notion of "natural group development" and of McGrath's (1991) "default" path of development that will occur in 'an average expectable environment' unless impeding factors intervene. It is thus built firmly on the foundation of sequential stage development.

Time is also important as an external variable. Psychotherapy has tended to be practiced as if time did not exist. The imposition of a predefined time-limit puts into motion important processes. The importance of working quickly without periods of avoidance of the task is underlined. The member must deal with the necessity of accepting that not enough therapy will be experienced. There is the task of facing termination with its themes of loss and grief according to an external timetable. Existential issues centering around ultimate responsibility for managing one's own life are raised. These pressures are likely to either accelerate the process of group development or derail it altogether. The impact of time limitation must be taken into account in comparing studies.

An Integrative Viewpoint of Group Development

The idea of group developmental stages is a higher order conceptualization that is built upon lower level processes. Given the complexity of the field of action, it seems important to struggle with how it is to be conceptualized. Only with a satisfactory larger frame of reference is it likely that individual pieces of the puzzle will make sense. With this perspective, the literature can be polarized around three views of group process over time.

One view holds that group process is of a repetitive cyclic nature. Consider the work of Altman, Vinsel, and Brown (1981), Bales (1950), Bennis and Shepard (1956), Bion (1961), Caple (1978), Gibbard, Hartman, and Mann (1974), Schutz (1958), Slater (1966). These authors stress that the group must continually come back to re-address certain basic process issues.

The second view maintains that groups progress over time in an orderly sequence that addresses group organizational tasks and ends with coming to

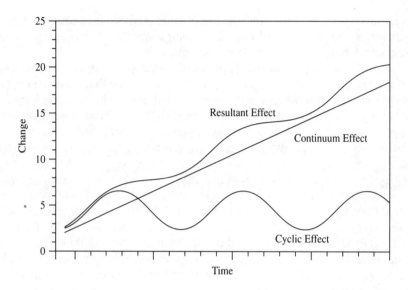

Figure 7.3. Theoretical appearance of cyclic effects superimposed on continuum effects.

terms with group termination. This life cycle tradition has borrowed many ideas from the literature concerning individual growth and development. Consider here Beck (1974), Gibbard, Hartman, and Mann (1974), Hare (1973), Kaplan and Roman (1963), MacKenzie and Livesley (1983), Martin and Hill (1957), and Tuckman (1965).

A third view sees a number of patterns both within the individual and in the interaction between individuals that systematically progress over time. Here we have Barker (1991), Butler (1981), Chelune, Robison, and Kommor (1984), Clark and Reiss (1988), Duck (1973), Dunphy (1972), Kivlighan and Jauquet (1990), Neimeyer, Banikiotes, and Fami (1979), and Perlmutter and Hatfield (1980).

These three views might be integrated and conceptualized in the following way: consider some processes to be progressive and others to be cyclical. When graphed on a time line, the combination of cumulative unidimensional change and cyclical change will produce the impression of stages (Figure 7.3). This approach offers a way of locating the effects of different variables. Without pretending to be inclusive, some of the applications of progressive and cyclic processes might look as follows.

Thematic Continuums

Thematic continuums that develop progressively over time as a group matures might include the following sorts of processes:

Self-revelation moving from factual information to personal reactions;
An steadily increasing level of group relatedness;

Progressive self initiation from dependence to autonomy;

Increasing interpersonal intimacy from social to personal relationships;

The quality of interpersonal themes shifting from power relationships to affiliation/affection; from competition to cooperation;

Interpersonal perception changing from unidimensional stereotypic roles to complex persons;

Interpersonal constructs shifting from general/abstract to detailed/specific knowledge;

Focus of attention changing from issues outside the group to issues inside the group; and

Increasing levels of group cohesion.

Recurrent Cyclic Issues

On the other hand, certain important group themes are likely to follow a recurrent cycle throughout the group's life:

From investment in the task to emotional displacement from the task;

From focus on being part of the group to focus on being autonomous;

From agreeing and becoming the same to disagreeing and becoming different;

From being defended to being open; and

From fearing isolation to fearing enmeshment.

Effective Group Development

Conceptually, groups that are developing effectively might be expected to show predictable features over time. Groups with interrupted or blocked development will not show such changes or will recycle back into earlier stage patterns. Such features may be:

Development will be regular and predictable: The sequence of changes within the group will follow a recognizable pattern, so that the observer can make accurate predictions of future developments.

The same developmental features will be evident in all groups: Development is a generic quality so that different kinds of groups with different goals and different types of members will show the same developmental features, though perhaps with differing tempos.

Developmental phenomena are epigenetic: Later development will be based on successful mastery of earlier developmental challenges, so that the sequence of changes will be invariant.

The group system will increase in interactional complexity: Development will be revealed in total group system characteristics, in interpersonal behaviors, and in internal psychological phenomena of individual members.

This review included comments on parts of the research literature that are not directly connected to the development of groups. This was done with the intent of illustrating aspects of methodology that might be relevant to the understanding of group developmental phenomenon. It would be helpful to see a greater application and integration of personality technology, for example through personal construct theory, measures of intimacy and construct complexity, or the use of a standard set of interpersonal dimensions. A focus on detecting specific change points and the nature of the events that induce them might be productive. Group system effects, such as the impact of early structure and the function of role types, offer other avenues of investigation. A better understanding of the complex term "cohesion" and its developmental components might be helpful.

The group psychotherapy research literature is currently at the stage of development of the individual psychotherapy research about a decade ago. There are many interesting and provocative findings, but the field has not yet become integrated. There is a need for the emergence and general acceptance of a limited number of standard instruments that have acceptable psychometric properties. These could then be used as a common language for describing group phenomena. Until that time, the fragmenting effects of idiosyncratic measures applied to small samples will hamper a general empirically based view of small group dynamics. This methodological development is particularly important because the group system is more complex than that of individual psychotherapy. Suitable measures must be found for the various levels in the group system. A consistent but not overwhelming number of established measures would promote a base of cumulative data against which individual studies could be compared.

REFERENCES

Altman, I., Vinsel, A. M., & Brown, B. B. (1981). Dialectic conceptions in social psychology: An application to social penetration and privacy regulation. In L. Berkowitz (Ed.), *Advances in experimental social psychology* (Vol. 14, pp. 108–161). New York: Academic Press.

Applegate, J. L., Kline, S. L., & Delia, J. G. (1991). Alternative measures of cognitive complexity as predictors of communication performance. *International Journal of Personal Construct Psychology, 4,* 193–213.

Bales, R. F. (1950). *Interaction process analysis: A method for the study of small groups.* Cambridge, MA: Addison-Wesley.

Bales, R. F. (1953). The equilibrium problem in small groups. In T. Parsons, R. F. Bales, & E. A. Shils (Eds.), *Working papers in the theory of action* (pp. 127–161). New York: Free Press.

Bales, R. F. (1970). *Personality and interpersonal behavior.* New York: Holt.

Bales, R. F., Cohen, S. P., & Williamson, S.A. (1980). *SYMLOG: A system for the multiple level observation of groups.* New York: Free Press.

Bales, R. F., & Slater, P. E. (1955). Role differentiation in small decision-making groups. In T. Parsons & R. F. Bales (Eds.), *Family, socialization, and interaction process* (pp. 259–306). New York: Free Press.

Bales, R. F., & Strodbeck, F. L. (1951). Phases in group problem solving. *Journal of Normal and Social Psychology, 46*, 485–495.

Barker, D. B. (1991): The behavioral analysis of interpersonal intimacy in group development. *Small Group Research, 22*, 76–91.

Beck, A. P. (1974). Phases in the development of structure in therapy and encounter groups. In D. A. Wexler & L. N. Rice (Eds.), *Innovations in client-centered therapy* (pp. 421–463). New York: Wiley.

Beck, A. P. (1981). A study of phase development and emergent leadership. *Group, 5*, 48–54.

Beck, A. P. (1983). A process analysis of group development. *Group, 7*, 19–26.

Beck, A. P., Dugo, J. M., Eng, A. M., & Lewis, C. M. (1986). The search for phases in group development: Designing process analysis measures of group interaction. In L. S. Greenberg & W. M. Pinsof (Eds.), *The psychotherapeutic process: A research handbook*. New York: Guilford Press.

Beck, A. P., Eng, A. M., & Brusa, J. (1989). The evolution of leadership during group development. *Group, 13*, 155–164.

Bednar, R. L., & Battersby, C. P. (1976). The effects of specific cognitive structure on early group development. *Journal of Applied Behavioral Science, 12*, 514–522.

Bednar, R. L., Melnick, J., & Kaul, T. J. (1974). Risk, responsibility, and structure: A conceptual framework for initiating group counseling and psychotherapy. *Journal of Counseling Psychology, 21*, 31–37.

Bennis, W. G., & Shepard, H. A. (1956). A theory of group development. *Human Relations, 9*, 415–437.

Berscheid, E., & Walster, E. H. (1978). *Interpersonal attraction* (2nd ed.). Reading, MA: Addison-Wesley.

Bibring, E. (1954). Psychoanalysis and the dynamic psychotherapies. *Journal of the American Psychoanalytic Association, 2*, 745–770.

Bion, W. R. (1961). *Experiences in groups*. New York: Basic Books.

Bloch, S., Reibstein, J., Crouch, E., Holroyd, P., & Themen, J. (1979). A method for the study of therapeutic factors in group psychotherapy. *British Journal of Psychiatry, 134*, 257–263.

Braaten, L. J. (1974/1975). Developmental phases of encounter groups and related intensive groups: A critical review of models and a new proposal. *Interpersonal Development, 5*, 112–129.

Broom, L., & Selznik, P. (1968). *Sociology*. New York: Harper and Row.

Brower, A. M. (1986). Behavior change in psychotherapy groups: A study using an empirically based statistical method. *Small Group Behavior, 17*, 164–185.

Budman, S. H., Demby, A., Feldstein, M., Redondo, J., Scherz, B., Bennett, M. J., Kippenaal, G., Daley, B. S., Hunter, M., & Ellis, J. (1987). Preliminary findings on a new instrument to measure cohesion in group psychotherapy. *International Journal of Group Psychotherapy, 37*, 75–94.

Butler, T. (1981). Level of functioning and length of time in treatment: Variables influencing patients' therapeutic experience in group psychotherapy. *Dissertation Abstracts International, 41,* 2749B.

Butler, T., & Fuhriman, A. (1980). Patient perspective on the curative process: A comparison of day treatment and outpatient psychotherapy groups. *Small Group Behavior, 11,* 371–388.

Butler, T., & Fuhriman, A. (1983). Curative factors in group therapy: A review of the recent literature. *Small Group Behavior, 14,* 131–142.

Caple, R. (1978). The sequential stages of group development. *Small Group Behavior, 9,* 470–476.

Cartwright, D., & Zander, A. (Eds.). (1960). *Group dynamics: Research and theory* (2nd ed.). Evanston, IL: Row, Peterson.

Catina, A., Gitzinger, I., & Hoeckh, H. (1992). Defense mechanisms: An approach from the perspective of personal construct psychology. *International Journal of Personal Construct Psychology, 5,* 249–257.

Chelune, G. J., Robison, J. T., & Kommor, M. J. (1984). A cognitive interactional model of intimate relationships. In V. J. Derlega (Ed.), *Communication, intimacy, and close relationships* (pp. 11–40). New York: Academic Press.

Cissna, K. (1984). Phases in group development: The negative evidence. *Small Group Behavior, 15,* 3–32.

Clark, M. S., & Reiss, H. T. (1988). Interpersonal processes in close relationships. In M. R. Rosenzweig & L. W. Porter (Eds.), *Annual Review of Psychology, 39,* 609–672.

Cooley, C. H. (1909). *Social organization: A study of the larger mind.* New York: Scribner's. Reprinted in Broom, L., & Selznik, P. (1968). *Sociology.* New York: Harper & Row.

Costa, P. T., & McCrae, R. R. (1990). Personality disorders and the five-factor model of personality. *Journal of Personality Disorders, 4,* 362–371.

Couch, A. S. (1960). *Psychological determinants of interpersonal behavior.* Unpublished doctoral dissertation, University of Chicago.

Crews, C. Y., & Melnick, J. (1976). Use of initial and delayed structure in facilitating group development. *Journal of Counselling Psychology, 23,* 92–98.

Crockett, W. H. (1965). Cognitive complexity and impression formation. In B. A. Maher (Ed.), *Progress in experimental personality research* (Vol. 2, pp. 47–90). New York: Academic Press.

Dewey, J. (1910). *How we think.* Boston, MA: Heath.

Drescher, S., Burlingame, G., & Fuhriman, A. (1985). Cohesion: An odyssey in empirical understanding. *Small Group Behavior, 16,* 3–30.

Duck, S. W. (1973). *Personal relationships and personal constructs: A study of friendship formation.* London: Wiley.

Dugo, J. M., & Beck, A. P. (1983). Tracking a group's focus on normative-organizational or personal exploration issues. *Group, 7,* 17–26.

Dugo, J. M., & Beck, A. P. (1984). A therapist's guide to issues of intimacy and hostility viewed as group-level phenomena. *International Journal of Group Psychotherapy, 34,* 25–45.

Dunphy, D. C. (1972). *The primary group: A handbook for analysis and field research*. New York: Appleton-Century-Crofts.

Evensen, E. P., & Bednar, R. L. (1978). Effects of specific cognitive and behavioral structure on early group behavior and atmosphere. *Journal of Counseling Psychology, 25,* 66–75.

Flowers, J. V., & Schwartz, B. (1980). Behavioral group therapy with clients with heterogeneous problems. In D. Upper & S. M. Ross (Eds.), *Handbook of behavioral group therapy.* New York: Putnam.

Francis, D. J., Fletcher, J. M., Stuebing, K. K., Davidson, K. C., & Thompson, N. M. (1991). Analysis of change: Modeling individual growth. *Journal of Consulting and Psychology, 59,* 27–37.

Freud, S. (1921/1955). Group psychology and the analysis of the ego. In J. Strachey (Ed. and Trans.), *The standard edition of the complete psychological works of Sigmund Freud* (Vol. 14, pp. 67–143). London: Hogarth Press.

Fuehrer, A., & Keys, C. (1988). Group development in self-help groups for college students. *Small Group Behavior, 19,* 325–341.

Garland, J. A., Jones, H. E., & Kolodny, R. L. (1965). A model for stages of development in social work groups. In S. Bernstein (Ed.), *Explorations in group work.* Boston, MA: Milford House.

Gersick, C. J. G. (1988). Time and transition in work teams: Toward a new model of group development. *Academy of Management Journal, 31,* 9–41.

Gersick, C. J. G. (1989). Marking time: Predictable transitions in task groups. *Academy of Management Journal, 32,* 274–309.

Gibb, J. R. (1951). The effect of group size and of threat reduction upon creativity in a problem solving situation. *American Psychologist, 6,* 324.

Gibbard, G., & Hartman, J. (1973) Relationship patterns in self-analytic groups. *Behavioral Science, 18,* 335–353.

Gibbard, G., & Hartman, J. (1973). The Oedipal paradigm in group development: A clinical and empirical study. *Small Group Behavior, 4,* 305–354.

Gibbard, G., Hartman, J., & Mann, R.D. (Eds.). (1974). *Analysis of groups.* San Francisco, CA: Jossey-Bass.

Gist, M., Locke, E., & Taylor, M. (1987) Organizational behavior: Group structure, process, and effectiveness. *Journal of Management, 13,* 237–257.

Gottschalk, L. A., & Gleser, C. G. (1969). *The measurement of psychological states through the content analysis of verbal behavior.* Berkeley, CA: University of California Press.

Graham, J. W., Collins, L. M., Wugalter, S. E., Chung, N. K., & Hansen, W. B. (1991). Modeling transitions in latent stage-sequential processes: A substance use prevention example. *Journal of Consulting and Clinical Psychology, 59,* 48–57.

Greene, C. (1989). Cohesion and productivity in work groups. *Small Group Behavior, 20,* 70–86.

Hall, J., & Williams, M. S. (1966). A comparison of decision-making performances in established and ad hoc groups. *Journal of Personality and Social Psychology, 3,* 214–222.

Hare, A. P. (1972). Four dimensions of interpersonal behavior. *Psychological Reports, 30,* 499–512.

Hare, A. P. (1973). Theories of group development and categories for interactional analysis. *Small Group Behavior, 4,* 259–304.

Hare, A. P. (1976). *Handbook of small group research* (2nd ed.). New York: Free Press.

Hare, A. P., Borgatta, E. F., & Bales, R. F. (Eds.). (1955). *Small groups.* New York: Knopf.

Hartman, J. J., & Gibbard, G. S. (1974). Anxiety, boundary evolution, and social change. In G. S. Gibbard, J. J. Hartman, & R. D. Mann (Eds.), *Analysis of groups* (pp. 154–176). San Francisco, CA: Jossey-Bass.

Harvey, O. J., Hunt, D. E., & Schroder, H. M. (1961). *Conceptual systems and personality organization.* New York: Wiley.

Heinicke, C. H., & Bales, R. F. (1953). Developmental trends in the structure of small groups. *Sociometry, 16,* 7–36.

Hill, W. F. (1965), *Hill Interaction Matrix* (rev. ed.). Los Angeles, CA: Youth Studies Center, University of Southern California.

Hill, W. F. (1977). Hill Interaction Matrix (HIM): The conceptual framework, derived rating scales, and an updated bibliography. *Small Group Behavior, 8,* 251–268.

Hill, W. F., & Gruner L. (1973). A study of development in open and closed groups. *Small Group Behavior, 4,* 355–381.

Jennings, H. H. (1936). *Control study of sociometric assignment.* Sociometric Review. New York: Beacon House.

Jensen, L. (1990). Guidelines for the application of ARIMA models in time series. *Research in Nursing and Health, 13,* 429–435.

Kaplan, S. R., & Roman, M. (1963). Phases of development in an adult therapy group. *International Journal of Group Psychotherapy, 13,* 10–26.

Karterud, S., & Foss, T. (1989). The group emotionality rating system: A modification of Thelen's method of assessing emotionality in groups. *Small Group Behavior, 20,* 131–150.

Kaul T. J., & Bednar, R. L. (1986). Experiential group research: Results, questions, and suggestions. In S. L. Garfield & A. E. Bergin (Eds.), *Handbook of psychotherapy and behavior change* (3rd ed., pp. 671–714). New York: Wiley.

Kelley, H., & Thibault, J. (1954). Experimental studies in group problem solving processes. In G. Lindzey (Ed.), *Handbook of social psychology* (Vol. 2, pp. 735–785). Reading, MA: Addison-Wesley.

Kelly, G. A. (1955). *The psychology of personal constructs.* New York: Norton.

Kelly, J. R., & McGrath, J. E. (1985). Effects of time limits and task types on task performance and interaction of four-person groups. *Journal of Personality and Social Psychology, 48,* 395–407.

Kennedy, J. L., & MacKenzie, K. R. (1986). Dominance hierarchies in psychotherapy groups. *British Journal of Psychiatry, 148,* 625–631.

Kirshner, B. J., Dies, R. R., & Brown, R. A. (1978). Effects of experimental manipulation of self-disclosure on group cohesiveness. *Journal of Consulting and Clinical Psychology, 46,* 1171–1177.

Kivlighan, D. M., & Jauquet, C. A. (1990). Quality of group member agendas and group session climate. *Small Group Research, 21,* 205–219.

Kivlighan, D. M., & Mullison, D. (1988). Participants' perception of therapeutic factors in group counseling: The role of interpersonal style and stage of group development. *Small Group Behavior, 19,* 452–468.

Klein, M. (1948). *Contributions to psycho-analysis: 1921-1945.* London: Hogarth.

Kline, S. L., Pelias, R. J., & Delia, J. G. (1991). The predictive validity of cognitive complexity measures on social perspective-taking and counseling communication. *International Journal of Personal Construct Psychology, 4,* 347–357.

Krayer, K. J., & Fiechtner, S. B. (1984). Measuring group maturity: The development of a process-oriented variable for small group communication research. *Southern Speech Communication Journal, 50,* 78–92.

Kuypers, B. C., Davies, D., & Glaser, K. (1986). Developmental arrestations in self-analytic groups. *Small Group Behavior, 17,* 269–302.

Kuypers, B. C., Davies, D., & Hazelwinkel, A. (1986). Developmental patterns in self-analytic groups. *Human Relations, 39,* 793–815.

Kuypers, B. C., Davies, D., & van der Vegt, R. (1987). Training group development and outcomes. *Small Group Behavior, 18,* 309–335.

Lacoursiere, R. (1980). *The life cycle of groups: Group developmental stage theory.* New York: Human Sciences Press.

Leary, T. F. (1957). *Interpersonal diagnosis of personality.* New York: Ronald Press.

LeBon, L. (1896). *The crowd: A study of the popular mind.* London: Fisher Unwin.

Lee, F., & Bednar, R. L. (1977). Effects of group structure and risk-taking disposition on group behavior, attitudes, and atmosphere. *Journal of Counseling Psychology, 24,* 191–199.

Leichty, G. (1989). Interpersonal constructs and friendship form and structure. *International Journal of Personal Construct Psychology, 2,* 401–415.

Lermer, S. P., & Ermann, G. (1976). Der Stuttgarter Bogen (SB) zur Erfassung des Erlebens in der Gruppe (The Stuttgarter Bogen: A questionnaire for describing group experience). *Gruppendynamik, 2,* 133–140.

Levin, E. M., & Kurtz, R. R. (1974). Structured and non-structured human relation training. *Journal of Counseling Psychology, 21,* 526–531.

Lewin, K. (1947). Frontiers in group dynamics: Concept, method and reality in social science; Social equilibria and social change. *Human Relations, 1,* 5–41.

Lewin, K., Lippitt, R., & White, R. (1939). Patterns of aggressive behavior in experimentally created "social climates." *Journal of Social Psychology, 10,* 271–299.

Lewis, C. M., & Beck, A. P. (1983). Experiencing level in the process of group development. *Group, 7,* 18–26.

Lieberman, M. A., Yalom, I. D., & Miles, M. (1973). *Encounter groups: First facts.* New York: Basic Books.

Lundgren, D. (1971). Trainer style and patterns of group development. *Journal of Applied Behavioral Science, 7,* 689–709.

Lundgren, D., & Knight, D. (1978). Sequential stages of group development in sensitivity training groups. *Journal of Applied Behavioral Science, 14,* 204–222.

MacKenzie, K. R. (1983). The clinical application of a group measure. In R. R. Dies & K. R. MacKenzie (Eds.), *Advances in group psychotherapy: Integrating research and practice* (pp. 159–170). New York: International Universities Press.

MacKenzie, K. R. (1987). Therapeutic factors in group psychotherapy: A contemporary view. *Group, 11,* 26–34.

MacKenzie, K. R. (1990). *Introduction to time-limited group psychotherapy.* Washington, DC: American Psychiatric Press.

MacKenzie, K. R., Dies, D. D., Coché, E., Rutan, J. S., & Stone, W. N. (1987). An analysis of AGPA institute groups. *International Journal of Group Psychotherapy, 37,* 55–74.

MacKenzie, K. R., & Kennedy, J. L. (1991). Primate ethology and group dynamics. In S. Tuttman (Ed.), *Psychoanalytic group theory and therapy: Essays in honor of Saul Scheidlinger.* New York: International Universities Press.

MacKenzie, K. R., & Livesley, W. J. (1983). A developmental model for brief group therapy. In R. R. Dies & K. R. MacKenzie (Eds.), *Advances in group psychotherapy: Integrating research and practice* (pp. 101–116). New York: International Universities Press.

MacKenzie, K. R., & Tschuschke, V. (in press). Relatedness, group work, and outcome in long-term inpatient psychotherapy groups. *Journal of Psychotherapy Practice and Research.*

Mann, R. D. (1966). The development of the member-trainer relationship in self-analytic groups. *Human Relations, 19,* 85–115.

Mann, R., Gibbard, G., & Hartman, J. (1967). *Interpersonal styles and group development.* New York: Wiley.

Martin, E. A., & Hill, W. F. (1957). Toward a theory of group development: Six phases of therapy group development. *International Journal of Group Psychotherapy, 1,* 20–30.

McDougall, W. (1920). *The group mind.* New York: Putnam.

McGrath, J. E. (1991). Time, interaction, and performance (TIP): A theory of groups. *Small Group Behavior, 22,* 147–174.

McGrath, J. E., & Kelly, J. R. (1986). *Time and human interaction: Toward a social psychology of time.* New York: Guilford Press.

McGuire, J. M., Taylor, D. R., Broome, D. H., Blau, B. I., & Abbott, D. W. (1986). Group structuring techniques and their influence on process involvement in a group counseling training group. *Journal of Counseling Psychology, 33,* 270–275.

Mennecke, B. E., Hoffer, J. A., & Wynne, B. E. (1992). The implications of group development and history for group support system theory and practice. *Small Group Research, 23,* 524–572.

Mills, T. M. (1964). *Group transformations: An analysis of a learning group.* Englewood Cliffs, NJ: Prentice-Hall.

Mills, T. M. (1978). Seven steps in developing group awareness. *Journal of Personality and Social Systems, 4,* 15–29.

Moos, R. H. (1974). *Evaluating treatment environments.* New York: Wiley. Moreland, R. L., & Levine, J. M. (1988). Group dynamics over time: Development and socialization in small groups. In J. E. McGrath (Ed.), *The social psychology of time* (pp. 151–181). Newbury Park, CA: Sage.

Moreland, R. L., & Levine, J. M. (1988). Group dynamics over time: Development and socialization in small groups. In J. E. McGrath (Ed.), *The social psychology of time*. Newbury Park, CA: Sage.

Moreno, J. L. (1931). *Who shall survive?* New York: Beacon House.

Moreno, J. L. (Ed.). (1960). *The sociometry reader.* New York: Free Press of Glencoe.

Neimeyer, G. J., Banikiotes, P. G., & Fami, L. E. (1979). Self disclosure and psychological construing: A personal construct approach to interpersonal perception. *Journal of Social Behavior and Personality, 7,* 161–165.

Neimeyer, G. J., & Merluzzi, T. V. (1982). Group structure and process: Personal construct theory and group development. *Small Group Behavior, 13,* 150–164.

O'Farrell, M. K. (1986). *The effect of timing of goal setting on outcome in personal growth groups.* Unpublished doctoral dissertation, University of Maryland, College Park, MD.

Orlinsky, D. E., & Howard, K. I. (1978). The relation of process to outcome in psychotherapy. In S. L. Garfield & A. E. Bergin (Eds.), *Handbook of psychotherapy and behavior change* (2nd ed., pp. 283–329). New York: Wiley.

Parsons, T., & Shils, E. A. (1951). *Toward a general theory of action.* New York: Harper & Row.

Perlmutter, M. S., & Hatfield, E. (1980). Intimacy, intentional metacommunication and second order change. *American Journal of Family Therapy, 8,* 17–23.

Peters, L. N., & Beck, A. P. (1982). Identifying emergent leaders in psychotherapy groups. *Group, 6,* 35–40.

Poole, M. S. (1983). Decision development in small groups: III. A multiple sequence model of group decision making. *Communications Monographs, 50,* 321–344.

Poole, M. S., & Roth, M. S. (1989). Decision development in small groups: V. Test of a contingency model. *Human Communications Research, 15,* 549–589.

Putman, L. L. (1979). Preference for procedural order in task-oriented small groups. *Communication Monographs, 46,* 193–218.

Rohde, R. I. (1988). The effect of structured feedback on goal attainment, attraction to group, and satisfaction with the group in small group counseling (Doctoral dissertation, Indiana University, 1988). *Dissertation Abstracts International, 49,* 2542A.

Rose, G. S., & Bednar, R. L. (1980). Effects of positive and negative self-disclosure and feedback on early group development. *Journal of Counseling Psychology, 27,* 63–70.

Saravay, S. M. (1978). A psychoanalytic theory of group development. *International Journal of Group Psychotherapy, 28,* 481–507.

Schein, E. H., & Bennis, W. G. (1965). *Personal and organizational change through group methods.* New York: Wiley.

Schroeder, M. L., Wormworth, J. A., & Livesley, W. J. (1992). Dimensions of personality disorder and their relationships to the big five dimensions of personality. *Psychological Assessment: A Journal of Consulting and Clinical Psychology, 4,* 47–53.

Schutz, W. C. (1958). *FIRO: A three-dimensional theory of interpersonal behavior.* New York: Holt, Rinehart and Winston.

Silbergeld, S., Koenig, G. R., Manderscheid, R. W., Meeker, B. F., & Horning, C. A. (1975). Assessment of environment-therapy systems: The group atmosphere scale. *Journal of Consulting and Clinical Psychology, 43,* 460–469.

Simmel, G. (1902-03). The number of members as determining the sociological form of the group. *American Journal of Sociology, 8,* 1–46, 158–196.

Slater, P. (1966). *Microcosm.* New York: Wiley.

Smuts, B., Cheney, D., Seyfarth, R., Wrangham, R., & Struhsaker, T. (1987). *Primate societies.* Chicago, IL: University of Chicago Press.

Stock, D., & Thelen, H. A. (1958). *Emotional dynamics and group culture.* New York: New York University Press.

Stockton, R., & Hulse, D. (1981). Developing cohesion in small groups: Theory and research. *Journal for Specialists in Group Work, 6*(3),188–194.

Stockton, R., Rohde, R. I., & Haughey, J. (1992). The effects of structured group exercises on cohesion, engagement, avoidance, and conflict. *Small Group Behavior, 23,* 155–168.

Stogdill, R. M. (1972). Group productivity, drive and cohesiveness. *Organizational Behavior and Human Performance, 8,* 26–43.

Thelen, H. A. (1954). *Dynamics of groups at work.* Chicago, IL: University of Chicago Press.

Tschuschke, V., & MacKenzie, K. R. (1989). Empirical analysis of group development: A methodological report. *Small Group Behavior, 20,* 419–427.

Tuckman, B. W. (1965). Developmental sequence in small groups. *Psychological Bulletin, 63,* 384–399.

Tuckman, B., & Jensen, M. (1977). Stages of small group development. *Group and Organizational Studies, 2,* 419–427.

Verdi, A. F., & Wheelan, S. A. (1992). Developmental patterns in same-sex and mixed-sex groups. *Small Group Research, 23,* 356–378.

Walster, E., Walster, G. W., & Berscheid, E. (1978). *Equity: Theory and research.* Boston, MA: Allyn & Bacon.

Waltman, D. E., & Zimpfer, D. G. (1988). Composition, structure, and duration of treatment: Interacting variables in counselling groups. *Small Group Behavior, 19,* 171–184.

Wheelan, S. A., & McKeage, R. L. (1993). Developmental patterns in small and large groups. *Small Group Research, 24,* 60–83.

Whitaker, D. S., & Lieberman, M. A. (1964). *Psychotherapy through the group process.* New York: Atherton.

Whitman, R. M., & Stock, D. (1958). The group focal conflict. *Psychiatry, 21,* 269–276.

Wiggins, J. S., & Pincus, A. L. (1989). Conceptions of personality disorders and dimensions of personality. *Psychological Assessment: A Journal of Consulting and Clinical Psychology, 1,* 305–316.

Yalom, I. D. (1985). *The theory and practice of group psychotherapy* (3rd ed.). New York: Basic Books.

CHAPTER 8

Therapeutic Factors: Interpersonal and Intrapersonal Mechanisms

ERIC C. CROUCH, SIDNEY BLOCH, and JANINE WANLASS

The notion that "therapeutic factors" operate in psychotherapeutic treatments is based on the assumption that it is possible to produce a classification of beneficial elements of therapy. In the case of group therapy, this classification includes many group-specific interpersonal factors as well as the intrapersonal factors frequently associated with individual therapy. For example, a person's sense of gain from the appreciation of being accepted "warts and all" by other members of a cohesive "working together" group is clearly an interpersonal element. In contrast, the realization that "I have learned an important lesson about myself today" may have arisen from interpersonal group events but has an intrapersonal focus similar to that observed in individual therapy.

How useful is the therapeutic factors framework in conceptualizing group therapy, and how well-established are specific therapeutic factors (TFs) appearing in the group therapy literature? In this chapter, we try to answer these questions by summarizing empirical research bearing on the subject. First, we briefly discuss the definition and the development of the therapeutic factor concept. Second, we report the empirical research to date on single interpersonal and intrapersonal factors. Third, we review empirical studies considering therapeutic factors as a set or group, particularly focusing on comparative evaluations. Last, we discuss limitations of the therapeutic factors framework and describe implications for future research and clinical practice.

Our review begins with studies conducted in the mid-1950s, since little investigative work on TFs occurred before this time. We have included group literature covering a variety of group treatments (e.g., educative, psychodynamic, sensitivity, "growth," cognitive-behavioral, research-based experimental), though most research bearing on TFs emerges from psychodynamic, interpersonal, and related group interventions. The quality of empirical work is extremely variable, and we have erred on the side of including less than satisfactory studies for two reasons. First, the view would be quite limited if it included only research that met exacting criteria of sample size, specified patient characteristics, clear description of therapy methods, valid and reliable measures of process and outcome, appropriate statistical methods, and relevant use of control subjects. Second, unsatisfactory studies may shed light on a topic, if only to suggest how future studies might be improved.

DEFINITION AND DEVELOPMENT OF THERAPEUTIC FACTORS

What is a therapeutic factor? The elements considered therapeutic by clinicians have been insufficiently investigated to establish a definitive clinical consensus. To provide some frame of reference for discussion, TFs are defined as *an element of group therapy that contributes to improvement in a patient's condition and can be a function of the actions of the group therapist, the other group members, and the patient himself.* Additionally, therapeutic factors may be categorized as predominantly interpersonal or intrapersonal in focus. Interpersonal factors depend primarily on interactional group processes and include cohesion (acceptance), learning from interpersonal action, guidance, vicarious learning, universality, altruism, and the instillation of hope. Insight (self-understanding), catharsis, and self-disclosure comprise intrapersonal factors, relying on internal, individual processes. Both sets of factors may promote therapeutic growth in the patient. For example, acceptance is a feeling that arises in the patient as a result of specific group forces, such as support, caring, validation, and friendliness. Their generation depends to a great extent on the therapist's actions in encouraging a cohesive group. On the other hand, self-disclosure is an individually oriented factor. The discloser gains from an activity he or she initiates and sustains, though the receptive nature of the group members is also important.

How did the concept of TFs develop? Early pioneers in group therapy made references to the TF idea. For instance, Joseph Pratt (1975) identified what we would now describe as the instillation of hope as a curative force in group treatment. Burrow (1927) alluded to vicarious learning and universality as contributing to patient improvement. Wender (1936) described four therapeutic factors operating in his groups: intellectualization, the effects exerted by one member on another, catharsis-in-the-family, and interaction. These early clinicians recognized the existence of growth promoting elements within the group setting, though their writing placed much more emphasis on technique.

During and after World War II, the application of psychoanalytic concepts to group therapy blossomed, with contributions from analysts such as Slavson and Wolf in the United States and Foulkes and Bion in the United Kingdom. Slavson (1979) emphasized that TFs in group therapy were identical to those in individual therapy (e.g., transference, catharsis, insight). In contrast, Foulkes identified group specific TFs such as acceptance, universality, vicarious learning, and the activation of the collective unconscious.

The watershed in the evolution of TFs came in 1955, when Corsini and Rosenberg published their review of the "dynamics leading to successful therapy." Examining some 300 articles, they constructed a list of 10 therapeutic elements (i.e., acceptance, altruism, universalization, intellectualization, reality testing, transference, interaction, spectator therapy, ventilation, miscellaneous), which could be further collapsed into three broad factors (i.e., intellectual, emotional, actional). Though Corsini and Rosenberg's categorization scheme has been criticized (Bloch & Crouch, 1985), it represents the "first and all important step in bringing some taxonomic order into the group psychotherapeutic scene" (Hill, 1975), ushering in a phase of substantial theoretical and empirical work.

Berzon, Pious, and Farson (1963) began asking group members what they regarded as significant, using the "most important event" questionnaire to elicit nine factors quite similar to those identified by Corsini and Rosenberg (1955). Another milestone was Yalom's 1970 publication, *The Theory and Practice of Group Psychotherapy.* Yalom makes his major theoretical contribution by exploring the therapeutic operation of interaction, marking his central TF as interpersonal learning. Additionally, he identifies instillation of hope, guidance, an existential factor, self-understanding, altruism, group cohesiveness, universality, catharsis, identification, and family re-enactment as therapeutic elements.

Our own classification system (Bloch & Crouch, 1985), guided by our belief that TFs should be atheoretical, includes self-understanding, catharsis (release of feelings), self-disclosure (revelation to the group of private material), learning from interpersonal interaction (relating constructively and adaptively by trying new behaviors), universality, acceptance, altruism, guidance, vicarious learning, and the instillation of hope.

Thus, some notion of TFs has existed since the beginnings of group intervention, though recent years have contributed specificity, theoretical debate, and empirically based research to early therapist speculations. The empirical research, which varies in quality, includes the examination of TFs in isolation and in combination, the latter allowing for more complex conclusions about the effects of TFs on group process and outcome.

RESEARCH ON SINGLE THERAPEUTIC FACTORS: COHESION (ACCEPTANCE)

The importance of cohesiveness has long been recognized. Corsini and Rosenberg (1955) noted that cohesion is the element most frequently described as therapeutic in the literature. However, cohesiveness as a concept has evaded clear definition and description. From our viewpoint, one definitional problem is the need to distinguish between a group's sense of "togetherness" or "esprit de corps" and the individual member's own feeling of belonging and being valued. The first element, termed group cohesiveness, is best regarded as a condition for change facilitating the operation of various TFs. In fact, it is often regarded as one of the most important conditions for change, reflected in Yalom's (1985) discussion of the therapeutic power of interpersonal learning occurring within a cohesive group context. However, it is the second element of cohesion, acceptance (the individual perceives a sense of belonging and gains benefit from the realization that this can happen to him), that seems more properly considered an actual TF.

Additionally, the multifaceted nature of cohesiveness contributes to the lack of clarity in the literature (Mudrack, 1989), prompting researchers to isolate more specific dimensions subsumed by this broad term. Cartwright's notable review from the 1960s attempts to distinguish between the forces that determine cohesiveness (e.g., group's prestige) and the consequences of cohesiveness (e.g., enhanced participation). Bednar and Kaul (1978) actually dispense with the term cohesiveness and replace it with the different specific elements it embodies. Braaten (1991) produced a five-factor model of cohesion comprising attraction and bonding, support and caring, listening and empathy, self-disclosure and feedback, and process performance and goal attainment. Evans and Jarvis (1980) review how the conceptualization of group cohesiveness has been linked to attempts at measurement, highlighting the failure to separate out attraction to the group from group cohesion. Drescher, Burlingame, and Fuhriman (1985) present a scholarly review dealing thoroughly with the lack of conceptual clarity and variable approaches to measurement in empirical studies of cohesiveness. They use a multidimensional process classification system to compare studies along the dimensions of Person ("who"), Variable ("what"), Measurement ("how"), and Time ("when"). They comment not only on the relevance of the four separate measurement parameters, but also on how such dimensions interact. For example, the group leader may contribute significantly to cohesiveness in the early hours of the group, but as time passes, member-to-member or member-to-group effects may become more important.

Empirical Research

A comprehensive review of empirical work on cohesiveness by Lott and Lott (1965) is now dated but does emphasize the importance of antecedent and consequential factors. Paralleling Cartwright's (1968) ideas about determinants and consequences, they suggest both antecedents to cohesion (e.g., a democratic atmosphere, interaction between members) and consequences of cohesion (e.g., tolerance for the expression of anger, increased attraction between members). Lott and Lott regard the interaction of these antecedent and consequential factors as pivotal in understanding cohesion as a therapeutic factor.

Piper, Marrache, Lacroix, Richardsen, and Jones (1983) focus on cohesiveness, constructing a strong study with laboratory groups. They set up nine groups of five participants each that met for eight sessions. Group procedures were carefully defined and measurements made by means of questionnaires (focusing on bonding items), behavioral ratings (focusing on cohesion), and self rating scales (focusing on learning). A factor analysis of the results suggested a multidimensional view of cohesiveness, including a circumscribed factor that might represent the core of cohesiveness and be distinguishable from related concepts. Three "group as a whole" factors were identified—mutual stimulation and effect (a level of arousal that may promote learning), commitment to the group (allegiance, identification with aims, etc.), and compatibility (mutual liking, enjoyment of the group's activities). The authors conclude that commitment represents the core component of cohesiveness.

Cohesiveness and Outcome

Clinicians typically describe the positive influence of cohesion on outcome, though there is some acknowledgment of an anti-therapeutic dimension. A few studies lend support to the positive contributions of cohesion, while one study relates cohesiveness to poor outcome.

Yalom, Houts, Zimmerberg, and Rand (1967) carried out an exploratory study aimed at identifying predictors of improvement among group therapy patients, and included among the measures a cohesiveness questionnaire. They studied 40 patients in five out-patient groups for a year, administering questionnaires before and during treatment, and conducting a semi-structured interview at the end of the year. They found a positive correlation between cohesiveness and self-ratings of symptom improvement and in overall functioning, but the correlation did not hold when interviewer ratings of outcome were included. Nevertheless, the specific factor of an individual's popularity in the group (more akin to acceptance) did correlate highly with both self- and interviewer-ratings on all outcome measures. The pattern of dropouts and the course of improvement in those who stayed suggested an initial, unstable phase followed later by a more cohesive and helpful period. This study was well-planned and executed, the one limitation being the lack of follow-up assessment beyond the termination of the group experience.

Weiss (1972) explored the relationships between cohesiveness, outcome, and aspects of group process in 12-hour marathon groups. Audiotaped segments of group sessions were rated for interaction while the participants completed questionnaires designed to measure cohesiveness on several occasions throughout the group's life. Cohesiveness developed in a linear fashion as the marathon proceeded, but no clear-cut relationship with interaction was discovered. One measure of cohesiveness was moderately correlated with outcome, but there were no clear indications of therapeutic gain. Although the study was well-designed, such a short-term group with student participants is unlikely to yield useful information about therapeutic outcome.

Budman and his colleagues (1989) completed the most impressive study from a design perspective. They investigated the multidimensional nature of cohesiveness (as suggested by theoretical speculation), the degree of correspondence between cohesiveness in group therapy and the therapeutic alliance in individual therapy, and the relationship between cohesion and outcome. The experimental sample consisted of 12 time-limited (15 sessions) psychotherapy groups for mostly anxious or depressed young adults. A range of outcome measures was used, including target problem measures and global scales. The selected cohesion measure was developed in an earlier study.

A scale for measuring alliance was adapted to measure the interrelationships of group members. Findings suggested that cohesiveness, while multidimensional in concept, acted as if related to a single underlying factor. Additionally, cohesion and alliance appeared closely connected. Furthermore, ratings of improvement correlated most strongly with cohesiveness measured early in the group's development. This finding suggests that therapy groups are more productive when group cohesion is quickly established. This study is notable not only for its rigorous design but also for the detailed specification of experimental variables and measures used. It warrants replication with different patient samples and therapy modalities to establish the generalizability of its results.

A study by Roether and Peters (1972) challenges the customary view that cohesiveness is advantageous. They examined cohesiveness, the expression of hostility, and the relationship of both to outcome in a group of sex offenders mandated to attend group therapy. Cohesiveness was associated with poor outcome. Successful treatment was linked to the expression of hostility to figures outside the group. Though interesting, this study has certain drawbacks and limits on generalizability. Cohesiveness was rated by the therapists rather than by members or independent observers, group membership was involuntary, and outcome was determined by offender rearrest rates—an important but idiosyncratic measure of improvement. The study reminds us that not all groups are similar, and that groups with unusual membership may have unusual characteristics.

Cohesiveness and TFs

If cohesiveness is a condition for change, it seems valuable to understand its relationship to other TFs. Janet (1969) investigated the relationship between feedback (excerpts of previous sessions viewed on videotape), interaction, and cohesiveness. Results suggested that videotape feedback and consequent interaction may increase cohesion, though the experiment must be criticized for its small numbers and poor design. Weiss (1972) sounds a note of caution in his study of marathon groups (six 12-hour groups), finding no relationship between cohesion and interaction. Braaten (1990) used his five-factor model to examine cohesiveness in 26 therapy and consulting groups (211 participants). Members regularly completed accounts of "critical events" from each session which were categorized by independent raters. Additionally, the total cohesiveness of specific sessions was measured with a group climate questionnaire, allowing for the comparison of sessions with high and low cohesiveness. Highly cohesive sessions were dominated by self-disclosure and feedback, attraction and bonding, listening and empathy. Less cohesive sessions were characterized by avoidance, defensiveness, conflict, and rebellion. Thus, the results of these studies lend moderate support to the positive effects of cohesion in promoting TFs.

The Therapist's Role

What can the therapist do to promote group cohesion? As confirmed by Liberman (1970a), the therapist can adopt a method of intervention specifically designed to increase cohesion. Liberman compared a control group to an experimental group where the leader was trained to reinforce and to prompt member statements reflecting cohesion. Observer ratings found higher levels of cohesion in the experimental group than in the control group. Liberman suggested that optimal levels of cohesion can be secured when the therapist responds quickly to the target behavior (i.e., cohesion), keeps the intervention simple in content, addresses the patient directly, uses reinforcement more than prompting, and avoids the satiation of the group through excessive comment. Though clearly stated, Liberman's conclusions may be a bit grandiose for one small experiment, supporting the importance of replication.

Another issue relevant to promoting cohesiveness is therapist style. Hurst (1978) studied 12 adolescent groups (6 each from two distinct cultural backgrounds) run by pairs of therapists, measuring leadership style, cohesiveness, and patients' attitudes towards self and others at various times during the 30-week program. Cohesiveness was associated with two aspects of leadership, therapist caring and self-expressiveness (i.e., transparency). Though therapist style is an important aspect of psychotherapy (Lieberman, Yalom, & Miles, 1973), the topic has received little empirical attention within the group therapy realm.

The way the therapist organizes the group may also affect cohesiveness. Group organization includes decisions about meeting times, group structure, and group composition. Dies and Hess (1971) showed that cohesiveness develops more rapidly in a marathon group (a single 12-hour session) than in a conventional group (one hour daily for 12 successive days). In an analogue study, Marshall and Heslin (1975) found that cohesion was higher in smaller groups of mixed gender.

The effects of group member compatibility on cohesion deserve comment. William Schutz (1958) developed the FIRO-B, a self-report questionnaire that assesses how the respondent behaves towards others and how the respondent wants others to behave towards him along the dimensions of inclusion (belonging), control (handling power), and affection (intimacy). A number of studies similar in design employed the FIRO-B to examine the relationship between cohesion and member compatibility. The FIRO-B was administered to members before the group began, and cohesiveness was rated by those same members at a later time. Although a positive relationship between compatibility and cohesiveness was noted by two research teams (Riley, 1971; Yalom & Rand, 1966), this conclusion was contradicted by Costell and Koran (1972). These inconclusive results and work by Bugen (1977) suggest that compatibility is neither a unitary concept nor stable over time, making its relationship with cohesion difficult to interpret.

Conclusion

The consideration of group cohesion as a therapeutic factor reflects Bednar and Kaul's (1978) comment, "there is little cohesion in the cohesion research." Despite this ambiguity (in part a result of definitional problems), we suggest some tentative conclusions. The core of cohesiveness (a condition for change) is the commitment of group members to the aims and the work of the group which can be distinguished from the compatibility of members (which may or may not be therapeutic) and from the satisfaction of being a group member. Additionally, we see a need to separate out a TF of acceptance, somewhat overshadowed by the large and engaging topic of cohesiveness. Cohesiveness is probably a primary condition that enables a group to function whereas acceptance may be a relatively less important TF. Certainly, cohesion is an important element of the group therapy experience. The therapeutic effect of cohesion appears more salient when established early in the group's development. The relationship of cohesion to outcome, group composition, other TFs, and therapist style warrants additional empirical attention.

LEARNING FROM INTERPERSONAL ACTION

Interpersonal interaction is clearly inherent in group psychotherapy and seems a necessary condition for change. The TF that arises from interaction is generally known as interpersonal learning or learning from interpersonal action (LIA). Its essence is a learning process arising from the experience of interaction and emphasizing the acquisition of new, more adaptive ways of relating to others.

Despite the fundamental nature of interpersonal learning, theoretical descriptions of its importance were curiously slow to develop. Much early writing on group therapy emphasized the importance of the therapist. Early didactic models stressed instruction by the group leader. The later psychoanalytic approach originally viewed interaction as the transference relationship between therapist and group members. In this way, group treatment was seen as comparable to individual analysis. Gradually, the idea grew that the dimensions of transference in group therapy were substantially wider than in individual work, and that transference between patients, or to the group as a whole, provided useful therapeutic material.

At the time Corsini and Rosenberg (1955) devised their classification of TFs, it was becoming clear that a distinct factor related to interaction needed definition. However, the nature of this factor remained vague and unspecified. A more precise definition highlighting the central importance of interpersonal learning in group therapy is most fully expressed by Yalom (1985). A comparative examination of his three editions illustrates that the ideas are still evolving. In the earlier edition of his text, a clear distinction is made between interpersonal learning-input (patient incorporation of feedback received from fellow group members) and interpersonal learning-output (an actional factor where the patient learns from her changed behavior in the group). The last edition brings the two elements together into one overarching factor of interpersonal learning (which also encompasses transference and insight).

Bloch and Crouch (1985) defined an actional factor related to interpersonal learning, adopting the term "learning from interpersonal action" (LIA). This view regards insight or self-understanding as separate, classifiable among the intrapersonal factors. LIA is the attempt to relate constructively and adaptively within the group, either by initiating some behavior or responding to group members. More important than the reaction of other group members is the patient's attempt to modify his or her own mode of relating. This factor operates when the patient tries out new, potentially positive ways of initiating behavior with other group members. These methods can include expressing oneself to co-members to clarify one's relationship with them, making an explicit and overt effort to develop a more open relationship with other members, expressing oneself in a constructively assertive fashion, and working to achieve intimacy with other group members. Additionally, the group member may demonstrate new ways of responding to others such as being more sensitive or accepting valid criticism.

Empirical Research

Theoretical discussions of interpersonal learning span a variety of orientations and have evolved over time (Astrachan, 1970; Bach, 1957; Coché & Coché, 1990; Cohn, 1969; Durkin, 1982; Farrell, 1962; Glad & Durkin, 1969; Slavson, 1966; Stein, 1970; Sullivan, 1953; Yalom, 1985). In great contrast to the theoretical work, systematic empirical research relevant to LIA has been limited in amount and quality. The few available studies have concentrated on measurements of interaction, the relationships between interaction and various personality factors of group members, and the connection between interaction and therapist behavior.

Measurements of Interaction

Though only indirectly related to LIA, measurement of interaction between patients provides a starting point for discussion. Most relevant are studies examining patients' interactional patterns. McPherson and Walton (1970) provided a useful review of the topic, reporting a study where experienced clinicians described group members' interactional patterns through a repertory grid technique. Analysis revealed three main independent dimensions of behavior: (1) assertive/dominant versus passive/submissive; (2) emotionally sensitive versus emotionally insensitive (to peers); and (3) aiding versus hindering the group's goals.

Empirically derived frameworks of this type provide a potentially valuable tool for observation and measurement of interaction in therapy groups. A more comprehensive classification of interpersonal behavior has been offered by Lorr (1966). He described a study of 45 groups containing nearly 200 neurotic or psychotic patients (in remission). Four meetings of mature groups were used as data by observers rating patients' interpersonal behavior on a schedule of 75 items. Factor analysis supported eight dimensions of relating: dominance, hostility, leadership role, supportive role, help-seeking, submissiveness, withdrawal, and disorganization. A second-order analysis yielded four higher level factors: activity level, submissiveness/disorganization, supportive role, and leadership role.

Another approach to the measurement of interpersonal behavior, the Fundamental Interpersonal Relations Orientation (FIRO) devised by William Schutz (1966), uses a self-report measure. Schutz regards humans' chief social needs as control, inclusion, and affection. The FIRO scales rate the need to control or be controlled, the wish to be included or excluded from the activities of others, and the wish for closeness or distance from others.

These measures are interesting but rudimentary. Lorr's work relies too much on the subjectivity of raters, and the self-administered FIRO was not derived for groups. However, these studies do at least draw attention to the difficulties of identifying and rating the key dimensions of interpersonal relatedness.

Interaction and Personality Factors

Two studies have examined the relationship between interaction and personality factors. Ryan (1958) focused on a quality he termed "capacity for mutual dependence" (CMD). CMD incorporates the capacity to "give" (empathize, form relationships, delay gratification, act altruistically) and the capacity to handle wishes for others to gratify one's needs. A Rorschach-based scale was used to assess whether individuals were giving, nongiving, dependence-flexible (i.e., able to handle both dependence and independence appropriately), dependence-accepting, or dependence-denying. A high CMD scale represents a giving, dependence-flexible individual. Ryan administered this measure to 25 group therapy patients, discovering that high CMD was associated with high group involvement (rated by group therapists). Although there are severe methodological limitations (small sample, nonindependent raters, questionable measuring instrument), this notion of CMD warrants more attention.

An analogue study by Lee (1976) investigated the link between interaction and preparedness to take risks, showing how these characteristics relate to gender and group structure. Ninety-six students with extreme scores on a risk-taking scale were randomly assigned to simulated first group therapy sessions. These sessions consisted of practice trials for training in three prescribed behaviors—self-disclosure, feedback, and confrontation. Group sessions were highly, moderately, or minimally structured. The results suggested that men and high-risk-taking subjects were most interactive in their behaviors and that interactive behaviors were most common in highly structured groups. These conclusions lend support to the idea that gender and specific personality characteristics may influence patterns of interaction.

Interaction and the Therapist's Role

Three studies consider the therapist's potential role in promoting interactive behavior. Heckel, Froelich, and Salzberg (1962) reported an experiment suggesting that therapists can directly manipulate the level and direction of group interaction. The therapist in a small group of psychiatric inpatients was trained to redirect members' comments back to the group. He employed this redirection in three sessions, then desisted this behavior. Analysis of audiotaped coding supported a clear relationship between the therapist's actions and the patients' interactional patterns. Redirection was associated with greater interaction among patients, though no outcome measures were employed to evaluate the result of such behavior.

In a similar study, Salzberg (1962) used four modes of relation between therapist and patients (i.e., silence, talking, redirecting, directing). Four combinations of these modes were deployed in 15-minute segments of each session. Patients' responses were coded by frequency, form (interactive or noninteractive), and content. As might be expected, therapist silence led to more interaction while therapist talking led to less interaction. Redirecting had no effect on the form of the patient's responses but did increase the frequency of patient responses. Salzberg concluded that the therapist should talk early in group development to provide structure, utilizing redirection as the group matures. Though a reasonable strategy, this seems to represent an overinterpretation of the data.

Land (1964) investigated the relationship between therapist style and outcome, comparing the effects of a more active, directive therapist stance to the effects of therapist silence and redirection. The sample consisted of 60 psychiatric inpatients divided into six groups (three groups of chronically ill and three groups of acutely ill). One group in each condition acted as an untreated control group. The discrepant findings emerging from these two clinical samples illustrate the complexity of the relationship between therapist behavior and group interaction. With acutely ill patients, interaction was more evident when the therapist employed silence and redirection. This effect was not noted among chronic patients. None of the patients showed any substantial improvement on outcome measures; however, 10 group therapy sessions do not represent an adequate intervention for seriously ill patients. Though Land's study adds nothing to discussions of interaction-outcome links, it makes a point that the relationship between therapist style and patient interaction is affected by group composition.

The Quality of Interaction

In the above studies, interaction is addressed as a unidimensional process worthy of encouragement. This raises a question about the nature and quality of group interaction, an issue investigated by Flowers (1978) through an ingenious, though somewhat intrusive, set of experiments. Patients and therapists were instructed to exchange tokens in response to statements made within the group—giving blue tokens to accompany positive statements and red tokens to accompany negative statements. This token exchange made explicit the perceived quality and effect of group interaction.

The first experiment was conducted with six "severely disturbed" outpatients participating in 18 group sessions. Flowers reports that the token exchange accurately reflected the proportions of positive and negative statements. Additionally their use was associated with an increase in interaction between patients, in overall interaction within the group, and in negative statements (critical feedback) made by therapists to patients. A second experiment with nine student volunteers attending 15 sessions employed a slightly different design. In this experiment, negative statements correlated with increased interaction between members, provided the negative statements were of low intensity. In other words, the gentle expression of critical comments by the group leader promoted interaction and trust between members. Another finding of interest was the reduction in positive interaction between members when the therapist delivered mostly negative statements. Thus, the therapist seemed to act as a model for negativity. These studies raise some questions about interaction quality, though the intrusiveness of the token strategy may confound the results.

Anecdotally, group size and stability is another issue that seems to influence the quality of interaction. Grosz, Stern, and Wright (1965) concluded that the level of group interaction did vary with the number of members (groups of six members were more interactive than groups of four members), though this study displays numerous methodological problems. Thomas and Fink (1963) reviewed the topic of group size, concluding that the number of group members does impact the quality of interaction. A later study by Grosz and Wright (1967) highlighted the effects of stable membership on group interaction. In addition to group size, they noted that stability of membership from session to session was associated with increased interaction.

Interaction and Outcome

The relationship between interaction and outcome has received little empirical attention. Land's (1964) inconclusive study has been mentioned. Kaye

(1973) investigated the interaction-outcome link in two sensitivity-training groups comprised of 27 academically unsuccessful students. These groups were compared to control groups of nonparticipating academically successful and unsuccessful students. Kaye used the Hill Interaction Matrix to measure the content and style of group interaction in a 10-day group experience and two outcome measures (the FIRO and an interpersonal checklist). Some group members showed evidence of positive change in response to member-centered, emotionally involving interaction. However, these positive changes were no longer evident during an eight month follow-up. Kaye suggested that long-term change would necessitate a more confrontational mode of group interaction. Despite the study's limitations (small, nonclinical sample and short-term group format), the positive design features of control subjects and long-term follow-up warrant replication.

Research by Swarr and Ewing (1977) observed an interaction-outcome association, with particular attention to timing issues. They studied 45 student patients with neurotic problems treated in interactional group therapy for an average of six months. Positive change was apparent in the first 10 sessions in specific areas such as low self-esteem and anxiety. Other problems such as poor interpersonal functioning, distrust, hostility, and lack of assertion showed significant improvement only at the end of treatment. Though this study lacks follow-up evaluation of treatment gains, it does lend support to the importance of interaction in treating various relationship-based problems and to the significance of timing and group development considerations.

Conclusion

Theoretical ideas about group therapy underline the importance of interactional process as a central therapeutic element. However, empirical study has been scanty and unsophisticated. What conclusions can be drawn from the combination of theoretical and empirical studies? The chief theoretical gulf is between psychoanalytic and dynamic-interactional approaches. The first emphasizes cognitive aspects of the interactional process with special attention to transference; the second is more concerned with behavioral change in the interpersonal domain. There are commonalities, a body of thought which suggests the relevance of both cognitive and behavioral dimensions in interactional learning.

Of the empirical studies, only Kaye's (1973) work sets out to clarify features of therapeutic interaction. Future research could be directed toward the experimental investigation of cognitive and behavioral aspects of interpersonal learning. For example, which aspects of interaction are associated with positive outcome in what type of patient? Do patients learn best from practicing new forms of interpersonal behavior or from understanding the source of their relationship difficulties? On the basis of current knowledge, it is possible to surmise that the therapist should not be unduly bound by theoretical models. Additionally, the therapist might consider research suggesting that therapist behavior influences interaction. The group therapist should adopt different intervention strategies for different types of groups to facilitate improved patient outcome.

VICARIOUS LEARNING

Group therapy provides obvious opportunity for learning through the observation of others. Nevertheless, vicarious learning is another rather neglected TF by theorists and researchers. Vicarious learning operates when a patient benefits by observing the therapy experience of another patient; identifies with a co-member to the extent that he or she gains from the co-member's therapy experience; recognizes some positive aspect of the behavior of the therapist or other group members to imitate; or finds models in the positive behavior of other group members and/or the group therapist.

The central processes in vicarious learning seem to be identification and modeling. Kissen (1974) asserts that identification with the therapist is particularly important and that therapist characteristics should influence the extent of this process. His review suggests a number of testable hypotheses, but in fact there has been little experimental work. Despite the suggestion by Bednar, Weet, Evensen, Lanier, and Melnick (1974) that modeling techniques have specific application in group therapy and provide a useful source of interpersonal learning, most of the empirical investigations of modeling have occurred in the individual therapy realm (see Rosenthal & Bandura, 1978).

A well-executed study by Falloon, Lindley, McDonald, and Marks (1977) compared the value of a discussion group to a group where modeling was a key feature for patients encountering interpersonal difficulties. In this group, the co-therapists modeled social interactions regarded as problematic for members. The group members were subsequently trained to practice the same interactions through the medium of role-play. Modeling proved of greater benefit than group discussion at the end of the program, although the difference diminished at follow-up. While explicit modeling may be much less appropriate in more conventional group therapy, the therapist and other group members are likely to be seen as models. It would be valuable to understand the effects of modeling within the group therapy context from an empirical perspective.

An ingenious experiment examining identification at the peer level is reported by Jeske (1973). On the assumption that identification involves not only mere imitation of the person being observed, but also the experiencing of the latter's "successes and defeats," Jeske devised a procedure to record episodes of identification. Individual patients in short-term group therapy pressed a button each time they noticed themselves identifying with a peer. Patients who improved recorded twice the number of such identifications than did nonimprovers. This suggested to Jeske that therapists should promote intermember identification in groups; however, the study appears too limited to warrant this conclusion.

Vicarious learning is explicitly promoted in one form of group treatment, namely psychodrama. The technique of "doubling," in which a group member stands behind the protagonist relating feelings or memories triggered by an element of the "drama," is a form of identification. In this situation, there is a bidirectional element, the protagonist perhaps learning something new about his or her situation from the double, and the double learning from identification with something in the protagonist's experience.

GUIDANCE

Group therapists only moderately emphasize guidance as a TF, but its history extends back to the pioneering work by Joseph Pratt (1975). Facilitating didactic groups to instruct patients with tuberculosis, Pratt recognized that the group setting itself had specific beneficial effects. Later therapists working with psychiatric patients created structured groups whose members were seen as "students" and tutored on aspects of mental health.

This model was short-lived, supplanted by the work of psychoanalysts, who strongly eschewed the didactic element. Thus, there is little reference to guidance in the pre-1955 literature. As a result, guidance does not appear in the Corsini and Rosenberg (1955) classification. Our own view is that guidance cannot be omitted from a list of TFs. Information is inevitably given in the course of group treatment, sometimes by the therapist and often by other group members. Admittedly, the emphasis placed on guidance differs from group to group. Guidance may represent a relatively weak TF in psychoanalytic groups and a relatively strong TF in cognitive/behavioral groups.

The definition of guidance highlights the imparting of information and the giving of direct advice. This factor operates when the group member receives useful information and instruction from the therapist (about mental health, mental illness, and general psychodynamics) or obtains explicit advice and suggestions from either the therapist or other patients. Three general areas in the group literature relate to the issue of guidance: specific didactic models of group therapy, self-help groups, and pretherapy training.

Maxmen (1978) made an important theoretical contribution in outlining a didactic model of group therapy emphasizing guidance, universality, and altruism. His model included other cognitive and behavioral factors, such as learning to accept appropriate help, recognizing maladaptive behavior, and avoiding stressful situations. The model was developed for work with short-term groups, especially on psychiatric inpatient units. Maxmen (1973), studying a sample of 100 inpatients treated according to this model, noted that hope, acceptance, altruism, and universality were the TFs most valued.

The limited empirical study of guidance reflects the clinical view that guidance is an unimportant TF, suggesting that direct advice is best avoided because it promotes dependence. Nevertheless, an illuminating study by Flowers (1979) makes the point that the value of guidance is demonstrable in defined circumstances. Flowers conducted a study in which compulsorily detained sex offenders were treated in small groups by psychiatric nurses trained to give advice of various types, including simple, direct advice, the offering of alternatives, and the provision of detailed instructions. When compared to a control group, patients attending guidance-focused groups showed greater improvement on specified treatment goals. Additionally, offering alternatives and detailed instructions proved to be of greater benefit than simple, direct advice. One limiting factor of this study revolved around the determination of outcome measures and treatment goals by the therapist rather than the patient. Nevertheless, one may conclude that certain forms of guidance do produce therapeutic effects.

Self-help groups are now a well-established phenomenon. After a rapid expansion on both sides of the Atlantic in the 1960s and 1970s, a wide variety of organizations offer supportive help of this kind. While it is probably inaccurate to regard these groups as providing psychotherapy, there is certainly an overlap between the effects of self-help and more traditional psychotherapy groups. It seems reasonable to assume that some TFs may operate in self-help settings. Lieberman (1980) has written convincingly about the change mechanisms in self-help groups. While Hurvitz (1970) concluded that self-help groups relied largely on guidance, Lieberman was able to show that considerable variation exists between groups run by different organizations. He suggested that some groups stress guidance, others avoid this focus. A further useful review was compiled by Killilea (1976), who includes guidance as one of the seven features common to self-help groups.

There is an obvious resemblance between the self-help group and the educative group conducted by Maxmen (1978). Psychoeducational groups are frequently employed on inpatient units to teach specific skills such as conflict resolution, assertiveness, and anger management. Descriptions of such methods can be found in the group literature. An illustrative paper by Rubin and Locascio (1985) describes a group for training long-term psychiatric patients in the skills required to adapt to community life. Operating much like a classroom, they used focused feedback and videotaped exercises in a supportive setting to teach specific skills.

A section on guidance would not be complete without reference to pretherapy training. Though this form of guidance is not a TF that arises from the group itself, there is little doubt that pretherapy training can influence the course of subsequent treatment (see review by Bloch & Crouch, 1985). The relationship between pretherapy training, other TFs, and final therapeutic outcome remains unclear.

UNIVERSALITY

Universality, gaining benefit from the realization that one is not alone with one's problems, is a TF receiving minimal attention in the literature. What explains this absence of empirical and theoretical comment? First, universality typically is experienced at the beginning of group therapy when the initial sharing of problems, thoughts, feelings, and fantasies dispels members' sense of uniqueness and aloneness. Second, universality is an experience implicitly felt and rarely articulated. Thus, its occurrence and effect may be unnoticed by the therapist or an external observer. Third, universality is more commonly featured in comparative studies of TFs rather than in explorations of single factors.

Corsini and Rosenberg (1955) did include universality in their early taxonomy of TFs. Additionally, universality has been identified in later descriptions of TFs (Bloch & Crouch, 1985; Yalom, 1985). More recent interest in universality has focused on the self-help group phenomenon. For example, Lieberman (1980) suggests that universality is maximized as a cardinal feature of the self-help group, creating a supportive atmosphere for group members. Robinson (1980) links the destigmatizing potential of self-help groups for those with psychological problems to the operation of universality. Members encounter other people similar to themselves, decreasing their sense of alienation.

Though clinical observation supports the value of universality, empirical studies of universality as an individual TF are virtually nonexistent. At present, judgments about its action and relative importance are drawn from comparative TF research and clinical practice.

ALTRUISM

Patients in group therapy clearly benefit from the discovery that their contributions can assist their peers. Though an individual in group therapy may avoid working on his or her own problems by being "therapist" to others, the human quality of altruism and its corresponding TF seem to be important aspects of group therapy. Altruism operates when the patient offers support, reassurance, suggestions, or comments to help other group members; shares similar problems with the purpose of helping other members; feels a sense of being needed and helpful; can forget self in favor of another group member; and recognizes the desire to do something for another group member.

Like universality, altruism was identified by Corsini and Rosenberg's taxonomy (1955) and has achieved prominence in the context of the self-help group. In a review of the self-help group literature, Marie Killilea (1976) included altruism as one of seven shared properties that typify such groups, where indeed altruism may be a more salient feature than in conventional therapy groups. Though the concept of altruism is readily addressed by social psychologists, empirical group research specifically directed at altruism is noticeably sparse. Similar to universality, altruism is cited in studies examining the comparative value of various TFs.

INSTILLATION OF HOPE

The establishment and maintenance of hope is an important aspect of most psychotherapeutic interventions. The instillation of hope may act as a condition for change, improving patient morale and promoting greater investment in tackling problems. The belief that one can "get better" and that life will improve in the future is a critical aspect of mental health treatment.

Hope has featured in lists of TFs from Corsini and Rosenberg (1955) onwards. Group therapy does provide an extra dimension that may confer TF status on the instillation of hope, though it is perhaps a weak factor. The extra dimension arises from the patient's opportunity to see that a co-group member is improving through therapy; this gives the patient hope of benefit from therapeutic interventions. There is a close link with vicarious learning in this respect; however, vicarious learning involves the patient learning something specific about his or her problems from the experience of another group member, whereas hope operates when the patient simply notes that improvement does occur.

Thus, the instillation of hope is a process which operates when the patient observes improvement in other group members and notes that the group can be helpful to its members in accomplishing their goals. Though clearly of therapeutic value, hope has not been empirically assessed as a single TF.

INSIGHT (SELF-UNDERSTANDING)

Insight, or some form of cognitive processing, is a central common feature of most psychotherapies. A strict behaviorist might view cognitive change as a secondary phenomenon, or an epiphenomenon of behavioral change. However, most contemporary therapists would unite in regarding change in self-concept and behavior as intimately related and would agree that causality may be bidirectional. In other words, behavior can cause shifts in self-concept, and self-concept can alter behavior. Several forms of self-understanding can potentially occur in the group setting: inter alia, recognizing defenses, understanding the origin of symptoms, appreciating the meaning of dreams, and becoming aware of how one's behavior affects other people.

In their early attempt to classify TFs, Corsini and Rosenberg (1955) used the term *intellectualization* to identify a process of learning or acquiring knowledge that leads to insight. This distinction between intellectualization and insight is problematic, because the former term has been used to reflect a defense mechanism. Yalom (1985) argued that interpersonal insight is the form of learning most relevant to group therapy, suggesting that psychogenetic insight (e.g., understanding the origin of symptoms) is subsidiary. He also places feedback within his factor of interpersonal learning rather than including it with self-understanding.

As a TF, insight can occur as a result of feedback (direct or indirect) and interpretation from other group members, both patients and therapists. Insight operates when patients (1) learn something important about themselves (understanding overt behavior, assumptions they hold about themselves, motivations that underlie their behavior, fantasies only recently uncovered), (2) learn how they come across to the group (comparable to Yalom's interpersonal learning input mainly achieved through feedback by other members), (3) learn more clearly about the nature of their problems (i.e., a more comprehensive understanding of a particular problem), and (4) learn why they behave as they do and how such behavior developed (psychogenetic insight).

Empirical Research

The research effort relevant to the TF of insight in group settings is scanty. Only a few studies have used insight as an experimental variable. Feedback, an aspect of insight readily accessible to observation, has received more attention. Examination of research directly addressing insight highlights inconsistent results. These inconsistencies can be attributed to the differences in experimental samples (ranging from patients with chronic schizophrenia to volunteer subjects with speech anxiety) and varying designs (ranging from an experiment comparing two treatment conditions, one stressing insight and the other stressing interaction, to an experiment comparing insight and an entirely separate form of therapy, such as assertiveness training). A brief summary of the three best studies illustrates why the findings are so inconclusive.

Roback (1972) compared the effectiveness of insight and interaction by randomly assigning patients to one of the following groups: an insight group focused on understanding links between current and past problems; an interaction group emphasizing patterns of relating; a combined treatment group; or a control group (an alternative activity). After 30 sessions, the only difference between the groups was a tendency for greater improvement in patients receiving combined treatment. However, the sample was comprised of hospitalized chronic patients, individuals unlikely to benefit greatly from insight-oriented therapy, especially over a brief period of 10 weeks. Nonetheless, the value of combined treatment is noteworthy.

Lomont, Gilner, Spector, and Skinner (1969) composed two groups of inpatients matched in terms of intelligence and personality pattern. They ran two treatment groups daily for six weeks, one an insight-oriented group (linking past and current behavior), the other an assertiveness training group. The latter showed slightly greater improvement on one outcome measure. However, the brief treatment, small sample size, and inadequate outcome measures cast doubt on conclusions drawn from this study.

In the best of these studies, Meichenbaum, Gilmore, and Fedoravicius (1971) argued the need for a specified form of insight-based treatment and a well-controlled test to examine the value of insight. They compared a derivative of rational-emotive therapy, where the patient learns how his own self-defeating thoughts contribute to maladaptive behavior, to a non-insight-oriented behavioral treatment, namely systematic desensitization. Volunteer subjects with a specific problem, speech anxiety, were assigned randomly to one of four groups: insight, desensitization, combined treatment, and a placebo treatment control. The groups met for eight weekly sessions. Participants were rated at termination and three months later, using a variety of self-report and objective ratings. The results are not straightforward. Overall, insight and desensitization were equally effective, ranking ahead of combined treatment and placebo. However, a retrospective analysis indicated that desensitization was particularly helpful for patients suffering from speech anxiety as an isolated problem. Subjects afflicted with speech anxiety encompassed by an overall pattern of shyness or generalized anxiety gained more from the insight and combined treatments.

The results of these three studies are consistent with the accepted view that insight is a relevant TF in certain clinical circumstances but not in others. Several related questions bear investigation, such as the circumstances surrounding and the nature of the insight offered. For example, timing is generally regarded as significant—an interpretation may prove meaningless at one point in therapy but be accepted and integrated when repeated months later. Two experiments demonstrate the multidimensional quality of insight, both from Abramowitz and colleagues and both employing a similar design. In one study, insight was examined in relation to "psychological mindedness" (Abramowitz & Abramowitz, 1974). Twenty-six student volunteers rated on psychological mindedness were randomly assigned to two insight-oriented and two noninsight-oriented groups. There were experimental shortcomings as the groups ran only for 10 weeks, the outcome measures were self-report, and the therapist was also the investigator (though independent raters validated the experimental conditions). The results found that psychological-mindedness was associated with greater improvement only in the insight-oriented groups, corresponding with the common clinical view that the capacity for insight is a salient selection criterion for group psychotherapy.

The second study (Abramowitz & Jackson, 1974) examined the relevance of the nature of the insight offered to group members. Twenty-eight students were randomly assigned to one of four groups, all led by the same therapist: a "here and now" group (focusing on intragroup feelings and behavior), a "there-and-then" group (focusing on the relationship between past events and present behavior), a combined group, and an attention-placebo group. All groups met for 10 sessions. As in the previous experiment, treatment conditions were validated and outcome measures were similar. The results were inconclusive, with no convincing differences between the treatment conditions and only a faintly discernible trend in favor of the combined group. The researchers conjectured that a combination of types of interpretation provided the students with greater opportunity for self-expression, which in turn enabled their problems to be approached in diverse ways. This interpretation corresponds to the view that group therapy is a forum for learning in which various paths to insight may be pursued. However, such conjectures may be an example of reading more into the results than is warranted.

Feedback by fellow members and therapist is distinct from interpretation but nevertheless pertinent to the acquisition of insight. Interpretation involves a level of inference from observation, whereas feedback involves reflecting back observed behavior. Feedback is easier to measure than interpretation, perhaps accounting for its empirical attention, particularly from one active group of researchers.

Jacobs and a number of his colleagues (Jacobs, 1974; Jacobs, Jacobs, & Gatz, 1973; Jacobs, Jacobs, Feldman, & Carior, 1973; Jacobs, Jacobs, Carior, & Burke, 1974) used a student sample to explore the various methods for providing feedback along two dimensions. First, they distinguished between positive feedback (e.g., paying a compliment) and negative feedback (e.g., criticism). Second, they considered behavioral feedback (pointing out an aspect of behavior), emotional feedback (expressing a personal reaction) and mixed behavioral-emotional feedback. Their studies focused on the process of feedback rather than its relationship to outcome. Though their sample was nonclinical, the complexity revealed by this research is likely to have relevance for clinical groups. When the source of feedback is known, recipients find positive feedback more credible than negative feedback, and behavioral feedback more credible than emotional feedback (though positive emotional feedback is the most credible type). In contrast, anonymous feedback produces different results with negative emotional feedback viewed as more credible than positive emotional feedback. Timing of the feedback was also examined, though with inconsistent results. The question about an optimal sequence for offering feedback—negative or positive first—remains unclear.

Finally, brief mention should be made regarding the value of videotaped feedback. Most accounts of the application of this technological approach are descriptive rather than experimental. In a well-planned investigation of psychiatric inpatients, Robinson and Jacobs (1970) employed short-term group therapy complemented by meetings where therapists used videotaped excerpts of therapy sessions to illustrate adaptive and maladaptive behaviors. Patients in the treatment condition showed greater improvement than patients in the control condition.

There is ample scope for further study of feedback, especially its association with outcome. Similarly, the TF of self-understanding warrants more empirical attention, though clarification of the concepts involved should precede additional research. Ambiguous definitions confound interpretations of research data, limiting generalizability and clinical implications.

CATHARSIS

The therapeutic value of the arousal and discharge of emotion has long been recognized. The term *catharsis* itself (from the Greek, "to clean") makes the metaphorical link with purgation of the bowels, a process regarded in popular imagination as a therapeutic emptying. Early writers such as Breuer and Freud (1955) applied the term *catharsis* in a narrow and specific manner (the expression simultaneously of previously repressed memories and associated affect). Generally, catharsis is used more loosely to indicate emotional arousal and a venting of feelings.

Corsini and Rosenberg (1955) labeled their ninth factor "ventilation," defining it as "the release of feelings and expression of ideas usually repressed in other nontherapeutic situations." Terms and phrases they gathered from the literature included catharsis, abreaction, ventilation of hostility, emotional release, release of hostility in a socially acceptable way, relief of guilt through confession, ventilation of guilt, ventilation of anxiety, release of emotional tension, release of unconscious material, and verbalization of fantasy.

Their approach to definition has the drawback of combining two different processes: the "release of feelings" (hostility, guilt, anxiety, tension, etc.) and the "expression of ideas" (usually the release of unconscious material). These two processes often occur together but are theoretically dissimilar as well as clinically separable. For example, a patient releases intense anger in reminiscing about childhood and also describes an emotionally impoverished family atmosphere. Through free association, she may begin to understand the origin of her strong feelings. But emotional ventilation and disclosure of personal information have different therapeutic effects. Discharge of anger often brings a sense of relief (e.g., "blowing off steam," "getting it off my chest," and "unbottling myself"), reflecting the resultant feeling of ease. This process is best regarded as the central element of catharsis. The revelation of early memories is potentially therapeutic for different reasons: it may constitute self-disclosure of private, personal information previously kept secret; it may be echoed by other group members, allowing the patient to feel that he or she is not alone (universality); and it may reflect the operation of self-understanding or insight by making the link between the feeling of anger and the memory of early deprivation.

Yalom (1985) retains this dual nature in his definition of catharsis, adding other aspects which further confound the definition. The category labeled *catharsis* in his TF questionnaire is composed of five items: getting things off one's chest, expressing negative or positive feelings toward a co-member; expressing such feelings toward the therapist, learning how to express feelings, and being able to say what is bothering oneself instead of holding it in. This contains the elements of discharging feelings, disclosing information, learning how to express feelings (i.e., developing a skill), and giving voice to here-and-now feelings about others.

Bloch, Reibstein, Crouch, Holroyd, and Themen (1979) deal with this issue by including a separate TF to address the expression of ideas and the revelation of bothersome issues, namely self-disclosure. They also regard the skill of being emotionally expressive as belonging to the TF, learning from interpersonal action (or interpersonal learning). This covers the patient's attempts to relate constructively and adaptively within the group, and includes by implication the expression of emotions to fellow members.

The definition for catharsis suggested by Bloch et al. (1979) highlights only the element of emotional release, creating an advantage by referring to one clearly recognizable process. Using this definition, catharsis operates when there is an emotional release, a ventilation of feelings (either positive or negative and about either life events or other group members) bringing about some measure of relief. Content may include both past and present material. These feelings include anger, affection, sorrow, and grief which have been previously difficult or impossible to discharge.

Empirical Research

Expression of Anger

Catharsis in group therapy, however defined, has received little attention in the research literature. Two investigators examined the expression of anger in therapy groups. Haer (1968) noted its effect on the frequency and style of the group's aggressive responses. Liberman (1970b) tested the hypothesis that group members would resolve their problems with authority and develop greater independence by expressing feelings of hostility and disappointment toward the therapist.

Haer (1968) led two groups for 20 sessions where he encouraged the ventilation of feelings. Taped sessions were then coded for member expression of anger and for the frequency of aggressive responses by co-members in the half-hour preceding and the half-hour following episodes of "cathartic anger." Expression of anger seemed to have a beneficial group effect, in that aggressive responses declined following cathartic events. The study was small scale, and the author participated as both researcher and therapist. Nevertheless, it illustrates that emotional discharge may influence, at least temporarily, patterns of interaction.

Liberman's (1970b) study was better executed, though also small scale. He focused on the therapist's role in promoting expression of anger by group members. His main hypothesis was that members would benefit by overtly expressing anger toward the therapist for failing to gratify their dependency wishes. This was based on three assumptions: (1) that the therapist as the central and most valued figure in the group can effectively prompt and reinforce specific types of member behavior, (2) that the therapist helps group members resolve their problems with dependency by accepting and encouraging hostility and disappointment directed toward himself and by deflecting onto himself undue hostility between members, and (3) that a therapist who systematically prompts and reinforces group members' behavior in this way induces more effective behavioral and personal change than a therapist using an intuitive, less planned approach.

Two matched groups of out-patients met weekly for nine months. The two group therapists were matched for experience and personality factors. One was trained to use methods increasing the expression of hostility and disappointment (about his nondirective role) directed toward himself—chiefly through verbal prompting and reinforcement. He also redirected toward himself potentially destructive hostility manifested between members. The other therapist led his group intuitively, using an analytic approach. With the aid of audiotapes and observers, the therapists' interventions were coded as reinforcement or prompting, and the group members' expressions of hostility to the therapist were rated. As predicted, therapist prompting and reinforcement promoted the expression of hostility, both in timing and amount. However, catharsis of this kind was not related to outcome as measured on behavioral and personality measures, including dominance-submissiveness and independence-dependence.

These two studies illustrate how elements of catharsis can be studied in groups. Although the Liberman study was carefully executed, if the experimental procedure had shown a positive outcome effect, it would have been impossible to exclude uncontrolled therapist variables. In retrospect, the idea that the expression of hostility to the therapist could lead directly to decreases in dependency and submissiveness is too mechanistic and omits the need for members to gain insight into their own behavior.

Emotionality and Duration of the Therapy Session

The marathon group was devised by Bach, Stoller, and others on the assumption that the longer format would lead to an intense emotional experience. Myerhoff, Jacobs, and Stoller (1970) examined this idea in their comparison of emotionality in marathon and traditional therapy groups. Psychiatric in-patients were assigned either to a group meeting for three two-hour sessions a week over three weeks or to a group meeting for three six-hour sessions over three days. Therefore, both groups participated in the same amount of therapy. All groups were led by the same therapist, whom observers rated as consistent. A checklist designed to measure emotional responses was administered to members after each two-hour interval of treatment. Emotionality, defined as the sum of the adjectives checked by each member on each occasion, did not develop to a higher degree in the marathon session except for the expression of negative feelings. The authors' own speculations are captured in the phrase "too tired to be polite." Perhaps time-extended sessions do not promote greater emotional experiences; moreover, the heightened negative expressiveness cannot necessarily be regarded as therapeutic.

Emotionality and Outcome

Only one study addresses the relationship between emotional expressiveness and outcome. In the Stanford encounter group study (Lieberman et al., 1973), students who underwent 30 hours of a group experience were followed up six months later and categorized as learners, unchanged, or negative outcomes. They ranked catharsis third out of 14 therapeutic mechanisms in terms of helpfulness, and a third of the "most important events" reported by participants covered emotional expressiveness. Nevertheless, there were no significant differences between the three outcome groups in the extent to which the expression of those feelings led to insight or other positive effects. An exception was that the ventilation of aggressive feelings was associated with negative effect. Negative outcome students had greater exposure to this form of catharsis than unchanged and learner groups. The authors concluded that "though people may feel good about getting up feelings and may believe that it is instrumental in their learning, no evidence yet supports the belief that expressivity per se is specifically associated with differences in individual growth."

Possible Adverse Effects of Catharsis

It is important to recognize that catharsis can exert negative effects. The ventilation of feelings may bring relief, and if self-understanding follows, there may be additional gain. But catharsis that is too intense for the patient to bear may create a distressing state of arousal that does not resolve and is plainly antitherapeutic. Yalom, Bond, Bloch, Zimmerman, and Friedman (1977) reported on this possible outcome in a study of the effects of an intense group experience on the process of individual therapy. Patients judged by their therapists to be "stuck" in long-term individual treatment were assigned to one of three matched groups, all of which met over a weekend. The two experimental groups, led by Gestalt therapists, were designed to arouse affect. The control group consisted of meditation and Tai Chi. The apparent impact of the group experience on individual therapy was reviewed 6 and 12 weeks later. At 6 weeks, patients in the experimental groups showed, on some measures, a significantly greater improvement in the quality of their individual therapy than control patients, but these differences were no longer present by 12 weeks. This gives credence to the notion that catharsis may not be beneficial by itself but needs to be accompanied by cognitive learning.

Conclusion

Catharsis, the ventilation of intense emotions which brings a sense of relief and may secondarily lead to greater self-understanding, has a distinct but circumscribed role in group therapy. Treatment inevitably entails the arousal of emotions in patients, probably a basic ingredient of all psychotherapies without which cognitive factors such as self-understanding and vicarious learning cannot operate effectively. It is commonplace in clinical practice to encounter patients who benefit from the discharge of bottled-up feelings in the group. However, catharsis itself is unlikely to lead to lasting change (Marshall, 1972) and the uncontrolled release of emotion may be hazardous. These conclusions arise mainly from clinical and theoretical considerations. The small quantity of research evidence is in line with this point of view. Weiner (1977) summarizes this position as follows:

> If, as therapists, we can clearly see the complexity of catharsis, we may have greater capacity to prescribe it intelligently and to understand it when it occurs spontaneously in the therapeutic situation. Our principal validation for catharsis as an important element in treatment continues to be the observation by patients that they feel better by virtue of it, provided it has occurred in an appropriate way in an appropriate context.

SELF-DISCLOSURE

The notion of self-disclosure in group therapy refers to a patient's direct communication of personal material about self to the group. This factor operates when the patient reveals information about life outside the group, past experiences, feared, embarrassing, or worrisome problems, or private fantasies. Such personal disclosures may be difficult and painful for the patient.

Empirical Research

Self-Disclosure and Cohesiveness

Studies of laboratory groups suggest a close relationship between self-disclosure and cohesiveness. Query (1970) studied short-term therapy groups composed of nurses allocated to groups that were rated as high, medium, or low in self-disclosure. Participants' ratings of cohesiveness and liking of fellow members showed that self-disclosure was associated with the former, but not the latter. Johnson and Ridener (1974) obtained a similar result using a different method. Volunteer students were assigned to one of three groups on the basis of Jourard's (1971) self disclosure questionnaire and met for four half-hour sessions of topic-based discussion. Again, group cohesiveness, but not perceived attraction of fellow members, was associated with self-disclosure.

Kirshner, Dies, and Brown (1978) also found a similar link between self-disclosure and cohesiveness using a different method. The study, involving encounter groups "led" by audiotapes, differs from the two studies above because the self-disclosure variable was manipulated experimentally.

Stokes, Fuehrer, and Childs (1983) showed intimacy of self-disclosure to be related to cohesiveness; however, the immediacy of self-disclosure (i.e., relating to the "here and now" rather than to the "there and then") was negatively related to cohesion. The experiment, though ingenious and carefully designed, was highly artificial. Students were shown videotaped scenes of actors simulating psychotherapy groups in which the experimental conditions were manipulated. Participants were then asked to imagine themselves as members of the groups they had witnessed and to complete questionnaires relating to their perceptions of these groups. "Here and now" self-disclosure was perceived as uncomfortable in this artificial situation, though this is not necessarily the case in a maturing therapy group.

The Leader's Role in Promoting Self-Disclosure

If we assume that self-disclosure is beneficial, the question arises about how therapists can enhance this process. For example, should therapists model self-disclosing behavior or should they set an explicit norm encouraging members to divulge personal information? The question is complex, and empirical research has produced inconsistent findings. Marked differences in the samples studied (e.g., volunteer students, inpatients and outpatients) and in the methodology applied have contributed to the variable results. Nonetheless, it would appear that the group leader can affect the pattern of self-disclosure, especially through the explicit setting of norms.

Ribner's (1974) study explored the effect of precise instructions designed to encourage self-disclosure. This was an analogue study in which 24 groups met for an hour; some groups received explicit instructions, others were merely told to "get acquainted." Audiotapes of the sessions confirmed that the instructions promoted both greater frequency and depth of self-disclosure. Another finding, in line with the work of Query (1970) and Johnson and Ridener (1974), was that mutual liking between subjects was greater in the control groups in which self-disclosure was less evident. However, there was a noticeable trend for subjects who were high self-disclosers to show greater mutual liking. Thus, the relationship between self-disclosure and interpersonal attraction is not straightforward and is a relationship that may change as a group evolves.

A study by Scheiderer (1977) supports Ribner's finding that explicit instructions promote self-disclosure. His subjects were self-referred students attending a counseling service. They were randomly assigned to one of four groups: (1) control (no instructions), (2) modeling (viewed a videotape of a "patient" exhibiting optimal self-disclosing behavior together with commentary), (3) given specific instructions about self-disclosing behavior, and (4) receiving both modeling and instruction. The instructional condition emerged as most effective. The finding that modeling was less effective than instruction is notable, but the experimental design (with a nine-minute instructional video) does not compare with the continuing presence of a therapist as model in a psychotherapy group.

This issue of the therapist as model has been investigated with interesting results. Weigel and Warnath (1968) found no differences in self-disclosure between two 10-session groups of students. One group was led by a self-disclosing leader and the other by an "opaque" leader. The more disclosing group leader was rated as less popular and less "mentally healthy." A similar study by Weiner, Rosson, and Cody (1974), but with clinical patients, also failed to detect any association between patient and therapist self-disclosure. On the other hand, Truax and Carkhuff (1965), who studied two larger clinical samples (40 patients each, psychiatric inpatients and institutionalized juvenile delinquents) in group therapy programs, demonstrated a clear correlation between therapist transparency and patient self-disclosure.

The Truax and Carkhuff (1965) study is more impressive in design than the others, but these inconsistent findings across studies suggest some difficulties with the research question. This question about therapist effects on self-disclosure is too general. Aspects of self-disclosure such as the content, form, and timing need more careful assessment. Dies (1973) attempted to tackle these issues in a series of investigations. First, he developed a scale to measure group members' attitudes toward therapist self-disclosure. Then he administered the scale to a sample of patients in group therapy (though unfortunately a small, and possibly biased sample). Therapists judged to be self-revealing were seen as friendlier and more trustworthy, but they were also regarded as less stable and strong than their less self-disclosing counterparts. These results echo the findings of Wiegel and Warnath (1968). Timing was of consequence. Patients in therapy for more than 10 sessions preferred that their therapists be self-disclosing, whereas those embarking on treatment wanted less therapist self-disclosure. Dies surmised that self-disclosure early in the course of therapy may provoke anxiety in patients because it occurs when they need support and structure. However, once the group matures, therapist self-disclosure becomes more appropriate and valued. The multifaceted nature of therapist self-disclosure is summarized by Dies (1977) in a review of the theoretical and experimental literature.

THE COMPARATIVE EVALUATION OF THERAPEUTIC FACTORS

The most common research strategy in studying TFs as a group relies on the member as "consumer." The group member is queried about what has been helpful in therapy, either by direct inquiry or more obliquely. The direct approach consists in asking members to rank in order of helpfulness a number of statements that cover the various factors. Yalom (1985) constructed a questionnaire of 60 statements covering 12 TFs. The respondent is asked to assign a TF to one of seven categories, from most to least helpful. This questionnaire is analyzed according to the Q-sort method.

A less direct approach is the "most important event" questionnaire (also referred to as the "critical incident questionnaire"), which has appeared in different wording variations and can claim the advantage of being less prone to bias than the direct enquiry. In this case, the respondent specifies the event (or events) he found most personally important and describes this event in detail. The responses are then categorized according to the TF involved in each event, ideally by trained raters using operational criteria such as those provided in this chapter.

The available research covers a range of groups and group therapies. Although this complicates the direct comparison of the results, it permits the beginning of an understanding about the differences between various types of therapy (and nontherapy) groups. Questions that have been examined within the framework of therapeutic factors as a group are (1) their comparative effectiveness in promoting clinical change, (2) their comparative evaluation by group members, (3) their relationship to group differences, and (4) their relationship to individual differences. By far the greatest number of studies has concentrated on the comparative evaluation of TFs, most likely because the experimental design is straightforward.

TFs and Outcome

Five studies have explored the relationship between a constellation of TFs and outcome. One concerns long-term outpatient group therapy, another short-term encounter groups, the third long-term institutional therapy of substance abusers, the fourth peer support groups, and the last short-term therapy groups.

Yalom and his colleagues (Yalom, 1985) administered their TF questionnaire on a single occasion to 20 outpatients who had recently terminated or were still in treatment—the average duration of treatment being 16 months. The sample was chosen by asking therapists to nominate successful patients so that the rank ordering indicated those factors particularly valued by such patients.

The three most helpful factors were interpersonal learning-input (mainly behavioral feedback), catharsis (in fact closer to self-disclosure), and acceptance. Least helpful were family reenactment (learning from the group as symbolic of one's family of origin), guidance, and identification (vicarious learning). The remaining six factors were rated in this order: insight, interaction, an existential factor, universality, hope, and altruism.

There are design problems with this study, the most obvious being the lack of a comparison group of less clinically successful outpatients. The criticism has also been leveled by Weiner (1974) that the questionnaire used is inherently biased toward interactional elements. The question about the TFs valued by improvers in long-term therapy is still wide open for study, perhaps using the most important event questionnaire and comparing groups with differing theoretical orientations.

Lieberman and his associates (1973) made use of both therapeutic factor and most important event questionnaires. The former measure was administered at the end of 30 hours of various forms of encounter groups (including

Gestalt, transactional analysis, psychoanalytically-orientated and psycho-drama). The student participants also recorded their most important events following each session. The study was designed prospectively, and the outcome was assessed across a number of measures. "High learners" (about one-third of the sample) were distinguished from "nonchangers" and "negative outcomes" chiefly on cognitive TFs. The first rated insight, acceptance, advice, and family reenactment significantly more than the second and third groups. The most important event analysis confirmed the direction of this trend.

Steinfeld and Mabli (1974) used a similar design to Yalom's, although on atypical subjects. Fifty male prison inmates, former drug abusers, and "successful" graduates of a group therapy program, completed Yalom's TF questionnaire immediately before release (most often many months after termination of the group). The subjects rated insight most highly followed by an existential factor, catharsis (self-disclosure), and feedback. Least important were altruism, guidance, universality, and identification. The high ranking of the existential factor seems to reflect the particular group. This factor that sits uneasily among the TFs may be particularly applicable in this group which consists mostly of poor black heroin users. The relevance can be seen from the top-ranking item: "Learning that I must take ultimate responsibility for the way I live my life no matter how much guidance and support I get from others."

Lieberman has continued to study encounter groups and self-help groups (SHGs) over many years. One fascinating and important study (Lieberman, 1990) looks at a specific sample of new mothers who did poorly in SHGs. The study is exemplary in design, measuring mental health, marital relationship, and motherhood role. The population was carefully delineated and compared with a random sample of new mothers. Completers, dropouts, and refusers were further compared. Participants and nonparticipants were similar both before the groups and one year later. The significant findings arise from a comparison of these groups with other, successful SHGs studied in the same way.

In successful SHGs (specifically women's consciousness-raising groups), the factors most emphasized were (adapting Lieberman's terminology) interpersonal learning, self-understanding, catharsis, and the instillation of hope. In the new mothers' groups, on the other hand, universality was most commonly cited, and other factors were hardly featured. The focus of these groups seemed very narrow, concentrating almost entirely on the mother-baby relationship and apparently avoiding the cognitive exploration that seems an aspect of other successful SHGs.

Lieberman also used his study to explore the concept of cohesiveness, particularly drawing attention to a discrepancy between expressed norms relating to group cohesion and actual measured behavior. Another telling result is the conclusion that a main reason for the discrepant characteristics of these groups was that these (largely middle-class) mothers had other sources of peer support, and the groups were not particularly important to them. Other SHGs studied by Lieberman presumably provide an important source of support to members. A corollary of this last observation is that care must be exercised in applying results obtained from nonclinical to clinical groups.

Last, an interesting paper from Flowers (1987) uses a research strategy that could bear repeating and extending. Twenty-four subjects in one of three short-term groups, (24 90-minute sessions) completed Yalom's questionnaire at termination. Most showed improvement on the measure used; three did not. A comparison of ratings between subjects revealed high agreement among improvers, not among the nonresponders.

The Comparative Evaluation of TFs by Outpatients

Several studies address this issue and the number is growing, but the extent to which knowledge accumulates is limited by the heterogeneity of subjects and types of therapy. Outpatient and inpatient studies, a few studies with nonpatient groups, and studies comparing TFs in different types of therapy are presented.

Six studies have examined the comparative evaluation of therapeutic factors in outpatient groups. Corder, Whiteside, and Haizlip (1981) studied 16 adolescents in four therapy groups which met weekly for 9 to 12 months. Participants completed Yalom's questionnaire after at least half a year's membership. Results require interpretation, because they are presented only as a ranking of the individual items, not in TF categories. Items selected as helpful came from self-disclosure and interaction, and those least helpful from insight (a combination of transference and learning about remote causes of current behavior) and vicarious learning (specifically modeling). The study reveals inconsistencies in Yalom's categories (notably items from catharsis being highly rated and unhelpful respectively).

Bloch and Reibstein (1980) chose the most important event questionnaire to obviate the methodological problems of Yalom's questionnaire. Thirty-three patients with neurosis or personality disorder, members of long-term groups, completed the questionnaire at intervals over the first six months of treatment. A team of independent judges then assigned the events to one of 10 factors by following explicit instructions set out in a manual designed for the study. Self-understanding emerged as most important, reflected in over one-third of reported events. Other factors frequently rated were self-disclosure (18%) and learning from interpersonal action (13%). Four factors, by contrast, did not seem important: guidance, catharsis, altruism, and universality. Acceptance, vicarious learning, and instillation of hope were of intermediate importance. Since the groups were insight-oriented, the emphasis on a cognitive factor and the unimportance of guidance were expected.

This study is also of interest in that therapists completed a version of the most important questionnaire (modified to request the therapist's estimation of the event most important for the patient) for each patient in their group during the study period. The accounts were then assigned to TF categories by the same judges who assigned patients' accounts. As with the patients, therapists cited self-understanding most frequently (38%), with learning from interpersonal action (25%) and self-disclosure (19%) considered important. Apart from acceptance, the remaining six factors were hardly cited at all. These results were consistent with predictions since the therapists were trained to follow a dynamic-interactional model.

MacKenzie (1987) reported a similar study of 34 members of four outpatient groups. The results were strikingly similar: self-understanding, self-disclosure and learning from interpersonal action were most highly rated. The order of other TFs was much the same, except that vicarious learning and catharsis were ranked higher than in previous studies.

In a study by Dickoff and Lakin (1963), 28 patients were interviewed on aspects of their experience after the end of treatment (between 18 and 24 months later). Their responses were transcribed and assigned to an idiosyncratic classification of TFs (support, suppression and tools for action). Support (mainly a combination of acceptance and universality) was valued by 60% of the sample, suppression (forgetting worries and self disclosure) by about 30% of the sample, and tools for action (insight leading to behavioral change) by only four patients (14%). Setting aside methodological concerns, the results are consistent with the nature of the groups, which were short-term (patients attending an average of only 11 sessions) and supportive rather than insight-oriented. Another finding, that "tools for action" were cited as important by the four patients with the highest scores on the Wechsler Adult Intelligence Scale, is also in line with expectations.

Kellermann (1985) studied 30 subjects of psychodrama groups who completed a Hebrew version of Yalom's questionnaire. Since the study was similar in design to Yalom's (1985) with clinically successful outpatients, the results can be compared. Although these represent two different types of therapy groups, the findings are broadly similar (Kellermann gives a figure of 0.84 for the correlation between the two sets of TF rankings), though the psychodrama group placed more emphasis on self-understanding and less emphasis on group cohesiveness than the traditional outpatient group.

Hobbs, Birtchnall, Harte, and Lacey (1989) studied patients who were members of a 10-week psychodynamic group, part of a treatment program for women with bulimia nervosa. Patients and therapists completed the most important event questionnaire at the end of sessions 3, 6, and 9; independent judges assigned the responses to TF categories. The most notable result was the low concordance between patient and therapist perceptions of helpful events operating in each three session period (29% for any concordance and 7% for full concordance). This may be a product of administering the questionnaire after every third rather than each session. Therapists regarded self-disclosure and acceptance as important, whereas the patients assigned little value to acceptance and none to self-disclosure. Patients assigned high value to universality, vicarious learning, and instillation of hope.

These investigators also comment on the shift in valuing of therapeutic factors during the course of the group. Self-disclosure and vicarious learning may be more important in the early phase, self-understanding in the middle phase, and instillation of hope in the final phase.

The Comparative Evaluation of TFs by Inpatients

We have referred to Maxmen's (1978) educational model of group therapy, devised specifically for working with short-term groups of inpatients. Associated with this theoretical model is experimental work on the comparative evaluation of therapeutic factors by members of such groups. The program consisted of daily, hour-long sessions run by two co-therapists. The membership was approximately six patients of mixed diagnosis requiring short-term hospitalization. On average, patients attended nine group sessions reflecting an interactional and "here and now" focus.

Maxmen (1973) administered a variant of Yalom's questionnaire to 100 consecutive participants in this program. Instillation of hope, cohesiveness (acceptance), altruism, and universality were judged most helpful. Least emphasized factors were insight, guidance (interestingly in view of the nature of Maxmen's model), family reenactment and identification (vicarious learning). Maxmen discusses these results (favoring affective over cognitive and behavioral factors) at some length. He suggests, for example, that hope may be crucial in a patient for whom admission to the hospital represents failure and whose awareness of improvement in peers may be encouraging. He also makes the point that these results have no clear bearing on outcome.

Several other studies have focused on inpatient groups, but the settings, samples, and methods differ considerably. Macaskill (1982) administered a version of Yalom's questionnaire to nine women with borderline personality disorder undergoing inpatient group therapy for an average of 11 months. Therapy (carried out by the investigator) was psychoanalytic in orientation. Members rated insight and altruism most highly; interaction, vicarious learning, guidance, acceptance, and universality were viewed as least helpful.

Marcovitz and Smith (1983) studied a population resembling Maxmen's sample (though treatment was psychodynamic rather than educative): 30 short-term inpatients with mixed diagnoses. Patients attending an average of eight group sessions completed Yalom's questionnaire immediately prior to discharge from the unit. Therapeutic factors ranked most helpful were catharsis (self-disclosure), cohesiveness, and altruism (the latter two were also stressed by Maxmen's sample). Factors identified as least helpful were vicarious learning, family reenactment, and guidance. Interaction, insight, instillation of hope, and universality received intermediate rankings.

Schaffer and Dreyer (1982) used the questionnaire developed by Lieberman and others (1973) with a sample of 100 inpatients on a crisis unit. Respondents were asked to specify on two occasions one week apart which two items were most relevant to their group experience. Choices did not change from one week to the next; "being responsible for oneself" and insight were regarded as most helpful. Least helpful were vicarious learning (interpersonal learning), self-disclosure, and family reenactment. Therapists were also asked to complete a similar questionnaire. The effect seen in the Bloch and Reibstein (1980) study was also noted here. Therapists focused more on interpersonal factors while patients emphasized intrapersonal factors. In this case, the therapists emphasized catharsis, vicarious learning, and interpersonal learning.

Brabender, Albrecht, Sillitti, Cooper, and Kramer (1983) used the most important event questionnaire to study therapeutic factors in short-term inpatient groups. Subjects were 84 mixed-diagnosis patients treated in small groups over two weeks, using an interactional approach. The results did not show any shift of TFs between the first four and second four sessions. The most valued factor was vicarious learning (23% of events), followed by acceptance (9%), learning from interpersonal action and universality (each 8%), hope (5%), altruism and self-understanding (4% each), self-disclosure (3%) and catharsis (2%). A notable feature was the high incidence of unassignable responses (26%).

Whalen and Mushet (1986) employed the same method with 46 mixed-diagnosis patients in an acute psychiatric unit who attended an open group based on Maxmen's (1973) model. The order in this case was altruism and universality (21% each), self-disclosure and guidance (14% each), hope (9%), acceptance and vicarious learning (7% each), self-understanding (5%), and interpersonal learning (1%).

TFs have also been examined in therapeutic communities. Whiteley and Collis (1987) administered the most important event questionnaire to patients in a residential therapeutic setting. Learning from interpersonal action, acceptance, and self-understanding were the most important TFs. Acceptance and hope were important early on, but learning from interpersonal action and self-understanding increased in importance over time. Stephen, van den Langenberg, and Dekker (1989), in a study of two therapeutic communities, found self-understanding most important followed by learning from interpersonal action and self-disclosure. In this study, acceptance was ranked as relatively unimportant.

TFs and Differences between Individuals and Groups

Butler and Fuhriman (1980) compared the evaluation of TFs by two contrasting samples: patients attending a day program and those participating in outpatient groups, the former considerably more impaired. Both samples completed the TF questionnaire used by Lieberman et al. (1973). There were substantial differences between the groups. The outpatients discriminated more subtly between TFs, with most emphasis placed on self-understanding, universality, feedback, and catharsis. In the day-patient sample, cohesiveness was the only highly rated factor. The authors relate these differences to the different focus of the two types of groups—the day-patient more supportive, and the outpatient more challenging.

Butler & Fuhriman (1983) went on to study 91 group therapy outpatients who completed Yalom's questionnaire and were rated by their therapists regarding the severity of their symptoms. The researchers found that higher functioning patients valued catharsis, self-understanding (including feedback), and interaction more than the remaining sample. Additionally, self-understanding, interaction, and cohesiveness were more valued by longer-standing group members.

Rohrbaugh and Bartels (1975) investigated the relationship between age, sex, education, and previous group experience and the perceptions of TFs by group members. The influence of group size and duration was also noted. The sample consisted of 72 subjects in 13 therapy or human relations groups. They completed Yalom's questionnaire on one occasion. Weaknesses of the study included variable timing of the questionnaire administration which was supervised by the therapists themselves. The results are useful, but the study was probably overambitious in its aims. Therapy groups valued insight more and "relatedness" (cohesiveness plus interaction) less than did human relations groups. More educated group members emphasized relatedness and placed comparatively little value on an existential factor and guidance. Group variables were more important than individual differences in respondents' evaluations. As in Yalom's study of improved patients, there was no relationship between age, sex, previous group experience, attraction to the group, verbal participation, and TF evaluation.

Kahn, Webster, and Storck (1986) compared two types of psychiatric inpatient groups. The awareness group was designed to facilitate psychodynamic change; the focus group was formed to help patients with chronic, severe problems reduce isolation and elicit support from others. The leaders administered Yalom's questionnaire at discharge, and outcome was rated by both patients and therapists. Patients who rated themselves improved valued all TFs (except family recapitulation) more highly than those who did not acknowledge benefit, but no particular TF improvers were specially valued. In addition, the rankings by the two types of groups were surprisingly similar, with universality, altruism, and hope among the top five for both groups.

Kapur, Miller, and Mitchell (1988) compared TFs in members of inpatient and outpatient psychotherapy groups. The two groups were diagnostically different: inpatients had affective disorders, psychotic illness, anorexia, personality disorders, and alcohol dependence; outpatients mostly had anxiety or affective disorders. Therapy with the inpatient group concentrated on interpersonal feedback concerning here and now behavior (Yalom, 1983), while outpatients received conventional dynamic-interactional therapy. Yalom's questionnaire was administered to inpatients who had completed three or more group sessions and to outpatients at the midpoint of their group experience. Both groups placed value on cohesiveness and universality; outpatients especially prized self-understanding, and inpatients emphasized altruism and existential issues surrounding their admission to the hospital.

An investigation by Colijn, Hoencamp, Snijders, van der Spek, and Duivenvoorden (1991) divided TFs into those that are helpful in all therapies, those that are helpful in all group therapies, and those that seem to be helpful in specific groups for particular group members. The authors' aim was to identify the last type of TF. They used Yalom's questionnaire in a study of 134 subjects in 22 mostly long-term groups across a variety of settings (inpatient, day patient, outpatient etc.). Diagnostically, the subjects had mostly anxiety, affective, and personality disorders. Highly ranked TFs included catharsis, self-understanding, interpersonal learning, and cohesiveness; family reenactment and identification were rated low. Interestingly, most factors did not differentiate between types of group or characteristics of members. The TFs were valued similarly across groups regardless of age, sex, months in treatment, or type of group, with the exception of the low-ranked factor of identification. This factor was ranked more highly by patients early on in therapy and by older patients, especially males.

In another experiment attempting to explore the relationship between TFs and individual differences, Bohanon (1982) studied 102 members of inpatient and outpatient groups. The author used cluster analysis to identify patients who responded differently to a curative factors instrument. Two clusters were found: subjects in the first cluster rated most TFs highly, whereas in the second cluster, only self-understanding was so rated. Patients who tended to give low ratings for most TFs had low affiliation scores, high harm-avoidance scores and substantial previous therapy. Affiliation and harm avoidance were among variables used to discriminate between the two clusters.

Conclusion

The reader tracking this discussion may feel somewhat confused about the comparative evaluation of TFs. There are numerous investigations, but a variety of groups have been studied using differing methods, and a range of results is not surprising. However, a careful comparison of the data yields some consistency, suggesting some tentative conclusions about comparative evaluation of TFs.

The studies can be divided into two broad categories reflecting patient and methodological characteristics. The studies can be organized along a patient dimension, allowing comparisons of less disturbed (usually outpatients) and more disturbed patients (usually inpatients). Additionally, the studies can be considered along a methodological dimension, separating those employing the most important event questionnaire from those utilizing a TF questionnaire (usually Yalom's).

Five studies with less disturbed subjects used the most important event method, including one therapeutic community study. In these studies, the most valued TFs are self-understanding and learning from interpersonal action. Self-disclosure is also important, except in the therapeutic community study, where acceptance is important. Only two studies with more disturbed patients used the most important event method, and these yielded inconsistent results.

The TF questionnaire method has been more popular. The studies of less disturbed patients give a wider range of results than do the most important event studies; however, self-understanding, learning from interpersonal action, and self-disclosure/catharsis are again most highly rated. The seven TF questionnaire studies of more disturbed patients reveal cohesiveness, altruism, and universality as most important. These studies also suggest that the instillation of hope is significant. Considering Maxmen's model for inpatient therapy, an interesting finding is that guidance seems almost universally unimportant in all types of therapy groups.

It is gratifying to discover that the two different methods of study (TF questionnaire and most important event questionnaire) concur about the relative importance of TFs operating in more functional, exploratory groups. Self-understanding (insight), learning from interpersonal action, and self-disclosure appear as particularly strong TFs for this type of group, a finding consistent with theoretical ideas about TFs in outpatient groups.

Inpatient groups most often have a rapidly changing membership and a "here and now" focus. The results of TF studies with this type of group therapy suggest that patients gain most from feeling accepted by others, from discovering that they are not alone with their problems, and experiencing their ability to help other members. The hope generated by seeing others improve also seems important.

As yet, few studies have examined the relationship between TFs and outcome, a question of considerable potential interest to researchers and clinicians. Additionally, the relationship between TFs and group development warrants further investigation, illuminating possible shifts in evaluations of TFs as the group matures. Though the complexity of such relationships presents methodological challenges, information gleaned from such potential studies may assist in the understanding of TFs.

LIMITATIONS AND IMPLICATIONS

Limitations of the TF Concept

Three main difficulties characterize the concept of TFs. First, TFs are unbalanced in their content. For example, many more phenomena are classifiable within self-understanding than altruism. Second, factors overlap, making it difficult to classify an event into one TF or another. This may be a particular drawback of the "most important event" questionnaire method.

Third, because of differing perspectives, patients are more likely to high-light cognitive and affective factors, whereas therapists will focus on more directly observable behavioral factors.

Therefore, a question arises regarding other means of classifying "helpful events" in group therapy. An ingenious Belgian study bears on this issue. Dierick and Litaer (1990) placed statements from group members and thera-pists into clusters on the basis of similar content themes. The purpose was to ascertain whether or not a more "natural" set of factors would ap-pear than the TF categories outlined in the original work of Corsini and Rosenberg (1955). Fourteen groups with a total membership of 115 were studied. Group configurations included two outpatient groups, one group for trainee therapists, and 11 growth groups for clinical psychology students. Leaders demonstrated a variety of orientations. Group members completed a questionnaire during the initial or middle phase of the group.

The questionnaire method is noteworthy in that it consisted of a global evaluation of the session together with an ingenious extension of the "most important event" questionnaire. Group members were requested to specify events that were helpful for themselves and for other members, and also events that were unhelpful or harmful. Therapists were asked to complete the questionnaire in relation to group members. Responses were broken down into meaningful segments, and a category system was de-signed to encompass these segments on the basis of similarity of meaning. By this method, a series of "main categories" was obtained. The cate-gories further subdivided into three sections:

- Section 1: Relational climate and structural aspects of the group: (1) group composition and structure; (2) group cohesion; (3) space and freedom (the group as a safe, tolerant place); (4) empathy and feeling understood; (5) confirmation, appreciation, support; (6) authenticity and self-revelation in others.
- Section 2: Specific interventions by group members or the therapist: (7) stimulating and structuring interventions; (8) clarifying and inter-pretive interventions; (9) feedback and confrontation.
- Section 3: Process aspects in the group member: (10) personal involve-ment, authenticity and self-revelation; (11) self-exploration; (12) inter-personal exploration; (13) becoming conscious of; (14) insight into oneself; (15) spectator therapy; (16) experiences with new behavior; (17) experiencing hope and progress, the capacity to help others, and relief; (18) experiencing the helpful potential of the group.

Comparing these categories with customary TFs, the researchers com-ment, "Most of the TFs found in the group psychotherapy literature are quite recognizable in the helpful events we reported. . . . We find the same processes appearing centrally, and the same ones to remain in the periphery." They add, "We have in some instances found a more finely differentiated content."

This research raises several questions. Is there value in breaking down the concept of insight into separate cognitive and affective aspects of self-discovery? Should deep, psychogenic insight be considered apart from budding recognition of something new? These "natural" categories collapse some factors considered individually by traditional listings of TFs. For example, "spectator therapy" includes both universality and vicarious learning. Should these two concepts be combined? Such questions prompt implications for future research.

Implications for Future Research

Some TFs have clearly received more research attention than others. Overall the endeavor is disappointing in extent and quality, suggesting ways that research in this area might be improved. Though far from exhaustive, some research recommendations are as follows:

1. Concepts need more clarity of definition. TF categories should be mutually exclusive and jointly exhaustive. Distinctions between TFs and conditions for change might lead to greater consistency, avoiding muddles such as the cohesiveness/acceptance debate.
2. New theoretical models need to be explored for group therapy-based on clinical observations which would facilitate the formulation of testable hypotheses.
3. Experimental variables should be specified in more detail, allowing for greater comparability of results. For example, greater specificity about the nature of the clinical sample, the type of therapy, and the therapist orientation would improve methodology. Some recent studies are impressive in this respect, suggesting that authors pointing out this requirement have been heeded.
4. There is a need for replication of studies, either exact or repeating an investigation with specific modifications. Certainly, replications would allow for greater generalizability of results.
5. The development of valid and reliable research measures relating to TFs seems essential. Additionally, such measures need to be paired with outcome data to expand the research base in this area. Despite these strictures, the quality of TF research is comparable to work in other areas of psychotherapy and seems to be leading toward a more secure empirical basis for the practice of group therapy.

The Belgian study by Dierick and Litaer (1990) raises the question whether the current classification of TFs is adequate. Though an important question, dramatic reclassification of TFs seems unwarranted at this time.

If techniques and conditions for change are excluded from their list, it becomes similar to previous classifications of TFs. The question becomes whether the differences are important and whether any advantage is served by a different division of TF phenomena. Certainly the alternative classification suffers from the same drawbacks as the TF effort in that some factors are more likely to be self-rated, others more observer-rated. Further study would be required to demonstrate whether a more "natural" taxonomy of TFs exists than current classification systems.

Implications for the Group Therapist

Empirical research on TFs suggests some clinical guidelines for intervention. First, the therapist should differentiate between conditions for change, TFs, and techniques. Second, the application of a working classification of TFs will similarly enhance treatment, allowing the therapist to emphasize certain factors in relation to particular patients or specific phases of a group's development.

Learning from interpersonal action and cohesiveness present as particularly salient interpersonal TFs for outpatient therapy groups. Therapists can increase interpersonal learning by promoting interaction among group members and by creating a safe environment for the exploration of new methods of relating. Cohesiveness seems particularly important during the early stages of group therapy. Group leaders can enhance cohesion through various means such as employing specific interventions like reinforcement, adopting a moderately self-expressive and caring style, and organizing the group in specific ways (e.g., small and mixed sex groups).

Intrapersonal TFs valued by outpatient groups include insight and self-disclosure. Also, moderate levels of catharsis when paired with cognitive reflections will likely benefit outpatient group members. Sources of insight within groups are diverse, allowing therapists to take advantage of opportunities for patient growth. Feedback is an important part of insight, especially in positive and behavioral forms. Self-disclosure can be encouraged in group members through direct instruction or therapy pretraining. The therapist's modeling of self-disclosure is best deferred until the group has established itself as a cohesive entity. Both patient self-disclosure and catharsis need to be carefully tracked and paced by the therapist, preventing the patient from overdisclosing or becoming overwhelmed by emotion.

Vicarious learning has received moderate rankings in comparative studies of TFs; however, some patients may benefit from identifying with the therapist or group peers. Therapists can encourage patients to acknowledge similarities between themselves and other group members. Guidance is regarded as an unimportant TF, but may have some limited usefulness in inpatient groups or psychoeducational groups. Universality, altruism, and the instillation of hope appear more significant for inpatient groups. Despite their limited empirical investigation, patient reports and clinical observations support the probable importance of these TFs, particularly during the early stages of group treatment.

REFERENCES

Abramowitz, S. I., & Abramowitz, C. V. (1974). Psychological-mindedness and benefit from insight-oriented group therapy. *Archives of General Psychiatry, 30*, 610–615.

Abramowitz, S. I., & Jackson, C. (1974). Comparative effectiveness of there-and-then versus here-and-now therapist interpretations in group psychotherapy. *Journal of Counseling Psychology, 21*, 288–293.

Astrachan, B. (1970). Towards a social systems model of therapeutic groups. *Social Psychiatry, 5*, 110–119.

Bach, G. R. (1957). Observations on transference and object relations in the light of group dynamics. *International Journal of Group Psychotherapy, 7*, 64–76.

Bednar, R. L., & Kaul, T. J. (1978). Experiential group research. In S. Garfield & A. Bergin (Eds.), *Handbook of psychotherapy and behavior change*. New York: Wiley.

Bednar, R. L., Weet, C., Evensen, P., Lanier, D., & Melnick, J. (1974). Empirical guidelines for group therapy: Pretraining, cohesion and modelling. *Journal of Applied and Behavioral Science, 10*, 149–165.

Berzon, B., Pious, C., & Farson, R. (1963). The therapeutic event in group psychotherapy: A study of subjective reports by group members. *Journal of Individual Psychology, 19*, 204–212.

Bloch, S., & Crouch, E. (1985). *Therapeutic factors in group psychotherapy*. Oxford: Oxford University Press.

Bloch, S., & Reibstein, J. (1980). Perceptions by patients and therapists of therapeutic factors in group psychotherapy. *British Journal of Psychiatry, 137*, 274–278.

Bloch, S., Reibstein, J., Crouch, E., Holroyd, P., & Themen, J. (1979). A method for the study of therapeutic factors in group psychotherapy. *British Journal of Psychiatry, 134*, 257–263.

Bohanon, L. M. (1982). Personality differences in the curative experience of group therapy. *Dissertation Abstracts International, 43*, 1606B.

Braaten, L. J. (1990). The different patterns of group climate critical incidents in high and low cohesion sessions of group psychotherapy. *International Journal of Group Psychotherapy, 40*, 477–493.

Braaten, L. J. (1991). Group cohesion: A new multidimensional model. *Group, 15*, 39–49.

Brabender, V., Albrecht, E., Sillitti, J., Cooper, J., & Kramer, E. (1983). A study of curative factors in short term group therapy. *Hospital and Community Psychiatry, 34*, 643–644.

Breuer, J., & Freud, S. (1955). *Studies on hysteria* (Vol. 2., standard ed.). London: Hogarth Press.

Budman, S. H., Soldz, S., Demby, A., Feldstein, M., Springer, T., & Davis, S. (1989). Cohesion, alliance and outcome in group psychotherapy. *Psychiatry, 52,* 339–350.

Bugen, L. A. (1977). Composition and orientation effects on group cohesion. *Psychological Reports, 40,* 175–181.

Burrow, T. (1927). The group method of analysis. *Psychoanalytic Review, 14,* 268–280.

Butler, T., & Fuhriman, A. (1980). Patient perspective on the curative process. A comparison of day treatment and out-patient psychotherapy groups. *Small Group Behavior, 11,* 371–388.

Butler, T., & Fuhriman, A. (1983). Level of functioning and length of time in treatment variables influencing patients' therapeutic experience in group psychotherapy. *International Journal of Group Psychotherapy, 33,* 489–504.

Cartwright, D. (1968). The nature of group cohesiveness. In D. Cartwright & A. Zander (Eds.), *Group dynamics: Research and theory.* London: Tavistock.

Coché, J., & Coché, E. (1990). *Couples group psychotherapy.* New York: Brunner/Mazel.

Cohn, R. C. (1969). Psychoanalytic or experiential group psychotherapy: A false dichotomy. *Psychoanalytic Review, 50,* 333–345.

Colijn, S., Hoencamp, E., Snijders, H., van der Spek, M., & Duivenvoorden, H. (1991). A comparison of curative factors in different types of group psychotherapy. *International Journal of Group Psychotherapy, 41,* 365–378.

Corder, B. F., Whiteside, M. S., & Haizlip, T. M. (1981). A study of curative factors in group psychotherapy with adolescents. *International Journal of Group Psychotherapy, 31,* 345–354.

Corsini, R., & Rosenberg, B. (1955). Mechanisms of group psychotherapy: Processes and dynamics. *Journal of Abnormal and Social Psychology, 51,* 406–411.

Costell, R. M., & Koran, L. M. (1972). Compatibility and cohesiveness in group psychotherapy. *Journal of Nervous and Mental Disease, 155,* 99–104.

Danet, B. N. (1969). Videotape playback as a therapeutic device in group psychotherapy. *International Journal of Group Psychotherapy, 19,* 433–440.

Dickoff, H., & Lakin, M. (1963). Patients' views of group psychotherapy: Retrospection and interpretations. *International Journal of Group Psychotherapy, 13,* 61–73.

Dierick, P., & Litaer, G. (1990). In G. Litaer, J. Rombauts, & R. van Balen (Eds.), *Client-centered and experiential psychotherapy in the nineties.* Leuven: Leuven University Press.

Dies, R. R. (1973). Group therapist self-disclosure: An evaluation by clients. *Journal of Counseling Psychology, 20,* 344–348.

Dies, R. R. (1977). Group therapist transparency: A critique of theory and research. *International Journal of Group Psychotherapy, 27,* 177–200.

Dies, R. R., & Hess, A. K. (1971). An experimental investigation of cohesiveness in marathon and conventional group psychotherapy. *Journal of Abnormal and Social Psychology, 77,* 258–262.

Drescher, S., Burlingame, G., & Fuhriman, A. (1985). Cohesion: An odyssey in empirical understanding. *Small Group Behavior, 16,* 3–30.

Durkin, H. E. (1982). Change in group psychotherapy: Therapy and practice: A systems perspective. *International Journal of Group Psychotherapy, 32,* 431–439.

Evans, N. J., & Jarvis, P. A. (1980). Group cohesion: A review and re-evaluation. *Small Group Behavior, 11,* 359–370.

Falloon, I., Lindley, P., McDonald, R., & Marks, I. (1977). Social skills training of out-patient groups. *British Journal of Psychiatry, 131,* 599–609.

Farrell, M. P. (1962). Transference dynamics of group psychotherapy. *Archives of General Psychiatry, 6,* 66–76.

Flowers, J. V. (1978). The effect of therapist support and encounter on the percentage of client-client interactions in group therapy. *Journal of Community Psychology, 6,* 69–73.

Flowers, J. V. (1979). The differential outcome effects of simple advice, alternatives and instructions in group psychotherapy. *International Journal of Group Psychotherapy, 29,* 305–316.

Flowers, J. V. (1987). Client outcome as a function of agreement or disagreement with the model group perception of curative factors in short term structured group psychotherapy. *International Journal of Group Psychotherapy, 37,* 113–117.

Glad, D. D., & Durkin, H. E. (1969). Summary of panel discussion on interaction and insight in group psychotherapy. *International Journal of Group Psychotherapy, 19,* 279–280.

Grosz, H. J., Stern, H., & Wright, C. S. (1965). Interactions in therapy groups as a function of differences among therapists and group size. *Psychological Reports, 17,* 827–834.

Grosz, H. J., & Wright, C. S. (1967). The tempo of verbal interaction in an open therapy group conducted in rotation by three different therapists. *International Journal of Group Psychotherapy, 17,* 513–523.

Haer, J. L. (1968). Anger in relation to aggression in psychotherapy groups. *Journal of Social Psychology, 76,* 123–127.

Heckel, R. V., Froelich, I., & Salzberg, H. C. (1962). Interaction and redirection in group therapy. *Psychological Reports, 10,* 14.

Hill, W. F. (1975). Further considerations of therapeutic mechanisms in group therapy. *Small Group Behavior, 6,* 421–429.

Hobbs, M., Birtchnall, S., Harte, A., & Lacey, H. (1989). Therapeutic factors in short term group therapy for women with bulimia. *International Journal of Eating Disorders, 8,* 623–633.

Hurst, A. G. (1978). Leadership style determinants of cohesiveness in adolescent groups. *International Journal of Group Psychotherapy, 28,* 263–279.

Hurvitz, N. (1970). Peer self-help psychotherapy groups and their implication for psychotherapy. *Psychotherapy: Theory Research and Practice, 7,* 41–49.

Jacobs, A. (1974). The use of feedback in groups. In A. Jacobs & W. Spradlin (Eds.), *Group as an agent of change.* New York: Behavioral Publications.

Jacobs, M., Jacobs, A., Carior, N., and Burke, J. (1974). Anonymous feedback: credibility and desirability of structured emotional and behavioral feedback delivered in groups. *Journal of Counseling Psychology 21,* 106–111.

Jacobs, M., Jacobs, A., Feldman, G., and Carior, N. (1973). Feedback II—"the credibility gap," delivery of positive and negative and emotional and behavioral feedback in groups. *Journal of Consulting and Clinical Psychology, 41,* 215–223.

Jacobs, M., Jacobs, A., and Gatz, M. (1973). Credibility and desirability of positive and negative structural feedback in groups. *Journal of Consulting and Clinical Psychology, 40,* 244–252.

Jeske, J. O. (1973). Identification and therapeutic effectiveness in group therapy. *Journal of Counseling Psychology, 20,* 528–530 (1973).

Johnson, D., & Ridener, L. (1974). Self-disclosure, participation, and perceived cohesiveness in small group interaction. *Psychological Reports, 35,* 361–363.

Jourard, S. (1971). *The transparent self.* New York: Van Nostrand.

Kahn, M. E., Webster, P. B., & Storck, M. J. (1986). Curative factors in two types of inpatient therapy groups. *International Journal of Group Psychotherapy, 36,* 579–585.

Kapur, R., Miller, K., & Mitchell G. (1988). Therapeutic factors within inpatient and outpatient psychotherapy groups. *British Journal of Psychiatry, 152,* 229–233.

Kaye, J. D. (1973). Group interaction and interpersonal learning. *Small Group Behavior, 4,* 424–448.

Kellermann, P. F. (1985). Participants' perception of therapeutic factors in psychodrama. *Journal of Group Psychotherapy, Psychodrama and Sociometry, 38,* 123–132.

Killilea, M. (1976). Mutual help organizations: Interpretations in the literature. In G. Caplan & M. Killilea (Eds.), *Support systems and mutual help: Multidisciplinary explorations.* New York: Grune & Stratton.

Kirshner, B. J., Dies, R. R., & Brown, R. A. (1978). Effects of experimental manipulation of self-disclosure on group cohesiveness. *Journal of Consulting and Clinical Psychology, 46,* 1171–1177.

Kissen, M. (1974). The concept of identification: An evaluation of its current status and its significance for group psychotherapy. In M. Rosenbaum (Ed.), *Group psychotherapy from the Southwest.* New York: Gordon & Breach.

Land, E. C. (1964). A comparison of patient improvement resulting from two therapeutic techniques. *Dissertation Abstracts, 25,* 628–629.

Lee, F. T. (1976). The effects of sex, risk-taking, and structure on prescribed group behavior, cohesion, and evaluative attitudes in a simulated early training phase of group psychotherapy. *Dissertation Abstracts International, 36,* 4695B–4696B.

Liberman, R. (1970a). A behavioral approach to group dynamics: I. Reinforcement and prompting of cohesiveness in group therapy. *Behavior Therapy, 1,* 141–175.

Liberman, R. (1970b). A behavioral approach to group dynamics: II. Reinforcing and prompting hostility to the therapist in group therapy. *Behavior Therapy, 1,* 312–327.

Lieberman, M. A. (1980). Analyzing change mechanisms in groups. In M. A. Lieberman & L. D. Borman (Eds.), *Self-help groups for coping with crisis.* San Francisco, CA: Jossey-Bass.

Lieberman, M. A. (1990). Understanding how groups work: A study of homogeneous peer group failures. *International Journal of Group Psychotherapy, 40,* 31–52.

Lieberman, M. A., Yalom, I. D., & Miles, M. D. (1973). *Encounter groups: First facts.* New York: Basic Books.

Lomont, J. F., Gilner, R. H., Spector, N. J., & Skinner, H. (1969). Group assertion training and group insight therapies. *Psychological Reports, 25,* 463–470.

Lorr, M. (1966). Dimensions of interaction in group psychotherapy. *Multivariate Behavioral Research, 1,* 67–73.

Lott, A. J., & Lott, B. E. (1965). Group cohesiveness and interpersonal attraction. *Psychological Bulletin, 64,* 259–309.

Macaskill, N. D. (1982). Therapeutic factors in group therapy with borderline patients. *International Journal of Group Psychotherapy, 32,* 61–73.

Marcovitz, R. J., & Smith, J. E. (1983). Patients' perceptions of curative factors in short-term group psychotherapy. *International Journal of Group Psychotherapy, 33,* 21–39.

Marshall, J. E., & Heslin, R. (1975). Sexual composition and the effect of density and group size of cohesiveness. *Journal of Personality and Social Psychology, 31,* 952–961.

Marshall, J. R. (1972). The expression of feelings. *Archives of General Psychiatry, 27,* 786–790.

MacKenzie, R. (1987). Therapeutic factors in group psychotherapy: A contemporary view. *Group, 11,* 26–34.

Maxmen, J. S. (1973). Group therapy as viewed by hospitalized patients. *Archives of General Psychiatry, 28,* 404–408.

Maxmen, J. S. (1978). An educative model for in-patient group therapy. *International Journal of Group Psychotherapy, 28,* 321–338.

McPherson, F. M., & Walton, H. G. (1970). The dimensions of psychotherapy group interaction: An analysis of clinicians; constructs. *British Journal of Medical Psychology, 43,* 281–290.

Meichenbaum, D. H., Gilmore, J. B., & Fedoravicius, A. L. (1971). Group insight versus group desensitization in treating speech anxiety. *Journal of Consulting and Clinical Psychology, 36,* 410–421.

Mudrack, P. E. (1989). Defining group cohesiveness: A legacy of confusion? *Small Group Behavior, 29,* 37–49.

Myerhoff, H. L., Jacobs, A., & Stoller, F. (1970). Emotionality in marathon and traditional psychotherapy groups. *Psychotherapy: Theory, Research and Practice, 7,* 33–36.

Piper, W. E., Marrache, M., Lacroix, R., Richardsen, A., & Jones, B. (1983). Cohesion as a basic bond in groups. *Human Relations, 36,* 93–108.

Pratt, J. H. (1975). The tuberculosis class: An experiment in home treatment. In M. Rosenbaum & M. Berger (Eds.), *Group psychotherapy and group function.* New York: Basic Books.

Query, W. T. (1970). An experimental investigation of self-disclosure and its effect upon some properties of psychotherapeutic groups. *Dissertation Abstracts International, 31,* 2263B.

Ribner, N. G. (1974). Effects of an explicit group contract on self-disclosure and group cohesiveness. *Journal of Counseling Psychology, 21*(2), 116–120.

Riley, R. (1971). An investigation of the influence of group compatibility on group cohesiveness and change in self-concept in a T-group setting. *Dissertation Abstracts International, 31*, 3277A.

Roback, H. B. (1972). Experimental comparison of outcomes in insight and non-insight-oriented therapy groups. *Journal of Consulting and Clinical Psychology, 38*, 411–117.

Robinson, D. (1980). Self-help health groups. In P. B. Smith (Ed.), *Small groups and personal change*. London: Methuen.

Robinson, M., & Jacobs, A. (1970). Focused videotape feedback and behavior change in group psychotherapy. *Psychotherapy: Theory, Research and Practice, 7*, 169–172.

Roether, H. A., & Peters, J. J. (1972). Cohesiveness and hostility in group psychotherapy. *American Journal of Psychiatry, 128*, 1014–1017.

Rohrbaugh, M., & Bartels, B. D. (1975). Participants' perceptions of 'curative factors' in therapy and growth groups. *Small Group Behavior, 6*, 430–456.

Rosenthal, T. L., & Bandura, A. (1978). Psychological modeling: Theory and practice. In S. L. Garfield & A. E. Bergin (Eds.), *Handbook of psychotherapy and behavior change*. New York: Wiley.

Rubin, J. H., & Locascio, K. (1985). A model for communication skills group using structural exercises and audiovisual equipment. *International Journal of Group Psychotherapy, 35*, 569–584.

Ryan, W. (1958). Capacity for mutual dependence and involvement in group psychotherapy. *Dissertation Abstracts, 19*, 1119.

Salzberg, H. C. (1962). Effects of silence and redirection of verbal responses in group psychotherapy. *Psychological Reports, 11*, 455–461.

Schaffer, J. B., & Dreyer, S. F. (1982). Staff and in-patient perceptions of change mechanisms in group psychotherapy. *American Journal of Psychiatry, 139*, 127–128.

Scheiderer, E. (1977). Effects of instruction and modeling in producing self-disclosure in the initial clinical interview. *Journal of Consulting and Clinical Psychology, 45*(3), 378–384.

Schutz, W. G. (1958). *The interpersonal underworld*. Palo Alto, CA: Science and Behavior Books.

Schutz, W. G. (1966). *The interpersonal underworld*. Palo Alto, CA: Science and Behavior Books.

Slavson, S. R. (1966). Interaction and reconstruction in group psychotherapy. *International Journal of Group Psychotherapy, 16*, 3–12.

Slavson, S. R. (1979). In M. Schiffer (Ed.), *Dynamics of group psychotherapy*. New York: Aronson.

Stein, A. (1970). The nature and significance of interaction in group psychotherapy. *International Journal of Group Psychotherapy, 20*, 153–162.

Steinfeld, G., & Mabli, J. (1974). Perceived curative factors in group therapy by residents of a therapeutic community. *Criminal Justice Behavior, 1*, 278–288.

Stephen, J. A. M., van den Langenberg, & Dekker, J. (1989). What is therapeutic in the therapeutic community. *International Journal of Therapeutic Communities, 10,* 81–90.

Stokes, J., Fuehrer, A., & Childs, L. (1983). Group members' self-disclosures: Relation to perceived cohesion. *Small Group Behavior, 14,* 63–76.

Sullivan, H. S. (1953). *The interpersonal theory of psychiatry.* New York: Norton.

Swarr, R. R., & Ewing, T. N. (1977). Outcome effects of eclectic interpersonal-learning-based group psychotherapy with college student neurotics. *Journal of Consulting and Clinical Psychology, 45,* 1029–1035.

Thomas, E. J., & Fink, C. F. (1963). Effects of group size. *Psychological Bulletin, 60,* 371–384.

Truax, C., & Carkhuff, R. (1965). Correlations between therapist and patient self-disclosure: A predictor of outcome. *Journal of Counseling Psychology, 12,* 3–9.

Weigel, R. G., & Warnath, G. F. (1968). The effects of group therapy on reported self-disclosure. *International Journal of Group Psychotherapy, 18,* 31–41.

Weiner, M. F. (1974). Genetic vs. interpersonal insight. *International Journal of Group Psychotherapy, 24,* 230–237.

Weiner, M. F. (1977). Catharsis: A review. *Group Process, 71,* 173–184.

Weiner, M. F., Rosson, B., & Cody, B. S. (1974). Studies of therapeutic and patient affective self-disclosure. In M. Rosenbaum (Ed.), *Group psychotherapy from the Southwest.* New York: Gordon & Breach.

Weiss, B. J. (1972). The development of cohesiveness in marathon growth groups. *Dissertation Abstracts International, 32,* 6065B.

Wender, L. (1936). Dynamics of group psychotherapy and its application. *Journal of Nervous and Mental Disease, 84,* 54–60.

Whalen, G. S., & Mushet, G. L. (1986). Consumers' views of the helpful aspects of an inpatient psychotherapy group. *British Journal of Medical Psychology, 59,* 337–339.

Whiteley, S. J., & Collis, M. (1987). The therapeutic factors in group therapy applied to the therapeutic community. *International Journal of Therapeutic Communities, 8,* 21–32.

Yalom, I. D. (1983). *Inpatient group psychotherapy.* New York: Basic Books.

Yalom, I. D. (1985). *The theory and practice of group psychotherapy* (3rd ed.). New York: Basic Books.

Yalom, I. D., Bond, G., Bloch, S., Zimmerman, E., & Friedman, L. (1977). The effects of a weekend group experience on the course of individual psychotherapy. *Archives of General Psychiatry, 34,* 399–415.

Yalom, I. D., Houts, P. S., Zimmerberg, S. M., & Rand, K. H. (1967). Prediction of improvement in group therapy. *Archives of General Psychiatry, 17,* 159–68.

Yalom, I. D., & Rand, K. (1966). Compatibility and cohesiveness in therapy groups. *Archives of General Psychiatry, 15,* 267–275.

PART FOUR

Special Applications and Populations

CHAPTER 9

Progress in Short-Term and Time-Limited Group Psychotherapy: Evidence and Implications

SIMON H. BUDMAN, PAUL G. SIMEONE, RICHARD REILLY, and
ANNETTE DEMBY

Brief group psychotherapy has been practiced in various forms for many years. Indeed, most research reports on group therapy have described relatively short-term or time-limited treatment (Dies, 1992). Recently, short-term and time-limited group therapy has taken on even greater importance.* This is due to the growing concern in this country regarding the rising cost of health care and strategies of cost-containment that include managed care, inpatient and outpatient case review, and a general move in the direction of briefer, more circumscribed, focal treatments.

THE HEALTH CARE CRISIS AND SHORT-TERM GROUP THERAPY

It is an often cited fact that there is a health care inflation crisis of major proportions in this country (Freudenheim, 1988; Karr, 1990; Kimball, 1990), and that the cost of medical services has risen significantly more than the cost of living. Whereas inflation (CPI) has been running between 2% to 4%, the medical price index (MPI) has averaged 7% to 8% (Berman, 1987). In its 1990 National Executive Poll on Health Care Costs and Benefits, *Business & Health* found that 9 out of 10 top executives around the country cited the rise of health insurance costs as the health care issue of greatest concern (*Business & Health,* 1990). Berwick, Godfrey, and Roessner (1990) astutely point out that, " . . . if the American health care industry were declared a

---

This chapter was supported in part by funds from NIMH Grants # 5 RO1 MH 43908 and # 3 RO1 MH 40151.
* Throughout this review, we will use the terms and abbreviations short-term group (STG) and time-limited group (TLG) interchangeably.

nation, it would have the sixth largest GNP of all of the nations on earth" (p. 5).

To restrain costs, insurance providers and employers have turned increasingly to managed health care programs. In 1989, 35.03 million people (14% of the U.S. population) belonged to health maintenance organizations (HMOs) and it is estimated that by the end of 1994 over 53 million Americans will receive their care through an HMO (Marion Laboratories, 1989; Marion Merrel Dow, 1990). While HMO enrollment has been slowing, the rate of growth of preferred provider organizations (PPOs) is currently accelerating. Although PPOs are a relatively new phenomenon, already over 30 million people receive their health care through PPO systems (DeLeon, VandenBos, & Bulatoa, 1991; Melnick, Zwanziger, & Verity-Guerra, 1989). Some estimates are that by the mid-1990s up to 70% of the U.S. population will receive health care through some type of managed care organization (Berkman, Bassos, & Post, 1988). The predominant mode of mental health treatment within all managed care programs is brief and time-effective therapy (Bennett, 1988, 1992; Budman, 1992; Budman & Gurman, 1988; Hoyt & Austad, 1992).

Within the current *Zeitgeist,* shorter and time-limited group treatments take on major importance as practical models of therapy that can be both economical and effective. In a recent survey of 75 experts who were asked to predict the future of psychotherapy, the panel overwhelmingly forecasted increases in the use and popularity of short-term treatment and of group therapies (Norcross, Alford, & DeMichele, 1992). This chapter will review some central issues in such therapies. First we will discuss the nature and characteristics of time-limited group therapy. We will then consider selected outcome data on time-limited groups, group member characteristics, and treatment factors in time-limited groups, including pregroup preparation, group composition, and group focus. We will pay particular attention to the significance of cohesion, the role of the leader, and the issue of time in time-limited groups, and conclude with some thoughts about the future of time-limited group psychotherapy.

The Nature of Short-Term and Time-Limited Group

Using the most common definition of short-term psychotherapy, as treatment that is under 20 to 25 visits (Koss & Butcher, 1986), most group treatment in this country (like most other therapies) is in practice relatively brief in nature. For example, Klein and Carroll (1986) surveyed over 700 patients at a university-based outpatient group therapy clinic. Groups at this clinic were supposed to be long-term and most had open memberships, with new members filling spots as they became available. Most of the patients referred to this clinic were fairly well-educated, working and/or middle class. Of the patients referred for groups, more than 40% dropped out during the evaluation and preparation process. Among the remaining patients who did ultimately join a group, 52.4% had 12 or fewer visits. Only 8% of those who began treatment attended a group for one year or longer. The therapists in the Klein and Carroll survey were mostly trainees. In groups led by inexperienced leaders nearly everyone stops treatment before 12 months have passed. Indeed, even in the practices of highly experienced and well-trained practitioners nearly half of those who begin, end before one year. In a similar survey done with a select private practice population, Stone and Rutan (1984), two highly experienced group clinicians, found that in their own practices nearly 40% of the patients who began treatment quit before the end of the first year. It appears that most people who begin group therapy leave well before their therapist would anticipate their ending. In keeping with these findings, other data on average length of outpatient treatment in varied settings and different modes of treatment (Garfield, 1986) suggest that most therapy that is carried out in the United States tends to be relatively short in nature (usually 4 to 8 sessions).

In our clinical research with short-term groups, we have noted a relatively low drop-out rate of 16.6% in 15-session young adult outpatient groups led by experienced therapists (Budman, Demby, & Randall, 1980). In 72-session outpatient therapy groups for more disturbed patients with personality disorders, 20% of the group members dropped out before six months and 41% dropped out before 12 months (Budman, Soldz, Demby, & Merry, in preparation). It does appear that group therapy is frequently short in practice, regardless of whether or not it is planned to be "short" or "long."

Our intent is to examine group treatment that is *planned* to be short-term or time-limited, rather than being so by default. We are not defining time-limited group therapy in terms of the number of sessions or length of treatment, but, instead, *by the presence of the notion of time being rationed* within the treatment. Generally, this translates into a planned limit to the number of sessions offered based upon the principle of parsimony.

We must also state another caveat regarding the type of therapy discussed. Many authors present their approaches to short-term group treatment in a vacuum. That is, theoretically and empirically the group treatment described is often offered without regard to previous, concurrent, or future therapies. In fact, it is clearly the case that most therapy utilizers seek out many different therapies over the course of their lives and that most of those treated in courses of (long-and short-term) therapy, return for additional treatment after a given episode of therapy is completed. Indeed, there are indications that between 50% and 60% of patients who terminate at any given time seek additional care within the following year (Budman & Gurman, 1988). Thus, viewing the index episode of therapy as being brief treatment is, in some ways, misleading. Although a particular episode of group therapy may be relatively short-term (compared to some "ideal" model in the therapist's mind regarding how long such therapy should take), any treatment takes place within a broader context of care that may include multiple courses of group, individual and/or couples therapy over a multi-year period. Short-term group treatment approaches are often only one component of a more expansive (and often lifelong) process of change. This is an important point because it changes the way in which we think about measuring outcome in time-limited therapy in general. Rather than thinking about "cure," we are thinking about limited improvement and changes. Therapy goals then become more realistic and achievable.

A number of the leading brief psychodynamic individual therapists (Davanloo, 1978; Mann, 1973; Sifneos, 1972) discuss their work in terms of treatment "cures"—definitive and complete courses of treatment. As noted previously, however, many patients return for treatment episodes intermittently. Consequently, it may be more appropriate to think in terms of limited and achievable goals for any given course of treatment. With respect to short-term groups in particular, Klein (1985) adopts fairly modest goals, noting that ". . . it may only be possible to meaningfully identify these core conflicts and begin to examine their interpersonal implications, but not to work them through and to achieve any lasting structural change"[*] (p. 321). McCallum and Piper (1990) view their patients in loss groups as having the opportunity to utilize the loss of the group as a way to begin dealing with unresolved conflicts and feelings from previous losses. Poey (1985) stresses the need to work in these groups primarily on an ego level, accentuating secondary over primary process and, in general, supporting rather than challenging defenses. He feels that with adherence to this level of work, patients can make significant gains in many areas, including symptom relief, re-establishment of psychological equilibrium, comfort in interpersonal relationships and enhanced self-understanding. Like many other brief therapists, he also believes that the work initiates a process that continues long after the direct clinical contact is completed.

We will be reviewing interactionally-oriented group therapy rather than psycho-educational, cognitive behavioral, and/or highly structured models of group treatment. It is our impression that many of these models do not make use of the unique aspects of group interaction, but operate in a group format because it is more economical and/or convenient. Often such models may be based on individual treatment practices and are manually driven. Under these circumstances, the group context adds little more to the treatment method than a broader venue for the therapy in question.

Does Short-Term and Time-Limited Group Therapy Work?

With several important recent exceptions, the outcome literature on short-term group therapy is limited. As recently as 1985, Poey suggested that there

---

[*] We feel somewhat uncertain as to what constitutes "true structural change" and have not yet seen convincing research that supports the ways in which such change differs from improvement in symptomatology. For a fascinating example of research dealing with this question, the reader is referred to Mintz (1981).

was a ". . . paucity of rigorous outcome research available on short-term dynamic group psychotherapy though many such groups are being run" (p. 332). Rather than a comprehensive review of the literature on outcome studies of time-limited groups, we will concentrate on a select group of studies that focus on interactionally oriented outpatient time-limited groups. The studies of note are those of LaPointe and Rimm (1980), Piper, Debbane, Bienvenu, and Garant (1984), Piper, McCallum, and Hassan (1992), and our own clinical research with the Harvard Community Health Plan.

LaPointe and Rimm (1980) and Piper et al. (1984) compared dynamic, interactional short-term group therapies to other types of treatment. In both studies, the authors found that the patients in the STGs improved on various outcome measures, but not more than patients in other active treatment conditions. In the four-way design study by Piper and his colleagues, STG was the least effective therapy examined, when compared to individual, long-term individual, and long-term group.

In a recent project that studied the efficacy of short-term dynamically oriented groups for patients dealing with recent losses, Piper et al. (1992) compared the STGs to a waiting list control condition. The effects of treatment in this carefully controlled, well-designed, and well-executed study were encouraging:

> The results of the clinical trial were clearly supportive of the effectiveness of time-limited, short-term dynamic therapy groups for patients experiencing difficulties following the loss of one or more persons. Treated patients improved significantly more on many outcome variables than did their matched counterparts who had been assigned to a wait-list control condition. The results were evident from both independent sample and own-control comparisons. (Piper et al., 1992, p. 167)

Budman, Demby, Feldstein, and Gold (1984) compared a small sample of patients, approximately half of whom had been randomly assigned to short-term interactional group treatment and half to a waiting-list control condition. The 16 immediate treatment patients, who entered a 15-session STG were significantly better on a multidimensional outcome battery at the end of the therapy period than were the waiting list patients. In particular, the STG patients had greater improvement in the area of target problem change. Six months after treatment ended for the STG patients, there were no longer any significant difference between the two populations. It must be remembered, however, that many of the waiting list and the STG patients received additional therapy during this half-year period, making it more likely that the original differences would be obfuscated.

Budman et al. (1988), in a randomized clinical trial, compared time-limited group psychotherapy and time-limited individual psychotherapy. This study involved ninety-eight nonpsychotic psychiatric outpatients and five experienced brief therapists. Significant improvement and maintenance of improvement occurred in both treatments, on a multidimensional outcome battery. There was, however, a clear preference by patients for the individual therapy, as evidenced by the individual patients *attributing* a higher benefit to their therapy than the group patients. On closer examination, only those patients in specific groups rated their benefit from group therapy as high or higher than the average individual patient.

This data led Budman and his colleagues to investigate further the elements that contributed to some groups being experienced by members as more effective or helpful than others. A series of studies of group cohesiveness in time-limited groups was begun at the Harvard Community Health Plan by Budman and his colleagues in 1981. Empirical investigation supported group cohesion as a central factor contributing to positive outcome in group psychotherapy (Budman et al., 1987; Budman et al., 1993). We will return to the discussion of cohesiveness in a later section.

In addition to the outcome research discussed thus far, Budman and his colleagues have studied the effectiveness of time-limited groups of 72 sessions for 50 patients with personality disorders. Although these groups clearly are not brief or "short," they do meet the criteria of groups that have a defined time limit, and they may be construed as parsimonious in their therapy approach to an especially difficult and complex patient population. Preliminary results of 25 patients who completed the groups reflect positive outcomes for these patients on a large multidimensional assessment battery (Budman, Soldz, Demby, & Merry, unpublished).

Taken together, the results would seem to generally support the efficacy of STG and time-limited group as a useful treatment modality. A more enthusiastic assessment must wait for an accumulation of additional data in this area.

SHORT-TERM GROUPS—FOR WHOM?

With the exception of the study involving patients with personality disorders, the patients studied in the projects cited were not severely disturbed and tended to be anxious and/or depressed. They were not generally individuals with DSM-IIIR Axis I pathology. Regarding patient exclusionary criteria, Burlingame and Fuhriman (1990) indicate:

> More consensus exists across writers on specific exclusionary criteria, irrespective of settings. Clients with particularly severe pathology (e.g., psychoses, character disorders, extreme paranoia, sociopathy) are typically excluded from short-term group treatment. A notable exception to this observation is models designed for inpatient setting where only the most severe cases are excluded, undoubtedly for logistic reasons . . . (p. 95)

There is sufficient data available to support the use of short-term and time-limited group therapy (generally under 20 visits) as an intervention modality. With one exception, the patients in the studies cited were anxious and/or depressed, but not severely disturbed, nor suffering from severe personality disorders. The evidence appears to indicate that for an appropriate outpatient population, such treatment is both time- and cost-effective. It should again be emphasized that many patients treated in such groups will go on for additional treatment. As one course of treatment in what will often be multiple courses of intervention, planned short-term group therapy can be recommended as efficacious and presumably cost-effective. Where time-limited groups have been attempted with a personality disorder population, the initial results are promising.

Important Treatment Factors in Short-Term Group Therapy

The factors widely recognized as curative or therapeutic (Yalom, 1975, 1985) in open-ended group treatment have general applicability to STGs as well (McCallum, Piper, Azim, & Lakjoff, 1991; Poey, 1985). There is, however, a somewhat distinct emphasis that has emerged from the work of those primarily investigating short-term group modalities. Several key components of successful STGs occur before the group's formal inception: pregroup preparation and screening, the articulation of a group focus or theme, and composition. Throughout treatment, cohesiveness assumes special import in short-term groups, along with two additional factors: the role of the leader and the orientation to time.

Pregroup Preparation and STG

In all types of group therapy adequate preparation is viewed as important for the enhancement of process and outcome. Nowhere is this as true as in STGs. When one is attempting to lead a short-term group it is important to "hit the ground running." A significant component of such a rapid start is the preparation that members have before beginning the group.

We refer the reader to Kaul and Bednar's chapter, in this volume, on the empirical evidence regarding pregroup preparation. Although clinical research regarding the efficacy of pregroup preparation has produced mixed results, nonetheless wisdom dictates to the STG therapist that time be taken to prepare patients adequately. While the impact upon outcome may be small (i.e., dropout rate reduced), the practice should still lead to less demoralization in the group and a greater likelihood of a productive process.

Budman and Gurman (1988) have offered structured models for pregroup preparation that can be applied to many different types of short-term groups. In this model, a pregroup workshop is held after the therapist has met individually with potential group members. In the individual pregroup session, the therapist helps the patient to reframe the presenting problems in a way that clarifies the relationship between the patient's issues and the focal theme of the group.

In the pregroup workshop, the members are engaged in dyadic, small group, and group-as-a-whole exercises that are designed to (1) decrease patient anxiety, (2) provide skills training in desirable group behaviors, and (3) provide both therapist and patient with an opportunity to make a more informed decision about the patient's suitability for the group.

Budman and Gurman's model for STG pregroup workshops contains the following components: (1) introductions, (2) subgroup tasks, and (3) whole group tasks. In the beginning of the workshops, members form dyads and introduce themselves to each other, and then introduce their dyad partner to the larger group. In a second structured exercise, members get together in three- or four-person groups and perform a task, at the direction of the leader, which is related to the central focus of the group. For example, in an interactionally oriented group focused on relationship issues, members are invited to role-play a recent problematic interaction with another person. Subgroup members are then instructed to suggest alternatives to the problematic interaction. In the large-group exercise, all members work together in a group task, the focus of which is again related to the group's theme. In a young adult group, for example, the members are invited to plan a party together. The leader observes the way in which the members go about achieving the task (i.e., which members take leadership roles, which members are passive, what roles are assumed by various participants, and how decisions are reached (or not reached)).

The group leader is provided with a rich amount of information about members' interactions, a chance to model and teach desirable group skills, and specific information about each member's appropriateness for the group. The leader then uses the workshop for screening purposes. If an individual appears to be inappropriate for the group, the leader communicates with that individual, who can be referred to a more appropriate group or to further individual therapy as appropriate.

The clinical and research literature is sufficiently supportive of pregroup preparation to indicate that it is very important for patients entering short-term groups to receive some type of thorough preparation. This may take the form of a special workshop, videotape, or the more traditional orientation interview, similar to the one described by Yalom (1985). It is unclear that these preparation processes will enhance outcome, nevertheless the data do strongly indicate that a good preparation process will reduce dropout rates in these groups.

Focus and Group Composition

A *sine qua non* in all models of brief and time-limited psychotherapy is the maintenance of a focus for the treatment (Budman, 1992; Budman & Gurman, 1988). Without such a focus, the treatment lacks a central theme and direction. Since the possible directions that therapy can take are so varied and multi-faceted, the focus provides the therapist and patient alike with some guide as to what the most important themes in the therapy will be. For example, in brief cognitive behavioral therapy the focus is on the irrational cognitions that dominate the patient's emotional responses to his or her life (Beck, Emery, & Greenberg, 1985; Ellis, 1992). Psychoanalytically oriented brief therapies often focus on transference and/or developmental factors (Butler, Strupp, & Binder, 1992). Interpersonal therapy focuses on interactions with other people in the patient's life (Klerman, Rounsaville, Chevron, & Weissman, 1984) and the impact of these involvements.

In short-term and time-limited group therapy, the issue of focus has been addressed in several ways. Many of these groups have a central theme or set of themes around which the group is organized. For example, Budman, Bennett, and Wisneski (1980; 1981) organize their STGs around the concept of adult developmental issues. Piper et al. (1992) focus their time-limited groups on the issue of dealing with personal loss. Donovan and his colleagues (Donovan, Bennett, & McElroy, 1981) help patients deal with intense crisis situations. Goldberg, Schuyler, Bransfield, and Savino (1983) suggest that the short-term group therapist use as a "central principle . . . broad based homogeneity including the development of a common theme" (p. 423).

Having a focus allows the leader to bring together a group of individuals who share a sense of similarity in regard to a particular concern or set of concerns. Although maintaining a focus in the STG is key, it is also imperative that the therapist understand the focus as only a tool and concept for organizing the group and not a rigid reality. In this regard, Budman (1993) in his review of *Adaptation to Loss* (Piper et al., 1992) writes:

. . . the focal theme of the group is really a heuristic around which members initially come together. In the clinical examples offered in the book it is obviously the case that members coming to the group are different from one another more than they are similar and that their stages of loss and clarity about how their losses are affecting them varies greatly. To illustrate, in the group from which excerpts are presented one member is dealing with the death of a supervisor at work 9-months prior to her entry into treatment, while another member is a 36-year-old man whose depression is seemingly precipitated by the tenth birthday of his son. It is assumed that this man became depressed at the time of his son's birthday because the patient's mother had died when he was a 10-year-old boy. Obviously, although both of these members are dealing with the issue of loss, the type of loss being dealt with, the stage of working the loss through, and the symptom pictures for each of these people varies greatly.

It has been my experience in working with short-term groups that the members need to have some way to rapidly view themselves as "in the same boat." If the leader starts with a common theme differences are de-emphasized by the members themselves. That is, members want to see themselves as similar so that they can quickly start working and use the time available most beneficially. This would be less possible under circumstances where such a central thematic focus was not offered. At the same time it is not necessary for the leader to just have members who rigidly fit a given set of focal issues. Members (if they are reasonably healthy) are interested in overcoming differences not in building barriers. The authors show clinical savvy and skill in recognizing that *rigid* adherence to a focal theme is not necessary nor desirable.

The issue of focus and homogeneity in STGs differs considerably from what is generally recommended for those leading long-term, open-ended therapy groups. In such groups, it is often the case that heterogeneity is recommended to allow the group microcosm to have the greatest degree of diversity (Whitaker & Lieberman, 1964; Yalom, 1985).

Research does not exist that systematically compares group development and treatment outcome in STGs that are unfocused and heterogeneous versus focused and homogeneous. Clinical experience indicates that homogeneity and focus is a very important element of most short-term group therapy. Since homogeneity allows members to see one another as sharing certain common characteristics, problems, or concerns, it may contribute to a more rapid cohesiveness in the group. The implication of the work cited is that more cohesiveness is related to better outcomes.

Our recommendation is that the STG therapist establish his or her groups around a particular focus or theme and bring together members who share in this particular focus or theme. At the same time, it is important that the therapist understand that the focus is only a heuristic and not a truth or a reality. Many individuals may be able to see aspects of themselves within a particular theme.

GROUP COHESION IN STGs

Cohesiveness in group psychotherapy is the conceptual counterpart to the therapeutic alliance in individual treatment. Both are considered central "curative factors" in psychotherapy broadly defined, and both have been the focus of extensive clinical and theoretical discussion (Kaul & Bednar, 1986; Kellerman, 1981; Yalom, 1985). The vital importance of cohesiveness to STG therapy lies in the fact that there is minimal time in a short-term group for the therapist to assist the group in pulling together as a safe, working unit. Short-term group treatment has a way of telescoping group processes such that the beginning, middle, and final phases take on an exaggerated significance. The task confronting the therapist in this case is to ensure that cohesiveness develops in a timely manner, and that the phases of cohesion development are not missed, delayed, or minimized. Thus, for the therapist doing STG, it is very important to understand the concept of cohesion, the related research, and to be able to think about how to foster cohesion as quickly as possible.

Unlike the concept of therapeutic alliance, a well-researched variable found to be a durable predictor of outcome, the phenomenon of cohesiveness does not enjoy nearly the same level of empirical examination and conceptual clarity. This is due not only to the complexity of the idea itself, but also to the immensely difficult undertaking of the measurement of cohesiveness.

In this section, we will review the evolution of cohesiveness as a compelling theoretical and clinical issue, and we will examine research efforts past and present that point to important and relevant clinical advances.

Historically, research on cohesiveness in group treatment has relied heavily upon self-report measures based on Frank's (1957) seminal definition of the concept as "the attraction of the group for its members" (p. 54). This notion of cohesiveness was later operationalized by Gross (1957) in his Cohesiveness Scale, which then went through two subsequent modifications, first by Yalom, Houts, Zimberg, and Rand (1967) and then again by Stokes (1983). Recently, Drescher, Burlingame, and Fuhriman (1985) reviewed the research in group cohesiveness and found that the vast majority of published studies measure cohesiveness with simple self-report measures typically completed at one point early in the group. In most instances, the Gross Scale or some modification of it was employed. While this strategy is a useful starting point, there are clear limitations which need to be addressed (Budman et al., 1989). At the broadest level of analysis, such an undimensional approach fails to enhance any clinical/theoretical understanding of the phenomenon in any fundamental way. Moreover, it does not allow for any tracking of group cohesiveness over a single session or, more interestingly, over the entire life span of the group. This limitation is especially constraining because it precludes the study of both patient and therapist influences on the development of group cohesiveness. Finally, and perhaps most problematic, this approach presumes cohesiveness to be a static, non-organismic (Werner, 1957) phenomenon. Such an assumption runs counter to the idea of cohesiveness as "process," and, as such, sanitizes it of its most intriguing and compelling clinical and theoretical aspects.

Not surprisingly, the approach outlined has yielded only marginal results. In recognition of this reality, Bloch and Crouch (1985) astutely argued that so called "curative factors" in group psychotherapy (of which cohesiveness in generally included as primary) might more defensibly be labeled "putative therapeutic factors." They do so because they quite accurately note that research linking these factors to outcome is sparse. In addition, these authors point out further that such factors have not been shown to be therapeutic. For example, regarding cohesiveness, they were able to find only four studies examining its relationship to outcome (Kapp et al., 1964; Roether & Peters, 1972; Weiss, 1972; Yalom et al., 1967). Of these, only two exclusively involved psychotherapy patients. Yalom et al. (1967) found a positive relationship between self-reported improvement and cohesiveness in a sample of outpatient group psychotherapy patients. Roether and Peters (1972) investigated the relationship between cohesion and outcome in compulsory groups for sexual offenders and found cohesion to be correlated with increased rates of recidivism! As is clear, these results are mixed at best, but, more alarming, they point to persistent and troubling problems with this area of research in general. Kaul and Bednar (1986), in bemoaning the sad state of cohesiveness research, perhaps put it best in a recent review of the field:

Despite their apparent utility in the practice of group work, however, cohesion and cohesiveness have been a spectacular embarrassment to group therapy and research. Over 30 years of effort has not enabled us to achieve an accepted definition of the terms. Literally hundreds of research attempts have made no demonstrable impact on our understanding of the concept. There is an interactability somewhere in the concept or in our approach to their comprehension. (p. 70)

More recently, Budman and his colleagues at Harvard Community Health Plan (HCHP) in Boston, Massachusetts have undertaken a new approach to the study of cohesiveness and outcome in group psychotherapy. In a radical departure from traditional conceptualizations and methodologies, they have developed a clinically relevant, observer rated process measure of group cohesiveness. At the conceptual level, Budman et al. (1989) have attempted to go beyond Frank's (1957) attraction-to-group conceptualization and revised cohesiveness as:

. . . the connectedness of the group, demonstrated by working together toward a common goal, constructive engagement around common themes, and an open, trusting attitude which allows members to share personal material. (p. 341)

This definition raises two points that need to be briefly addressed. First, this model of cohesion is broader in scope than its time honored predecessor, and, as such, recasts cohesiveness as a dynamic rather than static process. On the other hand, this definition is also narrower than "group attraction," because it is explicitly restricted to therapeutic groups (as opposed to any other group situation). The result of this reconceptualization has been the development and refinement of the Harvard Community Health Plan Group Cohesion Scale (HCHP-GCS; Budman et al., 1987), a process scale designed to measure cohesiveness in group psychotherapy.

The Harvard team has used versions I and II of the HCHP-GCS in a number of outcome studies over the past five years. The findings from these studies are quite promising. Perhaps most impressive is the general finding that group cohesiveness is not only highly correlated with therapeutic alliance (Budman et al., 1989), but, equally important, it is consistently related to improved self-esteem, reduced symptomatology, and increased satisfaction with treatment as rated by patients (Budman et al., 1987; Budman et al., 1989; Budman et al., 1992).

The last set of findings to be reviewed here concerns the phase specific aspects of group cohesiveness and its relationship to outcome. Here, Budman et al. (1993) focused on the early, middle, and final phases of group process, paying particular attention to what promotes cohesiveness (and thus good outcome) in each phase.

In order to examine group process and its relationship to outcome, Budman et al. (1993) developed an instrument measuring statement-by-statement group therapy process dimensions hypothesized to be associated with positive outcome in group therapy. This scale was used to rate 12 time-limited 15-session outpatient psychotherapy groups. It appears that various types of observable group member behaviors are related to group cohesion, which is in turn associated with outcome. The specific member behaviors associated with cohesion, however, vary according to the *phase* of the group therapy. That is, a particular type of member behavior, such as disclosures of personal material about life outside the group, is associated with favorable cohesiveness levels at a certain point in the course of the therapy, but not during other stages of the therapy.

Although these findings are preliminary in nature they are consistent with current stage-related theories of group development (Beck, Dugo, Eng, & Lewis, 1986; Budman & Gurman, 1988; Mackenzie, 1990) and may help to inform therapists' decisions about which specific interventions to employ to enhance group cohesion at different stages of group therapy. Some examples of *stage-specific behaviors* found by Budman et al., (1993) to be associated with favorable (high) group cohesion follow.

In the early stage (sessions 1–5 of 15-session groups), many group members presenting issues to one another about their lives *outside* the group is associated with higher cohesiveness. In the middle stage (sessions 6–10), discussions about both inside- and/or outside-the-group matters are associated with cohesiveness. In the final stage (sessions 11-15), inside-the-group content is associated with higher cohesiveness. These findings throw light on the theoretical issue of the relationship of inside-the-group versus outside-the-group material to cohesion. This is an important distinction given interactional group theory that postulates that the group becomes a social microcosm for the members where outside problematic behaviors are replicated within the group.

Continuing with additional examples of stage-specific relationships between group process and group cohesion, Budman et al. found that in the early group sessions, the correlations between cohesiveness and the number of different group member statements is significant. In the middle of the group, this relationship becomes stronger, and late in the group there is no significant relationship.

Group members discussing their own issues is not significantly associated with cohesion levels at any stage of the group. Members discussing other group members (asking questions of one another, making comments about other members) is positively related to cohesion throughout the group, but significant only in the beginning stage.

The extent to which members focus upon the therapist early in the group has a significantly negative correlation with cohesion, has no relationship to cohesion in the middle stage, and a weakly negative correlation with cohesion in the final stage. It may be that a protracted focus on the therapist during the early stage indicates member dissatisfaction with the therapy or the therapist, and that this dissatisfaction at the very beginning of a group indicates a potentially problematic course of treatment. This is less true in the middle phase, when it may be more stage-appropriate for members to express negative comments about the therapy and the therapist. In the final stage, as in the early stage, extensive discussion about the leader appears to be negatively associated with cohesion. This may be true because the group has not been able to address the group "crisis" stage adequately in the middle sessions.

Thus, for example, the disclosure of material regarding members' problems, behaviors, relationships, or feelings *outside* the group in the early sessions of the therapy group should be encouraged by a therapist. It may be that the converse is true as well—that the therapist should discourage disclosure of material regarding inside-the-group relationships or feelings until a later stage of the group. Also, the group therapist may be wise to encourage members to focus on other group members in the early and middle phases of a group, and to be aware that this behavior is less important during the late sessions. Similarly, group members discussing the therapist in early sessions may signal problems in the group. It may well be that a protracted focus upon the therapist during this stage is an indication of members' dissatisfaction with the therapy.

Although the data are preliminary, there is evidence to suggest that some behaviors or interventions (i.e., by both patients and therapists) which are cohesion-building at one stage of the group may later become cohesion-neutral or even cohesion-toxic at another. These findings underscore the contextual nature of cohesiveness as a dynamic phenomenon, and, as such, contribute to the generation of an emerging paradigm with implications for how group psychotherapy is conceptualized and carried out.

Cohesiveness in both short-term groups and time-limited groups has been shown to be critically and significantly related to therapeutic outcome, as well as to patient satisfaction with group as a treatment modality. To ensure the establishment of cohesiveness, one must not only achieve those conditions that are shown to yield effective group treatment, but, equally important, the therapist must appreciate how such conditions vary across the early , middle, and end phases of group therapy. Accordingly, cohesion must be viewed as a dynamic and complex clinical phenomenon, which, like all developmental processes, needs to be understood and worked with on a moment-to-moment basis.

LEADER'S ROLE IN THE TIME-LIMITED GROUP

The leader who has done an effective job in screening, selecting, and preparing, choosing a focus, and defining suitable group goals has already done a great deal toward providing the opportunity for a favorable group experience. But what of his or her role once the group is underway?

There is extant a general consensus that the STG leader needs to adopt an active style (Budman & Bennett, 1983; Dies, 1977; Klein, 1985; Poey,

1985). Klein (1985) emphasizes the need to tailor the therapist's activity level to the patients' levels of pathology—in essence, the greater the latter, the more the former is required. Regardless of diagnostic category, however, he believes that STG therapists must be comfortable in a supportive and sometimes directive role. Poey (1985) concurs, and advocates selective self-disclosure and modeling as well. He also recognizes the use of "homework" as appropriate in this modality. Most interpersonally oriented short-term group therapists would probably utilize some of these techniques, and in varying degrees might also incorporate cognitive and/or didactic elements, advice, and suggestions in their group work.

Much of the above has to be considered a departure from therapist neutrality, a principle increasingly being called into question from a variety of quarters. For a particularly illuminating discussion, see Wachtel (1986). If, as Wachtel argues, therapeutic neutrality simply is not possible, what then becomes the place of transference in these groups? Ideally, a rapidly developed, positive transference is sought, albeit its general significance is de-emphasized by most STG therapists. Poey is particularly lucid on this point:

> The anxiety such an ambiguous, distant posture (blank screen) produces is intolerably high when coupled with the crisis atmosphere that exists right from the beginning when the members realize just how much there is to do in such a short time. Rather, the keystone to successful group work is the immediate development of a trusting climate of understanding between the leaders and members. . . . (1985, p. 344)

In contrast, McCallum, Piper, and their colleagues (McCallum & Piper, 1988; McCallum et al., 1991) view transference interpretations as central to their work with loss patients. They argue that one of the benefits of group work is that it helps patients tolerate therapists' frustrating interventions (or lack of interventions), which are essential to maintenance of the "true" psychodynamic approach. In addition, these authors question, if the leader moves away from neutrality and the encouragement of regression, whether one is practicing persuasion rather than analytic treatment.

ORIENTATION TO TIME

Time sensitivity is a key, unifying constituent in all forms of brief therapy. Rather than an encumbrance, brief therapists view the limitation of time as having a potentially treatment-enhancing effect when used judiciously. As cited in Applebaum (1975), the utilization of "end-setting" during treatment has a long tradition in individual therapy practice (Dewald, 1965; Ferenczi, 1955; Freud, 1955; Orens, 1955; Rank, 1945). James Mann (1973) was among the first psychoanalytic practitioners to both set the end of treatment at the outset and to delimit the course of therapy to a specified number of (12) sessions. He believed that the use of a time limit, together with focus on a central issue led to a "telescoping of events and heightened affective state that makes for an intense in vivo experience" (p. 207). Mann emphasizes the mastery of separation anxiety, forced by the termination of treatment, as a model for dealing with subsequent anxieties. McCallum and Piper (1988) hold a similar view with respect to termination of their loss groups.

Applebaum (1975), again in reference to individual treatment, has written eloquently about the therapeutic use of time. In a paper entitled "Parkinson's Law in Psychotherapy," he suggests that the work in treatment will expand or contract to fill the time available for it. He accurately observes how hard work and enthusiasm (important variables in brief therapy) can be more readily sustained in most endeavors when the end is in sight. He comments:

> An understanding of endings requires that we consider the existential meaning of time, and that requires us to deal with death. As the therapist, literally or figuratively, flips the calendar's pages, the patient, unconsciously at least, hopes the therapist will never find the last page. Saying goodbye, surmounting loss, and bringing things to an inexorable conclusion are among the most difficult tasks we are asked to perform, as patients and as people. (p. 429)

Hoyt (1990) notes the "strangers on a train" analogue in brief therapy—that people who know the end is clearly defined and in sight may feel encouraged to become involved quickly and intensely. Budman and Gurman (1988) stress how the realization that a group will end evokes issues related to life stage, prior losses and the need to "act before it is too late." In their view, exploration of the issues raised by the group's time limit often brings into focus the existential issue of the limitation of time in one's life. A secondary benefit noted by Budman (1989) is the reduction in dropouts that accompanies a specified termination date.

With the possible exception of Piper and McCallum's groups, in which past losses may be highlighted, the focus in most STGs is on here-and-now or there-and-now interactions. The past is de-emphasized, and generally, historical material is used to illuminate the present, as well as to guide possible future actions.

The accumulated clinical and research evidence suggests that short-term group treatment is most effective when goals are limited and achievable, and time is viewed as catalytic rather than constraining. In general, the short-term group therapist must adopt a style which is active, supportive, and directive, all the while using homework, advice-giving, and extra-therapeutic resources as effective adjuncts to treatment. Transference work, while central to some short-term approaches, is generally de-emphasized as this is frequently regressive and counter progressive. In brief, short-term group treatment is found to be effective when these critical conditions are adequately and consistently achieved.

WHITHER SHORT-TERM AND TIME-LIMITED GROUP PSYCHOTHERAPY?

Survey data already exist which indicate the widespread use of groups in a variety of different mental health settings (Dies, 1992). Many of these groups are short-term, time-limited groups for adults in outpatient settings. In our view, this trend is likely to continue and to broaden. That is, pushed forward by a continued emphasis upon cost and time-effectiveness, short-term and time-limited group therapies are likely to become a dominant mode of mental health outpatient treatment in this country. The data that currently exist on outcome with relatively healthy patients are quite encouraging for these modalities and therefore their use will very likely be strongly supported by managed mental health companies.

It is also likely that more researchers and clinicians will move in the direction of experimenting with time-limited groups for patients with severe disorders. Budman and the Harvard Research Group (Demby & Budman, 1991) have been studying the impact of time-limited 18-month group treatment for patients with severe DSM-III, Axis II personality disorders. Although still preliminary, the early results from their study are encouraging. Linehan and Heard (1992) have also been testing a time-limited group model for patients with personality pathology and feel that these findings also support such intervention.

To date, the breadth of possible uses for short-term group treatments has been relatively unexplored. The next 5 to 10 years should see ever wider utilization of such therapies with broader and more severely impaired populations. Much of this expansion will be economically driven. We hope that what we anticipate to be great clinical and financial enthusiasm in this area is matched (even partially) by theoretical and empirical work.

REFERENCES

Appelbaum, S. A. (1975). Parkinson's law in psychotherapy. *International Journal of Psychoanalytic Psychotherapy, 4,* 425–435.

Beck, A. P., Dugo, J. M., Eng, A. M., & Lewis, C. M. (1986). Analysis of group development. In L. S. Greenberg & W. M. Pinsof (Eds.), *The psychotherapeutic process: A research handbook.* New York: Guilford Press.

Beck, A. T., Emery, G., & Greenberg, R. L. (1985). *Anxiety disorders and phobias.* New York: Basic Books.

Bennett, M. J. (1988). The greening of the HMO: Implications for prepaid psychiatry. *American Journal of Psychiatry, 136,* 1544–1549.

Bennett, M. J. (1992). Managed care as a framework for clinical practice. In J. Feldman & R. Fitzpatrick (Eds.), *Managed mental health care: Administrative and clinical issues* (pp. 203–217). Washington, DC: American Psychiatric Press.

Berkman, A., Bassos, C. A., & Post, L. (1988). Managed mental health care and independent practice: A challenge to psychology. *Psychotherapy, 25,* 434–440.

Berman, K. (1987). Health insurance rates keep climbing. *Business Insurance, 21*(1), 34.

Berwick, D. M., Godfrey, A. B., & Roessner, J. (1990). *Curing health care.* San Francisco, CA: Jossey-Bass.

Bloch, S., & Crouch, E. (1985). *Therapeutic factors in group psychotherapy.* New York: Oxford University Press.

Budman, S. H. (1993). [Review of *Adaptation to loss through short-term group psychotherapy*]. *International Journal of Group Psychotherapy, 43,* 379-382.

Budman, S. H. (1989). *Time-limited group psychotherapy for patients with personality disorders: A preliminary treatment manual.* Unpublished manuscript.

Budman, S. H. (1992). Models of brief individual and group psychotherapy. In J. Feldman & R. Fitzpatrick (Eds.), *Managed mental health care: Administrative and clinical issues* (pp. 231–248). Washington, DC: American Psychiatric Press.

Budman, S. H., & Bennett, M. J. (1983). Short-term group psychotherapy. In H. Kaplan & B. Sadock (Eds.), *Comprehensive group psychotherapy* (rev. ed., pp. 138–144). Baltimore, MD: Williams & Wilkins.

Budman, S. H., Bennett, M. J., & Wisneski, M. (1980). Short-term group psychotherapy: An adult developmental model. *International Journal of Group Psychotherapy, 30,* 63–76.

Budman, S. H., Bennett, M. J., & Wisneski, M. (1981). An adult development model of group psychotherapy. In S. H. Budman (Ed.), *Forms of brief therapy* (pp. 305–342). New York: Guilford Press.

Budman, S. H., Demby, A., Feldstein, M., & Gold, M. (1984). The effects of time-limited group psychotherapy: A controlled study. *International Journal of Group Psychotherapy, 34,* 587–603.

Budman, S. H., Demby, A., Feldstein, M., Redondo, J., Scherz, B., Bennett, M. J., Koppenaal, G., Daley, B. S., Hunter, M., & Ellis, J. (1987). Preliminary findings on a new instrument to measure cohesion in group psychotherapy. *International Journal of Group Psychotherapy, 37,* 75–94.

Budman, S. H., Demby, A., & Randall, M. (1980). Short-term group psychotherapy: Who succeeds, Who fails? *Group, 4,* 3–16.

Budman, S. H., Demby, A., Redondo, J. P., Hannan, M., Feldstein, M., Ring, J., & Springer, T. (1988). Comparative outcome in time-limited individual and group psychotherapy. *International Journal of Psychotherapy, 38,* 63–86.

Budman, S. H., & Gurman, A. S. (1988). *Theory and practice of brief therapy.* New York: Guilford Press.

Budman, S. H., & Gurman, A. S. (1992). A time-sensitive model of brief psychotherapy: The I-D-E approach. In S. H. Budman, M. Hoyt, & S. Friedman (Eds.), *The first session in brief therapy: A book of cases.* New York: Guilford Press.

Budman, S. H., Hoyt, M., & Friedman, S. (Eds.). (1992). *The first session in brief therapy.* New York: Guilford Press.

Budman, S. H., Soldz, S., Demby, A., Davis, M., & Merry, J. (1993). What is cohesiveness? An empirical examination. *Small Group Research, 24,* 199–216.

Budman, S. H., Soldz, S., Demby, A., Feldstein, M., Springer, T., & Davis, M.S. (1989). Cohesion alliance and outcome in group psychotherapy. *Psychiatry, 52,* 339–350.

Budman, S. H., Soldz, S., Demby, A., & Merry, J. (in preparation). *Outcome in time-limited group psychotherapy for patients with personality disorders.* Unpublished manuscript.

Burlingame, G. M., & Fuhriman, A. (1990). Time-limited group psychotherapy. *The Counseling Psychologist, 18,* 93–118.

Business & Health (1990). The 1991 National Executive Poll on Health Care Costs and Benefits. *Business & Health, 14,* 1–8.

Butler, S. F., Strupp, H. H., & Binder, J. L. (1992). Time-limited dynamic psychotherapy. In S. H. Budman, M. F. Hoyt, & S. Friedman (Eds.), *The first session in brief therapy* (pp. 87–110). New York: Guilford Publications.

Davanloo, H. (Ed.). (1978). *Basic principles and techniques in short-term dynamic psychotherapy.* New York: Spectrum.

DeLeon, P. H., VandenBos, G., & Bulatoa, E.O. (1991). Managed mental health care: A history of federal policy initiative. *Professional Psychology, 22,* 15–25.

Demby, A., & Budman, S. H. (1991). The Harvard Community Health Plan Mental Health Research Program. In L. Beutler & M. Crago (Eds.), *Psychotherapy research: An international review of programmatic studies* (pp. 41–47). Washington, DC: American Psychological Association.

Dewald, P. A. (1965). Reactions to the forced termination of therapy. *Psychiatric Quarterly, 39,* 102–126.

Dies, R. (1977). Group therapist transparency: A critique of theory and research.

Dies, R. R. (1992). The future of group therapy. *Psychotherapy, 29,* 58–64. *International Journal of Group Psychotherapy, 27,* 177–200.

Donovan, J. M., Bennett, M. J., & McElroy, C. M. (1981). The crisis group: Its rationale format and outcome. In S. H. Budman (Ed.), *Forms of brief therapy* (pp. 283–304). New York: Guilford Press.

Drescher, S., Burlingame, G., & Fuhriman, A. (1985). Cohesion: An odyssey in empirical understanding. *Small Group Behavior, 16,* 3–30.

Ellis, A. (1992). Brief therapy: The rational-emotive approach. In S. H. Budman, M. F. Hoyt, & S. Friedman (Eds.), *The first session in brief therapy* (pp. 36–58). New York: Guilford Press.

Ferenczi, S. (1955). In M. Balint (Ed.), *The selected papers of Sandor Ferenczi.* New York: Basic Books.

Frank, J. D. (1957). Some determinant manifestations and effects of cohesion in therapy groups. *International Journal of Group Psychotherapy, 7,* 53–63.

Freud, S. (1955). From the history of an infantile neurosis. *Standard Ed., 17,* 7–122. London: Hogarth Press.

Freudenheim, M. (1988, November 19). U.S. Health care spending continues sharp rise. *New York Times,* p. 1.

Garfield, S. L. (1986). Research on client variables in psychotherapy. In S. L. Garfield & A. E. Bergin (Eds.), *Handbook of psychotherapy and behavior change* (3rd ed., pp. 213–256). New York: Wiley.

Goldberg, D. A., Schuyler, W. R., Bransfield, D., & Savino, P. (1983). Focal group psychotherapy: A dynamic approach. *International Journal of Group Psychotherapy, 33,* 413–431.

Gross, C. F. (1957). *An empirical study of the concept of cohesiveness and compatibility*. Unpublished honors thesis, Harvard University, Cambridge, MA.

Hoyt, M. F. (1990). On time in brief therapy. In R. A. Wells & V. J. Gianetti (Eds.), *Handbook of the brief psychotherapies*. New York: Plenum Press.

Hoyt, M. F., & Austad, C. S. (1992). Psychotherapy in a staff model health maintenance organization: Providing and assuring quality care in the future. *Psychotherapy, 29,* 119–129.

Kapp, F. T., Gleser, G., Brissenden, A., Emerson, R., Winget, J. A., & Kashdan, B. (1964). Group participation and perceived personality change. *Journal of Nervous and Mental Disease, 139,* 255–265.

Karr, A. R. (1990, January 30). Employer medical costs up 20.4% in 1989 and still climbing. *The Wall Street Journal*, p. 1.

Kaul, T., & Bednar, R. (1986). Research on group and related therapies. In S. Garfield & A. Bergin (Eds.), *Handbook of psychotherapy and behavior change* (pp. 671–714). New York: Wiley.

Kellerman, H. (1981). *Group cohesion: Theoretical and clinical perspectives.* Grune & Stratton.

Kimball, M. C. (1990, January 8). Nation's health bill to rise 10.4% in 1990, U.S. says. *Health Week*, pp. 1, 52.

Klein, R. H. (1985). Some principles of short-term group therapy. *International Journal of Group Psychotherapy, 35,* 309–329.

Klein, R. H., & Carroll, R. A. (1986). Patient characteristics and attendance patterns in outpatient group psychotherapy. *International Journal of Group Psychotherapy, 36,* 115–132.

Klerman, G. L., Rounsaville, B., Chevron, E., & Weissman, M. (1984). *Interpersonal psychotherapy of depression.* New York: Basic Books.

Koss, M. P., & Butcher, J. N. (1986). Research on brief psychotherapy. In S. L. Garfield & A. E. Bergin (Eds.), *Handbook of Psychotherapy and Behavior Change* (3rd ed., pp. 627–670). New York: Wiley.

LaPointe, K. A., & Rimm, D. C. (1980). Cognitive, assertive and insight-oriented group therapies in the treatment of reactive depression in women. *Psychotherapy: Theory, Research and Practice, 17,* 312–321.

Linehan, M. M., & Heard, H. L. (1992). Dialectical behavior therapy for borderline personality disorder. In J. F. Clarkin, E. Marziali, & H. Munroe-Blum (Eds.), *Borderline personality disorder: Clinical & empirical perspectives* (pp. 248–267). New York: Guilford Press.

Mackenzie, K. R. (1990). *Introduction to time-limited group psychotherapy.* Washington, DC: American Psychiatric Association Press.

Mann, J. (1973). *Time-limited psychotherapy.* Cambridge, MA: Harvard University Press.

Marion Laboratories. (1989, October). *Marion managed care digest update.* Kansas City, MO: Author.

Marion Merrel Dow. (1990). *Marion managed care digest—HMO edition.* Kansas City, MO: Author.

McCallum, M., & Piper, W. E. (1988). Psychoanalytically oriented short-term groups for outpatients: Unsettled issues. *Group, 12*(1), 21–32.

McCallum, M., & Piper, W. E. (1990). The psychological mindedness assessment procedure. *Psychological Assessment: A Journal of Consulting and Clinical Psychology, 2,* 412–418.

McCallum, M., Piper, W. E., Azim, H. F. A., & Lakjoff, R. S. (1991). The Edmonton model of short-term group therapy for loss: An integration of theory, practice and research. *Group, 24,* 375–388.

Melnick, G., Zwanziger, J., & Verity-Guerra, A. (1989). The growth and effects of hospital selective contracting. *Hospital Care Management Review, 14,* 57–64.

Mintz, J. (1981). Measuring outcome in psychodynamic psychotherapy. *Archives of General Psychiatry, 38,* 503–506.

Norcross, J. C., Alford, B. A., & DeMichele, J. (1992). The future of psychotherapy: Delphi data and concluding observations. *Psychotherapy, 29,* 150–158.

Orens, M. H. (1955). Setting a termination date—an impetus to analysis. *Journal of the American Psychoanalytic Association, 3,* 651–665.

Piper, W. E., Debbane, E. G., Bienvenu, J. P., & Garant, J. (1984). A comparative study of four forms of psychotherapy. *Journal of Consulting and Clinical Psychology, 52,* 268–279.

Piper, W. E., McCallum, M., & Hassan, A. (1992). *Adaptation to loss through short-term group psychotherapy.* New York: Guilford Press.

Poey, K. (1985). Guidelines for the practice of brief, dynamic group therapy. *International Journal of Group Psychotherapy, 35*(3), 331–354.

Rank, O. (1945). *Will therapy and truth and reality.* New York: Knopf.

Roether, H. A., & Peters, J. J. (1972). Cohesiveness and hostility in group psychotherapy, *American Journal of Psychiatry, 128,* 1014–1017.

Sifneos, P. (1972). *Short-term psychotherapy and emotional crisis.* Cambridge, MA: Harvard University Press.

Stokes, J. P. (1983). Towards an understanding of cohesion in personal change groups. *International Journal of Group Psychotherapy, 33,* 449–476.

Stone, W. N., & Rutan, J. S. (1984). Duration of treatment in group psychotherapy. *International Journal of Group Psychotherapy, 34,* 93–109.

Wachtel, P. (1986). On the limits of therapeutic neutrality. *Contemporary Psychoanalysis, 22,* 60–70.

Weiss, B. J. (1972). Development of cohesiveness in marathon growth groups. *Dissertation Abstracts International, 32,* 6065–6068.

Werner, H. (1957). The concept of development from a comparative and organismic point of view. In D. B. Harris (Ed.), *The concept of development: An issue in the study of human behavior.* Minneapolis, MN: University of Minnesota Press.

Whitaker, D. S., & Lieberman, M. A. (1964). *Psychotherapy through the group process.* Chicago, IL: Aldine.

Yalom, I. D. (1975). *The theory and practice of group psychotherapy* (2nd ed.). New York: Basic Books.

Yalom, I. D. (1985). *The theory and practice of group psychotherapy* (3rd ed.). New York: Basic Books.

Yalom, I. D., Houts, P. S., Zimberg, S. M. & Rand, L. (1967). Prediction of improvement in group psychotherapy. *Archives of General Psychiatry, 17,* 159–168.

CHAPTER 10

Group Psychotherapy Research with Children, Preadolescents, and Adolescents

JOHN C. DAGLEY, GEORGE M. GAZDA, STEPHANIE J. EPPINGER, and
ELIZABETH A. STEWART

This chapter examines research related to group psychotherapy with children, preadolescents, and adolescents. The definitions of group psychotherapy employed by reviewers whose works are summarized in the first section of this chapter are quite liberal; the accepted definitions of group psychotherapy include group counseling, structured groups, and training groups, among others. The definition of psychotherapy used by Weisz, Weiss, Alicke, and Klotz (1987) in their review of studies of psychotherapy with children and adolescents perhaps best illustrates this inclusiveness. They define psychotherapy "as any intervention designed to alleviate psychological distress, reduce maladaptive behavior, or enhance adaptive behavior through counseling, structured or unstructured interaction, a training program, or a predetermined treatment plan" (p. 543). The coverage of the present review is equally broad, ranging from 1929, the time of the first study reviewed by Levitt (1957) to 1992, the date of several studies reviewed and presented herein. Most comprehensive reviews summarized span a decade; however, some, such as Gazda and Larsen (1968) span three decades (1938–1967).

The reviews of group psychotherapy with children, preadolescents, and adolescents are varied in purpose and methodology. The first two types include a qualitative or a combination of qualitative and quantitative reviews of treated cases with quantitative reviews using the so-called box-score model that applies some baseline criterion against which the cases are judged, such as greatly improved, improved, moderately improved, or unimproved. There is also the quantitative method of meta-analysis in which an effect size is obtained by subtracting the mean of the control group from the mean of the experimental group and dividing by a pooled within-group standard deviation or the control group standard deviation. Effect sizes are then averaged across studies.

The first section of this chapter consists of summaries of the qualitative and quantitative reviews cited above and concludes with a summary, pertinent conclusions, and recommendations. The remaining sections of this chapter include the authors' review of the current literature on group psychotherapy with children, preadolescents, and adolescents and a comparison with the reviews summarized in the first section of the chapter.

GROUP PSYCHOTHERAPY/TREATMENT WITH CHILDREN, PREADOLESCENTS, AND ADOLESCENTS

Only three reviews specifically address *group* psychotherapy with children, preadolescents, and adolescents. Abramowitz (1976) included "children" ages 4 to approximately 16 with the mode being about age 10. Kraft (1968) included only adolescents. Gazda and Larsen (1968) included children, preadolescents, and adolescents.

Abramowitz (1976) reviewed journal articles for the years 1964 through 1973. Her review includes articles that report scores before and after therapy on a quantitative measure of psychosocial or behavioral well-being. Forty-two articles met these criteria. Most of the research samples were drawn from school and psychiatric populations; research was rare on group therapy with the intellectually and physically handicapped and with children having severe symptoms such as autism. Kraft (1968) did not specify the extent of his review or the criteria used for inclusion of the articles. He indicated, however, that most evaluations of adolescent group psychotherapy tend to be more empirical and impressionistic than experimental, controlled, and statistical. The emphasis in the literature he surveyed is on the delinquent and neurotically disturbed adolescent. Gazda and Larsen (1968) reviewed the group and multiple counseling literature from 1938–1967. Their review includes studies of children (n = 2), preadolescents (n = 9), adolescents (n = 16), and adults. They required some kind of control group as well as a "true experimental design" for the studies included in their review. The majority of studies were samples obtained from school or predelinquent or delinquent populations.

Kraft (1968) reported that most researchers conclude adolescents in group therapy "gain" from the experience. Gazda and Larsen's (1968) review found that most studies of children, preadolescents, and adolescents show statistically significant changes in favor of treated subjects over untreated controls. However, in these cases, the significant changes did not occur for the majority of dependent variables.

Of the approximately 100 studies reviewed by Gazda and Larsen, 10 were process studies with children, preadolescents, and adolescents. Of these, 9 were with adolescents and 1 with preadolescents. Most of these process studies deal with underachieving and problem children from the schools—8 with underachieving ninth graders. These studies focus on nonverbal behavior of clients and counselors, roles played by clients, content analysis related to outcomes, and positive and negative affect related to outcome. Most of the studies do not show significant relationships between predictors and outcomes.

Abramowitz (1976) concluded that the available evidence of the outcome studies with children is "inconclusive, but nonetheless discouraging. About one-third of the studies yielded generally positive results, one-third generated mixed (i.e., some positive, some null, and some negative) results, and one-third produced null findings" (p. 321). Results of a few studies suggest that group therapy can have deleterious consequences.

In her implications, Abramowitz concluded that conclusions regarding the effectiveness of group psychotherapy with children must await further research even though the database does not promise a favorable prognosis. Abramowitz found that behavior modification groups were overrepresented among the positive and mixed outcome studies, but that gain maintenance or generalization of behavior modification-produced effects was established in only a small number of studies. "When group therapy does seem indicated, the feasibility of a behavioral approach might be considered first" (Abramowitz, 1976, p. 325); however, she recommends that the "comparative effectiveness of the various group modalities with children be held in abeyance pending the return of more decisive research" (Abramowitz, 1976, p. 324).

Regarding analysis of process, Abramowitz focused on group composition. She referred to Slavson's contentions that therapy groups of children should contain a well-chosen mix of personality and behavior styles, that is, heterogeneous groups. In one study reviewed, the authors found greater gains in sociometric status among low-status children who participated in a heterogeneous (high-status and low-status members) group than among their peers who had been exposed to a homogeneous (low-status members only) group. Another study reported gains in homogeneous groups with regard to leadership style, but deterioration in a heterogeneous group. Other investigations found heterogeneous therapy groups to be ineffective in modifying their poorest functioning members' behavior. Abramowitz concluded that more thorough examinations of group composition effects are necessary.

Reviews of group psychotherapy research with children, preadolescents, and adolescents are extremely limited; nonetheless, common findings are cited at the end of this chapter and compared with the authors' independent literature review of the most recent research. While the findings and issues presented here represent a summary perspective of commonly held beliefs among group researchers who have focused their work on children, preadolescents, and adolescents, there is less than 100% agreement on any given point.

- Most reviewers define group psychotherapy very broadly to include counseling groups as well as training groups.

- Most of the research samples reported in the literature are from institutions such as schools, juvenile correctional institutes, and psychiatric hospitals, rather than from a clinical practice population; therefore, the findings may not represent the more seriously disturbed youngsters.
- The majority of reviewers argue that childhood, preadolescent, and adolescent research should not be combined because it masks differences that are a function of age, developmental level, and type of treatment.
- Therapy typically is brief, between 8 to 10 sessions—a length that does not characterize longer treatment for children/adolescents from a clinical practice population.
- Therapy is more often provided by novice rather than experienced therapists.
- Most control groups are no-treatment controls.
- Boys rather than girls are more often the subjects of treatment.
- Behavioral treatments tend to be evaluated as more effective than nonbehavioral; however, most reviewers qualify these findings, suggesting that research measures and other variables somewhat favor behavioral treatment.
- Treatment gains increase from post-treatment evaluations to follow-up evaluation.
- There is a paucity of studies of children and adolescents when compared to studies of adults.
- There is an equally limited number of process studies; therefore, the causes and relationships of positive findings cannot be identified.
- Some groups have casualties.

Not surprisingly, such findings have led to calls for improvement in group therapy research with children, preadolescents, and adolescents. Reviewers of earlier research studies appear in agreement that more studies are needed involving cases with severe psychological problems. In addition, it is agreed that a wider range of outcome domains should be sampled and longer treatment periods studied. Furthermore, placebo control groups need to be included in all research designs of outcome studies.

Conclusions gleaned from previous research reviews about process dimensions dictate the provision of explicit descriptions of treatment modalities. Also, reliability checks on treatment consistency should be completed, and experienced or trained therapists should be used to avoid therapist bias. In virtually all comparative studies, differential outcomes are confounded by such variables as treatment populations, therapist personalities, treatment goals, and outcome measures. These variables demand control either in the research design or through statistical manipulation. Finally, there is a general consensus that child, preadolescent, and adolescent group psychotherapy research has not controlled for the developmental stage or maturational effects of the child or adolescent; controls are needed.

Although group process research with children and adolescent groups is limited, some common findings and recommendations include the following:

- The effects of group composition are inconclusive and more research is recommended.
- Structure dimensions have produced some tentative suggestions for practice. For example, perceptions, expectations, and beliefs have an immediate influence on members' experiences in the group. Positive expectations can lead to positive early group experience.
- Cohesion is a multidimensional and developmental phenomenon, but the research on cohesion is confusing and unclear. Researchers are advised to specify their meaning of cohesion and indicate the equivalence between their conceptual and operational definitions.
- Feedback can be manipulated in predictable ways. The effect of feedback is not always positive; however, people prefer positive feedback to negative feedback. Negative feedback seems more likely to be accepted if preceded by positive feedback; group members also find it easier to give positive rather than negative feedback.
- Self-disclosure can be manipulated in predictable ways. For example, self-disclosure begets self-disclosure.

The present review of research pertaining to group therapy with children, preadolescents, and adolescents represents an attempt to be exhaustive within the confines of computerized literature searches. The authors relied primarily on searches of the PsycLit database to identify salient studies for analysis. Such an approach has some limitations, but there is a good chance that the overwhelming majority of the pertinent studies have been reviewed. We have expanded our approach to the review of works published in the most recent decade by pursuing cross-referencing, using additional referent terms and phrases, and by reviewing other primary and secondary sources. We have extended the decade of coverage to include all studies reported on during the twelve-year period of 1980 to 1992. Analyses of research studies published in the last dozen years are presented in three summary sections: outcome research, process research, and clinical research.

Outcome Research

Of the approximately 800 studies on group therapy with children, preadolescents, and adolescents reviewed, only 27 of the studies published in the targeted decade can be considered experimental in nature. Our selection criteria consisted of the following: (1) The population served was to include only children, preadolescents, and adolescents, roughly translated as young people between the ages of 6 and 19, (2) the treatment had to consist of group therapy, as defined rather broadly to include counseling, guidance, or training groups, and involve group interaction and the potential for reciprocal influence of three members or more, (3) the research design had to include both an experimental group and a control group, whether it was a true control group or a comparison group or a placebo-attention control group, and (4) the study had to include a report of some kind of attempt to identify quantifiable outcomes. Table 10.1 presents a brief overview of the studies that meet these criteria, and therefore are included in this review.

Population

The ages of the children and adolescents in the groups range from 7 to 19. Twenty of the 27 studies deal with children, and 7 with adolescents. The most popular age range is from 9 to 12, roughly equivalent to grades 3 to 6, or upper elementary school. Most studies include both sexes and are fairly evenly matched, but two studies are of adolescent males only (categorized as delinquents in these particular studies) and one of adolescent females only (an empowerment group). Sample sizes range from an N of 11 to an N of 185, with a mean sample of 66. Multiple treatment groups are typically around 6 to 10 in size. Almost all of the studies were conducted in school settings, with no empirical studies reported on from in-patient hospital settings; however, one was completed in a wilderness program with patients from an adolescent psychiatric unit of a hospital. One study was conducted in a community counseling center, and another was conducted in a camp setting. When compared to a comprehensive review of an earlier decade's (1967–1977) psychotherapy research studies with adolescents (Tramontana, 1980), the present report highlights a significant shift to schools away from institutionalized delinquents (Kraft, 1968).

Design

A study had to include some type of control group to be considered in the present review. Approximately 89% of the designs were constructed to compare pretest/post-test results of at least two different groups. The favorite design reflected was the pretest/post-test comparison of randomly assigned members of an experimental group with members of a control group. Almost two-thirds (63%) of the studies include a no-treatment control group for comparison with the experimental group(s). An additional 30% of the research designs employ a placebo-attention control group, rather than a no-treatment control. The final 7% of the studies include both a true control and a placebo-attention control group. Of the 10 studies that employ a placebo group, two use films as a substitute group focus; two use story-telling sessions, and the remaining studies use such activities as planned recreation, drama lessons, and counseling. One other noteworthy feature of this collection of research designs is that 15% of the studies employed follow-ups to

TABLE 10.1. Experimental Studies of Group Therapy Outcome with Children and Adolescents (1980–1992)

Author(s)/Title	Design	Treatment	Measures	Outcomes
Alpert-Gillis, Pedro-Carroll, & Cowen (1989) The children of divorce intervention program	Pre-post design with exp. ($n = 52$), divorce control ($n = 52$), and "intact" comparison control group ($n = 81$). Exp. group included 9 mixed-sex groups of 2nd and 3rd graders from 8 urban schools. Divorce control matched exp. group in time since divorce.	Exp. groups met for 16 weekly 45-minute sessions. Control groups participated only in assessment. A revision of the Children of Divorce Intervention Program, focusing on feelings, problem-solving skill development, and enhancing positive perceptions of self and family.	*Children's Divorce Adjustment Scale, Child Rating Scale, Parent Evaluation Form, Teacher-Child Rating Scale,* and *Group Leader Evaluation Form.*	Results showed positive gains in all predicted directions and showed positive differences when compared to control groups.
Anderson, Kinney, & Gerler (1984) The effects of divorce groups on children's classroom behavior and attitudes toward divorce	Pre-post control; no placebo control ($n = 52$) 8 groups of 6–8 members. Grades 3–6, balanced for gender and ethnicity.	Effects of divorce groups on children's attitudes toward divorce, class behavior, & academic performance. 8 weeks 1-hour sessions.	Newly constructed scales, no reliability/validity. *The Attitude Toward Divorce and The Classroom Behavior Rating Form.*	Sign. different in "improved attitudes toward divorce and improved classroom conduct grades." No differences on academics.
Bundy & Boser (1987) Helping latchkey children	Pre-post with delay control; no placebo control ($n = 48$) exp. group ($n = 67$) control group.	Developmental guidance curriculum presented in six 45-minute sessions in classroom discussion format.	Content-centered *Knowledge Test* (author-created), Parental questionnaire.	Sign. gains (pre-post) and differences between exp. and control on test of self-care practices.
Chen (1984) Group therapy with Chinese schoolchildren	Exp./control; no placebo control ($n = 53$) 7 groups of students in grade 3–5.	50 sessions on a twice weekly basis.	Author's *Behavior Rating Scale.* Teachers rated changes.	Exp. showed sign. behavioral improvement compared to controls. No sign. differences on school achievement.
Crosbie-Burnett & Newcomer (1990) Group counseling children of divorce	Pre-post, exp./wait list control design. 11 subjects were divided randomly into the 2 groups (6 and 5). Controls later served.	8 session multimodal group counseling for 6 participants.	*Self-Perception Profile for Children, The Children's Beliefs about Parental Divorce Scale,* and *The Child Depression Scale.*	Pre-post comparison of exp. group showed sign. positive differences on all measures.

Study	Design	Treatment	Measures	Results
Denkowski & Denkowski (1984)	Exp./placebo control design. Forty-five 3rd, 4th, & 5th graders divided into 2 exp. groups (7–8 subjects) compared to a placebo group.	Systematic relaxation training & individualized biofeedback training for exp. treatment group and story groups for placebo.	*The Nowicki-Strickland Locus of Control Scale, The Gates-MacGinites Reading Tests, and Teaching Rating Scales.*	No sign. differences found between exp. methods when all dependent measures simultaneously considered. Alone, locus of control was more internal for progressive relaxation condition.
Gwynn & Brantley (1987) Effects of a divorce group intervention for elementary school children	Pre-post, control group design. Participants included 60 9–11 year-olds, paired by sex and time since parental separation. Yoked controls attended regular classes. No placebo group.	8 week educational support group for 5 groups of 6 children each.	*Children's Depression Inventory; What I Think and Feel, State-Trait Anxiety Inventory for Children,* and 2 author-constructed scales —*Children's Divorce Information Scale* and *Children's Affective Scale.*	Exp. groups made sign. changes on all measures showing less depression and anxiety, more knowledge, and fewer negative feelings about divorce than controls.
Hoover (1984) Peer culture development	Exp./control group design. No placebo group. Participants were 100 junior high and senior high, students randomly selected from a pre-selected list who qualified for participation in semester-long program.	Group sessions were held for small groups of 12 to 15 students over a period of a school semester.	Frequency counts of police contacts, school attendance, suspensions, grades, drop-outs, and questionnaires on substance abuse and *School Climate Inventory.*	PCD participants showed a 44% reduction in police contacts, while control group student showed a 36% increase; there were similar results on all other measures with the exception of suspensions.
Huey & Rank (1984) Effects of counselor and peer-led group assertive training on Black adolescent aggression	Pre-post exp./control design. In a true experimental design, 4 experimental groups were compared to each other and to a control group. 6 groups consisted of 6–8 black adolescent members.	Small groups (n of 6–8) met twice weekly for 4 weeks, except for control group which did not meet. Two experimental groups focused on assertiveness training and 2 on discussion groups.	*The Hand Test,* the Acting-out subscale of the *Walker Problem Behavior Identification Checklist, The Anger Index, The Behavioral Role Playing Test,* and a post-group satisfaction questionnaire.	Assertiveness training groups, both peer-led and counselor-led had greater effect on reducing aggression ratings than did the discussion group participants or the control group. No differences were found between counselor-led and peer-led assertiveness groups or satisfaction ratings for any group.
Johnson & Johnson (1991) Using short-term group counseling with visually impaired adolescents	Pre-post exp./control design. 14 visually impaired adolescents from ages 12–18 were split into 2 groups of 7. Groups were balanced on race, sex, age, and measured intelligence.	Exp. group taking part in a group therapy experience for 12 sessions over a 4 week period.	*The Tennessee Self-Concept Scale, The Attitudes Toward Blindness Scale,* and *The North Carolina Internal/External Scale (Short Form).*	Strong support for a positive impact on participants' self-concept, attitudes toward blindness, and an internal locus of control.

TABLE 10.1. (*Continued*)

Author(s)/Title	Design	Treatment	Measures	Outcomes
McLinden, Miller, & Deprey (1991) Effects of a support group for siblings of children with special needs	Pre-post exp./control design. No placebo group. 11 children ages 7–12, who were siblings of children with special needs were split into 2 groups, 6 and 5.	6 week sibling support group for 6 members, with weekly hour-long sessions.	*The Child Behavior Checklist for ages 4–16, The Piers-Harris Children's Self-Concept Scale, Who Helps Me,* and *Let's Grow Together.*	With one exception on the *Who Helps Me,* there were no sign. differences between the groups on any of the measures.
Milne & Spence (1987) Training social perception skills with primary school children	$2 \times 3 \times 3$ factorial design consisting of 2 schools, 3 exp. conditions including a placebo attention and no-treatment control group with pre-post and follow-up assessment.	Sessions focused on social perception training for the exp. group, and drama lessons for the attention placebo group. Sessions lasted 40 minutes, on a twice weekly basis for a total of 9 sessions (n = 48).	Sociometric ratings, positive and negative peer nominations, *The Children's Social Perception Test* (constructed by authors), *The Walker Problem Behavior Identification Checklist Revised,* and the *Children's Depression Inventory.*	Children receiving training in social perception skills did not significantly improve their scores on a measure of social perception & sociometric ratings than children in either placebo or no attention. 10-week follow-up showed no evidence for a differential treatment effect.
Morse & Bockoven (1987) The Oregon DUSO-R research studies series: Integrating a children's social skills curriculum in a family education/ counseling center	A true exp. pre- and post-test design with 2 exp. groups and placebo control group. Random assignment of 26 children, ages 7–9, to DUSO-R group (n = 8), DUSO group (n = 10), or placebo control (recreational activities) group (n = 8).	Children met in a family education/counseling center on 11 Saturday mornings for 3 hour session in 1 of the 3 groups.	*California Test of Personality* (Social Adjustment section) and the *Culture-Free Self-Esteem Inventory.*	Gain scores indicated sign. differences for DUSO-type intervention over placebo-attention group. DUSO-R gain scores were significantly higher than results of the DUSO and placebo groups.
Niehoff (1983) Psychological perceptions of special needs children: The gifted and talented	A pre-post assessment of 2 randomly assigned exp./control groups, with 5 month follow-up. Boys and girls ages 9–11 (28) designated as gifted by their school participated in a summer enrichment program. No placebo groups.	Treatment program included sessions emphasizing understanding and acceptance of self, with individual counseling up to 3 times weekly for 7 weeks. Controls received no counseling, but did participate in the enrichment program.	Pre-post administration of *The Maslow Security-Insecurity Inventory* and *The Rogers Personal Adjustment Inventory.*	Both exp. and control groups decreased in personal insecurity and maladjustment with no significant differences between the 2 groups. A 5-month follow-up did reveal between group differences.

Study	Design/Sample	Treatment	Measures	Results
Niles (1986) Effects of a moral development discussion group on delinquent and predelinquent boys	A pre-post test control group design, including placebo and no-treatment control groups. 59 delinquent or predelinquent adolescent males (ages 13–16) participated in the study. The placebo group (n = 19) received training in a values clarification program. A control (n = 21) group received no treatment.	The Moral Dilemma Group (MDG) emphasized problem-solving activities and consensus-seeking resolution efforts & included: Classroom behavior, spontaneous real-life, and hypothetical dilemmas. Treatment and placebo groups met for twice a week for 16 weeks.	The *Moral Judgment Interview* was used as both a blocking and outcome assessment means. The *Self-Control Rating Scale* was used to assess change in classroom behavior.	Sign. differences in moral maturity between the treatment group and the placebo group, and between the placebo group and the control group. No sign. differences were found between the groups on the Self-Control Ratings Scale.
Omizo, Cubberly, & Longano (1984) The effects of group counseling on self-concept and locus of control among learning-disabled children	Pre-post, control group comparison design, with no placebo group or follow-up; random assignment to conditions. Sample included 66 children, ages 8–11, who had been certified by the State as learning disabled.	Group treatment consisting of eight 60–90 minute sessions focusing on the elimination of self-defeating behaviors. The experimental group was subdivided into 3 groups of 11, according to school schedules.	*Dimensions of Self-Concept Scale* and the *Nowicki-Strickl and Locus of Control Scale.*	Significant differences between gps. included higher level of aspiration, locus of control (internal) for the experimental groups, and the anxiety score for the self-concept measure was lower.
Omizo, Cubberly, & Omizo (1985) The effects of rational-emotive education groups on self-concept and locus of control among learning-disabled children	Pre-post exp./placebo control design with X random assignment. No follow-up. Sample included 60 children, ages 8–11, who had been certified by the State as learning disabled.	Training sessions lasting approximately 1 hour took place twice weekly for 12 weeks. Children in placebo control met in small groups twice weekly to listen to short stories.	*Dimensions of Self-Concept Scale* and the *Nowicki-Strickl and Locus of Control Scale.*	Participants in the counseling gps. scored sign. higher on the locus of control and self-concept subscales and lower on anxiety than on control. Other subscales, academic interest, and satisfaction as well as identification—alienation, did not discriminate.
Omizo, Hershberger, & Omizo (1988) Teaching children to cope with anger	Pre-post exp./placebo control group (24) design. Participants were randomly selected from a list of students (44) who had been nominated by teachers because of aggressive behavior in class.	Ten weekly group counseling sessions that focused on cognitive-behavior techniques and modeling; placebo control watched films that did not depict aggression.	Teachers' ratings of class behaviors on the *School Behavior Checklist*; Aggression and Hostile Isolation subscales.	Exp. group members as being sign. less aggressive and hostile than those in the control group.

TABLE 10.1. *(Continued)*

Author(s)/Title	Design	Treatment	Measures	Outcomes
Omizo & Omizo (1987a) Group counseling with children of divorce	Pre-post, exp./placebo control design. Randomly selected 60 of the 93 children in grades 3–6 of an elementary school whose parents had been divorced for a year and who volunteered (along with their parents) to participate in the study. Each small group was comprised of 10 students.	The group counseling consisted of activities designed to clarify feelings about divorce, to strengthen coping skills, and to enhance self-concept. Groups met weekly for approximately an hour. Control groups met for the same amount of time and watched films that did not involve divorce issues.	*Nowicki-Strickland Locus of Control Scale* and the *Dimensions of Self-Concept Scale.*	The locus of control measure and several subscales (aspiration, anxiety, and identification versus alienation) of the self-concept measure were sign. discriminators between exp. and control groups.
Omizo & Omizo (1987b) The effects of eliminating self-defeating behavior of learning-disabled children through group counseling	A pre-post test control group design, with random assignment of children to exp. and control groups. A total of 55 students, almost all boys, ranging in ages from 12–15, diagnosed as learning disabled. No placebo control.	Weekly sessions of approx. 90 minutes in length were conducted for a period of 7 weeks.	*Locus of Control Inventory for Three Achievement Domains* and the *Coopersmith Self-Esteem Inventory.*	The self-esteem measure and several subscales (success-intellectual domain, failure-intellectual domain, and failure-social domain) of the locus of control measure were sign. discriminators between exp. and control groups.
Omizo & Omizo (1987c) The effects of counseling on classroom behavior and self-concept among elementary school learning-disabled children	Pre-post exp./placebo control group design. 60 children, ages ranging from approx. 6 to 8, and diagnosed as learning-disabled, randomly assigned to group.	Control group members watched neutral films for 50 minutes weekly, the same amount of time for a period of 12 weeks, the exp. groups' sessions focused on minimizing distractibility and acting out behaviors.	*The Primary Self-Concept Inventory*—Personal, Social, and Intellectual and the *Walker Problem Behavior Identification Checklist*—The Acting Out and Distractibility Scales.	Sign. differences on the social self-concept and on the distractibility and acting subscales.
Pedro-Carroll & Cowen (1985) The children of divorce intervention program	Pre-post, exp./control design, with no placebo group or follow-up. Small groups of 8–10 students in grades 4–6, matched by sex, age, and length of time since parents' divorce.	Small group counseling sessions. Exp. group (n = 41) met weekly for 10 weeks for 1-hour sessions.	Teacher Measures: *Classroom Adjustment Rating Scale. Health Resources Inventory.* Parent Measure: *Parent Evaluation Form.* Leader Measure: *Group Leader Evaluation Form.*	Sign. differences on all measures except *Harter's Scale* and the *Children's Attitudes and Self Perceptions.*

Study	Design	Treatment	Measures	Results
Pedro-Carroll & Cowen (*continued*)			*Child Measures: Harter's Perceived Competence Scale, State-Trait Anxiety Inventory for Children, Children's Attitudes and Self-Perceptions, and Comments.*	
Pedro-Carroll, Cowen, Hightower, & Guare (1986) Preventive intervention with latency-age children of divorce	Pre-post test exp. group (n = 54) with an "intact" family comparison control groups (n = 78). Exp. group included 8 groups of 4th–6th grade children in 6 schools. Comparisons were matched demographically.	Exp. groups met for 11 weekly 45-minute sessions. Control groups participated only in assessment. Treatment: (Children of Divorce Intervention Program) focused on feelings, problem-solving skill development, and enhancing positive perceptions of self and family.	*Teacher-Child Ratings Scale, Parent Evaluation Form: The STAIC A-Trait Scale, Child Rating Scale, Children's Attitudes and Self Perceptions, The Multidimensional Measure of Children's Perceptions of Control, Comments about Group, and Group Leader Evaluation Form.*	All measures (teacher, child, and global-cross perspective) reflected sign. group differences for exp. group when compared to comparison group.
Schectman (1991) Small group therapy and preadolescent same-sex friendship.	Pretest and a post-test comparison group design, with no placebo, but a one-year follow-up with some of the participants. Unisex exp. groups (n = 55) of six to ten members.	Exp. groups participated in weekly 40-minute nonstructured group treatment process based on a relationship-emphasis model. Control group was a wait-list delayed treatment group.	Each participant completed the *Sharabany Intimacy Scale* (pre and post) about his or her best friend, and the *Me and the Group Scale* about his or her group (also pre and post).	Divergent developments of intimacy for experimental and control groups, with the former showing a significant increase and the latter a significant decrease. Boys in treatment groups showed positive gains and boys in control showed sharp decreases, yet girls showed higher gains overall. Greatest gains in group intimacy were in boys' groups.
Simmons & Parsons (1983) Developing internality and perceived competence: The empowerment of adolescent girls	Pre/post comparison group design. Multi-cultural group of 11-year-old females: Group from working class (31), from lower class (34) and matching control (34). No placebo and no follow-up.	Workshop on "Life Choices" & Empowerment.	Multi-dimensional: *Perceived Competence Scale for Children* (o); *Measure of Children's Perceptions of Control*; self-report checklist on *Careers for Women.*	Mixed: Working class experimental group increased in attributing success internally and decreased attributing success to external and powerful others, and as well increased in perceived internal control over school achievement.

TABLE 10.1. (*Continued*)

Author(s)/Title	Design	Treatment	Measures	Outcomes
Sorsdahl & Sanche (1985) The effects of classroom meetings on self-concept and behavior	Pretest, post-test, placebo group design with no true control group or follow-up. Four intact fourth-grade classrooms identified as practicing democratic classroom principles were divided into exp. and placebo control, two groups each. Exp. groups (n = 45) and placebo groups (n = 46).	Experimental groups participated in classroom meetings, as a form of group counseling, twice a week for 20 weeks. Placebo groups were given special activity periods for same amount of time.	*Pupil Behavior Rating Scale* and the *Piers-Harris Children's Self-Concept Scale* were administered to all pre/post treatment. Also, two scales developed to assess behavior during classroom meetings (*The Classroom Meeting Behavior Rating Scale* and *The Classroom Meeting Self-Concept Rating Scale*) were administered to the exp. group pre/post treatment.	Positive gains by exp. group that were significantly different than controls on all measures other than the *Piers-Harris*.
Waksman (1984) A controlled evaluation of assertion training with adolescents	Pretest, post-test, and placebo control comparison group design, with a one-month follow-up. Fifty-eight 13-year-olds were members of two intact middle school classes that were randomly assigned to the treatment or control status.	Treatment consisted of eight sessions of 45 minutes each over a period of two weeks. The placebo-counseling group experienced group exercises.	The *Piers-Harris Children's Self-Concept Scale*, the *Intellectual Achievement Responsibility Questionnaire*, and the *State-Trait Anxiety Inventory for Children*; teachers completed the *AML Behavior Rating Scale* on each child.	Weak affirmation of treatment. Only difference found between groups was on *Piers-Harris Scale* and it held up at follow-up.

their outcome assessment. Time lapses after post-assessments vary from 4 weeks to 52 weeks. Follow-up data confirm pre/post results on all studies analyzed; one follow-up even found an increase in the pre/post gain to a level of significance in which the gain had not quite reached significance at the time of post assessment. No study reflects the ideal design of comparing multiple treatment groups to multiple control groups using pre/post and follow-up assessment.

Treatment

Three major treatment themes are reflected in the set of studies included in the past decade's database: divorce adjustment groups (26%), groups for children and adolescents with special needs (26%), and personal competency enhancement groups (37%). Treatment typically took the form of traditional group therapy or counseling for half of the studies (52%, or 14 of the 27). Structured groups, emphasizing specific training foci, such as assertiveness training, account for almost all of the rest (41%). The length of the group treatment sessions is typically that of a class period (45 minutes) or a therapy hour (50 to 60 minutes); however, the range of minutes devoted to group treatments vary from 40 minutes to 180 minutes per session. The duration of treatment ranges from 6 sessions (over a period of four weeks) to 50 sessions (over a period of 25 weeks); the mean duration of group treatment is 15 weeks, and the median is 9 weeks.

In the empirical studies reviewed, very little attention, if any at all, is given to comprehensive descriptions of such vital group dimensions as group composition, leader characteristics and leadership style, cohesion of the group, quality of interaction, satisfaction of members with group process, and process evaluation. Only those treatment plans that included structured group experiences are described sufficiently to replicate the study, and even then the descriptions consist mostly of curriculum outlines. There is an obvious need for future researchers to collect and to publish more specific data regarding group process variables. Most of the studies published on group research with children and adolescents during the last extended decade (1980–1992) started out as clinical interventions and not research studies. Research designs for the most part reflect efforts to test the impact of a therapeutic intervention.

Dependent Measures

A few studies report the use of author-constructed questionnaires and newly developed instruments that have no validity or reliability data, but the clear majority (85%; or 23 of the 27) employ multiple, established measures to assess pre/post differences. In many instances, the choice of instruments often seems to place researchers in less than favorable positions for showing gains; nevertheless, the studies still demonstrate differences. For example, it seems fairly presumptuous to assume that a four-week group counseling experience would affect one's self-concept or one's self-esteem. Nonetheless, several of the studies reported here do just that. Employing such self-concept and self-esteem measures as the Piers-Harris Children's Self Concept Scale, the Coopersmith Self-Esteem Inventory, the Tennessee Self-Concept Scale, and the Dimensions of Self Scale, researchers in this set of studies demonstrate significant pre/post gains on nearly half of the studies reported herein. The same success is evident in the use of locus of control measures as well. A few studies rely heavily on rating scales completed by teachers who knew about and sometimes were heavily involved in the studies themselves. Therefore, the data are undoubtedly biased. Nevertheless, when four-week interventions can make a difference on self-esteem measures and locus of control measures, they deserve attention.

Outcomes

A large percentage (85%) of the studies covered here report at least mildly positive pre/post gains on some of the dependent measures. While some of the measures do not reveal significant overall gains on all of the instruments or subscales, nearly all show some improvement on target dimensions. Only four studies (15%) report a lack of positive and discriminative results between experimental and control comparisons of pre/post assessments. Each of the seven studies on divorce adjustment groups report positive gains, as do each of the studies that can be classified as dealing with minorities and with delinquency intervention groups.

Summary

When the present studies are compared to earlier reviews of studies presented in the beginning of this chapter, it quickly becomes apparent that measurement strategies and instruments have changed little since Abramowitz's (1976) review. One obvious change that has occurred, however, is that sociometric devices are virtually non-existent in the current set of studies, whereas once these measures were apparently among the most popular. Behavior rating scales completed by teachers and others, and self-report measures of self-concept remain the most popular, as well as the most problematic. Rating scales potentially suffer from a likely bias of the rater, and self-report scales suffer from a similar built-in bias. Treatment interventions continue to be relatively brief (9 weeks currently versus 10 to 15 before), and still tend to include no-treatment control groups rather than placebo-attention groups. Abramowitz's finding of a prevalence of behavioral methodology and treatment may not hold true with the current set of research studies. A traditional approach to a group therapy or group counseling treatment seems as solid in the present as it was in the past, however. Behavioral strategies, techniques, and designs are still an important part of group therapy modalities, but structured groups seem to be gaining a position of increasing use in group work. These structured groups are not necessarily behavioral in nature; they simply are more time-limited and are set within a tighter set of parameters that dictate a delineation of pre-set general goals and strategies for goal-achievement. Specially designed intervention programs (e.g., divorce adjustment) seem to have gained in popularity today.

Abramowitz's conclusions from the earlier decade seem almost as tenable today, with very few exceptions. Too many designs still neglect placebo control groups. Too many still provide virtually no definitive information about the therapist or the therapeutic intervention, other than to present general outlines. And too many use novice therapists and loose measures. Nevertheless, regardless of the shortcomings associated with group research, several studies included in the present review deserve elaboration, primarily because of their design.

Niles (1986) designed a solid study to assess the effects of a moral development discussion group on delinquent and predelinquent boys. The particular value of this study is that the placebo-attention control group consisted of an activity (values clarification) that was especially similar to the treatment group (the Moral Development Group); the main difference was the emphasis on role-taking in the moral discussion group. Results between the two groups on moral maturity scores are significantly different and also predictably different from the no-treatment control group. Follow-up assessment 10 weeks later affirmed the results. The study includes a good description of the different treatment conditions—a rarity for outcome research studies—but falls disturbingly into the selection of untrained group leaders.

Another well-designed study conducted by Milne and Spence (1987) aimed to test the effectiveness of a social perception training curriculum. To do so they created a design that consists of three treatment conditions (a social perception training group, an attention placebo group that received drama lessons, and a no-treatment control group), and three assessment times (pretreatment, post-treatment, and a 10-week follow-up). Multiple outcome measures were used, including several sociometric devices as well as The Children's Social Perception Test and The Walker Problem Behavior Identification Checklist—Revised. Unfortunately, the small groups of randomly assigned 8- to 12-year-olds were led by relatively inexperienced graduate student therapists and little data are provided regarding group process or group leader characteristics or style. The results are inconclusive.

A third study worth mentioning is one conducted by Morse and Bockoven (1987) to test the relative effectiveness of the DUSO-R and the original DUSO on children's social skills and self-esteem. Both were found to be more effective than a placebo-attention control group that experienced planned recreational activities, and the revised version of DUSO was found to be significantly more effective than the original.

Finally, two series of studies deserve highlighting as examples of simple, but worthy programs of research. Pedro-Carroll and Cowen (1985) and Pedro-Carroll, Cowen, Hightower, and Guare (1986) studied the effectiveness of various length and content configurations of the Children of the Divorce Intervention Program; these authors have met with some success. Likewise, Omizo, Cubberly, and Longano (1984), Omizo, Cubberly, and Omizo (1985), Omizo and Omizo (1987), and Omizo, Hershberger, and Omizo (1988) carried out a series of simple, but effective studies that investigated the impact of small groups on learning disabled children.

Process Research

Process research on group therapy with children, preadolescents, and adolescents is inadequate, in terms of the quality and quantity. Unfortunately, little has changed since Roback, Abramowitz, and Strassberg (1979) characterized the quality of process research as quite poor. In our review of the relevant literature published during the last dozen years, only six studies were identified that were designed to assess process variables of groups comprised of children or adolescents. By "process" we mean the myriad of factors occurring throughout the group's life (e.g., membership characteristics and group composition, leadership style and effectiveness, goal clarity and ownership, members' perceptions of the curative factors, the quality of group interaction, the level of group cohesiveness).

Exclusive focus on outcome measurement at the expense of process assessment weakens the generalizability and replicability of research. Moreover, when too little attention is given to process assessment, there is a possibility of misreading the data. One could assume that the absence of a significant outcome might demonstrate the ineffectiveness of a certain group intervention, when in fact the result may have been impacted more by ineffective leadership or by the unique character of a particular adolescent group than by the nature of the planned intervention. In our judgment, the most unfortunate result of failing to assess process variables is that clinicians find less applied utility in the results; thus, the gap widens between researcher and clinician. One does not inform the other in a reciprocal fashion when too little attention is given to a detailed assessment of group process. Outcome research adds to our knowledge base only to the extent that we know about group process. Ideally, research designs should incorporate elements of both process and outcome. However, there is not a single study in this review that meets the criteria for a process-outcome study.

Zimpfer and Waltman's (1982) study of the correlates of effective group counseling comes as close to a process-outcome design as any reviewed, but it fails to include a control group. Nevertheless, it is an excellent process study. Assessments of multiple groups and multiple counselors were compared to process and outcome variables in an effort to identify process-outcome relationships. Results indicate that group composition and counselor variables relate significantly to group interaction, members' valuing of the group, and to members' self-images. Counselors scoring high in close-mindedness, as measured by a dogmatism scale, led groups whose members expressed more warmth, as measured by a system of interaction analysis. Likewise, counselors scoring high on probing/questioning as a leadership style, as measured by a counselor attitudes scale, led groups characterized by warm responses of members. Another interesting finding is that there seemed to be a relationship between age of member and group cohesiveness. Middle school students formed more cohesive groups than high school students; this finding is consistent with expectations that preadolescents are developmentally more oriented to peer influence and interaction.

The Zimpfer and Waltman study and other process studies are briefly described in Table 10.2. The clear majority of the studies can be considered relatively weak in research design, typically falling short on the use of appropriate outcome measures. Nevertheless, the authors are to be commended for at least attempting to study process variables. The series of studies by Corder and colleagues (Corder, Cornwall, & Whiteside, 1984; Corder, Russell, & Koehne, 1984–1985; Corder, Whiteside, & Haizlip, 1981), though plagued by the absence of decent outcome measures, shows promise for adding to our understanding of issues related to co-therapy.

Clinical Research

The literature is replete with clinical studies that relegate research design to a position of secondary importance under clinical intervention. A clinical study is defined as largely uncontrolled—a study in which an intervention approach or technique is assessed (pre/post comparisons or post only as compared to criteria) without comparing the independent variable to a control group, whether a placebo-attention group or a no-treatment control group. The overwhelming majority of the professional literature in group work is comprised of clinical studies, though it truly is a misnomer to refer to them as studies, because of their almost uniform disregard for objective assessment of process or outcome variables. There is value, however, in presenting a very brief overview of the clinical literature, if for no other reason than to identify issues of clinical importance to children, preadolescents, and adolescents that are currently being addressed in various forms of group therapy.

Divorce adjustment groups have become a very popular and important intervention for children and adolescents. When clinical studies (Bornstein, Bornstein, & Walter, 1988; Kalter, Pickar, & Lesowitz, 1984; Lesowitz, Kalter, Pickar, Chetnik, & Schaefer, 1987; Tedder, Scherman, & Wantz, 1987) are added to the outcome research studies described in Table 10.1, it becomes clear that clinicians have had good success in impacting this particular set of issues and concerns that confronts large numbers of today's children and adolescents. Group therapy with depressed adolescents (Fine et al., 1989), with suicidal adolescents (Shulman & Margalit, 1985), with adolescent psychiatric patients (Berman & Anton, 1988) and with clinically disturbed children (Lockwood, 1981) have shown mixed, but largely positive results on improvement of depressed moods, on decrease of targeted symptoms, on measures of psychological internality, and on assessments of overall psychological adjustment. The enhancement of children's and adolescents' pro-social mental health competencies has become an important target for group intervention (Kazdin, 1993). Using for the most part various cognitive-behavioral techniques and strategies, clinicians have led a number of groups that emphasize social skills training (Callias, Frosh, & Michie, 1987; Gresham & Nagle, 1980; Keat, Metzgar, Raykovitz, & McDonald 1985), and anger management training (LeCroy, 1988); others

TABLE 10.2. Group Therapy Process Research with Children and Adolescents (1980–1992)

Author(s)/Title	Design	Treatment	Measures	Outcomes
Bernfeld, Clark, & Parker (1984) The process of adolescent psychotherapy	Examination of the adolescent group therapy process in terms of change.	22 adolescents (11 male & 11 female) in an inpatient psychiatric center participated twice weekly in an open-ended group for approximately 7 months. The focus of the hour-long group sessions was on personal and interpersonal issues.	An independent observer, cross-checked for reliable assessment skill, recorded observations on a schedule of two five-minute segments per hour. The rating system was Dimock's tripartite model of group roles–task roles and individual roles. Clinical ratings of progress were also recorded.	Group roles increase (significantly) over time and individual roles decrease (nonsignificant) while task roles remain rather constant throughout the various stages of the group. Sharpest increase in clinical ratings occurred between the early stages and middle stages of the group.
Corder, Cornwall, & Whiteside (1984) Techniques for increasing effectiveness of co-therapy functioning in adolescent psychotherapy groups	Assessment of the utility of a newly developed scale designed to aid co-therapists working with adolescent groups.	10 sets of co-therapists providing co-therapy treatment to adolescents in inpatient mental health center, correctional center, and adolescent group residence settings used *The Co-Therapist Rating and Critical Incidents and Issues Form* over a two-year period.	Self-report assessments on effectiveness of the form.	Form helped: (1) lower anxiety about co-therapist's personality and related characteristics, (2) heighten understanding of predictable areas of difficulty identified early by the form, (3) improve the planning and review of each session, and (4) focus group progress.
Corder, Russell, & Koehne (1984–85) A format for evaluating group process and co-therapy functioning in adolescent therapy groups	A pilot study assessment of the utility of a newly developed co-therapy rating form.	Co-therapists in three adolescent group therapy settings (2 residential and 1 juvenile detention center) utilized an experimental evaluation form over a one-year period to structure their post-session collaborations.	*Corder Collaboration Process Record.*	Self-reports suggested that record form enhances the richness and smoothness of co-therapy collaboration.

Corder, Whiteside, & Haizlip (1981) A study of curative factors in group psychotherapy with adolescents	Assessment of adolescents' perceptions of curative factors in group psychotherapy	16 adolescents, ranging in age from 13 to 17, participated in weekly open-ended groups that focused on fostering an internal locus of control, social learning skills, and positive peer interaction.	Employing Q-sort methodology, adolescents ranked the curative factors previously identified by Yalom as present in effective therapeutic groups.	When compared to early rankings by adults as reported by Yalom in an earlier study, adolescents report similar rankings in the present study. Four of the adults' top-five-ranked categories were included by the adolescents, differing only on the item ranked highest by the adults, "insight."
Holmes (1983) "Dropping out" from an adolescent therapeutic group: A study of factors in the patients and their parents which may influence this process	Investigation of factors (including the personality characteristics of adolescent group members and their parents) that may influence an adolescent to stay in groups or drop out, with or without consultation	11 boys and 6 girls (ages 11–16) were referred to participate in an open-ended weekly group, 150 minutes in length, lasting for 5 school terms. Most participants were diagnosed as emotional disordered, conduct disordered, or mixed.	Retrospective assessment for personality types by use of the International Classification of Diseases.	Adolescents who dropped out prematurely seemed to do so in two ways: negotiated and unnegotiated. Younger age, paranoid personality of one of the parents, and being a member of a family without follow-up therapeutic attention marked some of the key differences.
Zimpfer & Waltman (1982) Correlates of effectiveness in group counseling	33 male & 37 female adolescents (ages 12–17) in school referred by teachers for behavior or learning problems; 9 groups.	Client-centered groups of two-hours in length met twice weekly for 10 weeks.	**Outcome:** A self-concept Q-sort and the *Syracuse Scale of Social Relations*, a sociometric device. **Process:** System of interaction analysis with Warmth, Hostility, and Flight categories for members' responses; also used counselor variables (e.g., experience, age) and group variables (e.g., age, sex) for comparison. *The Dogmatism Scale* and a counseling attitudes measure were also used.	Counselors high in closed-mindedness led groups whose members expressed more warmth; counselors high in probing were also high in warmth expressions; counseling experience had no relation to process or outcome; counselor and group composition variables related significantly to process and outcome.

have used educational/counseling approaches dependent on Adlerian principles in their self-esteem enhancement and social skills training groups (Clark & Seals, 1984; Morse, Bockoven, & Harman, 1987; Twardosz, Nordquist, Simon, & Bobkin, 1983). Other clinical groups have focused on such special populations as juvenile delinquents (Carpenter, 1984; Larson, 1990), sex offenders (Hains, Herrman, Baker, & Graber, 1986; Margolin, 1984), victims of family violence and abuse (Critchley, 1982; Downing, Jenkins, & Fisher, 1988; Hall, Kassees, & Hoffman, 1986; Hazzard, King, & Webb, 1986; Huebner, 1984; Jaffe, Wilson & Wolfe, 1988; Lubell & Soong, 1982; Mackay, Gold, & Gold, 1987; Wayne & Weeks, 1984). Additionally, popular clinical intervention topics include treatment programs for children and adolescents with eating disorders (Hendren, Atkins, Sumner, & Barber, 1987), chemical dependency, drug abuse, or alcoholism (Davis, Johnston, DiCicco, & Orenstein, 1985; Mason, 1988; Smith, 1985), and various forms of learning disability (Janus & Podolec, 1982; Lewis, 1984; McKibbon & King, 1983) or behavioral problems (Cobb & Richards, 1983; McNeil & Franklin, 1988). Some small groups have focused on minority issues (Freeman & McRoy, 1986; Lothstein, 1985; Hardy-Fanta & Montana, 1982; McFadden, Lee, & Lindsey, 1985), concerns of siblings of oncology patients (Bendor, 1990; Kinrade, 1985), special needs of foster children (Cordell, Cicely, & Krymow, 1985; Euster, Ward, Varner, & Euster, 1984; Pawley, 1985), and concerns of children of deployed military parents (Mitchum, 1991; Waldron, Whittington, & Jensen, 1985). Thus, it is apparent that there is a wide range of interest in providing small group experiences for children, preadolescents, and adolescents who represent a broad range of needs.

A Research Agenda

A comprehensive overview of the professional literature on group therapy research with children and adolescents can conclude with a brief summary statement that highlights some of the more salient issues and offers a few thoughts about directions of promise for the future. Group therapy has become a treatment of choice for a growing number of helping professionals who work with children and adolescents. It is clear that much is being done in the field to redress the oft-cited imbalance in the amount of attention given to individual and group therapy with young people. Nonetheless, it is readily apparent from a review of the literature that research has not kept pace with the expansion and innovation in group work that can be said to characterize clinical intervention. In general, there is a lack of sophistication in the research designs employed in group therapy research.

There are several cogent reasons for this state of affairs. First, group therapy research is a phrase that leads to an implicit assumption that there is such an entity as group therapy research. Each word in the phrase is sufficiently complex to warrant multiple definitions, so when the three words are put together, the phrase becomes exponentially fuzzy and increasingly less singular in nature. Even the word group presents some difficulties in definition (Aveline & Dryden, 1988, p. 3). What constitutes a group? How large can a small group be? Some extend this definition downward in size to include pairs, and others, particularly those in the person-centered movement of Carl Rogers, extend upward to include several hundred. In this chapter, the defined group meant at least three members who interact and influence each other, thus eliminating interventions that were designed for pairs or masses.

As for problems with the second word in the phrase, "therapy," it is simply no longer appropriate to speak of a single group therapy (Bloch, 1988). A singular interpretation of the term therapy contributes to a uniformity myth (Kiesler, 1971) that implies a given technique will affect most or all persons in the same way (Kazdin, 1993). Further, it is no longer accurate or necessarily appropriate to refer to therapy as though it were provided only in a hospital or clinical setting or only by medical, or health-care professionals (Aveline & Dryden, 1988). In actuality, little therapy is done with children, preadolescents, and adolescents in these settings. More often, the therapy takes place in school settings and might be more appropriately and accurately referred to as group guidance or group counseling. The clear majority of the studies reported in the literature deal with developmental or skill-building interventions rather than with crisis-oriented, remedial, or personality reconstruction groups. Regardless, group therapy may effectively serve as a rubric of accepted tradition, as long as we understand that there is no such entity. Therapy is to be viewed in a broader context as consisting of activities that are therapeutic, if not exactly therapy, and include such disparate forms as group guidance, group counseling, unstructured, and intentionally structured groups.

Group therapy research, in its present form, is relatively unsophisticated, probably because of the overwhelming complexities of all of the potential interactions of process and outcome variables that attach to group work. The current status of group therapy research is heartening in its growth as compared to earlier reviews, but disconcerting in terms of the lack of attention to (1) process research, (2) utilization of theoretical models (Stockton & Morran, 1982) for contextual and multiplistic interventions (e.g., too few studies involving multiple interventions from a variety of sources in the school, family, and community), and (3) the necessity of increasing the relative sophistication of research designs and instrumentation used in outcome studies. Adolescent intervention and research must shift from the remediation of single problems to more integrated approaches (Takanishi, 1993), and must extend intervention and research to underserved populations in more culturally sensitive ways (Kazdin, 1993). It is also clear that mental health intervention and research for children and adolescents need to be time-extended beyond the short-term focus of the present to become more developmental, contextual, and integrative (Jessor, 1993).

A recurrent assertion made by reviewers is that the general group psychotherapy literature often seems to lag behind the individual therapy literature in its substantive and methodological sophistication. In a similar vein, the group research with children and adolescents emerges as trailing in both substance and in comparison to the general group research literature. The level of maturity of the studies reviewed herein more often parallel studies in the general group literature that were published in the 1970s. If this observation has merit, there is reason for concern, given the increased emphasis on applying group therapy to this clinical population (Fuhriman & Burlingame, Chapter 1 this volume).

A Clinical Agenda

A synthesis of the literature on group work with children, preadolescents, and adolescents points out a clinical agenda in addition to a research agenda. While there are obvious similarities in the two, there are also some significant differences. At the top of both lists is a call for greater sophistication in design. As our understanding increases regarding the subtleties of psychological development through the life span, so too should our understanding of how to make effective use of group dynamics in different ways with different groups.

Group leaders cannot and should not act as though leadership practices are the same regardless of the developmental needs and stages of the group members (Grunebaum & Solomon, 1982). Group therapy should reflect what we know about human development as well as what we know about group work. Unfortunately, descriptions of clinical group interventions too often lack appropriate levels of complexity and specificity. Nowhere is the need for improved sophistication in group design more evident than in the age range of the preadolescent. Social and psychological development of the preadolescent involves many critically important tasks, including the development of new and different relationships with peers. There is probably no single period in life that includes a greater range of "normal" development than preadolescence. For example, there is a world of difference between a typical 14-year-old female and a male who is 11-years-old, particularly in areas of cognitive complexity, yet both unknowingly could be invited to join a middle school group. Some suggest that the differences in the social experiences of the genders is so great during preadolescence that such groups should consist of single-gender members and, moreover, that group leaders should be of the same gender as the members (Kennedy, 1989). Thus, it is apparent that differential consideration of possible variations in development stages is required when comprising a group. Likewise, group leaders need to consider members' normal developmental differences when planning group goals, structure, duration, and other group process dimensions and variables. There is a need for more sophisticated group interventions. For too long, group leaders have led all groups in the same way. Further, there is a need for a greater commitment to the use of theory-based techniques. Too many group interventions consist of atheoretical gimmicks and game-like strategies. If the case is that more than 230 different treatment techniques are used with children and adolescents (Kazdin, 1988), then there is an obvious need for conceptual frameworks to serve clinicians who use those techniques deemed appropriate in group intervention.

A second clinical agenda item is the need to broaden the scope of practice. While the range of groups described in the literature of the last dozen years extends beyond the topics (conduct/oppositional disorders, attention-deficit/hyperactivity, and anxiety disorders) identified by Kazdin (1991) as reflective of child therapy research and practice, there is still a need to focus on more developmental issues and concerns. The trend is moving in that direction, but too few groups currently deal with normal developmental issues.

A third important challenge is to integrate group interventions with the work of others in the child's life. Interventions coordinated and conducted jointly with families, community agencies, and school personnel have the potential to maximize effectiveness by taking advantage of the vast range of contextual variables that may impact the intervention (Kazdin, 1991). No doubt, such coordinated efforts have greater potential for impact, but also may take more of a time commitment than has been obvious to this point. Children suffering from alcoholism or abuse in the home demand more than eight or nine brief group sessions.

While it is evident that group work is an increasingly important treatment option in the helping professions, it is equally evident that group work has not yet become a preferred choice for helping young people meet the challenges of life. Preadolescents and adolescents are provided very few opportunities to participate in small groups that are not devoted to cognitive instruction. Schools have yet to embrace students' affective development as something of commensurate importance to cognitive development. Thus, few secondary school counselors lead groups on a regular basis. If any counseling is taking place in high schools, it is typically in the form of individual counseling.

The literature provides sufficient evidence to suggest that it is important to renew the call for a commitment to a developmental group counseling model (Gazda, 1989). A developmental framework for group work can serve as a vehicle for integrating the efforts to pursue the critical ingredients of the proposed clinical agenda. Although groups work, we have yet to implement all that is known to expand the power of group intervention in the lives of children, preadolescents, and adolescents, and to make more effective use of our knowledge of human development knowledge and of small group dynamics knowledge.

Group leadership needs to become a greater emphasis in training programs. At present, most graduate training programs focus training on work with adults; trainees are simply expected to adjust their interventions downward, as though one size fits all. Unfortunately, psychological development is more complex and requires more specific knowledge of process-outcome relationships. Clinical group work also needs to be age-appropriate.

In like fashion, what we know about group dynamics should be shared with those who participate with children in naturally occurring groups.

Teachers in particular need to know more about effective group leadership techniques and strategies. So do counselors, social workers, psychologists and other helping professionals who provide counseling and therapy on a routine basis. Only when we develop more than an occasional expert in group therapy will we live up to our potential in providing effective group interventions with children, preadolescents, and adolescents.

REFERENCES

Abramowitz, C. V. (1976). The effectiveness of group psychotherapy with children. *Archives of General Psychiatry, 33,* 320–326.

Alpert-Gillis, L. J., Pedro-Carroll, J. L., & Cowen, E. L. (1989). The children of divorce intervention program: Development, implementation, and evaluation of a program for young urban children. *Journal of Consulting and Clinical Psychology, 57*(5), 583–589.

Anderson, R. F., Kinney, J., & Gerler, E. R. (1984). The effects of divorce groups on children's classroom behavior and attitudes toward divorce. *Elementary School Guidance and Counseling, 18,* 70–76.

Aveline, M., & Dryden, W. (Eds.) (1988). Group therapy in Britain: An introduction. *Group therapy in Britain* (pp. 1–10). Philadelphia, PA: Open University Press.

Bendor, S. J. (1990). Anxiety and isolation in siblings of pediatric cancer patients: The need for prevention. *Social Work in Health Care, 14*(3), 17–35.

Berman, D. S., & Anton, M. T. (1988). A wilderness therapy program as an alternative to adolescent psychiatric hospitalization. *Residential Treatment for Children and Youth, 5*(3), 41–53.

Bernfeld, G., Clark, L., & Parker, G. (1984). The process of adolescent group psychotherapy. *International Journal of Group Psychotherapy, 34*(1), 111–126.

Bloch, S. (1988). Research in group psychotherapy. In M. Aveline & W. Dryden (Eds.), *Group therapy in Britain* (pp. 283–316). Milton Keynes/Philadelphia, PA: Open University Press.

Bornstein, M. T., Bornstein, P. H., & Walter, H. A. (1988). Children of divorce: Empirical evaluation of a group treatment program. *Journal of Clinical Child Psychology, 17*(3), 248–254.

Brandes, N. S., & Moosbrugger, L. (1985). A 15-year clinical review of combined adolescent/young adult group therapy. *International Journal of Group Psychotherapy, 35*(1), 95–107.

Bundy, M. L., & Boser, J. (1987). Helping latch key children: A group guidance approach. *The School Counselor, 35*(1), 58–65.

Callias, M., Frosh, S., & Michie, S. (1987). Group social skills training for young children in a clinical setting. *Behavioral Psychotherapy, 15*(4), 367–380.

Carpenter, P. (1984). "Green stamp therapy" revised: The evolution of twelve years of behavior modification and psychoeducational techniques with young delinquent boys. *Psychological Reports, 54,* 99–111.

Chen, C. (1984). Group therapy with Chinese school children. *International Journal of Group Psychotherapy, 34*(3), 485–501.

Clark, A. M., & Seals, J. M. (1984). Group counseling for ridiculed children. *Journal for Specialist in Group Work, 9*(3), 157–162.

Cobb, H. C., & Richards, H. C. (1983). Efficacy of counseling services in decreasing behavior problems of elementary school children. *Elementary School Guidance and Counseling, 17*, 180–187.

Cordell, A. S., Cicely, N., & Krymow, V. P. (1985). Group counseling for children adopted at older ages, *Child Welfare, 64*(2), 113–124.

Corder, B., Cornwall, T., & Whiteside, R. (1984). Techniques for increasing effectiveness of co-therapy functioning in adolescent psychotherapy groups. *International Journal of Group Psychotherapy, 34*(4), 643–654.

Corder, B. F., Russell, R., & Koehne, P. (1984-85). A format for evaluating group process and co-therapy functioning in adolescent therapy groups. *The Psychiatric Forum, 13*(1), 22–27.

Corder, B., Whiteside, R., Haizlip, T. M. (1981). A study of curative factors in group psychotherapy with adolescents. *International Journal of Group Psychotherapy, 31*(3), 345–354.

Critchley, D. L. (1982). Therapeutic group work with abused preschool children. *Perspectives in Psychiatric Care, 20*(2), 79–85.

Crosbie-Burnett, M., & Newcomer, L. L. (1990). Group counseling children of divorce: The effects of a multimodal intervention. *Journal of Divorce, 13*(3), 69–78.

Davis, R. B., Johnston, P. D., DiCicco, L., & Orenstein, A. (1985). Helping children of alcoholic parents: An elementary school program. *The School Counselor, 32*, 357–363.

Denkowski, K. M., & Denkowski, G. C. (1984). Is group progressive relaxation training as effective with hyperactive children as individual EMG biofeedback treatment? *Biofeedback and Self Regulation, 9*(4), 353–364.

Downing, J., Jenkins, S. J., & Fisher, G. L. (1988). A comparison of psychodynamic and reinforcement treatment with sexually abused children. *Elementary School Guidance & Counseling, 22*, 291–298.

Euster, S., Ward, V., Varner, J., & Euster, G. (1984). Lifeskills groups for adolescent foster children. *Child Welfare, 63*(1), 27–36.

Fine, S., Gilbert, M., Schmidt, L., Haley, G., Maxwell, A., & Forth, A. (1989). Short term group therapy with depressed adolescent outpatients. *Canadian Journal of Psychiatry, 34*(2), 97–102.

Freeman, E. M., & McRoy, R. G. (1986). Group counseling program for unemployed black teenagers. *Social Work with Groups, 9*(1), 73–89.

Gazda, G. M. (1989). *Group counseling: A developmental approach* (4th ed.). Boston, MA: Allyn & Bacon.

Gazda, G. M., & Larsen, M. J. (1968). A comprehensive appraisal of group and multiple counseling research. *Journal of Research and Development in Education, 1*(2), 57–132.

Gresham, F. M., & Nagle, R. J. (1980). Social skills training with children: Responsiveness to modeling and coaching as a function of peer orientation. *Journal of Consulting and Clinical Psychology, 48*(6), 718–729.

Grunebaum, H., & Solomon, L. (1982). Toward a theory of peer relationships: II. On the stages of social development and their relationship to group psychotherapy. *International Journal of Group Psychotherapy, 32*(3), 283–307.

Gwynn, C. A., & Brantley, H. T. (1987). Effects of a divorce group intervention for elementary school children. *Psychology in the Schools, 24*(2), 161–164.

Hains, A. A., Herrman, L. P., Baker, K. L., & Graber, S. (1986). The development of a psychoeducational group program for adolescent sex offenders. *Journal of Offender Counseling, Services & Rehabilitation, 11*(1), 63–76.

Hall, R. P., Kassees, J. M., & Hoffman, C. (1986). Treatment for survivors of incest. *Journal for Specialists in Group Work, 72*(2), 85–92.

Hardy-Fanta, C., & Montana, P. (1982). The hispanic female adolescent: A group therapy model. *International Journal of Group Therapy, 32*(3), 351–366.

Hazzard, A., King, H. E., & Webb, C. (1986). Group therapy with sexually abused adolescent girls. *American Journal of Psychiatry, 40*(2), 213–223.

Hendren, R. L., Atkins, D. M., Sumner, C. R., & Barber, J. K. (1987). Model for the group treatment of eating disorders. *International Journal of Group Psychotherapy, 37*(4), 589–602.

Holmes, P. (1983). "Dropping out" from an adolescent therapeutic group: A study of factors in the patients and their parents which may influence this process. *Journal of Adolescence, 6*(4), 333–346.

Hoover, T. (1984). Peer culture development a focus on the behavior problem student. *Small Group Behavior, 15*(4), 511–524.

Huebner, E. S. (1984). A group treatment approach for abused middle school students. *Techniques, 1*(2), 139–143.

Huey, W. C., & Rank, R. C. (1984). Effects of counselor and peer-led group assertive training on black adolescent aggression. *Journal of Counseling Psychology, 31*(1), 95–98.

Jaffe, P., Wilson, S. K., & Wolfe, D. (1988). Specific assessment and intervention strategies for children exposed to wife battering: Preliminary empirical investigations. *Canadian Journal of Community Mental Health, 7*(2), 157–163.

Janus, N. G., & Podolec, M. (1982). Counseling mentally retarded students in the public schools. *School Psychology Review, 11*(4), 453–458.

Jessor, R. (1993). Successful adolescent development among youth in high-risk settings. *American Psychologist, 48*, 117–126.

Johnson, C. L., Jr., & Johnson, J. A. (1991). Using short-term group counseling with visually impaired adolescents. *Journal of Visual Impairment and Blindness, 85*(4), 166–170.

Julian, A., & Kilmann, P. R. (1979). Group treatment of juvenile delinquents: A review of the outcome literature. *International Journal of Group Psychotherapy, 29*(1), 5–37.

Kalter, N., Pickar, J., & Lesowitz, M. (1984). School-based developmental facilitation groups for children of divorce: A preventive intervention. *American Journal of Orthopsychiatry, 54*, 613–623.

Kazdin, A. E. (1988). *Child psychotherapy: Developing and identifying effective treatments*. Elmsford, NY: Pergamon Press.

Kazdin, A. E. (1989). Developmental psychopathology: Current research, issues and directions. *American Psychologist, 44*(2), 180–187.

Kazdin, A. E. (1991). Effectiveness of psychotherapy with children and adolescents. *Journal of Consulting and Clinical Psychology, 59*(6), 785–798.

Kazdin, A. E. (1993). Adolescent mental health: Prevention and treatment programs. *American Psychologist, 48*(2),127–141.

Keat, D. B., Metzgar, K. L., Raykovitz, D., & McDonald, J.(1985). Multimodal counseling: Motivating children to attend school through friendship groups. *Humanistic Education and Development, 23*(4), 166–175.

Kennedy, J. F. (1989). Therapist gender and same-sex puberty age psychotherapy group. *International Journal of Group Psychotherapy, 39*(2), 255–263.

Kiesler, D. I. (1971). Experimental designs in psychotherapy research. In A. E. Bergin & S. L. Garfield (Eds.) *Handbook of psychotherapy and behavior change: An empirical analysis* (pp. 36–74). New York: Wiley.

Kinrade, L. C. (1985). Preventive group intervention with siblings of oncology patients. *Children's Health Care, 14*(2), 110–113.

Kraft, I. A. (1968). An overview of group therapy with adolescents. *International Journal of Group Psychotherapy, 18,* 461–480.

Larson, J. D. (1990). Cognitive-behavioral group therapy with delinquent adolescents: A cooperative approach with the juvenile court. *Journal of Offender Rehabilitation, 16*(1-2), 47–64.

LeCroy, C. W. (1988). Anger management or anger expression: Which is most effective? *Residential Treatment for Children and Youth, 5*(3), 29–39.

Lesowitz, M., Kalter, N., Pickar, J., Chetnik, M., & Schaefer, M. (1987). School based developmental facilitation groups for children of divorce: Issues of group process. *Psychotherapy, 24*(1), 90–95.

Levitt, E. E. (1957). The results of psychotherapy with children: An evaluation. *Journal of Consulting Psychology, 21*(3), 189–196.

Lewis, H. W. (1984). A structured group counseling program for reading disabled elementary students. *The School Counselor, 31,* 454–459.

Lockwood, J. L. (1981). Treatment of disturbed children in verbal and experiential group psychotherapy. *International Journal of Group Psychotherapy, 31*(3), 355–366.

Lothstein, L. (1985). Group therapy for latency age black males: Unplanned interventions, setting and racial transferences as catalysts for change. *International Journal of Group Psychotherapy, 35*(4), 603–623.

Lubell, D., & Soong, W. (1982). Group therapy with sexually abused adolescents. *Canadian Journal of Psychiatry, 27,* 311–315.

MacKay, B., Gold, M., & Gold, E. (1987). A pilot study in drama therapy with adolescent girls who have been sexually abused. *Arts in Psychotherapy, 14*(1), 77–84.

Margolin, L. (1984). Group therapy as a means of learning about the sexually assaultive adolescent. *International Journal of Offender Therapy and Comparative Criminology, 28,* 65–72.

Mason, C. M. (1988). Adolescent chemical dependency aftercare: A non-traditional approach to recovery through group dependence. *Alcoholism Treatment Quarterly, 4*(4), 43–51.

McFadden, J., Lee, C., & Lindsey, C. (1985). Black consciousness development: A group counseling model for black elementary school students. *Elementary School Guidance and Counseling, 19*(3), 228–236.

McKibbon, E., & King, J. (1983). Activity group counseling for learning-disabled children with behavior problems. *The American Journal of Occupational Therapy, 37,* 617–623.

McLinden, S. E., Miller, L. M., & Deprey, J. M. (1991). Effects of a support group for siblings of children with special needs. *Psychology in the Schools, 28,* 230–237.

McNeil, J. S., & Franklin, C. (1988). A university based alternative school for high school drop outs. *Residential Treatment for Children and Youth, 5*(4), 43–58.

Milne, J., & Spence, S. H. (1987). Training social perception skills with primary school children: A cautionary note. *Behavioral Psychotherapy, 15*(2), 144–157.

Mitchum, N. T. (1991). Group counseling for navy children. *The School Counselor, 38,* 372–377.

Morse, C. L., & Bockoven, J. (1987). The Oregon DUSO-R research studies series: Integrating a children's social skills curriculum in a family education/counseling center. *Individual Psychology, 43*(1), 101–114.

Morse, C. L., Bockoven, J., & Harman, M. A. (1987). DUSO-R and ACCEPTS: The differential effects of two social skills curricula on children's social skills and self-esteem. *Child Study Journal, 17*(4), 287–299.

Niehoff, M. S. (1983). Psychological perceptions of special needs children: The gifted and talented. *Individual Psychology, 39,* 402–408.

Niles, W. J. (1986). Effects of a moral development discussion group on delinquent and predelinquent boys. *Journal of Counseling Psychology, 33*(1), 45–51.

Omizo, M. M., Cubberly, W. E., & Longano, D. M. (1984). The effects of group counseling on self-concept and locus of control among learning disabled children. *Humanistic Education and Development, 23*(2), 69–79.

Omizo, M. M., Cubberly, W. E., & Omizo, S. A. (1985). The effects of rational-emotive education groups on self-concept and locus of control among learning disabled children. *The Exceptional Child, 32*(1), 13–19.

Omizo, M. M., Hershberger, J. M., & Omizo, S. A. (1988). Teaching children to cope with anger. *Elementary School Guidance and Counseling, 22*(3), 241–245.

Omizo, M. M., & Omizo, S. A. (1987a). Group counseling with children of divorce: New findings. *Elementary School Guidance and Counseling, 22*(1), 46–52.

Omizo, M. M., & Omizo, S. A. (1987b). The effects of eliminating self-defeating behavior of learning disabled children through group counseling. *The School Counselor, 34*(4), 282–288.

Omizo, M. M., & Omizo, S. (1987c). The effects of group counseling on classroom behavior and self-concept among elementary school learning disabled children. *Exceptional Child, 34*(1), 57–64.

Pawley, P. (1985). Family preparation group for children. *Adoption and Fostering, 9*(1), 41–44.

Pedro-Carroll, J. L., & Cowen, E. L. (1985). The children of divorce intervention program: An investigation of the efficacy of school based prevention program. *Journal of Consulting and Clinical Psychology, 53*(5), 603–611.

Pedro-Carroll, J. L., Cowen, E. L., Hightower, A. D., & Guare, J. C. (1986). Preventive intervention with latency-aged children of divorce: A replication study. *American Journal of Community Psychology, 14*(3), 277–289.

Roback, H. B., Abramowitz, S. I., & Strassberg, D. S. (1979). *Group psychotherapy research: Commentaries and selected reading.* Huntington, NY: Robert F. Krieger.

Shechtman, Z. (1991). Small group therapy and preadolescent same-sex friendship. *International Journal of Group Psychotherapy, 41*(2), 227–243.

Shulman, S., & Margalit, M. (1985). Suicidal behavior at school: A systemic perspective. *Journal of Adolescent, 8*(3), 263–269.

Simmons, C.H., & Parsons, R.J. (1983). Empowerment for role alternative in adolescence. *Adolescence, 18*(69), 193–200.

Smith, T. E. (1985). Group work with adolescent drug abusers. *Social Work With Groups, 8*(1), 55–64.

Sorsdahl, S. N., & Sanche, R. P. (1985). The effects of classroom meetings on self-concept and behavior. *Elementary School Guidance and Counseling, 20*(4), 49–56.

Stockton, R., & Morran, D. K. (1982). Review and perspective of critical dimensions in therapeutic small group research. In G. M. Gazda (Ed.), *Basic Approaches to Group Psychotherapy and Group Counseling* (3rd ed., pp. 37–85). Springfield: Thomas.

Takanishi, R. (1993). The opportunities of adolescence-research, interventions, and policy. *American Psychologist, 48,* 85–87.

Tedder, S. L., Scherman, A., & Wantz, R. A. (1987). Effectiveness of a support group for children of divorce. *Elementary School Guidance & Counseling, 22*(2), 102–109.

Tramontana, M. G. (1980). Critical review of research on psychotherapy outcome with adolescents: 1967-1977. *Psychological Bulletin, 88*(2), 429–450.

Twardosz, S., Nordquist, V., Simon, R., & Bobkin, D. (1983). The effect of group affection activities on the interaction of socially isolate children. *Analysis and Intervention in Developmental Disabilities, 3*(4), 311–338.

Waksman, S. A. (1984). A controlled evaluation of assertion training with adolescents. *Adolescence, 19*(74), 277–282.

Waldron, J. A., Whittington, R. R., & Jensen, S. (1985). Childrens single-session briefings: Group work with military families experiencing parent's deployment. *Social Work with Groups, 8*(2), 101–109.

Wayne, J., & Weeks, K. K. (1984). Group work with abused adolescent girls: A special challenge. *Social Work with Groups, 7*(4), 83–104.

Weiss, B., & Weisz, J. R. (1990). The impact of methodological factors on child psychotherapy outcome research: A meta-analysis for researchers. *Journal of Abnormal Child Psychology, 18*(6), 639–670.

Weisz, J. R., Weiss, B., Alicke, M. D., & Klotz, M. L. (1987). Effectiveness of psychotherapy with children and adolescents: A meta-analysis for clinicians. *Journal of Consulting and Clinical Psychology, 55*(4), 542–549.

Zimpfer, D., & Waltman, D. (1982). Correlates of effectiveness in group counseling. *Small Group Behavior, 13*(3), 275–290.

CHAPTER 11

Inpatient Group Therapy

ROBERT H. KLEIN, VIRGINIA BRABENDER, and APRIL FALLON

The use of inpatient group therapy is steadily increasing, as is the evidence for its efficacy. Virtually every contemporary psychiatric inpatient unit provides group therapy as part of treatment. For the behaviorally oriented approaches, there has been a large-scale empirical effort directed at evaluation and further refinement; for other approaches there has been relative inattention to this empirical endeavor. Although there is an accumulating research base, there is a need for much more rigorous research in this area. Over the past 15 years, three to four times as many publications have been devoted to theoretical or clinical expositions as compared to empirical studies or reviews of research (Klein, 1993a).

In this chapter, we focus on inpatient group therapy as practiced in the small group format. An examination of recent theoretical developments and a consideration of the efficacy of inpatient group therapy, including both outcome and therapeutic factor studies will be conducted. The chapter concludes with a discussion of the structure of the group and the use of various techniques.

Inpatient group therapy has been practiced since the early 1900s. Only within recent years, however, have therapists recognized that the special features of inpatient groups require modification of the methods originally developed for conducting long-term outpatient groups. More specifically, effective inpatient group work requires changes in group goals and structure, on the one hand, and leadership style and technique on the other. A comprehensive account of the history of inpatient group therapy that addresses the broader social, cultural, and philosophical influences that shaped the treatment of mental illness in relation to which inpatient group therapy evolved can be found elsewhere (e.g., Klein, 1983a; Rice & Rutan, 1987; Yalom, 1985).

THEORETICAL DEVELOPMENTS

The past 15 years have seen the efflorescence of theory development in inpatient group psychotherapy. Two sets of factors necessitated advances upon existing theory. The first was practitioners' awareness of research findings from the late 1960s and early 1970s demonstrating that methods derived from outpatient groups are ineffective with inpatient groups (Kibel, 1992). The second set of factors were changes within the inpatient setting itself. Driven by attempts to control the rising costs of psychiatric treatment, the influence of managed-care has led to a change in hospital composition in the direction of more severe psychopathology as well as a diminishing length of stay (Kiesler & Simpkins, 1991). These changes have made untenable the therapist's commitment to the long-term goals of outpatient therapy (e.g., resolution of psychological conflict or modification of maladaptive ways of relating to others). Finally, specialized psychiatric units emerged designed to accommodate populations that are homogeneous along some dimension such as age (e.g., an adolescent unit) or symptom pattern (e.g., an eating disorders unit).

Together these factors inspired the development of approaches designed specifically for short-term inpatient settings and, in some instances, particular types of inpatient settings or populations. Inpatient group psychotherapy approaches have emerged from most of the major schools of personality theory and psychopathology. Four theoretical orientations to personality and psychopathology from which inpatient group approaches have developed are psychodynamic, interpersonal, cognitive, and behavioral.

Psychodynamic Approaches

In recent years, a movement has occurred toward the creation of short-term dynamic models of group therapy that has paralleled a similar but earlier movement within individual therapy. Existing short-term psychodynamic models of inpatient group treatment vary greatly depending on the school of psychodynamic thought to which they are most closely aligned—object relations, self psychology, and so on. However, many of these models have been influenced by general systems theory in either their conceptualization of the relationship of the group to the unit, or in their use of group-level phenomena to affect change in the individual. Although a number of psychodynamic approaches have emerged (e.g., Brabender, 1985; Marcovitz & Smith, 1983; McGuire, 1988), this section focuses on the object relations/systems and self-psychological approaches, in part because they are based upon widely disparate notions of the nature of psychopathology. Whereas the object relations/systems approach views inpatients and their problems from a conflict perspective, the self-psychological model regards psychological problems as deficits (Kibel, 1990; Klein, Bernard, & Singer, 1992). This theoretical difference gives rise to intervention strategies that diverge greatly from one another.

For the object relations/systems model proposed by Kibel (1978, 1981), the theoretical point of departure is the Kernbergian object relations' view of the need for hospitalization as a consequence of the breakdown of the defense mechanism of splitting. Splitting is used in healthy development for the purpose of protecting positively toned representations of self and other until they can be integrated with negatively toned representations without being overwhelmed by the latter. In the course of normal development, splitting is abandoned once a successful integration of oppositely toned self and object images is achieved. However, in persons with severe characterological disturbances, failure to integrate diverse self and object representations leads to an ongoing reliance on splitting for the maintenance of a sense of well-being. Hospitalization occurs when events (often losses) in the individual's life lead to a collapse in the tenuous boundaries between positive and negative representations. The consequence of this collapse is that individuals are overrun by the affects of anger, envy, sadness, and so on which then dominate their perception of themselves and others. This model sees the goal of hospitalization as the restoration of splitting. Through this reacquisition, hospitalized patients are able to gain access to the positive affects that make themselves, others, and their lives tolerable and are once again able to perform adaptive tasks necessary for life in the community.

From the standpoint of this model, while the goal of hospitalization is to help patients to reconstitute, there are many features of hospital life (e.g., loss of privacy and familiar surroundings and roles) that intensify the negative feelings that brought patients into the hospital and create tensions on the unit (Kibel, 1981; Klein, 1977, 1983b; Rice & Rutan, 1981). The model further holds that the group is likely to reflect the tensions of the unit. This supposition has considerable empirical support from studies showing that the emotional climate, tensions, and values of the unit have parallels in the group process and atmosphere (Astrachan, Harrow, & Flynn, 1968; Karterud, 1988). The inpatient psychotherapy group rather than simply reflecting unit concerns also provides a forum for their examination. Through the acknowledgment of such feelings within the group and their attribution to circumstances on the unit, members are able to contain and direct these feelings in a way that restores their access to the splitting defense. Members' negative reactions to unit life are explored primarily on a group-as-a-whole basis because group-level interventions promote cohesiveness, avoid the narcissistic hurt often stimulated by individually directed comments, and convey the notion that negative reactions are acceptable given that they are well within the scope of shared human experience. Through such explorations and interpretations, the intensity and pervasiveness of members' negatively toned experiences are lessened. The value of such explorations is supported by a study showing that the more members are permitted to express hostility in a group, the more benefit they derive from the group (Koch, 1983).

While the object relations/systems model sees psychopathology as conflict-based, the newly emerging self-psychological approaches regard psychopathology as the result of a deficit. More specifically, self-psychology sees psychopathology as the result of arrested development in the establishment of a cohesive self due to early and repeated empathic failures of the parent (Kohut, 1977, 1984). The self psychological approach is seen as having particular advantage for inpatients because it takes into account their great vulnerability to fragmentation of sense of self, a fragmentation stimulated by any perception of themselves as being attacked, ignored, or dismissed. Such a perception can be precipitated by interventions (such as those advocated by the object relations/systems model) that focus upon the negative or aggressively-toned aspects of their experience. What the self psychological approach advocates is empathic affirmation of inpatients' needs and attempts to adapt, while assiduously avoiding the stimulation and interpretation of negative transference. Within this here-and-now approach, the therapist emphasizes the healthy, self-affirming aspects of members' communications. For example, members' engagement in small talk early in the life of a group is not construed as defensive withdrawal. Rather, it is regarded as an effort to, at once, protect the self and maintain relations with others (Josephs & Jhuman, 1985).

Self psychology writers (Baker, 1993) emphasize the nurturant potential of the psychotherapy group in that it creates manifold opportunities for members to satisfy self-object transference needs (i.e., needs stimulated by early deprivation of developmentally appropriate needs). Such transference needs can be satisfied through their relations with other individual members, a subgroup of members, the therapist, or the group-as-a-whole. However, the self psychological approach does not merely gratify transference needs, but assists them in building the necessary structure to tolerate narcissistic hurt without disintegration. This occurs when the group responds with empathy to the inevitable frustration of self-object needs in the group.

In general, the psychodynamic approaches have been untested in terms of efficacy. A major step in the process of evaluation would be the development of operational means to test abstract concepts such as "splitting" or "mirroring self-transference" and so on. There is indication from the literature that such effort is underway (Greene, Rosenkrantz, & Muth, 1986).

Interpersonal Approaches

Over the last three decades of the history of inpatient group psychotherapy, the interpersonal approach has had an important role. The literature reflects the fact that inpatient group therapists were highly influenced by the seminal work of Irvin Yalom. In applying the interpersonal theory of Harry Stack Sullivan to group psychotherapy, Yalom takes as a point of departure the notion that most if not all forms of psychopathology have an interpersonal dimension. That is, difficulties in relating to others lead to the development, maintenance, or intensification of symptoms.

In 1983, Yalom proposed a set of interpersonal approaches which, unlike earlier less structured applications, took into account certain realities of inpatient groups—the brevity of members' stay, the severity of psychopathology, the presence of the group within a broader treatment context. These realities require the therapist to embrace goals that are somewhat more conservative than the traditional goal of interpersonal approaches of modifying members' styles of relating. These newer models were directed toward reducing patients' immediate levels of distress and cultivating a positive attitude toward psychotherapy. A model which enabled members to see that psychotherapy is helpful and which gave members some tools to pursue psychotherapy (such as being able to identify certain problem areas) would enhance the likelihood that members would continue with treatment on an outpatient basis. The interpersonal agenda model is designed for higher functioning patients who can tolerate the anxiety associated with certain therapeutic processes such as the giving and receiving of feedback. This model entails the use of a highly structured session in which members through a "go-around" establish concrete, here-and-now agenda that can be accomplished in the session. The focus group model, directed toward the needs of lower functioning patients and, in particular, their low anxiety tolerance, involves members' performance of a series of brief interpersonal exercises. Both the interpersonal agenda and focus group models of the interpersonal approach are amenable to use if a patient participates in even a single group therapy session.

The major research effort on the interpersonal approach has been directed toward the identification of the therapeutic factors that members see as relevant to their progress (e.g, Leszcz, Yalom, & Norden, 1985). Some results indicate that inpatients value the leadership functions of focus and integration (Leszcz, Yalom, & Norden, 1985). With respect to outcome, the application of the unstructured interpersonal approach has been found to help chronic patients show more flexible behaviors in relation to a goal and to correct distorted perceptions relative to no group subjects (Beard & Scott, 1975). Beutler, Frank, Schieber, Calvert, and Gaines (1984) found that an interpersonally oriented group produced more symptomatic change than an emotional/expressive or behavioral group, or a no-group condition. Coché, Cooper, and Petermann (1984) found that female group members seemed to gain more from the interpersonal approach and male members more from the problem-solving training. Jones and McColl (1991) found no difference between the members of an interactional agenda group and a social skills training group in their willingness to participate in other groups.

Cognitive Approaches

The cognitive school seeks to treat psychopathology through modification of cognitive processes or contents (Hollon & Beck, 1986). The set of approaches that have emerged from cognitive theory has been readily adaptable from the individual therapy settings where they were originally applied with depressed individuals to inpatient groups because of the short-term, problem-oriented character of these approaches (Freeman, Schrodt, Gilson, & Ludgate, in press). Nonetheless, most applications require that members be present in the group for at least three or four sessions. This is a demand that many settings, with near-daily turnover, cannot accommodate.

Perhaps the best-known, commonly utilized application of the cognitive approach to inpatient groups has been developed by Freeman and associates (Freeman, 1987; Freeman et al., 1989; Greenwood, 1987). In this approach, members are taught the tenets of cognitive therapy, particularly the notion that cognitions control affects and behaviors. Once members have had an exposure to these concepts, they are given practice in identifying negative cognitions in the group and in homework assignments on the unit. There has been only one reported study to evaluate the cognitive therapy approach with an inpatient population. Relative to a waiting list and no treatment control groups, adolescent males in cognitive group therapy became less aggressive and exhibited more self-control (Feindler, Ecton, Kingsley, & Dubey, 1986).

A different type of cognitive approach is problem-solving therapy that focuses on the process of solving problems rather than the content of the solutions. This approach is based upon a large fund of research showing that psychiatric patients are frequently deficient in addressing and solving problems in daily life (Nezu, 1986; Platt & Spivack, 1972a, 1972b, 1974), and the more severe the psychopathology, the greater the problem-solving deficiency (Gilbride & Hebert, 1980).

The goal of this model is to improve problem solving and thereby enhance members' abilities to perform life's daily tasks. The problem-solving model has generated a considerable fund of research. Problem-solving therapy has been shown to improve members' performance at various stages of problem solving (Coché & Douglass, 1977; Coché & Flick, 1975; Intagliata, 1978; Siegel & Spivack, 1976), to increase impulse control (Coché & Douglass, 1977) and to decrease depression and psychotic thinking (Coché & Douglass, 1977). However, D. E. Jones (1981) failed to find a problem-solving group to be more effective than two comparison groups in either increasing members' adaptive behaviors or reducing their identified problems in daily living. McLatchie (1982) failed to find that problem-solving therapy ameliorates psychotic symptomatology in a chronic schizophrenic group.

Behavioral Approaches

Although behavioral approaches have been available to the inpatient group therapist for many years, they have not been broadly used. Insufficiently appreciated by group therapists is the extent to which contemporary behavioral approaches have evolved to make use of the factors unique to group life such as group cohesiveness (Liberman, DeRisi, & Mueser, 1989), and the emphasis such approaches place on how affective and cognitive mechanisms must be deployed for change to occur. Current behavioral approaches are also likely to be comprehensible to most group therapists in that they embrace assumptions that have long been identified with the interpersonal school of group therapy. For example, the behavioral approach, and particularly the popular social skills variant, sees the cultivation of effective interpersonal relating as important to enhancing post-hospital adjustment.

Behavioral group therapy is unique in its detailed, concrete, and behavioral delineation of basic social skills such as greeting others, making requests, and terminating interactions, and sorting these behaviors into their constituent parts. This analysis enables skills to be taught systematically, in manageable units to severely disordered patients. Application of the behavioral approach, and particularly the social skills variant, involves assessment of the member's skill level both before and throughout the member's participation in the group. Once a skill is chosen for each member and his or her level of skill deficit has been assessed, members proceed through a series of training sessions involving: modeling of the skill; behavioral rehearsal with coaching; positively oriented feedback from the therapist and other group members; repeated practice during the session and through homework assignments; and continual monitoring of progress by self-report, observations by staff and family members, and overt indicators such as success in finding employment.

Inpatient research on social skills training groups has been extensive with a great variety of patient populations and particular skills studied. As will be discussed next, the vast majority of these studies have demonstrated successfully the efficacy of the social skills approach with inpatient populations (e.g., Douglas & Mueser, 1990; Wong & Wooley, 1989).

OUTCOME RESEARCH

In 1983, Yalom noted that methodological problems associated with outcome research (e.g., the necessity for large groups of patients randomly assigned to various types of therapy groups led by skilled therapists while the remaining aspects of the patients' treatment are held constant) are so overwhelming, that relatively few rigorous studies have been conducted on inpatient group therapy. Indeed, the inpatient setting presents problems of which the researcher must be mindful: each inpatient group is embedded in a unique system whose prejudices, emphases, and interdependent treatment components can differentially enhance or attenuate its impact. Thus, it is necessary to articulate the important contextual variables and be wary about the generalization from one setting to another in the same manner that researchers would be cautious about generalizing a particular model or treatment to a different population.

As with other types of treatment, how to define and measure outcome, from whose perspective, and at what points in time is of fundamental concern to the study of outcome. In order to conclude that group is a valuable treatment modality, it must be shown that the individuals have changed significantly in the positive or predicted direction. In other words, there must be a comparison between: two or more types of groups conducted, the group and "standard care," or pre- and post-group. The variable chosen to measure this difference or change must be observable, measurable, and reproducible. Whether a study shows that inpatient group is efficacious in part hinges upon the particular variable chosen to represent outcome. How improvement should be defined is dependent upon the model of psychopathology embraced. For example, should the goal be to reduce symptomatology while in the hospital or reduce relapse rate by changing the vulnerability of the individual via improving his ability to manage his stressors more effectively? Or should the primary goal be to improve life quality by enabling appreciation of the rewards of social relationships (Donahoe & Driesenga, 1988)? The definition of improvement may also be determined by the severity of psychopathology and dysfunction. What can be accomplished in a group where patients will shortly return to the community is very different from what can be addressed in a state hospital group where many individuals may never function independently; the reduction of symptomatology or improvement in social relationships may be an appropriate goal for the former whereas the reduction of aggressive behavior or "soiling" behavior on the unit may be appropriate for the latter. Thus, only those studies that included one of the above comparisons and produced a significant difference on a reasonable measurable outcome variable were included in this review. However, positive findings should not be interpreted as equivalent across patients and settings. With these constraints, a review of the outcome literature a decade after Yalom's statement reveals considerable empirical support for the efficacy of inpatient group therapy with a range of diagnostic categories in a variety of treatment settings using various theoretical approaches.

Group Therapy in Short-Term Acute Care Treatment

Diagnostically Heterogeneous Groups

There is much evidence that inpatients can benefit from participation in short-term diagnostically heterogeneous groups. Positive results have been found with groups that have utilized a social skills model (Douglas & Mueser, 1990; Fiedler, Orenstein, Chiles, Fritz, & Breitt, 1979; Fromme & Smallwood, 1983; Gutride, Goldstein, & Hunter, 1973; Katz, 1986; Monti et al., 1979; Mueser, Bellack, Douglas, & Wade, 1991; Mueser, Kosmidis, & Sayers, in press; Mueser, Levine, Bellack, Douglas, & Brady, 1990; Powell, Illovsky, O'Leary, & Gazda, 1988; Zappe & Epstein, 1987), a psychodynamic model (Greene & Cole, 1991), an interpersonal or interactional model (Beard & Scott, 1975; Beutler et al., 1984; Coché, Cooper & Petermann, 1984; Cohen, 1982; Leszcz, 1986), and a problem-solving model (Coché & Flick, 1975; Coché et al., 1984; Coché & Douglass, 1977; Cohen, 1982; Toseland & Rose, 1978).

While some studies compared one approach with another (Beutler et al., 1984; Coché & Douglass, 1977; Coché & Flick, 1975; Coché et al., 1984; Cohen, 1982; Gutride, Goldstein, & Hunter, 1973; Monti et al., 1979), others utilized a no treatment comparison (i.e., standard hospital care) with random assignment of individuals (e.g., Powell et al., 1988; Katz, 1986) or a pre and post within subject comparison (e.g., Douglas & Mueser, 1990;

Fromme & Smallwood, 1983; Leszcz, 1986; Mueser et al., 1990; Zappe & Epstein, 1987). Only a few studies have presented negative findings (Beutler et al., 1984; Jones, 1981), for example, that patients failed to benefit from short-term inpatient group therapy.

Within a short-term treatment program, a broad range of goals can be accomplished depending upon the techniques employed and the patient mix. Various interpersonal skills using social skills training are the most commonly researched, such as assertion training (Katz, 1986; Zappe & Epstein, 1987), expression of negative feelings (Douglas & Mueser, 1990; Mueser et al., 1990), compromise and negotiation (Douglas & Mueser, 1990; Mueser et al., 1990; Mueser et al., 1991), empathic listening and self-disclosure (Fromme & Smallwood, 1983), vocational skills (Powell et al., 1988), and initiating interactions, giving and receiving feedback, and response to criticism (Fiedler et al., 1979). Other types of goals accomplished in a short-term mixed diagnostic setting include: interpersonal problem solving (Coché & Douglass, 1977; Coché & Flick, 1975; Coché et al., 1984; Cohen, 1982; Toseland & Rose, 1978); behavioral flexibility (Beard & Scott, 1975); increased ability to reality test (Beard & Scott, 1975), decreased symptomatology that precipitated hospitalization (Beutler et al., 1984; Coché & Douglass, 1977; Coché et al., 1984), decreased subjective anxiety (Coché et al., 1984), improved self-esteem (Coché & Douglass, 1977; Greene & Cole, 1991), improved general psychological health (Coché et al., 1984; Cohen, 1982) and greater impulse control (Coché & Douglass, 1977).

Several problems can be identified with the research on mixed psychiatric populations. First, many of the outcome measures are self-report or paper and pencil indications of interpersonal change (e.g., mean-ends test for interpersonal problem solving). While self-ratings are important, individuals are often not good judges of their own behavior and paper and pencil tasks may not accurately reflect behavior. In a departure from that format, Mueser and his colleagues used therapists' ratings and role play assessment (Douglas & Mueser, 1990; Mueser et al., 1990; Mueser et al., 1991). Only two of the studies reviewed included measures of generalization such as ward behavior (Beutler et al., 1984) or length of hospital stay (Coché & Flick, 1975). A few studies presented follow-up assessments, (e.g., Beutler et al., 1984 at one year, Mueser et al., 1991 at one month). Powell et al. (1988) showed that his social skills program (30 hours of training) resulted in fewer hospitalizations and greater employment than a control group. Despite the flawed nature of the individual studies, they consistently support the efficacy of a diagnostically heterogeneous inpatient group.

A recent trend throughout the empirical outcome literature is interest in the differentiating effectiveness of treatments in terms of patient characteristics (e.g., gender, symptoms, personality organization, and level of functioning), as well as by the salient dimensions of the treatment context (Brabender & Fallon, 1993; Erickson, 1987). A few studies exist in which gender has impacted on outcome. For example, while the problem-solving and the interpersonal psychoanalytic approach showed no differences in effectiveness, women gained more from the interpersonal approach, whereas men benefited more from the problem-solving training (Coché et al., 1984). The authors interpreted these results to suggest that men are more comfortable with a rational problem-oriented approach, while women prefer an interpersonal approach that encourages the expression of affect and focuses on unstructured interpersonal interaction (Coché et al., 1984). However, Leszcz (1986) noted the gender differences in the co-therapy teams; problem-solving group leaders were mixed gender, whereas the interactional group had female therapists. Leszcz (1986) suggests that female patients may have benefited more from the interactive group because the female therapists felt more comfortable with that format. Similarly, the ease with which each of the sexes can improve may be dependent upon the particular behavior that requires change. When compromise and negotiation and learning to express negative feelings were taught in a social skills training format, males improved more than females (Douglas & Mueser, 1990; Mueser et al., 1990).

Diagnostically Homogeneous Groups with Substance Abusers

Several empirical investigations have corroborated the belief that group therapy is important in the treatment of addictions. When social skills training was compared to cognitive restructuring (Jackson & Oei, 1978; Oei & Jackson, 1982) and to supportive group psychotherapy (Oei & Jackson, 1980; 1982) in a 24-session (12-week) program, social skills training was found to be superior to traditional supportive psychotherapy in social skills ratings and nurses' ratings (Jackson & Oei, 1978; Oei & Jackson, 1980, 1982). The group setting was superior to individual therapy for social skills training (Oei & Jackson, 1980). When social skills training is compared to cognitive restructuring, the former is superior at post-treatment (Jackson & Oei, 1978). The combination of social skills training and cognitive restructuring does not improve the result (Oei & Jackson, 1982). At follow-up, however, (3–12 months later depending upon the study), cognitive restructuring was superior to social skills and the cognitive restructuring-social skills combination was superior to social skills alone in alcohol consumption and social skills (Jackson & Oei, 1978; Oei & Jackson, 1982). Unfortunately, these studies utilized a 12-week program, which has become less and less feasible in our cost-cutting economy. However, a study by Eriksen, Bjornstad, and Gotestam (1986) utilizing 8 sessions (once per week for 90 minutes) supports the superiority of social skills training (instruction, modeling, roleplaying, feedback, in vivo homework) with nonpsychotic alcoholics over a discussion group for the acquisition of assertiveness and other social skills. Furthermore, at one-year follow-up, those receiving social skills training had fewer hospital days, consumed less alcohol, and had more sober days and more working days than those who had been in the discussion group treatment.

Problem-solving training that focuses on potential relapse precipitating events (e.g., anger and frustration, negative mood states, interpersonal pressure, and intrapersonal temptation) has also been shown to be effective

with alcoholics. Two studies have reported on male alcoholics who participated in either a problem-solving group, a discussion group (dealing with
the emotional nature of alcohol asking questions like why and what keeps
you an alcoholic), or a standard hospital treatment control group for six
(twice weekly) 90-minute sessions (Chaney, O'Leary, & Marlatt, 1978;
Jones, Kanfer, & Lanyon, 1982). At the end of treatment, the problem-
solving group showed improved performance in their ability to role play
problematic situations in both studies. At one-year follow-up, the problem
solving group had decreased duration and severity of relapse episodes compared to the standard hospital treatment. However, the results are equivocal
with regard to the utility of the discussion group. In the Jones et al. study
(1982), the problem-solving group and discussion group at post-treatment or
at one-year follow-up were not distinguishable. In the Chaney et al. (1978)
study, the problem-solving group was superior at post-treatment and at one-
year follow-up. Level of patient functioning may have a role in explaining
the discrepancy. The Jones et al. study had higher functioning (e.g., higher
socioeconomic class and more likely to be married) patients than did the
Chaney study. It may be that the lower functioning alcoholics require more
specific and concrete direction than the discussion group provides, whereas
the higher functioning alcoholics do not require the specific instructions
in order to maintain sobriety. Similarly, a problem-solving group that focused specifically on discharge planning (10 sessions) was superior to standard hospital treatment in helping participants to anticipate, plan, and cope
for post discharge problems (Intagliata, 1978). They also showed more improvement on paper and pencil measures of problem solving thinking than
the controls, irrespective of verbal proficiency. These skills were maintained at one-month follow-up.*

These studies took place on units devoted to the treatment of addiction.
However, experts in the addictions field note that the coexistence of a psychiatric illness with a substance abuse disorder results in a poor response to
primary substance abuse treatment alone; these patients often become the
responsibility of general psychiatric units (Kofoed & Keys, 1988). Despite
the common belief that alcoholics should be in a separate treatment program, when part of a mixed diagnostic group, they make comparable gains
to other diagnostic categories on a range of outcome measures (Albrecht &
Brabender, 1983). Similarly, a study on the use of a persuasion group on a
mixed diagnostic unit for dual-diagnosis patients, where member interaction was used to have patients admit to their addiction and to seek further

---

* All of the these studies investigated an alcoholic population. For other substances abused most of
what is reported is the descriptive use of whole treatment programs (e.g., Joughin, Tata, Collins,
Hooper, & Falkowski, 1991, reported on a treatment program which included group to help patients
withdrawn from long-term benziodiazepine use). There is one report on the use of a problem solving
skills training program with incarcerated heroin addicts (Platt reported in Intagliata, 1978). Although subjects were not randomly assigned to group treatments, a significant relationship between
completing problem-solving skills training program and successful parole performance did emerge
and suggested the potential effectiveness of this approach.

substance abuse treatment, found that patients from the persuasion group more frequently received and more frequently accepted discharge plans specifically addressing their addiction than a control group (Kofoed & Keys, 1988).

These studies provide evidence for the effectiveness of a structured, more cognitively or behavioral focused group with male alcoholics. More studies utilizing other theoretical frameworks and other substance abuse problems with patients of both sexes are needed. Although it is a common notion that addictions be treated in a homogeneous group, there is no empirical evidence for the superiority of this partitioning.

Homogeneous Groups of Developmentally Disabled Patients

While level of education has been shown to be a positive predictor of outcome in higher functioning outpatients (Lipsky, Kassinove, & Miller, 1980), virtually no evidence exists as to whether individuals with limited intellectual endowment can benefit from inpatient group therapy. Since many of the group models require a certain level of cognitive processing (e.g., problem-solving training, cognitive-behavioral therapy) or an ability to abstract from what is presented and to apply it to interactions in the group (interpersonal models) or to events on the unit (e.g., object relations systems model), it is important to know whether intellectually limited individuals can benefit from an inpatient group. A few studies with mentally retarded adults attending vocational training programs suggest that problem-solving training may aid in improving social functioning (e.g., improving ability to solve problems, improving social skills, and decreasing aggressive responses), but it is not clear that such training is more effective than other types of training or even than the nonspecific effects of attention to the problem (Benson, Johnson, & Miranti, 1986; Castles, 1983; Otsby, 1983).

Homogeneous Groups of Patients with Antisocial Tendencies

There is some evidence that individuals with antisocial tendencies can benefit from a group in an inpatient setting regardless of whether the group is heterogeneous (Coché et al., 1984) or homogeneous in terms of symptomatology (Jones & McColl, 1991; Laben, Dodd, & Sneed, 1991; Rice & Chaplin, 1979).

Jones and McColl (1991) found that when adult male (nonpsychotic) offenders participated either in an open-ended twice weekly social skills training group (life skills) specifically designed to increase prosocial behaviors or an interactional agenda group, both groups were effective in increasing the patients' desire to participate in social groups (self-report). However, the members of the life skills group were able to take a greater range of roles than those in the interpersonal group.* Similarly, male arsonists participated in a cross-over design of social skills training (with

---

* One problem with this study is that behavioral assessment for generalization and follow-up were not obtained and these patients may have been motivated by legal reasons to present themselves in a more socially desirable manner without actually changing their behavior.

instructions, modeling, coaching, role playing, and feedback) and a nondirective control group discussion (Rice & Chaplin, 1979). Pre- and post-treatment assessment indicated significant improvement in assertiveness with the social skills training but not the control condition. One-year follow-up revealed no fire-setting incidences. In a third study, imprisoned felons with long histories of antisocial behavior as well as heterogeneous psychiatric diagnoses attended a weekly group designed to help participants examine their prior behavior, accept responsibility for their actions and develop social skills necessary for successful reentry into the community. Goal attainment was frequently reviewed. Results indicated that "write-ups" within the institution and physical altercations diminished. Individuals became more outgoing and verbal within the group. Follow-up indicated that none of the members who were released had committed any major offenses (Laben et al., 1991).

These studies suggest that individuals with antisocial characteristics can benefit from group treatment. Their social skills and assertiveness improve while their antisocial tendencies decrease in the immediate setting as well as in the larger community.*

Schizophrenic Patients in Diagnostically Heterogeneous and Homogeneous Groups

During the past four decades, a number of studies have attempted to evaluate the effectiveness of group treatment with schizophrenics in a short-term setting (see Kanas, 1986 for a review of this literature). Early reviews of this literature failed to support the use of inpatient group therapy with schizophrenics (c.f., Bednar & Lawlis, 1971; O'Brien, 1975), although this may in part be due to the particular patients sampled. In contrast, the majority of subsequent outcome studies have found group psychotherapy to be helpful (Beal, Duckro, Elias, & Hecht, 1977; Jones & Peters, 1952; Kanas & Barr, 1982; Serok & Zemet, 1983; Sheppard, Olson, Croke, Lafave, & Gerber, 1990; Vitalo, 1971), regardless of whether patients have manifested acute (e.g., Serok & Zemet, 1983) or more chronic and unremitting schizophrenic symptoms (e.g., Beal et al., 1977). A few studies found no benefit of group therapy over a control group (Doty, 1975; Feifel & Schwartz, 1953†), and one found group therapy to have a detrimental effect on schizophrenics (Kanas, Rogers, Kreth, Patterson, & Campbell, 1980). Of the three studies which did not have positive findings, one provided only brief group therapy for chronically ill patients (Doty, 1975), while two relied upon group treatment that promoted insight or conflict analysis where the goal was to increase self-understanding through developmental and dynamic exploration via the use of uncovering and transference analysis. Open-ended (Beutler et al., 1984) and closed-ended groups (Coché & Flick, 1975) that embrace an

---

* It should be noted that most participants in these studies were male.
† Although the authors conclude that therapy group improved patients' behavior more than a matched group receiving no group treatment, the difference was not statistically significant.

interactional approach in which members relate to each other by discussion of interpersonal problems or other here-and-now issues, or groups that are more task-oriented appear more likely to yield positive results (e.g., Beal et al., 1977; Coché & Douglass, 1977; Coché & Flick, 1975; Coché et al., 1984; Jones & Peters, 1952; Kanas et al., 1980; Sheppard et al., 1990; Vitalo, 1971).

Behavioral (Vitalo, 1971), psychodrama (Jones & Peters, 1952), remotivation (Beal et al., 1977), and gestalt approaches (Serok & Zemet, 1983) have all been reported to be effective in a short-term inpatient setting. However, little is known about the particular treatment context and patient characteristics under which these approaches may be differentially effective. The one exception is Vitalo (1971) who found that when a more behavioral approach (instructional, feedback, and shaping) was used, group members were able to improve their interpersonal functioning in the group and on the ward (exhibit higher levels of empathy, positive regard, and genuineness) more than patients treated in a nondirective group that emphasized sharing of experiences and the development of concrete plans. However, improvement on the MMPI was more likely to occur among patients in the nondirective group than those in the behavioral group. These differential findings emphasize the role that a particular outcome measure can have in determining whether the group is seen as a success or failure.

While several studies have suggested that schizophrenic patients can benefit from groups that have some diagnostic heterogeneity (Beutler et al., 1984; Coché & Flick, 1975), the issue of group composition clearly requires further investigation.* One problem with research in this area is that despite diagnostic homogeneity, there is tremendous variation in terms of degree of psychosis, diagnostic subtype, chronicity, and the presence of positive versus negative symptoms. It is likely that patients with certain characteristics may be better able to benefit from particular kinds of groups. For example, Kanas and Barr (1982) found that patient perception of usefulness depended on age and the presence of paranoia; nonparanoid patients were more likely to find sessions useful than paranoid patients, and younger patients were more likely to see the sessions as useful than were older subjects (Kanas & Barr, 1982). An additional problem is that almost all of these studies have been done in a VA hospital; of the two that were not, only Serok and Zemet (1983) included females. Thus, the conclusions can be safely applied only to male schizophrenics.

Homogeneous Groups of Patients with Symptoms of Social Anxiety and Avoidance

There is consistent evidence that nonpsychotic inpatient populations suffering from social anxiety benefit from social skills training (Lomont, Gilner, Spector, & Skinner, 1969; Monti et al., 1980; van Dam-Baggen

---

* Coché and his colleagues also found schizophrenics to benefit equally from an interpersonal problem solving approach (Coché & Douglass, 1977; Coché & Flick, 1975; Coché et al., 1984).

& Kraaimaat, 1986). Specific social skills taught include assertiveness (Lomont et al., 1969), starting, continuing, and ending conversations, and giving and receiving compliments and criticism (Monti et al., 1980; van Dam-Baggen & Kraaimaat, 1986). Group social skills training appears superior to both an insight oriented approach that focused on catharsis, group transference, and understanding past and present behaviors in the context of recapitulation of a punitive conflict (Lomont et al., 1969) and sensitivity training (Monti et al., 1980). Success of the social skills training was measured by significant decreases in the clinical scales of the MMPI (Pa, Sc, Pd), increases in the dominance-submission dimension of the Learly ICL (Lomont et al., 1969), self-report and role-play measures (Monti et al., 1980; van Dam-Baggen & Kraaimaat, 1986).

It should be noted that while the van Dam-Baggen and Kraaimaat study (1986) conducted group sessions once a week for 17 weeks, Lomont et al. (1969) and Monti et al. (1980) achieved successful outcomes running their groups five days per week for 30 and 20 sessions respectively. Thus, with this population, these skills were acquired over a relatively large number of sessions. Furthermore, follow-up measures indicated that social skills were maintained (Monti et al., 1980; van Dam-Baggen & Kraaimaat, 1986). These studies provide strong support for acquisition and maintenance of social skills, but no measures of generalization were reported.

There is some evidence that individuals suffering from more general anxiety can also benefit from groups. Using a nondirective eclective approach with a symptomatically heterogeneous male veteran population, Haven and Wood (1970) found that those who were suffering primarily from an anxiety disorder had a decreased incidence of rehospitalization.

Group Therapy in Long-Term Treatment

There is a growing body of evidence that group therapy in a long-term setting such as a state hospital, residential treatment, or day hospital is an effective treatment modality (Brabender & Fallon, 1993; Kanas, 1986). A recent review of the literature indicated that group therapy was superior to a control group in 71% of the outcome studies in intermediate or long-term settings (Kanas, 1986). This conclusion is supported by the burgeoning of studies investigating approaches in the behavioral spectrum (see Brabender & Fallon, 1993 for a more complete review of these studies).

In a long-term setting, there are studies to support the use of psychoanalytic group therapy (Fairweather et al., 1960; MacKenzie & Tschuschke, 1993; Sacks & Berger, 1954; Semon & Goldstein, 1957), interpersonal or interactional group therapy (Cadman, Misbach, & Brown, 1954; Cowden, Zax, Hague, & Finney, 1956; Cowden, Zax, & Spoles, 1956; Olson & Greenberg, 1972; Sacks & Berger, 1954; Semon & Goldstein, 1957; Yehoshua, Kellerman, Calev, & Dasberg, 1985), interpersonal problem-solving therapy (Pierce, 1980), social skills training (Bellack, Turner,

Hersen, & Luber, 1984; Booraem & Flowers, 1972; Brown & Munford, 1983; Fecteau & Duffy, 1986; Field & Test, 1975; Finch & Wallace, 1977; Holmes, Hansen, & Lawrence, 1984; Kelly, Laughlin, Claiborne, & Patterson, 1979; Kelly, Urey, & Patterson, 1980; Liberman, Mueser, & Wallace, 1986; Liberman et al., 1984; Magaro & West, 1983; Mueser, Kosmidis, & Sayers, in press; Spenser, Gillespie, & Ekisa, 1983; Wallace, Liberman, Mackain, Blackwell, & Eckman, 1992; Williams, Turner, Watts, Bellack, & Hersen, 1977), attention focusing skill training (Massel, Corrigan, Liberman, & Milan, 1991; Wong et al., in press; Foxx, McMorrow, Bittle, & Fenlon, 1985), and a variety of eclectic approaches (Tucker, 1956; Vernallis & Reinert, 1961; Kraus, 1959; Roback, 1972).*

The specific goals accomplished vary widely. They can be broadly defined as improved ability to communicate (Cadman et al., 1954; Yehoshua et al., 1985), decreased psychopathology on psychological testing (Coons & Peacock, 1970; Fairweather et al., 1960), and improved ward behavior (Cowden, Zax, Hague, & Finney, 1956; Cowden, Zax, & Spoles, 1956; Fairweather et al., 1960; Olson & Greenberg, 1972; Pattison, Brissenden, & Wohl, 1967; Sacks & Berger, 1954). More specific goals have included decreased soiling behavior (Tucker, 1956), days out of the hospital (Vernallis & Reinert, 1961), assertion training (Booraem & Flowers, 1972; Field & Test, 1975; Williams et al., 1977), improved verbal and nonverbal conversational elements (Fecteau & Duffy, 1986; Finch & Wallace, 1977; Liberman et al., 1984; Yehoshua et al., 1985; Williams et al., 1977; Wong et al., in press), increased independence (Goldstein et al., 1973), more appropriate self-disclosure (Foxx et al., 1985; Holmes et al., 1984; Kelly et al., 1980), expression of negative feelings, compromise and negotiation (Mueser, Kosmidis, & Sayers, in press), listening (Fecteau & Duffy, 1986), ability to formulate questions and express interest (Holmes et al., 1984), using compliments (Kelly et al., 1980), improved problem-solving ability (Pierce, 1980), acquisition of life skills such as medication management, recreation, and grooming (Wallace et al., 1992), and health, nutrition, finance, and time management (Brown & Munford, 1983).

Researchers studying this chronic population have been sensitive to the issues of generalization and maintenance of gains. About half the studies have attempted to assess whether newly acquired behaviors generalize to either a community or ward environment (e.g., Kelly et al., 1979; Liberman et al., 1984; Massel et al., 1991; Olson & Greenberg, 1972). There have also been efforts to assess progress at 3 months (Finch & Wallace, 1977; Holmes et al., 1984; Liberman et al., 1984; Wong et al., in press), at one year (Wallace et al., 1992) and as long as 18 months (MacKenzie & Tschuschke, 1993). Follow-up data, when reported, are consistently positive.

---

* There have been a few studies that have not found group therapy to be a more effective treatment modality than its comparison group in this setting with this population (Doty, 1975; Evangelakis, 1961; Anker & Walsh, 1961; Katzenstein, 1954; Gorham & Porkorny, 1964; McLatchie, 1982; Pattison, Brissenden, & Wohl, 1967).

Summary Comments

While it is clear from this review that published positive findings far out-weigh negative findings, the conclusion that inpatient group therapy is helpful with a variety of patients and in a variety of settings is too vague to be meaningful to most researchers and practitioners alike. Many of the studies specify the patient population in terms of diagnosis, but the specifics of therapists' background and interventions are often vague, and the dimensions of the setting (e.g., the theoretical orientation of milieu and mission of the hospital) are rarely articulated. These latter variables can often play a major role in the success or failure of a group. Thus, we echo the call of Erickson (1987) and Parloff and Dies (1977) for greater specificity of the group, setting, and patient parameters. It should be noted that efficacy of group therapy is relevant only to the extent that patients agree to attend sessions in the hospital, perceive its value, and then follow through with the recommended treatment after hospitalization. While a few studies have evaluated patients' perceptions of the relative value of group therapy while in the hospital (Holcomb & Meacham, 1991; Lemberg & May, 1991; Leszcz, 1986), no study to date has attempted to evaluate the relationship of perceived value to follow-up compliance. Data on this would certainly be a valuable addition to the outcome literature.

RESEARCH ON THERAPEUTIC FACTORS IN INPATIENT POPULATIONS

The findings from studies of inpatient group therapy merit consideration here; more specifically, 11 studies have reported data regarding therapeutic factors evaluated by inpatient group participants (Brabender, Albrecht, Sillitti, Cooper, & Kramer, 1983; Chase, 1991; Colijn, Hoencamp, Snijders, van der Spek, & Duivenvoorden, 1991; Kahn, Webster, & Storck, 1986; Leszcz, Yalom, & Norden, 1985; Macaskill, 1982; Marcovitz & Smith, 1983; Maxmen, 1973; Mushet, Whalan, & Power, 1989; Schaffer & Dryer, 1982; Whalan & Mushet, 1986), and two others have provided data from a correctional institution (Steinfeld & Mabli, 1974) and a long-term day hospital (Butler & Fuhriman, 1983b). Of these 10, only two studies (Chase, 1991; Leszcz et al., 1985) presented data separately for high- and low-functioning patients, and only one compared the perceptions of group members with those of their inpatient therapists (Schaffer & Dreyer, 1982). In addition, the results from two of these studies are difficult to integrate with other relevant data because of significant methodological differences (e.g., the nature and duration of group treatment provided) acknowledged by the authors (Brabender et al., 1983; Colijn et al., 1991).

Not surprisingly, a wide range of therapeutic factors has been identified as helpful in these investigations. However, if these factors are considered interdependent and we are prepared to identify clusters of factors which probably operate in consort, then we may begin to make some sense of the findings reported. In their review of the literature, Butler and Fuhriman (1983a) suggested that catharsis, self-understanding, interpersonal learning, universality, and cohesiveness were valued most, while family reenactment and identification were regarded as least helpful in inpatient groups. In contrast, they note that outpatients reported the same factors as least helpful, but evaluated hope, cohesiveness, altruism, and universality as most helpful. Yalom (1985) points out that, with the exception of higher functioning inpatients, most hospitalized patients do not select the same constellation of factors (interpersonal learning, catharsis, and self-understanding) as do outpatients. He indicates that because inpatients tend to feel so demoralized and dysfunctional, and because they may have exhausted available resources in the form of friends, family, and therapists, many more inpatients than outpatients highlight the value of the instillation of hope and the assumption of responsibility as important therapeutic factors. Similarly, Chase (1991) found that children and adolescents value hope, cohesiveness, and universality. His higher functioning subjects appeared to place greater weight on the exploratory processes of feedback and understanding than did lower functioning subjects. Results from two studies (Brabender et al., 1983; Mushet et al., 1989) also point to the relative importance ascribed to vicarious learning by inpatients, as compared with outpatients. Indeed, Mushet et al. (1989) have suggested that inpatients seem to place greater importance on supportive morale-boosting factors such as universality, acceptance, hope, and altruism, whereas outpatients emphasize the value of self-understanding and learning from interpersonal interaction, factors that appear to be more related to doing psychological work. The influence of these latter factors might well take longer to evolve and might be of much more relevance for outpatients who, in comparison to inpatients, are not as likely to be so demoralized, dysfunctional, and intent upon crisis resolution.

In a comparison of acute inpatients' and their behaviorally oriented therapists' views about effective therapeutic factors, Schaffer and Dryer (1982) report significant disagreements. Consistent with their theoretical orientations, therapists overestimated the importance of modeling, behavioral experimentation, and catharsis, and underestimated the importance of advice, altruism, self-understanding, universality, insight, and family reenactment.

More recently, Hoge and McLoughlin (1991) attempted to integrate findings from previous research by averaging the rank orders reported in other studies in an effort to "minimize the effects that might be attributable to particular program or patient characteristics in each individual study." They identify a cluster of seven factors—self-responsibility, self-understanding, hope, cohesiveness, catharsis, altruism, and universality—as critical to promoting patient change, and, like others before them (e.g., Maxmen, 1978; Yalom, 1983) recommend that therapists adopt specific techniques to enhance the operation of these factors. However, it should be noted that their process of data analysis, simple averaging of the ranks reported for specific factors, runs the risk of obscuring important differences found across studies which may be a function of type of patient, group, or setting, or may result from the particular procedure and timing followed during data collection.

While these efforts to identify the crucial therapeutic factors that underlie inpatient group therapy are laudable, this area of investigation has been subject to a variety of criticism. Several reviewers (e.g., Colijn et al., 1991) have noted that this research has been, for the most part, intermittent and noncumulative (Bloch & Crouch, 1985; Coché & Dies, 1981; Kaul & Bednar, 1986), and has relied upon unsophisticated methods of statistical analysis (Bloch & Crouch, 1985; Fuhriman et al., 1986; Dies, 1987). Different therapeutic factors have been investigated across studies, using different data collection procedures, yielding results that are not always comparable. Results from different patient populations exposed to differing models of group therapy have varied in accord with patients' diagnoses and their levels of functioning, their length of time in the group, and the type of group treatment provided. Often the results have not been clearly linked with therapeutic outcome; patients who are successfully treated may provide us with different information from those who are not. Also, little attention has been devoted to the relationships between each of these variables and: (1) the patients' ego strength, goals, level of motivation for change, and phase of illness/recovery, (2) the developmental phase of the group, and (3) the overall mission and therapeutic philosophy of the unit on which the group is being held.

The operation of therapeutic factors needs to be considered part of a dynamic process that includes patient, therapist, group, and overall therapeutic context as important interacting variables. Their comparative potency poses a complex question since "different factors are valued by different types of therapy group, by the same group at different developmental stages, and by different patients within the same group depending upon individual needs and strengths" (Yalom, 1985, p.111). Thus, this literature may serve to sensitize us to those aspects of the inpatient group therapy experience that most patients evaluate as helpful, may enable us to better focus our efforts to enhance the effects of these therapeutic factors during various phases of group life, and may provide a set of guidelines for making empirically based decisions about therapeutic models and techniques. However, current attempts to delineate a generic model for inpatient group therapy based upon the results from these studies may be somewhat overzealous and even misguided. The one-size-fits-all idea seems premature. Yet this area of research holds enormous promise, and, as Maxmen (1978) cautioned, patients must be assisted to benefit from and to survive our theories, many of which are not firmly anchored to any empirical database.

STRUCTURE OF THE GROUP

The structure of the group refers to all of the features that define a group in a treatment context, including format and the frame of the group. The format of the session refers to how the session is conducted. An important aspect of session format that has received attention in the empirical literature is the degree of structure that the therapist builds into the session. While some therapists design a group with a very prescribed, articulated format, others allow events in the group to unfold more freely and spontaneously. Among the structural elements which therapists commonly incorporate into the format of a session are an orientation, the formulation of agenda, the systematic reporting on homework, and the provision of a summary at the end of the session. Certainly, the wide variation within the field on degree of structure may leave the individual therapist wondering what level of structure is appropriate for his or her group.

Existing research suggests that the decision on degree of structure should be in part driven by the consideration of the level of functioning of the group members. Leszcz (1986) found that high- and low-functioning patients more highly valued relatively unstructured and structured groups respectively. Moreover, several studies (e.g., Goldstein, 1971; Gruen, 1977; Jensen & McGrew, 1974) suggest that with extremely disturbed patients, a high level of structure increases the likelihood that members' interactions will be positively toned. However, Greene and Cole (1991) demonstrated that level of functioning must be considered in the light of the patient's dynamics. They found that lower functioning patients functioned better in a highly structured, task-oriented activity, but only if the patient exhibited the kind of anaclitic pathology characterized by a felt difficulty in maintaining close, stable relationships with others. If the individual's psychopathology was more introjective and therefore characterized by a problem in achieving a consistently positive view of self, then the patient was less sensitive to degree of structure regardless of level of functioning.

The developmental level of the group also must be considered. A high level of structure appears to be most appropriate in the earliest stages of the life of a group (Bednar, Melnick, & Kaul, 1974; Kinder & Kilmann, 1976). Hence, while groups with rapid membership turnover may profit from a well-defined sequence of group events, in longer term inpatient groups, a somewhat looser format may be desirable.

An important aspect of session format concerns the focus of the group. The therapist could focus on problems arising outside the group and the historical underpinnings of these problems (i.e., a there-and-then focus) or on the phenomena emerging within the group itself (i.e., a here-and-now focus). Existing research suggests that archaeological excavations of the there-and-then, and systematic attempts to expose for purposes of interpretation, unresolved transference reactions in an effort to promote structural change, generally prove to be unproductive and ill-advised (Coons, 1957; Kanas et al., 1980; Lomont et al.,1969; Roback, 1972; Watson & Lacey, 1974).

The frame of the group refers to the specific organizational features that define the group, such as time, place, frequency of meeting, locus of the group in the setting, selection criteria, and leadership structure. Most of the research pertaining to the organization of the group has focused on the relationship between group composition and outcome, as reviewed in the outcome section. The following focuses on the more limited research on noncompositional organizational features and their effect on either group process or outcome.

Time

The temporal variables that define a group include: (a) the length of a member's participation in the group, (b) whether the group is closed-ended or open-ended, (c) the duration of group sessions, and (d) the frequency of group sessions. The authors are aware of no inpatient studies in which temporal parameters are used as independent variables. However, one relevant question particularly in view of ever-declining lengths of hospitalization is whether there is some minimal number of sessions below which positive outcomes cannot be realized.

Existing outcome studies indicate that for some approaches, positive outcomes can be demonstrated over a very small number of sessions. For example, Mueser et al. (1990) found that in a short-term setting a minimum of two sessions was necessary to enhance social skills among acute psychiatric patients. Mueser et al. (1991) reported similar findings with severely disturbed patients being treated for acute exacerbations (e.g., persons with schizophrenic or schizoaffective disorders) who participated in social skills training groups for an average of six sessions. Members showed improvement in the targeted skills at the end of treatment and at a one-month follow-up. However, the study also shows the necessity of considering the characteristics of the subjects in evaluating the adequacy of the temporal frame. They found that subjects with good memory, as measured by the Wechsler Memory Scale, made greater gains during this period than subjects with poor memory. However, neither diagnosis nor medication dosage was predictive of outcome. Katz (1986) demonstrated that relative to controls, patients who had social skills training in assertiveness showed greater improvement in self-reported assertiveness over the course of seven sessions. Zappe and Epstein (1987) demonstrated an improvement in conflict resolutions skills in an acute-stay, mixed population of patients who received group assertiveness training over four to six sessions.

These studies focused on patients with acute disturbances. With chronic state hospital patients, successful treatment probably requires longer duration. Thus, the briefest reported length of successful treatment with a chronic population has been 12 hours (Field & Test, 1975; Finch & Wallace, 1977). However, in some studies, realization of treatment goals has taken longer than 150 hours (Liberman et al., 1984; Sacks & Berger, 1954; Yehoshua et al., 1985).

Another potentially limiting variable on the efficacy of group is the number of sessions per week. Yalom (1983) argues for scheduling inpatient group meetings as frequently as possible, ideally on a daily basis. However, there are outcome studies showing that gains can be realized with relatively few sessions per week. For example, Beutler et al. (1984) reported positive symptomatic change in an interpersonal group that met only twice weekly. Nevertheless, in this same study, the behavioral group showed no change. Hence, the minimum number of sessions necessary for a positive outcome may depend, at least in part, upon the approach used. Eriksen et al. (1986) had nonpsychotic inpatients with a DSM-III diagnosis of alcohol dependence participate in only a single session per week of a social skills group over an eight-week period. They found that, relative to a control discussion group, subjects in the experimental group showed, at one-year follow-up, fewer hospital days, a greater number of working days, and the consumption of less alcohol. Zerhusen, Boyle, and Wilson (1991) provided twice weekly cognitive-behavioral group therapy for residents of a nursing home over a 10-week period. Compared to participants in a music group or control group, the members of the psychotherapy group reported less depression.

While the results of these studies suggest that patients can indeed benefit from an infrequently meeting group or a brief group experience, they do not indicate that all approaches are likely to be equally effective, nor that all types of patients are able to profit from groups conducted under these temporal restrictions. Moreover, because these studies did not use frequency or number of sessions as independent variables, they do not show whether any positive effects of a particular group approach are enhanced by more frequent meetings or a greater total number of sessions.

In addition, there is the issue of duration of group sessions and total time spent in group. No systematic research data are available to answer the question of what length of session is most desirable for what type of patients using what type of group approach. Clinical experience, however, suggests that while some inpatient groups have involved a 90-minute session typical of outpatient groups (Brabender et al., 1983; Coché et al., 1984; Powell et al., 1988), shorter durations are more commonly reported in the literature. Nor is there available research data to indicate how much time needs to be spent in group therapy sessions to accomplish particular changes. Once again, clinical experience dictates that the goals of the group must be appropriately scaled to fit the patients' needs and capacities, as well as the total time available to address these issues.

A third temporal variable concerns the open versus closed nature of the group. In fact, positive outcomes have been associated with both close-ended (e.g., Coché et al., 1984; Zappe & Epstein, 1987) and open-ended (e.g., Beutler et al., 1984; Douglas & Mueser, 1990) formats. Essentially, the dimension that is being tapped is the stability of group membership. That stability may indeed affect the group process if not its outcome was demonstrated by Schopler and Galinsky (1990) who surveyed the leaders of 115 open-ended groups, including both inpatient and outpatient populations. They asked the therapists to what extent the group had completed certain formative tasks such as agreeing on the purpose of the group or bonding among members. They found that the degree to which groups had accomplished these goals was directly related to membership stability: the greater the membership stability, the greater the group's progress in completing these formative tasks. The importance of this finding is that the completion of the formative tasks would seem, at least at face level, to facilitate the group's work within virtually any approach. Hence, while studies show that some groups with rapid turnover can accomplish their goals, it is probably of benefit to the group to have as much membership stability as possible.

Size

There are two studies in the literature which address the relationship between group size and process or outcome. The first study (Castore, 1962), based on the observation of 55 inpatient groups, examined the number of verbal interrelationships among members as a function of group size. A verbal interrelationship was defined as a response that a member directed toward a particular other member. Castore found that the number of verbal interrelationships dropped when a group had more than eight members, and concluded that the optimal size of a group is between five and eight members.

In a second study, Schroeder, Bowen, and Twemlow (1982) studied dropout rates from an inpatient alcoholism treatment program over a 12-year span as a function of the size of the groups in the program. Psychotherapy groups were among the groups studied. They found that as the size of the group increased, dropout rate increased concomitantly. Since the group size varied from 5 to 10 members, the investigators concluded that the optimal group size is 5 members. In explaining their results, the investigators cite Hare's (1976) review of the small group literature which points to the general finding that as size of the group increases, the affectional ties among members diminish and inhibition increases. They suggest that when it is necessary to work with larger groups, leaders should actively promote members' development of affectional ties.

These studies sought to determine the optimal size for the inpatient group. The importance of patients' diagnoses and levels of functioning for optimal group size has been subjected to limited empirical investigation. The question of optimal group size, however, may have little relevance because typically the group therapist must accommodate to the waxing and waning census of the unit. A more practical question is whether there is some number of members below which and above which a given approach is rendered ineffective.

In a highly structured treatment that emphasizes individually-directed interventions, small size does not seem to preclude the demonstration of a positive effect. The behaviorally oriented social skills approach appears to be compatible with a small-sized group. Matson et al. (1980) provided social skills training to children with difficulties managing their aggression (ages 9–11). There were four subjects in the group. They found that "treatment enhanced verbal and nonverbal components (e.g., verbal response, affect, eye contact, and body posture) of effective responding across a variety of positive situations, including giving compliments, giving help and making appropriate requests" (p. 529). Liberman et al. (1984) provided social skills group therapy to a group of three schizophrenics over an eight-week period, six times a week. They found that gains were revealed on the Behavioral Assessment Test immediately following the treatment and were sustained by two of the three members at a three-month follow-up. Rice and Chaplin (1979) compared the effects of social skills group psychotherapy (n = 5) versus a control group (n = 5) in a cross-over design in which each group ultimately received the experimental treatment. They found that participants in the social skills training performed in a superior fashion on a role-playing assessment. Furthermore, they found that in the one-year follow-up, none of the group members had engaged in any further fire-setting behavior.

While these studies show the possibility of obtaining a positive effect with a small number of group members, it must be emphasized that in all cases, the treatment was more structured and the therapist more directive than is often the case in inpatient groups. These technical features as well as the more highly operationalized goals of the social skills and problem-solving models may make less necessary the range of interpersonal resources that is often seen as essential to an effective working group.

Fewer studies are available on relatively large-sized groups. Monti et al. (1979) compared the effects of social skills training, bibliotherapy, and no group therapy in groups of 20 subjects. Sessions lasted for one hour. They found that subjects in the social skills training group showed greater improvement on the Bathers Assertiveness Scale and on simulated interaction at the conclusion of the two-week intervention and again 10 months later, relative to the other two groups.

Ghuman and Sarles (1989) provided anecdotal data on a more interpersonally oriented long-term adolescent group of 12 members. Therapists complained that the large size of the group precluded their attending to all members. The group was "large enough to permit some members to remain silent or hidden. It was difficult for some patients to open up in such a large group and instead they continued to act out" (p. 162).

Leadership Structure: Single Therapist versus Co-Therapy

While in the outpatient literature lively debate continues regarding the desirability of solo leadership versus co-therapy (e.g., Klein & Bernard, in press), there is considerable agreement that the presence of more than one therapist in an inpatient group has a number of advantages (e.g., Block, 1961; Kibel, 1992; Yalom, 1983). Many writers emphasize the great emotional demand inpatients place upon therapists and the usefulness of having a co-worker in the group to both provide support and assist in the exploration of members' reactions (e.g., Klein, Hunter, & Brown, 1986, 1990). It is also frequently noted in the literature that inpatient settings are training sites and it is useful for a junior group therapist to have a senior therapist available for supervision and modeling. Indirect empirical support for the co-therapy model comes from a study by Greene, Rosenkrantz, and Muth (1986) showing that the presence of a difference between group therapists in their countertransference reactions to a co-led group can be diagnostic of the defenses being used by the group. In a solo leadership group, such diagnostic information would be unavailable through this means.

The issues that pertain to inpatient group psychotherapy concern the relationship of the group therapists to the treatment team and the ideal number of group leaders. The leadership structure of an inpatient group often reflects the lines along which patients are organized into groups. Yalom (1983) distinguishes between team-group and level-group formats. The team group format involves organizing patients into groups depending upon what treatment team is responsible for their care. In such a circumstance, the leaders are drawn from the treatment team and it is not unusual to have more than two leaders. Typically, there are representatives of different disciplines (e.g., Ghuman & Sarles, 1989; Klein, 1977, 1983b) with the specific representatives frequently varying from session to session (Cory & Page, 1978). In the levels groups, members are organized according to level of functioning (or it could be another compositional variable such as symptom pattern). In such cases, the leaders may not be members of the treatment team and may not be interdisciplinary (e.g., Brabender, 1985).

The authors are aware of no systematic comparisons of these types of leadership formats aside from a study in which members reported preferring the level group over the team group (Leszcz et al., 1985). However, whether this patient reaction pertained to the leadership structure of the group is unclear. Future research should address whether outcome is enhanced by leaders drawn from the treatment team or independent of the treatment team, and whether there is a certain number of therapists that is optimal for the group. Certainly, these factors must be addressed in their interaction with the types of patients being treated and the group approach used. For example, the application of the object relations/systems approach which specifically examines the interconnections between the group and the unit may be catalyzed by the presence of representatives of the treatment team. Conversely, a model which focuses more intensively on the dynamics of the group (e.g., the developmental model) may be run more effectively by leaders who are independent of the treatment team.

The Techniques of the Therapist

Although it is widely recognized that modifications in traditional outpatient therapist technique are required in order to conduct effective inpatient group therapy, relatively few techniques have been subjected to comprehensive investigation. For the most part, more specific behavioral techniques, in contrast to the more traditional psychodynamically-based techniques, have received much of the attention, specifically the use of homework, role playing, modeling, therapist reinforcement, and formalized feedback.

Homework

There is widespread use of the assignment of homework (i.e., giving patients specific tasks to complete outside the group session before the group reconvenes). The function of homework varies depending upon the group approach embraced: to empirically test or demonstrate the veracity of a particular belief; to aid in developing a more functional set of responses; to provide additional practice for a behavior or belief; or to increase the likelihood of generalization of a newly acquired skill to a setting outside the group. As a treatment technique, its importance varies depending upon the model used, ranging from a vital component of the treatment (Beck, Rush, Shaw, & Emery, 1979) to a rather adjunct and sometimes haphazard procedure.

However, despite its widespread use in the cognitive (Beck et al., 1979), cognitive-behavioral (Freeman et al., in press), problem solving (Coché 1987), and social skills training (Liberman et al., 1989) models of group, little systematic research has been done to determine the importance, parameters, and efficacy of homework (Primakoff, Epstein, & Covi, 1986). In an inpatient setting, Wong et al. (in press) recently reported that the addition of homework to a social skills training package with very regressed chronic schizophrenics increases generalization of the skills to be learned. When patients initially were acquiring the social skills, these often did not spontaneously transfer to the unit. However, when homework was then introduced, generalization of the skill to the unit setting improved significantly. While no studies have investigated homework as an independent variable in an inpatient group, there is some empirical evidence suggesting that homework results in a more substantial improvement in symptomatology in an outpatient group setting (Kazdin & Mascitelli, 1982; Neimeyer & Feixas, 1990; Neimeyer, Twentymen, & Prezant, 1985). However, its long-term effect is equivocal in that the differential substantive gains made initially may not be maintained after a 6–8 month period (Neimeyer & Feixas, 1990).

Despite the dearth of empirical evidence for its differential efficacy, the importance of homework in certain approaches is demonstrated by the myriad of group outcome studies that incorporate it as a component of treatment. In general, such studies have found that including homework as part of the group treatment has significantly improved patients' functioning over their baseline, or a control/discussion group condition. Homework has been used as part of successful group treatment for patients suffering from acute psychiatric disturbances (Douglas & Mueser, 1990; Katz, 1986; Monti et al., 1979; Mueser et al., 1990), alcoholics (Eriksen et al., 1986; Oei & Jackson, 1982), aggressive adolescents (Feindler et al., 1986), and chronic schizophrenics (Bellack et al., 1984; Brown & Munford, 1983; Liberman et al., 1984; Wallace & Liberman, 1985).

Bibliotherapy, a specific and unique type of homework, is often given to inpatients that participate in a cognitive-behavioral group therapy and is sometimes used in other social skills treatment packages, as well. It involves a reading assignment—usually either an explanation of a particular symptom, problem or syndrome, or instructions on how to change attitudes, affects, or behaviors. However, there are no studies demonstrating its efficacy as a significant component of a treatment package with inpatients in a group setting. Its use as a sole treatment has been found to improve functioning among anxious and depressed patients in an outpatient setting (Kassinove, Miller, & Kalin, 1980). But, the use of bibliotherapy as the sole treatment has been shown to have deleterious effects with inpatients in teaching such social skills as giving and receiving compliments and criticisms and starting conversations, when compared to a group therapy that combined instruction with role playing and discussion (Monti et al., 1979). This finding is consistent with most of the research on the use of bibliotherapy (Glasgow & Rosen, 1979). This kind of homework requires a good deal of concentration and self-motivation, attributes which inpatients at the time of their hospitalization often cannot access. However, these negative results should not be taken to mean that this technique as a component within the context of a broader treatment approach in a group setting could not have a significant impact on the efficacy of the treatment; it is worthy of further empirical exploration.

Role Playing

Role playing, also known as behavioral rehearsal, is a technique that is often used in cognitive-behavioral groups (Freeman et al., in press), problem-solving groups (Coché, 1987), social skills training groups (Douglas & Mueser, 1990). Whereas in some models such as the social skills training, it is considered an essential component to the treatment package in improving interpersonal skills (Mueser et al., 1990), in other models such as the problem-solving model, it is considered optional (Coché, 1987). Performance on a role play task is highly correlated with competence in social functioning for psychiatric patients (Bellack, Morrison, Mueser, Wade, & Sayers, 1990). Thus its utility as a legitimate activity in the group setting is twofold: as a reflection of social competence and a method to assess it, and as a technique to develop, modify, fine tune, and strengthen social behaviors likely to improve social functioning. Roleplaying is similar to homework in that its unique contribution to efficacy and outcome has not been teased out from the other components of the treatment. Yet it is clear that most studies that attempt to effect a specific behavioral change utilize role-playing technique. (See Brabender & Fallon, 1993 for a more complete listing of these studies.) There is evidence that groups that use role playing within the context of either the problem-solving approach or the social skills training have been found to be superior to discussion groups that do not use role playing in the treatment of patients with acute psychiatric conditions (Gutride et al., 1973; Lomont et al., 1969; Monti et al., 1979; Monti, Curran, Corriveau, DeLancey, & Hagerman, 1980), aggressive male adolescents (Feindler, et al., 1986) and chronic schizophrenics (Bellack et al., 1984; Brown & Munford, 1983; Fecteau & Duffy, 1986; Fiedler et al., 1979; Field & Test, 1975; Finch

& Wallace, 1977; Gutride et al., 1974; Liberman et al., 1984; Liberman et al., 1986; Peters & Jones, 1951; Wallace & Liberman, 1985; Williams et al., 1977; Wong et al., in press).

Mueser and his colleagues (Douglas & Mueser, 1990; Mueser et al., 1990) found that for diagnostically mixed patients in an acute care setting, outcome was influenced by role playing; the success of the group social skills training was related to the number of role plays that the patient engaged in during the group, but not to the number of sessions attended. That is, those patients that completed 5 or more role plays had significantly better outcomes than those that completed less than 5 role plays.

One diagnostic group, inpatient alcoholics, appear to have an equivocal response to role-playing technique. While most studies report that an approach involving role playing is superior to a discussion group (Eriksen et al., 1986; Chaney et al., 1978; Jackson & Oei, 1978; Oei & Jackson, 1980), Jones et al. (1982) found that both social skills training with role playing and a discussion group did better than control groups in terms of members' abstinence. The approach that involved role playing, however, was not superior to a discussion group. Comparison of two different active treatments—cognitive restructuring (no role playing) and social skills training (with role playing)—revealed that, on follow-up, cognitive restructuring was more effective than social skill training in decreasing alcohol consumption (Jackson & Oei, 1978; Oei & Jackson, 1982).

Modeling

Whether therapists intend it or not, their behaviors serve as a model for members and potentially influence their behaviors. Elsewhere it has been empirically demonstrated that outpatient group leaders' behaviors can have a significant impact on the group-as-a-whole and the behavior of its individual members (Dies, 1977; Dies, 1983). Many fewer studies address the effect that therapists' behaviors have on inpatient members. These studies can be placed into two categories. The first involves a visual demonstration of particular behaviors to the group, which is known as modeling. The model can be live (therapist or designate) or in the form of a videotape. Focusing the patients' attention on certain aspects of social interaction is usually done by verbal instruction and then demonstration. This technique is often associated with behavioral group approaches. The second involves the more subtle presence of a particular behavior or aspect of the therapist and is often intimately intertwined with the therapist's reinforcement of particular behaviors. This form occurs either with intent or inadvertently in all group approaches. Two examples are the therapists' personal disclosures to the group and the verbal presentation to the group of various explanations or formulations of problems. For instance, Roback (1972) in his insight group condition modeled interpretive procedures by presenting hypotheses about the relationship between current feelings, attitudes, or behavior and past sociopsychological experiences.

In most efficacy studies, when a modeling technique is used, it is usually accompanied by verbal instruction, suggesting that the best results require both. However, the research on the relative importance of instruction and modeling together and separately is somewhat more equivocal. Goldstein et al., (1973) found that with a group of chronic schizophrenics either modeling or verbal instruction was superior to groups that had neither in increasing independent behavior; there was no advantage to providing both modeling and instructions. Some evidence suggests, however, that modeling alone is not effective in producing changes in many interpersonal behaviors such as the development of empathy (Vitalo, 1971). The development of more complex and subtle social behaviors may require modeling in conjunction with other techniques such as direct instruction and feedback (Vitalo, 1971). Indeed modeling has been shown to improve some behaviors such as the kind and amount of affective display, but that additional instruction and feedback may be necessary to develop certain kinds of nonverbal gestures and appropriate amounts of eye contact (Edelstein & Eisler, 1976).

Within the context of a more comprehensive treatment package, the use of therapist modeling and instructions in a group setting has produced a significant improvement in outcome with alcoholics (Chaney et al., 1978; Eriksen et al., 1986), acute psychiatric states (Douglas & Mueser, 1990; Mueser et al., 1990), and chronic schizophrenics (Bellack et al., 1984; Brown & Munford, 1983; Fecteau & Duffy, 1986; Field & Test, 1975; Finch & Wallace, 1977; Goldstein et al., 1973; Liberman et al., 1984; Magaro & West, 1983; Wallace & Liberman, 1985; Williams et al., 1977). Most instruction and modeling focuses on specific social skills such as assertiveness (Eriksen et al., 1986; Field & Test, 1975; Finch & Wallace, 1977), conversational skills (Bellack et al., 1984; Fecteau & Duffy, 1986; Goldstein et al., 1973; Liberman et al., 1984; Magaro & West, 1983; Wallace & Liberman, 1985; Williams et al., 1977), handling difficult situations (Chaney et al., 1978), compromise and negotiation (Mueser et al., 1990; Douglas & Mueser, 1990), and life skills, such as finance, time management, and community networking (Brown & Munford, 1983).

Videotapes have also been used for modeling purposes. Teaching conversation skills to groups of chronic schizophrenics (Gutride et al., 1974, Gutride et al., 1973; Kelly et al., 1980) and teaching adolescent males how to handle anger (Feindler et al., 1986) have both been successfully implemented with the use of videotaped models.

Two studies have attempted to look at the relative importance of role playing, instructions, and modeling. In a study comparing the use of a remedial drama group (role playing, but no instruction or feedback), with a social skills group (role playing, instruction, and modeling) and with a discussion group control, chronic schizophrenic patients in the social skills group had a significantly better outcome than those in the remedial drama group or in the discussion group (Spencer, Gillespie, & Ekisa, 1983). Role playing alone was insufficient to improve these patients' social skills. Eisler, Blanchard, Fitts, and Williams (1978) attempted to further tease apart these components with homogeneous groups of psychotic and nonpsychotic patients. Some patients were involved in role playing with positive reinforcement, but no instruction or coaching. Some received coaching and feedback along with the role playing. A third condition had groups with modeling, role playing, coaching, and feedback. Eisler et al. (1978) found that, in general, role playing with coaching and feedback was sufficient to teach patients what to say verbally. The addition of modeling improved the style of delivery as reflected in nonverbal measures. For nonpsychotic patients, modeling produced little supplemental improvement, and role playing alone produced almost as much improvement as role playing with feedback. However, for psychotic patients, modeling was critical in producing consistent improvement.

The Role of Therapist Reinforcement and Formalized Feedback

The use of concrete reinforcement with inpatient groups has produced some limited, but positive results, particularly with the more chronic populations. Doty (1975), using a social skills training approach, compared the presence and absence of a small monetary incentive ($2.50/session) for group attendance. He found that patients in the monetary incentive condition showed greater improvement on ward behavior and more social responsiveness in group discussion than those not in the incentive condition. Hauserman, Zweback, and Plotkin (1972) also achieved positive results by distributing tokens to facilitate verbal exchange in a group of adolescents. They found that many nonverbal adolescents who generally are considered poor candidates for group were able to participate in the group sessions and that once the initiations increased, peer social reinforcement aided in decreasing inappropriate and irrelevant verbalizations. Using food and drink as primarily reinforcers, Wong et al. (in press) were able to teach chronic schizophrenics who had previously failed at social skills training to improve their social skills in the session and on the ward. On the other hand, Lopez, Hoyer, Goldstein, Gershaw, and Sprafkin (1980) did not find that a monetary incentive promoted social skills training with a group of geriatric state hospital patients.

With recent technological advances, the technique of formalized feedback by way of videotaping group sessions and/or members can now be offered. The immediacy and objectivity of the videotape can potentially optimize self-exploration (Stoller, 1967). Videotape feedback appears to result in less defensiveness than verbal feedback (Pinney, 1963), and more recognition of particular traits previously resisted (Kidorf, 1963). It has been used as part of the procedure in a number of outcome studies that have improved social skills. It has been successfully used in studies with adolescents (Fiedler et al., 1979), acute psychiatric states (Monti et al., 1980), chronic schizophrenics (Gutride et al., 1973), and alcoholics (Oei & Jackson, 1982). In each of these studies, the video viewing is not a passive process since the therapist or other members can prescreen the material and direct the individual's attention to specific segments of behavior considered important. Thus, while videotaping may offer certain advantages, it is unclear whether its use results in an improvement in social interchange that is superior to verbal feedback. Robinson (1970) compared video feedback to verbal feedback in a study with hospitalized patients. Half the groups were videotaped. After each group, patients participated either in a discussion group or a discussion that focused on the videotape. During the videotape discussion, the therapist reinforced specific strengths and appropriate behavioral patterns. Independent raters then evaluated patient interactions in the group setting. Patients who received the focused video feedback engaged in more adaptive responses and fewer maladaptive responses than those in the discussion sessions, with the greatest difference between the groups being in the adaptive responses. Interestingly, there were no group differences in the way that subjects perceived their improvement; all subjects saw themselves as moderately improved as a result of their group experience (Robinson, 1970). There results suggest that visual feedback can be more helpful in furthering appropriate interpersonal interaction than verbal feedback.

Pretraining

In some settings, an effort is made to enhance members' awareness of the group structure through the use of pretraining. While specific pretraining formats can vary greatly, they generally involve orienting members to the goals, temporal and spatial aspects, group rules, and some exposure to the process of the group. Sometimes the preparation leads to the patient's acceptance of a therapeutic contract in which the patient agrees to abide by the group rules and to attempt to engage in those behaviors that are regarded as consistent with the group goals (Rice & Rutan, 1987). The topic of pretraining seems to have been of greater interest to researchers of the inpatient group in the 1960s and 1970s than it is currently. This reduced level of interest may be due to a perception that there is not sufficient time for pretraining to occur (Yalom, 1983).

The results of early research on pretraining leads to a cautiously optimistic conclusion about its usefulness. The clearest positive effect of pretraining appears to be to encourage a higher level of activity early in the member's participation in the group. For example, in a particularly well-designed study, Heitler (1973) used an anticipatory socialization interview with an experimental group. The purpose of the interview was to develop appropriate expectations about the group therapy situation. He found that "the prepared patients tended to have lower latencies for voluntary participation, to communicate more frequently, to spend more clock time communicating, to communicate more frequently on a self-initiated basis, to engage in self-exploratory efforts more frequently, and to do so in a greater percentage of their communications" (p. 259). Similarly, Pastushak (1978), using videotaped preparation, found that prepared subjects exhibited greater interpersonal openness and a higher level of self-disclosure. However, Jacobs, Trick, and Withersty (1976) found that although prepared inpatients evidenced greater knowledge of role expectancies, they did not exhibit a greater tendency toward behavior consistent with this knowledge.

A second area which may be affected by pretraining is whether or not the member prematurely leaves the group. Heitler (1973) found that the dropout rate for prepared patients was less than that for unprepared patients.

A third area is outcome. Truax and Carkhuff (1965) studied the effects of an audiotaped pretraining in which state hospital patients got to hear excepts of "good" patient therapy behavior. The investigators found that the pretrained subjects, relative to the control subjects, obtained larger positive changes on Scales 7 and 8 of the MMPI than did the controls. All other MMPI comparisons were nonsignificant. Truax, Wargo, Carkhuff, Kodman, and Moles (1966) studied the effects of this same audiotaped pretraining on institutionalized juvenile delinquents and hospitalized mental patients. They found that pretrained subjects are more likely, as a function of group therapy, to construct ideal selves that are more consonant with a consensually validated view of the ideal person. However, their actual perception of themselves did not change with treatment. Similar results were obtained by Truax, Shapiro, and Wargo (1968). Hilkey, Wilhelm, and Horne (1982) studied the effects of pretraining on inmates in a medium-security federal penitentiary. While this is not an inpatient population, they found that prepared subjects made more progress toward individual goals as perceived by both therapists and peers than unprepared subjects.

Advice

Advice, often conceived as supportive in nature, if used judiciously can aid patients in attaining their goals. Flowers (1979) has posited that the use of certain kinds of advice in psychotherapy can enhance therapeutic outcome. He found that therapists' use of alternatives (statements about two or more possible ways of handling a situation) and instructions (statements explaining a step-by-step procedure for how to handle a situation) enabled patients to improve more on their goals than the therapists' use of simple advice (statements about what to do without an explanation on how to do it).

Summary

It must be emphasized that the topic of structure has particular importance given the nature of inpatient populations. While inpatient writers may disagree on specific structural issues, there is general agreement that it is essential that the structure of the inpatient group be well-defined for two reasons. First, a clearly delineated structure is critical given the fact that many members have lost access to the organizing structures available to them on a premorbid basis. Whereas a well-defined group structure serves as a model for internalization, an ambiguous structure is likely to promote further regression (Klein & Kugel, 1981; Rice & Rutan, 1987). Second, the success of any group is in large part determined by its endorsement by unit staff. If the staff see the group negatively, it has been demonstrated that group members are likely to acquire and reflect this attitude (Leonard, 1973). In order to develop a "progroup climate" (Rice & Rutan, 1981), the therapist must clearly specify the group's role in the overall treatment package and differentiate its contribution from that of other modalities (Klein, 1977, 1983b; MacKenzie, 1990; Maxmen, 1978).

Given the importance of the therapist's development of a clear structure, it is unfortunate that the research literature provides the therapist with very little direction on the effects of specific structural decisions on outcome. What is the impact on group outcome of having long versus short, frequent versus infrequent sessions, or a single therapist versus a co-therapy team? What are the effects of a closed- versus open-ended structure? The research literature is silent on these questions and a host of other issues that inevitably arise in the design of a group. One reason for this silence is that frequently the therapist does not have control over the many variables that define a group. For example, the overall treatment program may be organized so that all activities, including group therapy, are held three times a week. While more frequent sessions may be desirable, the therapist cannot implement this change without disrupting the overall program. Even more difficult would be to design a study in which frequency of sessions was manipulated.

Because the therapist rarely has control over all of the structural features of the group, the mission of the group and its structural features must be selected to be in concert with those of the treatment setting. That is, the pre-existing features inherent in the particular hospital setting limit the kinds of goals that can be pursued. For example, if members' participation is necessarily brief because hospitalization is brief, then certain goals which are inherently long-term in nature, such as intrapsychic conflict resolution, are likely to be unrealistic. On the other hand, rarely are all organizational features of the group fixed so that once the therapist has established goals which are congruent with pre-existing hospital features, the remaining structural features of the group can be selected with a view toward which ones will best promote its goals.

CONCLUSIONS

That group psychotherapy can be useful with an inpatient population has been clearly established. Numerous outcome studies indicate that patients benefit more from group treatment than no treatment or various alternate interventions. However, the existing outcome research is biased in that it is almost exclusively based upon the study of more behaviorally oriented approaches and is directed primarily to the examination of the short-term effects of group participation. Outcome research on the psychodynamic and interpersonal approaches, and the study of more long-term, post-hospital effects of group treatment would be welcome expansions of the literature. As demands for accountability (financial and clinical) increase, we will be called upon to demonstrate the unique contributions of group therapy to the complicated arsenal of treatment interventions available for inpatient care.

Nonetheless, from the outcome research that does exist, we can delineate certain features of those group approaches which have been demonstrated to hold benefit for their members. Successful approaches appear to have highly specific objectives and intervention strategies that are well-articulated and congruent with the established goals. Effective approaches appear to have a here-and-now rather than a historical focus. They also provide members with a clear cognitive framework for organizing the affective stimulation provoked by the group. Consistent with guidelines derived from research on effective leadership in short-term groups (e.g., Dies, 1983; Kanas, 1986; Klein, 1993b; MacKenzie, 1990), the inpatient group therapist, compared to his/her outpatient counterpart, apparently needs to assume a more active, directive, managerial, and flexible role. The development of treatment manuals may permit greater specificity and replicability of treatment approaches, and may enable us to determine which therapist behaviors and techniques reliably augment the operation of those therapeutic factors associated with successful outcome.

What needs to be done at this point is to study how outcome is affected by different approaches, interacting with various patient populations and treatment settings. While researchers have ready means for classifying patients, methods for identifying and classifying the salient parameters of treatment environments require further development.

Another area requiring empirical attention is group structure. Currently, decisions about the features of the group such as size, frequency of sessions, length of sessions, group format and agenda are made on the basis of practical considerations and happenstance. Systematic studies of these variables would enable more informed clinical decision making. These variables would also have to be considered in their interaction with patient and setting variables.

While the challenges to conducting rigorous research in the inpatient arena are many (Yalom, 1983), existing studies confirm that it is possible. Such efforts may be aided by the collaboration of clinicians and researchers working in different settings, thereby enabling the direct comparison of different patient populations and different settings within the same study.

REFERENCES

Albrecht, E., & Brabender, V. (1983). Alcoholics in inpatient, short-term interactional group psychotherapy: An outcome study. *Group, 7*(2), 50–54.

Anker, J. M., & Walsh, R. P. (1961). Group psychotherapy, a special activity program, and group structure in the treatment of chronic schizophrenics. *Journal of Consulting Psychology, 25,* 476–481.

Astrachan, B. M., Harrow, M., & Flynn, H. R. (1968). Influence of the psychiatric setting on behavior in group therapy meetings. *Social Psychiatry, 3*(4), 165–172.

Baker, M. (1993). Self psychology and group psychotherapy. In H. I. Kaplan & B. J. Saddock (Eds.), *Comprehensive group psychotherapy* (3rd ed., pp. 176–185). Baltimore, MD: Williams & Wilkins.

Beal, D., Duckro, P., Elias, J., & Hecht, E. (1977). Increased verbal interaction via group techniques with regressed schizophrenics. *Psychological Reports, 40,* 319–325.

Beard, M. T., & Scott, P. Y. (1975). The efficacy of group therapy by nurses for hospitalized patients. *Nursing Research, 24*(2), 120–124.

Beck, A. T., Rush, A. J., Shaw, B. F., & Emery, G. (1979). *Cognitive therapy of depression.* New York: Guilford Press.

Bednar, R. L., & Lawlis, C. F. (1971). Empirical research in group psychotherapy. In A. E. Bergin & S. L. Garfield (Eds.), *Handbook of psychotherapy and behavior change.* New York: Wiley.

Bednar, R. L., Melnick, J., & Kaul, T. J. (1974). Risk, responsibility, and structure: A conceptual framework for initiating group counseling and psychotherapy. *Journal of Counseling Psychology, 21,* 31–37.

Bellack, A. S., Morrison, R. L., Mueser, K. T., Wade, J. H., & Sayers, S. L. (1990). Role play for assessing the social competence of psychiatric patients. *Psychological Assessment: A Journal of Consulting and Clinical Psychology, 2*(3), 248–255.

Bellack, A. S., Turner, S. M., Hersen, M., & Luber, R. F. (1984). An examination of the efficacy of social skills training for chronic psychiatric patients. *Hospital and Community Psychiatry, 35,* 1023–1028.

Benson, B. A., Johnson, M., & Miranti, S. V. (1986). Effects of anger management training with mentally retarded adults in group therapy. *Journal of Consulting and Clinical Psychology, 54*(5), 728–729.

Beutler, L. E., Frank, M., Schieber, S. C., Calvert, S., & Gaines, J. (1984). Comparative effects of group psychotherapies in a short-term inpatient setting: An experience with deterioration effects. *Psychiatry, 47,* 66–76.

Bloch, S., & Crouch, E. (1985). *Therapeutic factors in group psychotherapy.* London: Oxford University Press.

Block, S. L. (1961). Multi-leadership as a teaching and therapeutic tool in group psychotherapy. *Comprehensive Psychiatry, 2,* 211–218.

Booraem, C. D., & Flowers, J. V. (1972). Reduction of anxiety and personal space as a function of assertion training with severely disturbed neuropsychiatric inpatients. *Psychological Reports, 30,* 923–929.

Brabender, V. (1985). Time-limited inpatient group therapy: A developmental model. *International Journal of Group Psychotherapy, 37*(3), 377–387.

Brabender, V., Albrecht, E., Sillitti, J., Cooper, J., & Kramer, E. (1983). A study of curative factors in short-term group psychotherapy. *Hospital and Community Psychiatry, 34,* 643–644.

Brabender, V., & Fallon, A. (1993). *Models of inpatient group psychotherapy.* Washington, DC: American Psychological Association.

Brown, M. A., & Munford, A. M. (1983). Life skills training for chronic schizophrenics. *The Journal of Nervous and Mental Disease, 171,* 466–470.

Butler, T., & Fuhriman, A. (1983a). Curative factors in group therapy: A review of the recent literature. *Small Group Behavior, 15,* 427–440.

Butler, T., & Fuhriman, A. (1983b). Level of functioning and length of time in treatment variables influencing patients' therapeutic experience in group psychotherapy. *International Journal of Group Psychotherapy, 33,* 489–505.

Cadman, W. H., Misbach, L., & Brown, D. V. (1954). An assessment of roundtable psychotherapy. *Psychological Monographs, 68*(13), 1–48.

Castles, E. E. (1983, March). Training in social skills and interpersonal problem-solving skills for mildly and moderately mentally retarded adults. *Dissertation Abstracts International, 3*(9), 3023-B.

Castore, G. F. (1962). Number of verbal interrelationships as a determinant of group size. *Journal of Abnormal and Social Psychology, 64*(6), 456–458.

Chaney, E. F., O'Leary, M. R., & Marlatt, G. A. (1978). Skill training with alcoholics. *Journal of Consulting and Clinical Psychology, 46,* 1092–1204.

Chase, J. L. (1991). Inpatient adolescent and latency-age children's perspectives on the curative factors in group psychotherapy, *Group, 15,* 95–108.

Coché, E. (1987). Problem-solving training: A cognitive group therapy modality. In A. Freeman & V. Greenwood (Eds.), *Cognitive therapy: Applications in psychiatric and medical settings.* New York: Human Sciences Press, Inc.

Coché, E., Cooper, J. B., & Petermann, K. J. (1984). Differential outcomes of cognitive and interactional group therapies. *Small Group Behavior, 15*(4), 497–509.

Coché, E., & Dies, R. R. (1981). Integrating research findings into the practice of group psychotherapy. *Psychotherapy: Theory, Research and Practice, 18*(4).

Coché, E., & Douglass, A. A. (1977). Therapeutic effects of problem-solving and play reading groups. *Journal of Clinical Psychology, 33,* 820–827.

Coché, E., & Flick, A. (1975). Problem-solving training group for hospitalized psychiatric patients. *Journal of Psychology, 91,* 19–29.

Cohen, S. R. (1982, January). A comparison of the effects of interpersonal problem-solving training groups and social interaction training groups on hospitalized psychiatric patients. *Dissertation Abstracts International, 42*(7), 2981-B.

Colijn, S., Hoencamp, E., Snijders, H. J., van der Spek, M. W., & Duivenvoorden, H. J. (1991). A comparison of curative factors in different types of group psychotherapy. *International Journal of Group Psychotherapy, 41,* 365–378.

Coons, W. H. (1957). Interaction and insight in group psychotherapy. *Canadian Journal of Psychology, 11,* 1–8.

Coons, W. H., & Peacock, E. P. (1970). Interpersonal interaction and personality change in group psychotherapy. *Canadian Psychiatric Association Journal, 15,* 347–355.

Cory, T. L., & Page, D. (1978). Group techniques for effecting change in the more disturbed patient. *Group, 2*(3), 149–155.

Cowden, R. C., Zax, M., Hague, J. R., & Finney, R. C. (1956). Chlorpromazine: Alone and as an adjunct to group psychotherapy in the treatment of psychiatric patients. *American Journal of Psychiatry, 112,* 898–902.

Cowden, R. C., Zax, M., & Spoles, J. A. (1956). Group psychotherapy in conjunction with a physical treatment. *Journal of Clinical Psychology, 12,* 53–56.

Dies, R. R. (1977). Group therapist transparency: A critique of theory and research. *International Journal of Group Psychotherapy, 27,* 177–200.

Dies, R. R. (1983). Clinical implications of research on leadership in short-term group psychotherapy. In R. R. Dies & K. R. Mackenzie (Eds.), *Advances in group psychotherapy,* (Chapter 2, pp. 27–78). New York: Universities Press.

Dies, R. R. (1987). Clinical application of research instruments: Editor's introduction. *International Journal of Group Psychotherapy, 37,* 31–38.

Donahoe, C. P., & Driesenga, S. A. (1988). A review of social skills training with chronic mental patients. In M. Hersen, R. Eisler, & P. M. Miller (Eds.), *Papers in behavior modification.* Newbury Park, CA: Sage.

Doty, D. W. (1975). Role playing and incentives in the modification of the social interaction of chronic psychiatric patients. *Journal of Consulting and Clinical Psychology, 43*(5), 676–682.

Douglas, M. S., & Mueser, K. T. (1990). Teaching conflict resolution skills to the chronically mentally ill. *Behavior Modification, 14*(4), 519–547.

Edelstein, B. R., & Eisler, R. M. (1976). Effects of modeling and modeling with instructions and feedback on the behavioral components of social skills. *Behavior Therapy, 7,* 382–389.

Eisler, R. M., Blanchard, E. B., Fitts, H., & Williams, J. G. (1978). Social skill training with and without modeling for schizophrenic and non-psychotic hospitalized psychiatric patients. *Behavior Modification, 2*(2), 147–171.

Erickson, R. (1987). The question of casualties in inpatient small group psychotherapy. *Small Group Behavior, 18,* 443–458.

Eriksen, L., Bjornstad, S., & Gotestam, G. (1986). Social skills training in groups for alcoholics: One-year treatment outcome for groups and individuals. *Addictive Behaviors, 11,* 309–329.

Ettin, M. F. (1988). Group building: Developing protocols for psychoeducational groups. *Group, 12*(4), 205–255.

Evangelakis, M. G. (1961). De-institutionalization of patients. *Diseases of the Nervous System, 22,* 26–32.

Fairweather, G. W., Simon, R., Gibhard, M. E., Weingarten, E., Holland, J. L., Sanders, R., Stone, G. B., & Reahl, J. E. (1960). Relative effectiveness of psychotherapeutic process: A multicriteria comparison of four programs for three different patient groups. *Psychological Monographs, 74*(1, Whole No. 492).

Fecteau, G. W., & Duffy, M. (1986). Social and conversational skills training with long-term psychiatric inpatients. *Psychological Reports, 59,* 1327–1331.

Feifel, H., & Schwartz, A. D. (1953). Group psychotherapy with acutely disturbed psychotic patients. *Journal of Consulting Psychology, 17,* 113–121.

Feindler, E. L., Ecton, R. B., Kingsley, D., & Dubey, D. R. (1986). Group anger control training for institutionalized psychiatric male adolescents. *Behavior Therapy, 17,* 109–123.

Fiedler, P. E., Orenstein, H., Chiles, J., Fritz, G., & Breitt, S. (1979). Effects of assertive training on hospitalized adolescents and young adults. *Adolescence, 14*(5), 523–528.

Field, G. D., & Test, M. A. (1975). Group assertive training for severely disturbed patients. *Journal of Behavioral Therapy and Experience in Psychiatry, 6,* 129–134.

Finch, B. E., & Wallace, C. J. (1977). Successful interpersonal skills training with schizophrenic inpatients. *Journal of Consulting and Clinical Psychology*, *45*(5), 885–890.

Flowers, J. V. (1979). Behavioral analysis of group therapy and a model for behavioral group therapy. In D. Upper & S. M. Ross (Eds.), *Behavioral group therapy 1979: An annual review*. Champaign, Ill: Research Press.

Foxx, R. M., McMorrow, J., Bittle, R. G., & Fenlon, S. J. (1985). Teaching social skills to psychiatric inpatients. *Behavioral Research Therapy*, *23*(5), 531–537.

Freeman, A. (1987). Cognitive therapy: An overview. In A. Freeman & V. Greenwood (Eds.), *Cognitive therapy: Applications in psychiatric and medical settings*. (pp. 19–35). New York: Human Sciences Press, Inc.

Freeman, A. Schrodt, G. R., Gilson, M., & Ludgate, J. (in press). Cognitive group therapy with inpatients. In J. Wright, A. Beck, M. These, & J. Ludgate (Eds.), *Cognitive therapy with inpatient populations*. New York: Guilford Press.

Fromme, D. K., & Smallwood, R. E. (1983). Group modification of affective verbalizations in a psychiatric population. *British Journal of Clinical Psychology*, *22*, 251–256.

Fuhriman, A., Drescher, S., Hanson, E., Henrie, R., & Rybicki, W. (1986). Refining the measurement of curativeness: An empirical approach. *Small Group Behavior*, *17*, 186–201.

Ghuman, H. S. & Sarles, R. M. (1989). Three group psychotherapy settings with long-term adolescent inpatients: Advantages and disadvantages. *The Psychiatric Hospital*, *19*(4), 161–164.

Gilbride, T. V., & Hebert, J. (1980). Pathological characteristics of good and poor interpersonal problem-solvers among psychiatric outpatients. *Journal of Clinical Psychology*, *36*, 121–127.

Glasgow, R. E., & Rosen, G. M. (1979). Self-help behavior therapy manuals: Recent developments and clinical usage. *Clinical Behavior Therapy Review*, *1*, 1–20.

Goldstein, A. P., Martens, J., Hubben, J., Van Belle, H. A., Schaff, W., Wiersma, H., & Goedhart, A. (1973). The use of modeling to increase independent behavior. *Behavior Research and Therapy*, *11*, 31–42.

Goldstein, J. A. (1971). Investigation of doubling as a technique for involving severely withdrawn patients in group therapy. *Journal of Consulting and Clinical Psychology*, *37*, 155–162.

Gorham, D. R., & Pokorny, A. D. (1964). Effects of a phenothiazine and/or group psychotherapy with schizophrenics. *Diseases of the Nervous System*, *25*, 77–86.

Greene, L. R., & Cole, M. B. (1991). Level and form of psychopathology and the structure of group therapy. *International Journal of Group Psychotherapy*, *41*(4), 499–521.

Greene, L. R., Rosenkrantz, J., & Muth, D. (1986). Borderline defenses and countertransference: Research findings and implications. *Psychiatry*, *9*(3), 253–264.

Greenwood, V. B., (1987). Cognitive therapy with the young adult chronic patient. In A. Freeman & V. Greenwood (Eds.), *Cognitive therapy: Applications in psychiatric and medical settings* (pp. 103–116). New York: Humans Sciences Press, Inc.

Gruen, W. (1977). The effects of executive and cognitive control of the therapist on the work climate in group therapy. *International Journal of Group Psychotherapy*, *27*, 139–152.

Gutride, M. E., Goldstein, A. P., & Hunter, G. F. (1973). The use of modeling and role playing to increase social interaction among asocial psychiatric patients. *Journal of Consulting and Clinical Psychology, 40*(3), 408–415.

Gutride, M. E., Goldstein, A. P., Hunter, G. F., Carrol, S., Clark, L., Furia, R., & Lower, W. (1974). Structured learning therapy with transfer training for chronic inpatients. *Journal of Clinical Psychology, 30*(3), 277–279.

Hare, A. P. (1976). *Handbook of small group research* (2nd ed.). New York: Free Press.

Hauserman, N., Zweback, S., & Plotkin, A. (1972). Use of concrete reinforcement to facilitate verbal initiations in adolescent group therapy. *Journal of Consulting and Clinical Psychology, 38,* 90–96.

Haven, G. A., Jr., & Wood, B. S. (1970). The effectiveness of eclectic group psychotherapy in reducing recidivism in hospitalized patients. *Psychotherapy: Theory Research and Practice, 7,* 153–154.

Heitler, J. B. (1973). Preparation of lower-class patients for expressive group psychotherapy. *Journal of Consulting and Clinical Psychology, 41*(2), 251–260.

Hilkey, J. H., Wilhelm, C. L., & Horne, A. M. (1982). Comparative effectiveness of videotape pretraining versus no pretraining on selected process and outcome variables in group therapy. *Psychological Reports, 50,* 1151–1159.

Hoge, M. A., & McLoughlin, K. A. (1991). Group psychotherapy in acute treatment settings: Theory and technique. *Hospital and Community Psychiatry, 42,* 153–158.

Hollon, S., & Beck, A. T. (1986). Cognitive and cognitive-behavioral therapies. In S. L. Garfield & A. E. Bergin (Eds.), *Handbook of psychotherapy and behavior change* (pp. 443–482). New York: Wiley.

Holmes, M. R., Hansen, D. J., & Lawrence, J. S. (1984). Conversational skills training with aftercare patients in the community: Social validation and generalization. *Behavior Therapy, 15,* 84–100.

Intagliata, J. C. (1978). Increasing the interpersonal problem-solving skills of an alcoholic population. *Journal of Consulting and Clinical Psychology, 46*(3), 489–498.

Jackson, P., & Oei, T. P. (1978). Social skills training and cognitive restructuring with alcoholics. *Drug and Alcohol Dependence, 3*(5), 369–374.

Jacobs, M. K., Trick, O. L., & Withersty, D. (1976). Pretraining psychiatric inpatients for participation in group psychotherapy. *Psychotherapy: Theory, Research and Practice, 13*(4), 361–367.

Jensen, J. L., & McGrew, W. L. (1974). Leadership techniques in group therapy with chronic schizophrenic patients. *Nursing Research, 23,* 416–420.

Jones, D. E. (1981, November). Interpersonal cognitive problem-solving training—A skills approach with hospitalized psychiatric patients. *Dissertation Abstract International, 42*(5), 101.

Jones, E. J., & McColl, M. A. (1991). Development and evaluation of an interactional life skills group for offenders. *Occupational Therapy Journal of Research, 11*(2), 81–92.

Jones, F. D., & Peters, H. N. (1952). An experimental evaluation of group psychotherapy. *Journal of Abnormal and Social Psychology, 47,* 345–353.

Jones, S. L., Kanfer, R., Lanyon, R. I. (1982). Skill training with alcoholics: A clinical extension. *Addictive Behaviors, 7*(3), 285–290.

Josephs, L., & Jhuman, L. (1985). The application of self psychology principles to long-term group therapy with schizophrenic patients. *Group, 9*(3), 21–30.

Joughin, N., Tata, P., Collins, M., Hooper, C., & Falkowski, J. (1991). In-patient withdrawal from long-term benzodiazepine use. *British Journal of Addiction, 86,* 449–455.

Kahn, E. M., Webster, P. B., & Storck, M. J. (1986). Curative factors in two types of inpatient psychotherapy groups. *International Journal of Group Psychotherapy, 36,* 579–585.

Kanas, N. (1986). Group therapy with schizophrenics: A review of controlled studies. *International Journal of Group Psychotherapy, 36*(3), 339–351.

Kanas, N., & Barr, M. A. (1982). Short-term homogeneous group therapy for schizophrenic inpatients: A questionnaire evaluation. *Group, 6*(4), 32–38.

Kanas, N., Rogers, M., Kreth, E., Patterson, L., & Campbell, R. (1980). The effectiveness of group psychotherapy during the first three weeks of hospitalization. *Journal of Nervous and Mental Diseases, 168,* 487–492.

Karterud, S. (1988). The influence of task definition, leadership and therapeutic style on inpatient group cultures. *International Journal of Therapeutic Communities, 9*(4), 231–247.

Kassinove, H., Miller, N., & Kalin, M. (1980). Effects of pretreatment with rational-emotive bibliography and rational-emotive audiotherapy on clients waiting at community health centers. *Psychological Reports, 46,* 851–857.

Katz, G. (1986). Group assertive training with psychiatric inpatients. *The Psychiatric Journal of the University of Ottawa, 22*(2), 62–67.

Katzenstein, A. (1954). An evaluation of three types of group psychotherapy with psychiatric patients. *International Journal of Group Psychotherapy, 4,* 409–418.

Kaul, T. J., & Bednar, R. L. (1986). Experimental group research: Results, questions, and suggestions. In S. L. Garfield & A. E. Bergin (Eds.), *Handbook of psychotherapy and behavior change.* New York: Wiley.

Kazdin, A. E., & Mascitelli, S. (1982). Covert and overt rehearsal and homework practice in developing assertiveness. *Journal of Consulting and Clinical Psychology, 50*(2), 250–258.

Kelly, J. A., Laughlin, C., Claiborne, M., & Patterson, J. (1979). A group procedure for teaching job interviewing skills to formerly hospitalized psychiatric patients. *Behavior Therapy, 10,* 299–310.

Kelly, J. A., Urey, J. R., & Patterson, J. (1980). Improving heterosocial conversational skills of male psychiatric patients through a small group training procedure. *Behavior Therapy, 11,* 179–188.

Kibel, H. D. (1978). The rationale for the use of group psychotherapy for borderline patients on a short-term unit. *International Journal of Group Psychotherapy, 28*(3), 339–358.

Kibel, H. D. (1981). A conceptual model for short-term inpatient group psychotherapy. *American Journal of Psychiatry, 181*(1), 74–80.

Kibel, H. (1990). The inpatient psychotherapy group as a testing ground for theory. In B. E. Roth, W. N. Stone, & H. D. Kibel (Eds.), *The difficult patient in group: Group psychotherapy with borderline and narcissistic disorders* (pp. 245–264). Madison, CT: International Universities Press.

Kibel, H. (1992). Inpatient group psychotherapy. In A. Alonso & H. Swiller (Eds.), *Group therapy in clinical practice* (pp. 93–112). Washington, DC: American Psychiatric Press.

Kidorf, I. W. (1963). A note on the use of tape recording during the therapy sessions. *International Journal of Group Psychotherapy, 13,* 211–213.

Kiesler, C. A., & Simpkins, C. (1991). The de facto national system of psychiatric inpatient care: Piecing together the national puzzle. *American Psychologist, 46*(6), 1–6.

Kinder, B. N., & Kilmann, L. P. R. (1976). The impact of differential shifts in leader structure on the outcome of internal and external group participants. *Journal of Clinical Psychology, 32,* 845–863.

Klein, R. H. (1977). Inpatient group psychotherapy: Practical considerations and special problems. *International Journal of Group Psychotherapy, 27*(2), 201–214.

Klein, R. H. (1983a). Group psychotherapy. In M. Hersen, A. E. Kazdin, & A. S. Bellack (Eds.), *The clinical psychology handbook* (pp. 593–610). New York: Permagon Press.

Klein, R. H. (1983b). A therapy group for adult inpatients on a psychiatry ward. In R. A. Rosenbaum (Ed.), *Handbook of short-term therapy groups* (pp. 291–320). New York: McGraw-Hill.

Klein, R. H. (1993a). Inpatient group psychotherapy: Old wine in new bottles? Paper presentation, American Group Psychotherapy Association,

Klein, R. H. (1993b). Short-term group therapy. In H. I. Kaplan & B. J. Sadock (Eds.), *Comprehensive group psychotherapy* (3rd ed.). Philadelphia, PA: Williams & Wilkins.

Klein, R. H., & Bernard, H. S. (in press). Using co-therapy in group therapy with borderline and narcissistic patients. In V. Schermer & M. Pines (Eds.), *The ring of fire.* London: Routledge & Paul.

Klein, R. H., Bernard, H. S., & Singer, D. L. (1992). *Handbook of contemporary group psychotherapy.* Madison, CT: International Universities Press.

Klein, R. H., Hunter, D. E. K., & Brown, S. L. (1986). Long-term inpatient group psychotherapy: The ward group. *International Journal of Group Psychotherapy, 36*(3), 361–380.

Klein, R. H., Hunter, D. E. K., & Brown, S. L. (1990). Long-term inpatient group psychotherapy. In B. E. Roth, W. N. Stone, & H. D. Kibel (Eds.), *The difficult patient in group.* Madison, CT: International Universities Press.

Klein, R. H., & Kugel, B. (1981). Inpatient group psychotherapy from a systems perspective: Reflections through a glass darkly. *International Journal of Group Psychotherapy, 31*(3), 311–328.

Koch, H. C. H. (1983). Correlates of changes in personal construing of members of two psychotherapy groups: Changes in affective expression. *British Journal of Medical Psychology, 56,* 323–327.

Kofoed, L., & Keys, A. (1988). Using group therapy to persuade dual-diagnosis patients to seek substance abuse treatment. *Hospital and Community Psychiatry, 39*(11), 1209–1211.

Kohut, H. (1977). *The restoration of the self.* New York: International Universities Press.

Kohut, H. (1984). *How does analysis cure?* Chicago, IL: University of Chicago Press.

Kraus, A. R. (1959). Experimental study of the effect of group psychotherapy with chronic psychotic patients. *International Journal of Group Psychotherapy, 9,* 293–302.

Laben, J. K., Dodd, D., & Sneed, L. (1991). King's theory of goal attainment applied in group therapy for inpatient juvenile sexual offenders, maximum security state offenders, and community parolees, using visual aids. *Issues in Mental Health Nursing, 12,* 51–64.

Lemberg, R., & May, M. A. (1991). What works in inpatient treatment of eating disorders: The patient's point of view. *British Review of Bulimia and Anorexia Nervosa, 5*(1), 29–38.

Leonard, C. V. (1973). What helps most about hospitalization. *Comprehensive Psychiatry, 14,* 365–369.

Leszcz, M. (1986). Interactional group psychotherapy with nonpsychotic inpatients. *Group, 10*(1), 13–20.

Leszcz, M., Yalom, I. D., & Norden, M. (1985). The value of inpatient group psychotherapy: Patients' perceptions. *International Journal of Group Psychotherapy, 35*(3), 411–433.

Liberman, R. P., DeRisi, W. J., & Mueser, K. T. (1989). *Social skills training for psychiatric patients.* New York: Pergamon Press.

Liberman, R. P., Lillie, F., Falloon, I. R. H., Harpin, R. E., Hutchinson, W., & Stoute, B. (1984). Social skills training with relapsing schizophrenics: An experimental analysis. *Behavior Modification, 8*(2), 155–179.

Liberman, R. P., Mueser, K. T., & Wallace, C. J. (1986). Social skills training for schizophrenics at risk for relapse. *American Journal of Psychiatry, 143,* 523–526.

Lipsky, M. J., Kassinove, H., & Miller, N. J. (1980). Effects of rational-emotive therapy, rational role reversal, and rational-emotive imagery on the emotional adjustment of community mental health center patients. *Journal of Consulting and Clinical Psychology, 48,* 366–374.

Lomont, J. F., Gilner, F. J., Spector, N. J., & Skinner, K. K. (1969). Group assertion training and group insight therapies. *Psychological Reports, 25,* 463–470.

Lopez, M. A., Hoyer, W. T., Goldstein, A. P., Gershaw, M. J., & Sprafkin R. P. (1980). Effects of overlearning and incentive on the acquisition and transfer of interpersonal skills with institutionalized elderly. *Journal of Gerontology, 35,* 403–408.

Macaskill, N. D. (1982). Therapeutic factors in group therapy with borderline patients. *International Journal of Group Psychotherapy, 32,* 61–73.

MacKenzie, K. R. (1990). *Time-limited group psychotherapy.* Washington, DC: American Psychiatric Association.

MacKenzie, K. R., & Tschuschke, V. (1993). Relatedness, group work, and outcome in long-term inpatient psychotherapy groups. *Journal of Psychotherapy Practice and Research, 2*(2), 147–156.

Magaro, P. A., & West, A. N. (1983). Structured learning therapy: A study with chronic psychiatric patients and level of pathology. *Behavior Modification, 7*(1), 29–40.

Mann J., & Semrad, E. V., (1948). The use of group therapy in psychoses. *Social Casework, 29*(5), 176–181.

Marcovitz, R. J., & Smith, J. E. (1983). An approach to time-limited dynamic inpatient group psychotherapy. *Small Group Behavior, 14*(3), 369–376.

Massell, H. K., Corrigan, P. W., Liberman, R. P., & Milan, M. A. (1991). Conversation skills training of thought-disordered schizophrenic patients through attention focusing. *Psychiatry Research, 38,* 51–61.

Matson, J. L., Esvelt-Dawson, K., Andrasik, F., Ollendick, T. H., Petti, T., & Herson, M. (1980). Direct, observational, and generalization effects of social skills training with emotionally disturbed children. *Behavior Therapy, 11,* 522–531.

Maxmen, J. S. (1973). Group therapy as viewed by hospitalized patients. *Archives of General Psychiatry, 28,* 404–408.

Maxmen J. S. (1978). An educative model for inpatient group therapy. *International Journal of Group Psychotherapy, 28*(3), 321–338.

McGuire, T. L. (1988). A time-limited dynamic approach to adolescent inpatient group psychotherapy. *Adolescence, 23,* 373–382.

McLatchie, L. R. (1982). Interpersonal problem-solving group therapy: An evaluation of a potential method of social skills training for the chronic psychiatric patients. *Dissertation Abstracts International, 42*(7), 2995-B

Monti, P. M., Curran, J. P., Corriveau, D., DeLancey, A. L., & Hagerman, S. M. (1980). Effects of social skills training groups and sensitivity training groups with psychiatric patients. *Journal of Consulting and Clinical Psychology, 48*(2), 241–248.

Monti, P. M., Fink, E., Norman, W., Curran, J., Hayes, S., & Caldwell, A. (1979). Effect of social skills training groups and social skills bibliotherapy with psychiatric patients. *Journal of Consulting and Clinical Psychology, 1,* 189–191.

Mueser, K. T., Bellack, A. S., Douglas, M. S., & Wade, J. H. (1991). Prediction of social skill acquisition in schizophrenic and major affective disorder patients from memory and symptomatology. *Psychiatry Research, 37,* 281–296.

Mueser, K. T., Kosmidis, M. H., & Sayers, S. (in press). Symptomatology and the prediction of social skills: Acquisition in schizophrenia. *Schizophrenia research.*

Mueser, K. T., Levine, S., Bellack, A. S., Douglas, M. S., & Brady, E. U. (1990). Social skills training for acute psychiatric inpatients. *Hospital and Community Psychiatry, 41*(1), 1249–1251.

Mushet, G. L., Whalan, G. S., & Power, R. (1989). In-patients' views of the helpful aspects of group psychotherapy: Impact of therapeutic style and treatment setting. *British Journal of Medical Psychology, 62,* 135–141.

Neimeyer, R. A., & Feixas, G. (1990). The role of homework and skill acquisition in the outcome of group cognitive therapy for depression. *Behavior Therapy, 21,* 281–292.

Neimeyer, R. A., Twentymen, C. T., & Prezant, D. (1985). Cognitive and interpersonal group therapies for depression: A progress report. *The Cognitive Behaviorist, 7,* 21–22.

Nezu, A. M. (1986). Efficacy of a social problem-solving therapy approach for unipolar depression. *Journal of Consulting and Clinical Psychology, 54*(2), 196–202.

O'Brien, C. P. (1975). Group therapy for schizophrenics: A practical approach. *Schizophrenia Bulletin, 13,* 119–130.

Oei, T. P., & Jackson, P. (1980). Long-term effects of group and individual social skills training with alcoholics. *Addictive Behaviors, 5*(2), 129–136.

Oei, T. P., & Jackson, P. R. (1982). Social skills and cognitive behavioral approaches to the treatment of problem drinking. *Journal of Studies on Alcohol, 43*(5), 532–547.

Olson, R. P., & Greenberg, D. J. (1972). Effects of contingency-contracting and decision-making groups with chronic mental patients. *Journal of Consulting and Clinical Psychology, 38,* 376–383.

Otsby, S. S. (1983). Social problem-solving training with mildly and moderately retarded individuals. *Dissertation Abstracts International, 43*(7), 2320-B.

Parloff, M. B., & Dies, R. R. (1977). Group psychotherapy outcome research, 1966–1975. *International Journal of Group Psychotherapy, 27,* 281–319.

Pastushak, R. (1978). The effects of videotaped pretherapy training on interpersonal openness, self-disclosure and group psychotherapy outcome (Doctoral dissertation, Temple University). *Dissertation Abstract International, 39,* 2.

Pattison, E. M., Brissenden, A., & Wohl, T. (1967). Assessing specific effects of inpatient group psychotherapy. *International Journal of Group Psychotherapy, 17,* 283–297.

Peters, H. N., & Jones, F. D. (1951). Evaluation of group psychotherapy by means of performance tests. *Journal of Consulting Psychology, 15,* 363–367.

Pierce, C. V. M. (1980). Interpersonal problem-solving training for psychiatric patients. *Dissertation Abstracts International, 41*(10), 4339-A.

Pinney, E. L. (1963). The use of recorded minutes in group psychotherapy the development of a readback technique. *Psychiatric Quarterly Supplement, 37,* 263–269.

Platt, J. J., & Spivack, G. (1972a). Problem-solving thinking of psychiatric patients. *Journal of Consulting and Clinical Psychology, 39*(1), 148–151.

Platt, J. J., & Spivack, G. (1972b). Social competence and effective problem-solving thinking in psychiatric patients. *Journal of Clinical Psychology, 28*(1), 3–5.

Platt, J. J., & Spivack, G. (1974). Means of solving real-life problems: I. Psychiatric patients vs. controls and cross-cultural comparisons of normal females. *Journal of Community Psychology, 2*(1), 45–48.

Powell, M., Illovsky, M., O'Leary, W., & Gazda, G. M. (1988). Life-skills training with hospitalized psychiatric patients. *International Journal of Group Psychotherapy, 38*(1), 109–117.

Primakoff, L., Epstein, N., & Covi, L. (1986). Homework compliance: An uncontrolled variable in cognitive therapy outcome research. *Behavior Therapy, 17,* 433–446.

Rice, C. A., & Rutan, J. S. (1981). Boundary maintenance in inpatient therapy groups. *International Journal of Group Psychotherapy, 31*(3), 297–309.

Rice, C. A., & Rutan, J. S. (1987). *Inpatient group psychotherapy: A psychodynamic perspective.* New York: Macmillan.

Rice, M. E., & Chaplin, T. C. (1979). Social skills training for hospitalized male arsonists. *Journal of Behavior, Therapy and Exp. Psychiatry, 10,* 105–108.

Roback, H. B. (1972). Experimental comparison of outcome in insight- and non-insight-oriented therapy groups. *Journal of Consulting and Clinical Psychology, 38,* 793–796.

Robinson, M. B. (1970). A study of the effects of focused video-tape feedback in group counseling. *Comparative Group Studies, 1,* 45–75.

Sacks, J. M., & Berger, S. (1954). Group therapy techniques with hospitalized chronic schizophrenic patients. *Journal of Consulting Psychology, 18,* 297–302.

Schaffer, J. B., & Dryer, S. F. (1982). Staff and inpatient perceptions of change mechanisms in group psychotherapy. *Clinical and Research Reports, 139,* 127–128.

Schopler, J. H., & Galinsky, M. J. (1990). Can open-ended groups move beyond beginnings? *Small Group Research, 21*(4), 435–449.

Schroeder, D. J., Bowen, W. T., & Twemlow, S. W. (1982). Factors related to patient attrition from alcoholism treatment programs. *The International Journal of the Addictions, 17*(3), 463–472.

Semon, R. G., & Goldstein, N. (1957). The effectiveness of group psychotherapy with chronic schizophrenic patients and an evaluation of different therapeutic methods. *Journal of Consulting Psychology, 21,* 317–322.

Serok, S., & Zemet, R. M. (1983). An experiment of Gestalt group therapy with schizophrenics. *International Journal of Group Psychotherapy, 34,* 431–450.

Sheppard, J., Olson, A., Croke, J., Lafave, H. G., & Gerber, G. J. (1990). Improvisational drama groups in an inpatient setting. *Hospital and Community Psychiatry, 41*(9), 1019–1021.

Siegel, J. M., & Spivack, G. (1976). Problem-solving therapy: The description of a new program for chronic psychiatric patients. *Psychotherapy: Theory, Research and Practice, 13*(4), 368–373.

Spencer, P. G., Gillespie, C. R., & Ekisa, E. G. (1983). A controlled comparison of the effects of social skills training and remedial drama on the conversational skills of chronic schizophrenic inpatients. *British Journal of Psychiatry, 143,* 165–172.

Steinfeld, G. J., & Mabli, J. (1974). Perceived curative factors in group therapy by residents of a therapeutic community. *Criminal Justice and Behavior, 1*(3), 278–289.

Stoller, F. H. (1967). Group psychotherapy on television. *American Psychologist, 22,* 158–162.

Toseland, R., & Rose, S. D. (1978). A social skills training program for older adults: Evaluation of three group approaches. *Social Work Research Abstracts* (pp. 873–874).

Truax, C. B., & Carkhuff, R. R. (1965). Personality change in hospitalized mental patients during group psychotherapy as a function of the use of alternate sessions and various therapy pretraining. *Journal of Clinical Psychology, 21,* 225–228.

Truax, C. B., Shapiro, J. G., & Wargo, D. G. (1968). The effects of alternate sessions and vicarious therapy pretraining on group psychotherapy. *International Journal of Group Psychotherapy, 18,* 186–198.

Truax, C. B., Wargo, D. G., Carkhuff, R. R., Kodman, J., & Moles, E. A. (1966). Changes in self-concepts during group psychotherapy as a function of alternate sessions and vicarious therapy pretraining in institutional mental patients and juvenile delinquents. *Journal of Consulting Psychology, 30,* 309–314.

Tucker, J. E. (1956). Group psychotherapy with chronic psychotic soiling patients. *Journal of Consulting Psychology, 20,* 20–30.

van Dam-Baggen, R., & Kraaimaat, F. (1986). A group social skills training program with psychiatric patients: Outcome, drop-out rate and prediction. *Behavioral Research and Therapy, 24*(2), 161–169.

Vernallis, F. F., & Reinert, R. E. (1961). An evaluation of a goal-directed group psychotherapy with hospitalized patients. *Group Psychotherapy, 14,* 5–12.

Vitalo, R. L. (1971). Teaching improved interpersonal functioning as a preferred mode of treatment. *Journal of Clinical Psychology, 27,* 166–171.

Wallace, C. J., & Liberman, R. P. (1985). Social skills training for patients with schizophrenia: A controlled clinical trial. *Psychiatry Research, 15,* 239–247.

Wallace, C. J., Liberman, R. P., Mackain, S. J., Blackwell, G., & Eckman, T. A. (1992). Effectiveness and replicability of modules for teaching social and instrumental skills to the severely mentally ill. *American Journal of Psychiatry, 149*(5), 654–658.

Watson, J. P., & Lacey, J. H. (1974). Therapeutic groups for psychiatric inpatients. *British Journal of Medical Psychology, 47,* 307–312.

Whalan, G. S., & Mushet, L. L. (1986). Consumers' views of the helpful aspects of an in-patient psychotherapy group: A preliminary communication. *British Journal of Medical Psychology, 59,* 337–339.

Williams, M. T., Turner, S. M., Watts, J. G., Bellack, A. S., & Hersen, M. (1977). Group social skills training for chronic psychiatric patients. *European Journal of Behavioural Analysis and Modification, 4*(4), 223–229.

Wong, S. E., Martinez-Diaz, J. A., Edelstein, B. A., Wiegand, W., Bowen, L., & Liberman, R. P. (in press). Conversational skills training with schizophrenic inpatients: A study of generalization across settings and conversants.

Wong, S. E., & Wooley, J. E. (1989). Re-establishing conversational skills in overtly psychotic, chronic schizophrenic patients: Discrete trials training on the psychiatric ward. *Behavior Modification, 13,* 431–447.

Yalom, I. D. (1983). *Inpatient group psychotherapy.* New York: Basic Books.

Yalom, I. D. (1985). *The theory and practice of group psychotherapy* (3rd ed.). New York: Basic Books.

Yehoshua, R., Kellerman, P. F., Calev, A., & Dasberg, H. (1985). Group psychotherapy with inpatient chronic schizophrenics. *Israeli Journal of Psychiatry and Related Sciences, 22*(3), 185–190.

Zappe, C., & Epstein, D. (1987). Assertive training. *Journal of Psychosocial Nursing, 25*(8), 23–26.

Zerhusen, J., Boyle, K., & Wilson, W. (1991). Out of the darkness: Group cognitive therapy for depressed elderly. *Journal of Psychosocial Nursing, 29*(9), 16–21.

CHAPTER 12

Group Treatment for Eating Disorders

J. KELLY MORENO

According to the American Psychiatric Association (1987), eating disorders are identified by dramatic disturbances in eating behavior. Anorexia and bulimia nervosa are the most commonly diagnosed eating disorders. Anorexia nervosa is characterized by subnormal body weight, fear of fat, body image distortion, and amenorrhea (in females). Other features commonly found in anorexia include hair loss, lanugo, hypothermia, bradycardia, edema, poor concentration, and fatigue. Bulimia nervosa is characterized by binge eating, purging (e.g., vomiting, diuretic and laxative abuse, fasting, compulsive exercise), body/weight preoccupation, and out-of-control feelings when binging. Other features found in bulimia include tooth decay, esophageal tears, tachycardia, electrolyte imbalance, swollen parotid glands, depression, and substance abuse.

In addition, the American Psychiatric Association (1987) has noted that anorexia and bulimia nervosa are primarily found in females, with only 0.4% to 5% of the male population diagnosed with such disorders. Age of onset in anorexia mostly occurs during adolescence, while onset in bulimia is more often found in late adolescence or early adulthood. Anorexia and bulimia also appear to be more widely represented in middle/upper middle class Caucasian families. The mortality rate in anorexia has been estimated at 5% to 18%. The prevalence of anorexia and bulimia among college age women has been estimated between 1% to 5%. There is some contention that the prevalence of eating disorders has increased over time (Inbody & Ellis, 1985).

Etiological factors in eating disorders are not well-understood and continue to be investigated. There is considerable agreement, however, that a complex interplay of biological, psychological, and sociocultural factors is involved in the development of an eating disorder (Garner & Garfinkel, 1985; Johnson & Connors, 1987). This approach to the etiology and treatment of eating disorders has been referred to as the "biopsychosocial" model (Garner & Garfinkel, 1985; Johnson & Connors, 1987). Consequently, approaches to treatment are commonly multidisciplinary (e.g., endocrinology, psychiatry, psychology, and nutrition), multidimensional (e.g., cognitive, behavioral, psychoeducational, psychodynamic, and psychopharmacologic interventions), and multimodal (e.g., individual, group, and family therapy).

Group therapy is commonly prescribed in the treatment of eating disorders (Oesterheld, McKenna, & Gould, 1987). Its popularity is based on the presupposition that it affords opportunities for universality, community, and observational and interpersonal learning, among other things, less pronounced in other treatment modalities. Group therapy is also believed to be more cost effective than other approaches. Research on the group treatment of eating disorders has increased dramatically in the last 25 years in order to validate empirically these and other treatment assumptions. For instance, the first paper on group therapy for eating disorders was an anorexia study reported by Lafeber and Lansen (1967) at a psychotherapy congress in West Germany. The next paper on group therapy for eating disorders was a bulimia study published by Boskind-Lodahl and White (1978) 11 years later. Over 80 papers were either published or presented on the subject in the 1980s, and by 1991 97 reports on group therapy for anorexia and bulimia could be found in the literature.

A list of the literature on group therapy with eating disorders is presented in Table 12.1. These reports include treatment models, surveys, case studies, controlled studies, correlational studies, multiple baseline designs, and reviews of the literature. Seventy-four of these reports were empirical in nature, with the majority being case studies. Case studies were included because of their richness in clinical details that as yet are not identified, operationalized, controlled for, and/or investigated in more experimental designs. These studies also provide observations on a much broader range of issues occurring in group than heretofore has been represented in the experimental literature. "Empirical," therefore, was liberally defined as any article, chapter, presentation, or other report with one or more qualitative and/or quantitative observations that resulted from one or more groups with eating disordered persons. Each report was reviewed and coded for information on the following variables: recruitment; assessment; preparation; inclusion/exclusion; composition; size; therapist gender, expertise, technique, and countertransference; cotherapy; patient prognosis, attendance, attrition, and outcome; group content, interaction, affect, development, and therapeutic factors; treatment setting, duration, modality, and orientation; and methodological limitations. The text that follows is a summary of what clinicians and researchers alike have "found" on the aforementioned features of the eating disorders group.

PATIENT AND THERAPIST VARIABLES

Patient Prognosis

A number of patient demographic and diagnostic features have been found to relate to participation and outcome in group psychotherapy for anorexia

TABLE 12.1. The Literature on Group Therapy for Eating Disorders

	Position Paper/Model[a]	Survey	Case[b]	Quasi-Experimental/Experimental	Review	Correlational
Anorexia	Hall (1985)		Yellowless (1988) Lieb & Thompson (1984) Polivy (1981) Maher (1984) Edelstein & Moguilner (1986) Marner & Westerberg (1987) Lansen (1986) Lafeber & Lansen (1967) Piazza et al. (1983) Hall (1985) Cox & Merkel (1989)			Merrill et al. (1987)
Bulimia[c]	Reed & Sech (1985) Yudkovitz (1983) Browning (1985) Fernandez (1984) Mitchell et al. (1985) Kearney-Cooke (1988) Barth & Wurman (1986) Asner (1990) Pyle et al. (1984) Laube (1990) MacKenzie et al. (1986) Hamilton (1988)	Malenbaum et al. (1988) Fernandez (1984) Mitchell et al. (1988)	Johnson et al. (1983) Stevens & Salisbury (1984) Roy-Berne et al. (1984) Hobbs et al. (1989) Bauer (1984) Brisman & Siegal (1985) Dedman et al. (1988) Brotman et al. (1988) Frommer et al. (1987) Schneider & Agras (1985) Weiss & Katzman (1984) White & Boskind-White (1981) Stuber & Strober (1987) O'Neil & White (1987) Pyle et al. (1984) Gerstein & Hotelling (1987) Connor-Greene (1987)	Kirkley et al. (1985) Wolchik et al. (1986) Lacey (1983) Huon & Brown (1985) Berry & Abramowitz (1989) Yates & Sambrailo (1984) Freeman et al. (1988) Boskind-Lodahl & White (1978) Gray & Hoage (1990) Leitenberg et al. (1988) Lee & Rush (1986) Mitchell et al. (1990) Pyle et al. (1990) Mitchell et al. (1989) Mitchell et al. (1987) Freeman et al. (1985) Telch et al. (1990)	Cox & Merkel (1989) Freeman & Munro (1988) Oesterheld et al. (1987) Griffiths et al. (1987) Garner et al. (1987) Hudson & Pope (1986)	

Kirkley et al. (1988)
Weinstein & Richman (1984)
Hinz & Ragsdall (1990)
Kearney-Cooke (1988)
Brotman et al. (1985)
McNamara (1989)
Hornak (1983)
Bohanske & Lemberg (1987)

Gordon & Ahmed (1988)
Dixon & Kiecolt-Glaser (1984)
Wilson et al. (1986)
Laessle, Waadt, & Pirke (1987)
Laessle, Zoettl, & Pirke (1987)

Hendren et al. (1987)
Inbody & Ellis (1985)
Edmands (1986)
Piran et al. (1989)
Franko (1987)
Block & Llewelyn (1987)
Loganbill & Koch (1983)
Weber & Gillingham (1984)
Lenihan & Sanders (1984)
Roth & Ross (1988)
Moreno & Hileman (1991)
Moreno et al. (1992)

Yager (1988)
Richards et al. (1990)

Glassman et al. (1990)
Vanderlinden &
    Vandereycken (1988)
Scheuble et al. (1987)

Yager et al. (1989)

Anorexia   Gary (1986)
/Bulimia   Lonergan (1991)
Mixed   Shisslak et al. (1986)
            Roth & Ross (1988)

[a] Papers noted here may also be represented under other designs if they included process/outcome observations on a group.
[b] Includes papers with process/outcome observations on one group, several groups, or a program of groups.
[c] An additional multiple baseline study by Connors et al. (1984) exists using a bulimia population.

and bulimia. With respect to attrition, personality disorder (particularly borderline) (Merrill, Mines, & Starkey, 1987; Roy-Byrne, Lee-Benner, & Yager, 1984), hostility (Kirkley, Schneider, Agras, & Bachman, 1985; Lee & Rush, 1986), dependence on family (Polivy, 1981; Weinstein & Richman, 1984), depression (Kirkley et al., 1985; Roy-Byrne et al., 1984), younger age (Kirkley et al., 1985; Merrill et al., 1987; Polivy, 1981), and substance abuse (Dixon & Kiecolt-Glaser, 1984; Scheuble, Dixon, Levy, & Kagan-Moore, 1987) are associated with high dropout rates. There is also some evidence to suggest that low motivation (Roy-Byrne et al., 1984), symptom severity at pretreatment (Kirkley et al., 1985), recent inpatient treatment, social phobia (Piran, Langdon, Kaplan, & Garfinkel, 1989), high social desirability (Dixon & Kiecolt-Glaser, 1984), early onset, conjoint treatment (different therapists for individual and group therapy) (Scheuble et al., 1987), unemployment, minimal sexual activity, little difficulty going to sleep, single marital status, and respiratory/muscle tension (Merrill et al., 1987) are also related to premature termination in eating disorder groups.

On the other hand, Merrill et al. (1987) and Leitenberg, Rosen, Gross, Nudelman, and Vara (1988) did not find depression or low age to differ significantly in treatment completers and dropouts, respectively. Likewise, severity of eating disorder at pretreatment did not discriminate between completers and dropouts in studies by Merrill et al. (1987), Dixon and Kiecolt-Glaser (1984), Wilson, Rossiter, Kleifield, and Lindholm (1986), and Leitenberg et al. (1988). Dixon and Kiecolt-Glaser (1984) and Leitenberg et al. (1988) also did not find single marital status and general psychopathology to discriminate between completers and dropouts, respectively. Interestingly, Merrill et al. (1987) found that patients were more likely to persist in group psychotherapy if they complained of cardiovascular/gastrointestinal tension and had negative cognitions of themselves, the world, and the future.

Eight reports provide data on why eating disordered patients drop out of group psychotherapy (Brotman, Alonso, & Herzog, 1985; Freeman, Sinclair, Turnbull, & Annandale, 1985; Hinz & Ragsdell, 1990; Lee & Rush, 1986; Merrill et al., 1987; Polivy, 1981; Scheuble et al., 1987; Telch, Agras, Rossiter, Wilfley, & Kenardy, 1990). Problems with other group members and dissatisfaction with group results were by far the most commonly reported reasons why anorexics and bulimics terminated prematurely. Other reasons for termination given by these patients included changes in residence, schedule, finances, treatment modality (e.g., OA, family), group norms and therapist techniques. Several studies concluded that better assessment/screening procedures and better preparation of patients for group therapy might have prevented the attrition observed (Dixon & Kiecolt-Glaser, 1984; Freeman et al., 1985; Hall, 1985; Moreno & Hileman, 1991; Scheuble et al., 1987; Telch et al., 1990; Wilson et al., 1986). Specifically, the prediction of interpersonal difficulties in the group may have helped patients contain (not to mention explore) future group tensions, and the anticipation of future lifestyle changes may have helped screen for unsuitable patients over time.

With respect to outcome, personality disorder, particularly borderline and histrionic personality disorder (Brotman, Herzog, & Hamburg, 1988; Browning, 1985; Glassman, Rich, Darko, & Clarkin, 1990; Maher, 1984; Polivy, 1981, p. 106), was found to yield less favorable results than dependent personality disorder (Glassman et al., 1990) or no personality disorder. There is some evidence to suggest that borderline personality disorder is particularly contraindicated for short-term treatment (Brotman et al., 1988; Glassman et al., 1990), although Wolchik, Weiss, and Katzman (1986) noted that several patients with fairly severe "characterological" disturbance made good progress in their short-term psychoeducational group. There is also mounting evidence to suggest that patients with a history of anorexia (Bauer, 1984; Brotman et al., 1985; Browning, 1985; Glassman et al., 1990; Hall, 1985; Lacey, 1983) and patients precariously underweight (Brotman et al., 1985; Glassman et al., 1990; Piran et al., 1989; Wilson et al., 1986) fare less well in group psychotherapy. One study (Hendren, Atkins, Sumner, & Barber, 1987), however, did not find low body weight to affect outcome in eating disorder group psychotherapy negatively. Likewise, higher binge/purge frequencies at pretreatment were associated with poor outcome in one study (Mitchell et al., 1988) and favorable outcome in another (Frommer, Ames, Gibson, & Davis, 1987). Other food/weight related features implicated in poor group psychotherapy outcome include high body/weight preoccupation, history of great weight fluctuation (Mitchell et al., 1988), menstrual dysfunction (Glassman et al., 1990), and employment in a career (e.g., modeling, entertainment) that encourages thinness (White & Boskind-White, 1981).

Other psychosocial features related to unfavorable outcome in group include poor treatment adherence (Roy-Byrne et al., 1984), high social desirability (thereby leading to defensiveness and low self-disclosure), social support (thereby decreasing motivation/pressure to change) (White & Boskind-White, 1981), other (versus self) referral (Gray & Hoage, 1990), childhood trauma (Glassman et al., 1990), dependence on family (Maher, 1984; Polivy, 1981), and social/occupational dysfunction at pretreatment (Maher, 1984). Young age (e.g., Dedman, Numa, & Wakeling, 1988) was associated with poor outcome in two reports (Gray & Hoage, 1990; Polivy, 1981), however, age was not a factor in outcome in another (Connors, Johnson, & Stuckey, 1984). There is also some evidence to suggest that marginal psychological mindedness is related to negative outcome in group psychotherapy (Maher, 1984); nevertheless, Brotman et al. (1985) suggested that this is less of a contraindication for cognitive-behavioral groups than psychodynamic ones. Likewise, substance abuse and mood disorder were associated with poorer outcome (Brotman et al., 1988; Browning, 1985; Lacey, 1983), but there is other evidence to suggest that these disturbances are unrelated to outcome (Glassman et al., 1990; Mitchell et al., 1988; Piran et al., 1989; Wolchik et al., 1986). Other features found unrelated to outcome include family history of mood disorder, highest percent overweight in the past (Wilson et al., 1986), and previous treatment (Brotman et al., 1985).

Therapist Expertise

No controlled research exists on the direct comparison of outcomes between patients in group therapy with expert versus nonexpert therapists. A host of retrospective and survey data, however, offer a variety of suggestions as to how therapist expertise affects process and outcome in group psychotherapy with eating disorders. With respect to availability, Yellowlees (1988) found that group therapy for anorexics (and, to a lesser extent, bulimics) was often not even initiated, due to a perceived lack of availability of qualified eating disorder group therapists. Kirkley, Battaglia, Earle, Gans, and Molloy (1988) reported that nonexperts with frequent and close supervision could conduct a psychoeducational eating disorder group quite satisfactorily, and Yager, Landsverk, and Edelstein (1989) discovered no significant differences in symptom change for patients receiving professional help versus patients receiving no treatment at all. On the other hand, Yager et al. (1989) also found that experienced leaders facilitated more openness and symptom improvement in their patients than inexperienced ones. Groups with lower dropout rates tend to be run by more experienced leaders (Merrill et al., 1987) and 94% of eating disorder patients surveyed found a need for professional input in a self-help group (SHG) for eating disorders (Franko, 1987). Block and Llewelyn (1987) found that trained leaders spoke significantly more often but of less duration, were significantly more caring and emotionally stimulating, were less cognitive, and facilitated more altruism (versus guidance) and satisfaction in their members than untrained leaders.

Gender

There is virtually no controlled research on the impact of therapist gender on process and outcome variables in group therapy with eating disorders. On the other hand, a host of observational and case studies report that male therapists—particularly with female cotherapists—are useful to anorexic and bulimic patients in group treatment (Brotman et al., 1985; Inbody & Ellis, 1985; Lieb & Thompson, 1984; Lonergan, 1991; Moreno & Hileman, 1991; Roth & Ross, 1988; Roy-Byrne et al., 1984; Shisslak, Crago, Schnaps, & Swain, 1986; Weber & Gillingham, 1984; Weinstein & Richman, 1984; Yellowlees, 1988). Specifically, the conventional lore is that in group, male therapists generate useful discussions around sex, competition, fathers/parents, and sex roles, and elicit transference material and promote reality testing in eating disordered patients as well. Similarly, female therapists elicit constructive interactions around identity, mothers, self-care, competition, and success. Only two investigators expressed reservations with respect to the presence of a male therapist in the eating disorders group (Hall, 1985; McNamara, 1989), claiming that male group therapists evoked resistance to discussing certain subjects (e.g., sex) and inhibited self-disclosure in their eating disordered patients. Nearly all of the above studies that found male therapists useful to the eating disorders group were long-term (e.g., greater than 6 months), interpersonally oriented groups. In contrast, one of the two studies cautioning against male therapists in group was short-term and highly structured. Hence, perhaps the presence of a male therapist is less advantageous in short-term groups that are dependent on rapid self-disclosure for maximal effectiveness.

Cotherapy

Again, although there is no controlled research on the subject, there is wide agreement in the case literature that cotherapy is advantageous in the group treatment of eating disorders (Brotman et al., 1985; Inbody & Ellis, 1985; Lieb & Thompson, 1984; Lonergan, 1991; Moreno & Hileman, 1991; Roth & Ross, 1988; Roy-Byrne et al., 1984; Shisslak et al., 1986; Weber & Gillingham, 1984; Weinstein & Richman, 1984; Yellowlees, 1988). Specifically, male/female cotherapy teams effectively and usefully model healthier forms of cooperation and conflict than heretofore has been the case for many eating disordered persons. Additionally, investigators describe coleadership as useful for dealing with other issues around dependency, resistance, splitting, reality testing, and affect management. Coleaders also have been reported to be particularly useful to one another after individual group sessions, especially with respect to the management of anger, frustration, exhaustion, confusion and other difficulties associated with leading this kind of group. Only two studies discussed disadvantages or difficulties of coleadership (e.g., competition, inequalities in experience and/or status in the organization, differences in theoretical orientation); yet, in both of these studies, the overall evaluation was that coleadership was beneficial (Brotman et al., 1985; Moreno & Hileman, 1991).

Countertransference and Other Difficulties

Perhaps one of the more unique features of the eating disorder group literature is the frequency with which investigators reported that it was a difficult, unrewarding, and/or draining experience for the therapist (Brisman & Siegel, 1985; Hall, 1985; Inbody & Ellis, 1985; Lansen, 1986; Maher, 1984; Moreno & Hileman, 1991; Roth & Ross, 1988). Low levels of patient interaction, affective experience, affective expression, cohesion, progress, insight, attachment, and energy were common reasons why groups with this population were said to be so difficult. Only Lee and Rush (1986) suggested that therapists did not feel taxed during their stewardship of the group. Interestingly, the group approach in this study was cognitive-behavioral which, in contrast to the more interactional/psychodynamic approaches taken by the studies above, may have required less of the therapist with respect to the identification, elicitation, facilitation, and tolerance or containment of affect *as it occurred in group*. In addition, 6 of the 7 studies above were conducted with groups of anorexics, or anorexics and bulimics, whereas the study by Lee and Rush (1986) was conducted with bulimics. Hence, it may also be that group psychotherapy with anorexics is especially difficult for the group therapist. Indeed, Hall (1985) was particularly forthright about the greater difficulties involved for the therapist in conducting anorexic versus bulimic groups. According to her, group therapy with anorexics "may be one of the most demanding, and anxiety provoking, and least rewarding of the psychotherapies in general . . ." (p. 214).

Research on patient prognosis thus far suggests that eating disordered persons with personality disorders, particularly borderline personality disorder, are more likely to drop out of group, and slower to improve in group, than nonpersonality disordered members. In addition, patients with a history of anorexia and precariously low body weight at pretreatment appear to fare less well in group than others. A host of other variables have been mentioned as prognostic of patient participation and outcome in group, but await further investigation before (even tentative) conclusions may be made. An association worth highlighting in this research is the frequency with which logistical problems, interpersonal tension, and dissatisfation with group treatment were reported by patients to be reasons for premature termination. The implications of this observation for preparation and assessment of the eating disordered patient for group are most important and are discussed in more detail later.

Experienced therapists appear to yield less attrition and more favorable outcome with their patients than inexperienced ones, however, inexperienced therapists with supervision may function satisfactorily in more structured psychoeducational approaches. The male therapist may be most useful to longer, interpersonally-oriented groups where patients have the luxury of exploring resistances and resolving transferences with him that they don't have in shorter groups with more of a symptom and/or extragroup relationship focus. Male/female cotherapy teams that model healthy competition, cooperation, and other adaptive behavior appear to be particularly useful to eating disordered patients starving for internal representations of more palatable relationships between the sexes. Finally, conducting groups with eating disordered persons appears to be more physically draining, psychologically taxing, and less immediately rewarding than it is with many other clinical populations.

SELECTION AND COMPOSITION

Recruitment

The relationship of patient recruitment to process and outcome variables has received scant attention in the eating disorder group psychotherapy literature. There is some evidence to suggest, however, that referred subjects are more disturbed, are more likely to receive individual as opposed to group treatment, and have less favorable outcomes than subjects recruited through advertisements (Garner, Fairburn, & Davis, 1987). Forty-two studies disclosed the methods used to recruit their patients/subjects. Overall, patients in 15 studies were secured through clinical referrals, while patients in 13 studies were obtained via advertisements of sorts. Another 12 studies recruited patients through a combination of referral and advertisement methods. Interestingly, in the studies on group therapy for bulimia, the median number of binges/purges per week at pretreatment for referral versus advertisement subjects was 14.3 and 9.6, respectively, while the median attrition rate for these two groups was 36% and 15%, respectively. The median reduction in weekly binging episodes at post-treatment for referral and advertisement subjects was 83% and 69%, respectively.

These figures suggest that referred subjects are, indeed, more disturbed than those responding to a treatment advertisement. This is understandable given that more disturbed individuals are more likely to come to the attention of health care providers. The higher attrition rate in the referred subjects is also understandable since we might expect more disturbed patients to drop out of treatment prematurely; indeed, the evidence on patient variables and attrition suggests that this is the case. The discrepancy in outcome between the two groups is a little more surprising due to earlier observations that more disturbed patients do less well in treatment.

On the other hand, since most of the outcome data across all studies was conducted on treatment completers (a big bruise on the methodological skin of many controlled, as well as uncontrolled studies), perhaps the more disturbed patients who remain in treatment are more motivated by their pain and make better use of the therapy. Indeed, there is some evidence to suggest that disturbed patients improve more than less disturbed ones (Frommer et al., 1987). Part of the discrepancy in outcome between referred and solicited subjects in these studies, however, could be spurious since more severely disturbed patients have more room to improve, or because most of the studies who advertised for subjects were controlled rather than case investigations. Overall, however, these figures suggest a relationship between recruitment method and pretreatment severity that warrants more attention in outcome research on group therapy with eating disorders than heretofore has been the case.

Assessment

Five types of assessment procedures were used across studies, with clinical interviews being the most common. There was a considerable amount of variation in the interview structure, however, with many of them being a single session, and some taking place over several sessions. Some interviews were conducted over the phone, while most interviews were done in person. The content of the interviews also appears to vary, with some interviews focused mostly on food and weight related issues, others on psychosocial issues, and some on both. At times, the function of the interview is to help educate and prepare the patient for group therapy. In general, however, the details of the clinical interview across most studies are not provided, and cookbooks for conducting the clinical interview with eating disordered persons do not seem to be forthcoming.

Psychological testing was the next most common method of assessment. Most of the time, measurement consisted of eating disorder, mood, self-esteem, and, to a lesser extent, social, anger, anxiety, and general personality or psychopathology measurement. Some of the most commonly used measures were the Eating Disorders Inventory, Eating Attitudes Test, Binge Eating Scale, Beck Depression Inventory, State-Trait Anxiety Inventory, SCL-90, and Rosenberg Self-Esteem Inventory. In general, however, there is considerable variability in tests used, thereby making comparisons between studies very difficult. In addition, in some studies, these measures are simply part of the standard inpatient or outpatient pretreatment assessment; in others, the tests seemed to be tailored more to the specific purpose of the study. In some cases, the testing is used primarily for screening and determination of inclusion/exclusion, while in others testing was conducted to make inferences about treatment outcome and/or response. In several studies, a considerable amount of attrition was observed between the first and second contacts when subjects were to return completed psychological test batteries, suggesting that the process of participation in pretreatment assessment may be just as useful as the content of the assessment in determining motivation and suitability for group treatment.

A third, and considerably less common form of pretreatment evaluation, was behavioral assessment. Typically, this involved patients in bulimia studies who were asked to record binge/purge episodes prior to treatment. There was considerable variation in self-monitoring, however, with some requiring only binge/purge frequencies, and others recording events, thoughts, feelings, places, times, foods, calories, and other associated features on the record form. Moreover, some studies required only several days of self-monitoring, most required 1 to 2 weeks, and a couple required 3 weeks. Given that binging/purging is the primary complaint in this population, it was surprising to find only 13 studies using this form of assessment. In addition, some have suggested that this method of assessment is more reliable than self-report data obtained during the clinical interview (Wilson et al., 1986). As with psychological testing, several studies reported a sizable amount of attrition between self-monitoring assignments, thereby suggesting that pretreatment behavioral assessment is another good indicator of patient motivation and commitment to treatment.

One of the least common forms of assessment was medical evaluation. For instance, only 7 of the 74 empirical reports included in this review noted that a physical exam was required of subject-patients. This is somewhat disconcerting given the number of (sometimes serious) medical complications associated with anorexia and bulimia. Moreover, the studies that required a medical exam at pretreatment did not mention any such

TABLE 12.2.   Attrition, Outcome, and Degree of Assessment

	Number of Assessment Procedures Reported			
	0–1	2	3	4+
Attrition[a]	26	33	16	14
Outcome[b]	50	71	82	91

[a]Median percent in anorexia and bulimia studies.
[b]Median percent reduction in binging and/or purging for subjects in bulimia
studies only.

measurement at post-treatment. This is unfortunate since it is certainly
possible that medical condition may have been another variable affected
by group participation over time. In general, medical condition appears to
be a neglected and untapped area in group treatment and research that
warrants more attention and examination.

Only one study (Glassman et al., 1990) reported on the use of collateral
assessment. This is somewhat surprising, given the generally accepted limitations with self-report data. There is some evidence to suggest, in fact, that
anorexic patients view their progress more favorably than their therapists or
fellow patients (Vanderlinden & Vandereycken, 1988). Collateral methods,
like medical ones, appear to be an underused assessment procedure.

Another very interesting and important aspect of assessment is its relationship to attrition and outcome. Indeed, numerous reports either commented on the importance of assessment in this regard, or concluded that
treatment adherence and outcome may have been much more pronounced in
their studies with better screening and assessment procedures. Attrition and
outcome data across levels of assessment are presented in Table 12.2.
Clearly, studies employing 3 or more methods of assessment at pretreatment
evidenced lower levels of attrition and more favorable outcomes that those
using 2 or less. Such figures suggest that multimodal assessment at pretreatment may be worthwhile given the benefits accrued by the patient—not
to mention the group, the group therapist, and/or the group investigator—
when group treatment proceeds with fewer disruptions.

Preparation

Interest in pregroup preparation for group psychotherapy has continued to
increase (Yalom, 1985); nevertheless, the literature on pregroup preparation in the group treatment of eating disorders, however, remains thin. Certainly no controlled investigations on the relationship between pregroup
preparation and process and outcome in this area have been undertaken.
Moreover, of the 74 reports reviewed, only 10 mentioned preparing the patient for group, and even then their descriptions of precisely how the patient
was prepared were short and vague. It could be that one reason why studies
with more pretreatment assessment evidenced lower attrition and better
outcome was because a fair amount of preparation/psychoeducation for

group was embedded, but not reported, in the assessment. In any case, recipes for preparing eating disordered patients for group psychotherapy are not in the clinical drawer.

The lack of controlled investigations notwithstanding, a number of investigators have informally observed a negative association between preparation and attrition and/or unfavorable outcome in eating disorder groups (Dixon & Kiecolt-Glaser, 1984; Hall, 1985; Hinz & Ragsdell, 1990; MacKenzie, Livesley, Coleman, Harper, & Park, 1986; Moreno & Hileman, 1991; Roy-Byrne et al., 1984; Scheuble et al., 1987; Wilson et al., 1986), and have made some recommendations. For instance, Hall (1985) suggested that the prospective anorexic patient not only anticipate difficulties in the group but review strategies for how she might deal with them. Roy-Byrne et al. (1984) recommended that the patient be educated with respect to the association between relationships, feelings, and food and how the interface of these phenomena might emerge within the "social microcosm" of the group. Brotman et al. (1985) suggested that the eating disordered patient be educated with respect to the theoretical orientation of various groups available to them and then be invited to select a particular approach to treatment. Likewise, Hinz and Ragsdell (1990) recommended that undue resistance to new interventions later in treatment may be lessened by appropriate preparation for such techniques at pretreatment. A number of ideas exist for preparing the eating disordered patient for group and only await integration and investigation with respect to their effect on group process and outcome.

Inclusion/Exclusion

Just under half of the studies reported on other inclusion/exclusion criteria besides diagnosis for group participation. Of the 39 studies that reported this information, minimum binging/purging, contracting, age, psychosis, medical condition, concurrent treatment, low body weight, anorexia (past and/or present), substance abuse, and suicidality were noted most often (Table 12.3). In addition, studies involving bulimics seemed to pay more attention to inclusion/exclusion criteria than did studies using anorexics. In fact, it was relatively uncommon for a study on anorexia to report on many other inclusion criteria besides diagnosis, medical condition, and body weight. Interestingly, other variables (e.g., personality disorder) found to be important prognostic indicators in eating disorder groups or important inclusion criteria for group therapy in general (e.g., rapport with pregroup interviewer, motivation, capacity for attachment, success in previous treatment [Yalom, 1985]) are mentioned in only a few studies.

Attrition and outcome data at post-treatment were similar for persons participating in studies employing low versus high criteria for inclusion/exclusion. Specifically, the median attrition rate in studies reporting one-or-fewer criterion and those reporting four-or-more was 20% and 25%, respectively. Likewise, the median percent reduction in binging at post-treatment between these two groups was 75% and 79%, respectively. These

TABLE 12.3.   Number of Studies Reporting
Various Types of Inclusion/Exclusion Criteria

Inclusion/Exclusion Criteria	Number of Studies Employing Criteria
Minimum binging/purging[a]	17
Contracting/commitment	9
Age	9
Psychosis	9
Medical condition	9
Concurrent treatment[b]	9
Low body weight	8
Anorexia[c]	6
Substance abuse	6
Suicidality	6
Motivation	4
Social functions	4
Personality disorder	2
Hostility	2
Competitiveness	2
Purging	2
Laxatives	2
Clean goals	2
Independent living	2

Note: Other inclusion/exclusion criteria such as development
level, previous hospitalization, mood disorder, gross
psychopathology, kleptomania, binge urges, out-of-
control eating, obesity, gender, pregnancy, and current
medical care were only mentioned once across studies.

[a]Mostly reported in controlled studies.
[b]Mostly used as an exclusion criterion in controlled studies.
[c]Mostly used as an exclusion criterion in bulimia studies.

figures suggest that the marginal utility of adding other inclusion/exclusion criteria beyond psychiatric diagnosis is minimal.

On the other hand, it could be that investigators are not attending to other potent indicators for inclusion/exclusion. For example, as noted earlier, the comorbidity of personality disorder—particularly borderline personality disorder—in eating disorder group members is frequently associated with premature termination and unfavorable outcome. Yet, in this review, only two studies used personality disorder as a consideration for exclusion from their group(s). Similarly, it also could be that there is a lack of attention, as noted above, to strengths or more positive patient features found to be good indicators for group inclusion. Yalom (1985), for instance, observed that some of the best indicators for favorable participation and outcome in more traditional heterogenous psychotherapy groups include factors such as rapport with the pregroup interviewer, capacity for attachment, psychological mindedness, and success in previous treatment. However, little attention is given to these criteria for inclusion into the eating disorder therapy group thus far. Consequently, greater attention to some of these other eating disorder group selection criteria may yield more favorable attendance and outcome than the figures above suggest.

Size

The literature on group size with anorexics and bulimics is mixed. With respect to anorexia, some investigators found that anorexics function better in small groups (Hall, 1985; Polivy, 1981). Hall (1985) recommended, however, that 8 to 10 anorexics be admitted to the group with the expectation that poor attendance and attrition will eventuate in a more desirable size of 4 to 6 members. Franko (1987), on the other hand, found anorexics to function well in a mixed eating disorder self-help group of 25 members. With respect to bulimia, Laessle, Waadt, and Pirke (1987) concluded that one reason why their results were as favorable as those reported by investigators of other treatment modalities was because their groups were smaller (e.g., 2 to 4 patients). Gray and Hoage (1990), however, found that their exposure-response prevention group for bulimia was as effective with groups of 8 as other exposure-response prevention group studies conducted on groups of 2 to 3. Stuber and Strober (1987) recommended that bulimia groups be conducted with more than 6 members because of poor attendance and attrition. Changes in the size of the eating disorder group are thought to be particularly difficult for group members (Moreno & Hileman, 1991; Roth & Ross, 1988) although Roy-Byrne et al. (1984) and Hendren et al. (1987) disagree especially once a cohesive core has been established.

Fifty-eight studies reported on group size. The mean group size across all studies was 8.38, with a range of 2 to 25 members. The majority of studies reported group size between 6 to 10 patients. The smallest groups (2 to 3 patients) tended to be exposure-response prevention ones (e.g., where a high degree of individual attention in the group was an important part of the treatment plan). The largest group was a self-help group of 25 patients with open membership (Franko, 1987). Interestingly, there did not appear to be any appreciable differences in the size of psychoeducational, cognitive-behavioral, eclectic, or psychodynamic groups. It was somewhat surprising to find that psychoeducational groups were not noticeably larger than more therapy-based ones. Theoretically, one might expect these groups to look more like classrooms, where patients participate like students, and clinicians like teachers. Despite alleged approaches, there was considerable overlap in techniques among studies that may have minimized expected differences in group size. Finally, there does not appear to be any appreciable difference in size with respect to homogenous anorexic groups, homogenous bulimic groups, or mixed eating disorders groups. This is somewhat surprising given common clinical lore that groups for anorexics should be smaller because of their deficits in desire and ability to interact with others (Hall, 1985).

The relationship between size, attrition, and outcome across studies is summarized in Table 12.4. Interestingly, attrition is somewhat lower in

TABLE 12.4. Size, Attrition, and Outcome in
Group Therapy for Eating Disorders

Group Size	Attrition[a]	Outcome[b]
≤ 7	16	67
≥ 8	23	76

[a]Median percent for subjects in anorexia and bulimia groups.
[b]Median percent reduction in weekly binging/purging at post treatment for bulimia subjects.

eating disorder groups with smaller membership; yet, in bulimia groups (unfortunately, outcome data on anorexia groups was insufficient to make similar comparisons), outcome appears to be somewhat more favorable in groups with larger membership. Some eating disordered patients, therefore, may not be able to tolerate membership in a larger group and quit; those patients (at least bulimic ones) who remain, however, may glean somewhat more from the experience than they would in a smaller group with less variety in observation and/or interaction. This is particularly interesting given some observations that vicarious learning is an inconspicuously potent source of therapy in the eating disorders group (Moreno, Hileman, & Fuhriman, 1992).

Composition

Several controversies exist around the issue of composition in the eating disorders group. Probably the least controversial issue is whether or not the eating disordered person should participate in a traditional heterogeneous (with respect to disorders) psychotherapy group. There appears to be some consensus that this type of arrangement is contraindicated given the inanition and extreme isolation of the anorexic, and the secrecy and shame of the bulimic. Moreover, in a mixed symptom group there is some concern that the eating disordered patient's symptoms and resources may be so different from those of other patients that the probability for deviancy and scapegoating is increased (Hall, 1985; Hendren et al., 1987). Consensus on this issue notwithstanding, process and outcome comparisons of eating disordered persons in heterogeneous psychotherapy groups versus homogeneous (with respect to eating disorder) psychotherapy groups is virtually nonexistent. Only Hall (1985) found that an eating disordered person benefited from a mixed symptom psychotherapy group, and only then once the patient was far along in her recovery and less of a standout in group.

A second controversy in the literature concerns the homo/heterogeneity of the group with respect to eating disorder. Some investigators suggest that separate groups for anorexic, bulimic, and obese persons are best because differences in eating, personality, and behavior among the eating disorders interfere with the development of cohesion and therapeutic interaction in group (Brotman et al., 1985; Franko, 1987; Lonergan, 1991; MacKenzie et al., 1986; Polivy, 1981; Roy-Byrne et al., 1984; Stevens & Salisbury, 1984; Weinstein & Richman, 1984). Others, however, found that anorexic, bulimic, and obese persons worked well together and benefited from the very differences that those above found problematic (Moreno & Hileman, 1991; Shisslak et al., 1986; Weber & Gillingham, 1984). Shisslak et al. (1986), in fact, argued that homogeneity with respect to eating disorder is contraindicated for anorexics because of the ways in which their extreme isolation, denial, intellectualization, and avoidance of affect limit their ability to learn from one another. In addition, a host of other investigators reported that homogeneity/ heterogeneity of eating disorder was less important a consideration than age or developmental level (Hendren et al., 1987; Shisslak et al., 1986; Stevens & Salisbury, 1984; Stuber & Strober, 1987). In other words, these investigators found that similarities in developmental tasks and concerns were at least as important, if not moreso, in the success of the group than homo/heterogeneity with respect to eating disorder. Indeed, several investigators (Hall, 1985; Hendren et al., 1987; Shisslak et al., 1986) found older eating disorder groups to differ in content (e.g., sexuality) and process (e.g., ability to generate insight and provide feedback) than younger ones.

Across studies, attrition was higher in homogeneous anorexia groups (median = 36%) than homogeneous bulimia groups (median = 23%), and both homogeneous groups had higher attrition rates than heterogeneous eating disorder groups (median = 16%). This suggests that there may be something about the mixed eating disorder group that is associated with greater perseverance than is otherwise found in the homogeneous anorexia or, to a lesser extent, bulimia group. Perhaps anorexics are so restricting in group and bulimics are so demanding, that homogeneous groups for each create less tolerable atmospheres for sustained participation. In other words, perhaps the energy supplied by the bulimic, and the control supplied by the anorexic, provide the group with a balance of energy that otherwise is absent in the understimulated or overstimulated homogeneous anorexia or bulimia group, respectively.

Gender is a third issue of concern in the composition of the eating disorder group. On the one hand, some argue that male patients (and therapists) in the group inhibit interaction, openness, and cohesion. Consequently, homogeneity with respect to gender is recommended. Roy-Byrne et al. (1984) and Brotman et al. (1985), however, suggest that a mixed gender eating disorder group is not contraindicated theoretically, and might potentiate useful relationship work. Only two studies (Edmands, 1986; Hendren et al., 1987) reported including males in their eating disorder groups, and neither one described any impediments to process or outcome for this reason. One study noted that some eating disordered males refused group treatment because they did not want to be the only male in the group (Shisslak et al., 1986). Empirical research on the homogeneous male eating disorder group does not exist.

Referred patients tend to be more disturbed, likely to drop out of treatment and, yet, likely to improve more in group than patients responding to an announcement or advertisement. Recruitment method, consequently, may be a useful source of information in the assessment of the patient, and an important prognostic feature worthy of consideration in the selection and composition of the group. Both the content *and process* of multidimensional assessment at pretreatment is useful for identifying patient features suitable to group therapy. The degree of assessment appears to have a negative effect on attrition and a favorable impact on outcome. Medical, behavioral, and collateral assessment procedures are underutilized, not only as pretreatment screening measures but as outcome measures at post-treatment as well. Educating the patient on group therapy, particularly with respect to how problems in her everyday life will manifest themselves in group *and that this is welcomed,* may also have a favorable effect on participation, outcome, and patient satisfaction in group. Exclusion criteria such as severe personality disorder, and inclusion criteria such as rapport, sociability, and success in previous treatment are conspicuously absent in the literature and also may have a favorable effect on participation and outcome. Smaller groups may yield less attrition than larger ones; however, outcome may not be quite as favorable in the small group due to less variety in the available opportunities for observation and interaction. Age and/or developmental level of the patient may be more important a consideration in the composition of the eating disorder group than type of eating disorder alone. Finally, patients with a current eating disorder diagnosis probably will fare less well in a group of patients with other psychiatric diagnoses, but, there is some evidence to suggest that eating disordered persons may be able to function in a mixed eating disorder group more effectively than commonly has been believed.

TREATMENT OUTCOME OBSERVATIONS

Setting

Controlled research on inpatient versus intensive outpatient or daypatient group treatment of eating disorders is nonexistent. A handful of reports, however, address the various merits and demerits of inpatient and outpatient group-oriented treatment. For instance, Hall (1985) commented that outpatient group therapy doesn't lead to weight gain in anorexia as quickly as inpatient treatment and recommended that outpatient group therapy for anorexia be indicated only when the patient is not suffering from extreme inanition. Hendren et al. (1987) found concurrent individual and group outpatient treatment more effective than inpatient treatment for anorexics and bulimics. Likewise, Mitchell et al. (1988) noted that improvement in 91 bulimics followed up 2 to 5 years after intensive outpatient group therapy for bulimia was comparable to earlier reports by Swift, Ritholz, Kalin, and Kaslow (1987) on long-term outcome in 30 bulimics treated on an inpatient basis. Mitchell et al. (1988) thus concluded inpatient treatment was no better than intensive outpatient group treatment of bulimia with respect to outcome.

Duration

Duration or length of group therapy with eating disorders has received considerable attention in the literature; most is retrospective in nature and largely favors longer treatment regardless of theoretical orientation. For instance, Bauer (1984) said 30 weeks of eclectic group therapy for bulimics was slightly more effective than 15 weeks. Gerstein and Hotelling (1987) found that bulimics participating in a 9-month therapy group were generally healthier and less symptomatic than those in a 4-month therapy group, even though their scores on selected eating disorder measures were not significantly different at post-treatment. Weinstein and Richman (1984) observed that 30 weeks of psychodynamic group therapy for bulimics was more effective than 20 weeks, and that 20 weeks was more effective than 10, concluding that even more benefits could have been accrued by patients if the group were longer than 30 weeks.

In addition, Lenihan and Sanders (1984) found successful patients participated in 2 or more consecutive time-limited (12 to 14 weeks) cognitive-behavioral/interpersonal groups for anorexics and bulimics, whereas less successful patients participated in only one. Roth and Ross (1988) noted that most patients in their cognitive/interpersonal group for anorexics and bulimics needed at least 6 months of treatment to experience any significant improvement. Continuing in the litany of requests for increased duration, Hendren et al. (1987) found that patients who didn't improve attended less than 10 group therapy meetings, while those who did improve attended greater than 25 group meetings. Hall (1985) thought short-term group therapy for anorexics to be unhelpful, and recommended longer group treatment with this subgroup. Laessle, Waadt, and Pirke (1987) reasoned that their cognitive-behavioral group for bulimics yielded better results than other groups using similar interventions because their treatment was longer. Finally, a host of other studies concluded that their results might have been more favorable with longer group treatment (Edelstein & Moguilner, 1986; Gordon & Ahmed, 1988; Lee & Rush, 1986; Reed & Sech, 1985; Schneider & Agras, 1985; Telch et al., 1990), or that "maintenance groups" were needed following formal group therapy to sustain treatment gains and prevent relapse (Kirkley et al., 1985; Telch et al., 1990). Additional group treatment was also indicated in some studies due to patient interest in continuing in group beyond the scheduled termination (Franko, 1987; Lieb & Thompson, 1984; Roy-Byrne et al., 1984).

Two semi-controlled investigations found no significant differences in outcome for bulimics participating in two different lengths of group treatment. Huon and Brown (1985), for instance, found that a 6-week, 5-hour-a-day, 5-day-a-week "multifaceted" group for bulimics was just as effective as a 12-week, 2½-hour-a-day, 5-day-a-week group using the same procedures. Likewise, a weekly maintenance group following a short-term intensive group treatment program for bulimia was unrelated to outcome at 6 months follow-up (Pyle et al., 1990). Pyle et al. (1990) noted, however, that post-treatment maintenance group therapy appeared to be more useful to severely disturbed subjects than less disturbed ones. The utility of longer group treatment for severely disturbed eating disordered patients also has been documented by Brisman & Siegel (1985), Brotman et al. (1988), and Roy-Byrne et al. (1984). On the other hand, Frommer et al. (1987) and Wolchik et al. (1986) found that severely disturbed eating disordered patients benefited considerably in their short-term groups for bulimics.

The above observations notwithstanding, an examination of outcome data across all studies providing such information suggests that longer treatment may be more effective than shorter treatment in attenuating bulimic symptomotology. For instance, the median weekly reduction in binging/vomiting for bulimia groups meeting weekly up to 12 weeks was 58%, while this figure for groups meeting weekly for 13 or more weeks was 75%. Intensive short-term groups (groups meeting roughly 2½ hours or more per session, 2 or more times per week, for up to 12 weeks), however, yielded median outcomes identical to longer groups meeting 13 or more weeks. In other words, intensive (multiple weekly) short-term group treatment appears to be as effective as longer (weekly) group treatment in promoting outcome in bulimics. Whether or not these differences hold over time, generalize to other psychosocial disturbances commonly found in bulimia, and/or apply to groups with anorexics, however, remains to be seen. In the meantime, there is some evidence to suggest that longer group treatment for bulimics is warranted unless one has the resources to offer a shorter, more intense, group psychotherapy experience.

Modality

Group Therapy versus No Treatment

There is an abundance of controlled research to suggest that group therapy is superior to no therapy in the treatment of bulimia (Berry & Abramowitz, 1989; Boskind-Lodahl & White, 1978; Connors et al., 1984; Freeman et al., 1985; Freeman, Barry, Dunkeld-Turnbull, & Henderson, 1988; Gray & Hoage, 1990; Huon & Brown, 1985; Lacey, 1983; Laessle, Waadt, & Pirke, 1987; Lee & Rush, 1986; Leitenberg et al., 1988; Mitchell et al., 1990; Pyle et al., 1990; Telch et al., 1990; Wolchik et al., 1986). Over half of these investigations are of cognitive-behavioral therapy groups, while the rest are of psychoeducational or eclectic approaches that include cognitive, behavioral, and other treatment strategies. In general, bulimic patients in these studies consistently are found to be significantly more improved on eating disorder and other measures of psychosocial functioning (e.g., mood, self-esteem, social) than patients in waitlist, attention-placebo, or no treatment conditions at post-treatment. In addition, many of the studies providing follow-up data reported group subjects to be significantly more improved on most dependent measures than no-treatment subjects. Only Boskind-Lodahl and White (1978) reported that significant differences between group treatment and no-treatment subjects at post-treatment were not maintained at follow-up. In several studies, follow-up data were either not collected or not reported. Regrettably, there is an absence of controlled comparisons of group therapy versus no-treatment control conditions for anorexia.

Group Therapy versus Individual Therapy

Several controlled/semi-controlled investigations compare individual versus group modalities in treating bulimics. For instance, Freeman et al. (1985) found subjects in individual cognitive, individual behavioral, and group therapy did not significantly differ with respect to binging and purging at post-treatment; they concluded group therapy was the most economical treatment condition. Likewise, Dixon and Kiecolt-Glaser (1984) found non-significant differences in binging at 9- to 12-months follow-up for patients in group therapy versus individual therapy. Group subjects, however, showed significantly more improvement at follow-up than individual ones on measures of binge-free days, psychopathology, and locus of control. On the other hand, Freeman et al. (1988) reported that individual behavior therapy and individual cognitive-behavior therapy improved eating attitudes and behavior a little more quickly than group therapy in their sample of bulimic patients. They added that due to a higher dropout rate, lower patient satisfaction, and somewhat slower symptom improvement, group was a little less "satisfactory" than individual therapy. These investigators concluded, however, that group therapy was "remarkably effective" for completers, and more cost effective than individual therapy.

Several uncontrolled observations have been made with respect to individual versus group therapy for anorexia as well as bulimia. Leitenberg et al. (1988) found that although their group therapy results were significantly superior to those of a waitlist condition, these results were not quite as pronounced as those reported in other individual therapy studies using the same treatment methods. Group therapy led to a significant improvement in bulimia and other psychosocial features at post-treatment and follow-up (Dedman et al., 1988), but these results were not quite as favorable as those reported in similar individual treatment studies on bulimia. In an earlier review on the treatment of bulimia, Freeman and Munro (1988) concluded that individual therapy was more clinically effective than group therapy, but that group was more cost effective. In another review, Cox and Merkel (1989) reported that 40.4% and 47.4% of bulimic subjects in group therapy and individual therapy, respectively, were abstinent at post-treatment, and that 37.6% and 41.5% of group therapy and individual therapy subjects, respectively, were abstinent at follow-up. Although Weber and Gillingham (1984) observed that group was superior to individual therapy in the treatment of both eating disorders, Piazza, Carni, Kelly, and Plante (1983) suggested that group therapy was superior to individual therapy in the treatment of anorexia. Well-controlled comparisons of individual versus group therapy in the treatment of anorexia, however, have not been conducted.

Group Therapy versus Family Therapy

While there are reports of both group and family therapy as a treatment modality, controlled comparisons of family therapy versus group therapy in the treatment of anorexia and bulimia have not been made. Several uncontrolled comparisons, however, offer mixed results on the relative treatment value of these two modalities for anorexics. For instance, Piazza et al. (1983) asserted the superiority of group therapy to family therapy in the treatment of anorexics. Marner and Westerberg (1987) found that anorexics communicated more openly in group therapy than family therapy; however, they and Hall (1985) concluded that, overall, family therapy was a more powerful treatment modality with anorexics than was group therapy. Polivy (1981) also observed that family therapy was more effective with younger anorexics who were still dependent on their families, but that group therapy may be more effective with older anorexics living independently.

Group Therapy versus Drug Therapy

One controlled comparison of group versus drug therapy in the treatment of bulimia exists. Mitchell et al. (1990) found intensive outpatient cognitive-behavioral group therapy superior to drug therapy with respect to binging, purging, and other measures of eating and mood disorder at post-treatment and 6-month follow-up. These investigators noted, however, that subsequent medication trials with their drug treatment subjects yielded results comparable to those found in group subjects. A meta-analysis (Laessle, Zoettl, & Pirke, 1987), an earlier review of the treatment literature (Freeman & Munro, 1988), and an uncontrolled observation (Brisman & Siegel, 1985) also concluded that group therapy was superior to drug therapy in the treatment of bulimia. Moreover, there is some agreement in these reports that group therapy is superior to drug therapy not only with respect to improvement in target behaviors, but also in cost effectiveness, patient preference, and safety. Comparisons—controlled or otherwise—of group versus drug therapy in the treatment of anorexia are yet to be reported in the literature.

Concurrent Treatment

A number of reports comment on the value of concurrent therapy in the treatment of eating disorders. Hendren et al. (1987) found outpatient individual and group therapy to be more effective than inpatient treatment with anorexics and bulimics, while Brisman and Siegel (1985) reported no differences in outcome between patients in individual and group treatment versus those in group therapy only. Lieb and Thompson (1984) asserted that group therapy expedited individual therapy with anorexics because it lessened denial of the disorder. Hall (1985) proposed concurrent treatment for anorexia as the needs of the anorexic are greater than any single treatment modality affords. Scheuble et al., (1987) and Stuber and Strober (1987) all concluded that concurrent individual and group therapy was beneficial in the treatment of bulimic adolescents. Other studies (Barth & Wurman,

1986; Bohanske & Lemberg, 1987; Connor-Greene, 1987; Franko, 1987; Kirkley et al., 1988; Reed & Sech, 1985) lend voice to the utility of group therapy as a useful prelude, adjunct, and/or follow-up to other treatment.

There is only one controlled comparative investigation of concurrent treatment with eating disorders. Mitchell et al. (1990) found that drug plus group therapy was no more effective than group therapy alone in treating binging, purging, and other eating disordered behavior in a sample of bulimics. Mitchell, et al. (1990) added, however, that concurrent treatment did result in more improvement with respect to anxiety and mood than group or drug treatment alone. Other evidence suggests that individual appointments or contact with the group therapist during the tenure of the group and/or during follow-up minimize relapse and potentiate outcome (Freeman & Munro, 1988; Wilson et al., 1986) and that combined treatment (same individual and group therapist) is associated with lower attrition and better outcome than conjoint treatment (different individual and group therapists) in bulimia (Roy-Byrne et al., 1984; Scheuble et al., 1987). Finally, there is considerable agreement that frequent and cooperative contact between the individual and group therapists is necessary to avoid splitting, patient confusion, incongruent treatment goals and methods, and other factors found to undermine a multimodal treatment program (Brotman et al., 1985; Hall, 1985; Hendren et al., 1987; Wilson et al., 1986; Yellowlees, 1988).

Global Outcome

Outcome data on bulimic patients-subjects participating in all controlled as well as uncontrolled group therapy studies providing such information are presented in Table 12.5. The median weekly percent reduction in binging at post-treatment and follow-up across studies was 75 and 86, respectively; the median weekly percent reduction in vomiting, 70 and 83; the median percent of subjects abstinent from binging and vomiting at post-treatment across studies was 33 and 38; at follow-up, also 33 and 38. Many of these studies also reported statistically significant improvement in other areas of functioning following treatment, with improvement in mood, self-awareness/esteem, and other eating disordered behavior being the most common. Several studies, however, noted that despite statistically significant improvement within and between treatment groups, bulimic patients

TABLE 12.5.   Global Outcome Following Group Therapy for Bulimia

Binging/Vomiting[a]	Post-Treatment[b]	Follow-Up[b]
Weekly % reduction in binging	75	86
Weekly % reduction in vomiting	70	83
% Abstinent from binging	33	38
% Abstinent from vomiting	33	38

[a]Data presented in some reports as purging is represented here as vomiting.
[b]Expressed as median.

still remained in clinically significant territory on measures of eating, mood, and other disorders. Finally, a number of studies reported nonsignificant changes in weight following group treatment of bulimia; in other words, not one study found that bulimic subjects gained a statistically significant amount of weight following group. This is particularly interesting given the bulimic dreaded fear of uncontrollable weight gain following normalization of eating and abstinence from binging and purging.

Although there is little evidence showing statistically significant improvement in weight within or between groups of anorexics treated with group versus no therapy, some studies (Hall, 1985; Hendren et al., 1987; Inbody & Ellis, 1985; Lansen, 1986; Lenihan & Sanders, 1984; Lieb & Thompson, 1984; Marner & Westerberg, 1987; Piran et al., 1989; Roth & Ross, 1988; Yellowlees, 1988) provided outcome information sufficient to make some rough estimates of the clinical significance of group therapy for this population (Table 12.6). About one-third of the subjects in the aforementioned studies showed no improvement (weight loss or no weight gain), another third showed mild-moderate improvement (some weight gain but still outside of normal parameters for age and height), and one-third showed marked improvement (substantial weight gain, actualization of treatment target weight, or post-treatment weight within normal limits) following group therapy for anorexia. A number of other studies implied that group therapy was an effective treatment of anorexia (Edmands, 1986; Franko, 1987; Gary, 1986; Lafeber & Lansen, 1967; Loganbill & Koch, 1983; Lonergan, 1991; Piazza et al., 1983; Polivy, 1981; Weber & Gillingham, 1984; 106), but did not provide enough information to be included in the estimates above. Two other studies (Edelstein and Moguilner, 1986; Maher, 1984) reported that group therapy was not particularly effective with anorexics, but did not offer any explanatory data. One study (Lafeber & Lansen, 1967) reported deterioration effects in some patients following group therapy for anorexia. Finally, most studies reported anorexic patients

TABLE 12.6. Global Outcome in Percent Following Group Therapy for Anorexia[a]

Investigator	No Improvement	Mild-Moderate Improvement	Marked Improvement
Yellowlees (1988)	33	33	33
Hendren et al. (1987)	33	33	33
Lieb & Thompson (1984)	0	100[b]	—
Inbody & Ellis (1985)	0	0	100
Piran et al. (1989)	26	74[b]	—
Hall (1985)	40	60[b]	—
Marner & Westerberg (1987)	12	50	38
Lansen (1986)	43	57[b]	—
Lenihan & Sanders (1984)	12	24	64
Roth & Ross (1988)	33	67[b]	—

[a]Some of these figures represent transpositions of information presented in another form.
[b]Represents a combination of both mild-moderate and marked improvement categories.

to be improved in other areas of psychosocial functioning following group therapy, with improvement in social functioning (e.g., less isolated, more assertive, more satisfied in relationships with others) noted considerably more often than improvement in mood, general psychopathology, or self-awareness/esteem.

Inpatient treatment may be indicated over intensive outpatient group treatment for severe disturbances in anorexia or bulimia, however, the evidence for bulimics on this issue is less favorable than it is for anorexics. Short-term group treatment of eating disorders yields statistically and clinically significant results, while long-term group treatment appears to be even more effective, particularly for severely disturbed patients. Short-term intensive group psychotherapy, however, may be as effective as longer treatment provided in the traditional weekly format. Group therapy is statistically and clinically superior to no therapy in the treatment of eating disorders, and there is some evidence to suggest that attrition and outcome is a little less favorable in group than individual therapy. There is considerable agreement, however, that group therapy is the most cost effective of the various treatment regimens, and that concurrent treatment is more effective than any one modality alone. Clinically, roughly one-third of all anorexic and bulimic patients evidence marked improvement or abstinence, respectively, following group therapy for an eating disorder.

Theoretical Orientation and Technique

A handful of investigators have conducted controlled comparisons of various theoretical orientations and techniques in the group treatment of eating disorders. Gordon and Ahmed (1988) and Kirkley et al. (1985) reported nonsignificant differences between cognitive-behavioral group therapy and nondirective or supportive group therapy on eating disorder and other psychosocial measures at follow-up, and in like fashion Yates and Sambrailo (1984) found cognitive-behavioral group therapy plus behavioral instruction to be equal to cognitive-behavioral group therapy alone on eating disorder and other measures of psychosocial functioning at follow-up. On the other hand, Leitenberg's et al. (1988) exposure-response prevention group subjects treated in multiple as well as single settings vomited significantly less than cognitive-behavioral group subjects at follow-up. These differences were of minimal clinical significance, however, and the two groups evidenced nonsignificant differences on other measures of depression and self-esteem. Wilson et al. (1986) noted nonsignificant differences between cognitive restructuring/exposure-response prevention group subjects, and cognitive restructuring only group subjects on measures of binging, purging, mood, psychopathology, and social behavior at post-treatment. However, cognitive restructuring/exposure-response prevention group subjects were significantly more improved than cognitive restructuring only subjects on several other eating disorder measures at post-treatment. Moreover, although nonsignificant statistically, the clinical significance of the

**TABLE 12.7.   Outcome Across Theoretical Orientation in Bulimia Group
Therapy Studies**

Theoretical Orientation	Weekly % Reduction in Binging at Post-Treatment[a]	Weekly % Reduction in Vomiting at Post-Treatment[a]
Cognitive-behavioral	91	81
Psychodynamic	75	—
Eclectic[b]	74.5	69
Psychoeducational	70	70

[a]Expressed as median.
[b]Defined as a combination of two or more approaches.

differences between the two groups on measures of binging and purging at
post-treatment and follow-up favored the cognitive restructuring/exposure-
response prevention subjects. Dozens of other uncontrolled studies,
particularly with bulimics, report statistically significant within group differences between pre/post-treatment assessment. Unfortunately, several
studies, however, did not find group therapy to be particularly helpful to
eating disordered patients (Edelstein & Moguilner, 1986; Hinz & Ragsdell,
1990; Lafeber & Lansen, 1967; Polivy, 1981).

Outcome data across theoretical perspectives reported in the controlled
and uncontrolled bulimia studies noted above are presented in Table 12.7.
Cognitive-behavioral approaches appear to yield somewhat more favorable
outcomes at post-treatment than psychodynamic, eclectic, and psychoeducational ones. Whether or not these differences are statistically significant
or hold up over time, however, remains to be seen. Moreover, there is a
dearth of outcome data on psychodynamic approaches to eating disorder
groups, despite the contention by some investigators that psychodynamic
approaches are the most widely prescribed (Hudson & Pope, 1986).

Specific Techniques

Overall, controlled as well as uncontrolled investigations suggest that group
therapy yields statistically and clinically significant changes in eating disordered persons. Investigators, however, remain at a loss to explain precisely what factors operating in group subsequently lead to patient change.
For instance, several researchers (e.g., Lee & Rush, 1986) acknowledged
the impossibility of determining whether cognitive-behavioral procedures
or other nonspecific factors associated with talking in a group promotes
patient change. Consequently, some investigators speculate on what was
particularly impactful; others survey patients for their perceptions on what
was most useful. A review of these retrospective observations from patients, therapists, and/or investigators was conducted in the spirit of shed-
ding further light on what works in group therapy for eating disordered
persons and why. These observations may be classified into the following
three categories: leader activity and structure, leader technique, and therapeutic factors.

Leader Activity and Structure

There seems to be considerable agreement that groups for the eating disordered function more effectively with greater structure than what may be useful to other populations in group. Specifically, eating disorder patients are so anxious, isolated, and impulsive that groups without much structure have met with high levels of resistance, absenteeism, and attrition. Three investigators (Brotman et al., 1985; Moreno & Hileman, 1991; Roy-Byrne et al., 1984) found that firm ground rules for attendance, tardiness, payment, acting-out, confidentiality, and out-of-group contact were associated with better attendance and cohesion, and less attrition and acting out, than more permissive ones. In 2 of these studies (Moreno & Hileman, 1991; Roy-Byrne et al., 1984), a sharp increase in attendance and cohesion was observed once concrete ground rules around attendance, commitment, and payment were established after a less structured and more lenient group beginning. Likewise, two studies containing groups with perfect patient attendance (Fernandez, 1984; Gray & Hoage, 1990) suggested that this was partially due to a high degree of structure in their groups. Supporting data from another study (Dixon & Kiecolt-Glaser, 1984) noted that a lack of structure was responsible for a 63% attrition rate. Franko (1987) reported that 84% of the patients in a large self-help group wanted more structure, and Block and Llewelyn (1987) found that leaders who spoke often but briefly were valued more by eating disordered patients in group than those who spoke less often but for longer duration. There exists some thought that high group structure is more important at the beginning of the eating disorders group (Hall, 1985; Roth & Ross, 1988) and with younger patients (Hendren et al., 1987).

There is some evidence to suggest that too much structure threatens the autonomy of the eating disordered patient and interferes with group participation (Roy-Byrne et al., 1984); indeed, several investigators conclude that some degree of leader flexibility is as important as structure in the eating disorder group (Fernandez, 1984; Hall, 1985; Roy-Byrne et al., 1984). Perhaps the most frequently addressed issue involving the coupling of structure and flexibility, however, has to do with policies around out-of-group contact. Most investigators commenting on this issue (Bauer, 1984; Bohanske & Lemberg, 1987; Brotman et al., 1985; Franko, 1987; Hall, 1985; Hornak, 1983; Roy-Byrne et al., 1984) have found extragroup contact valuable for the eating disorder patient. Specifically, these reporters suggested that out-of-group contact helped patients cope with eating disordered symptoms, anxiety, depression, and other problems between groups. Several investigators also noted that extragroup contact seems to increase attendance, lower attrition, and increase self-disclosure during group. Only two reports found extragroup contact to interfere with group effectiveness (Brotman et al., 1985; Yellowlees, 1988), with Brotman et al. indicating that this was more of a problem for the psychodynamic group than the cognitive-behavioral one.

Leader Technique

With respect to skills associated with the therapeutic alliance, several studies (Hall, 1985; Inbody & Ellis, 1985; Lonergan, 1991; Shisslak et al., 1986) suggest that therapist warmth, probing, encouragement, clarification, empathy, and acceptance are particularly useful in the identification, tolerance, expression, and acceptance of heretofore forbidden thoughts, feelings, impulses, and needs. With respect to behavioral techniques, several studies (Hornak, 1983; Johnson et al., 1983; Lacey, 1983; Loganbill and Koch, 1983) suggest goal setting, contracting, meal planning and normalization, and/or the cultivation of alternative coping behaviors as especially useful interventions for helping patients directly control symptoms. Two behavioral interventions, self-monitoring and/or role-playing, are also mentioned (Johnson et al., 1983; Lacey, 1983; Marner & Westerberg, 1987; Roy-Byrne et al., 1984; Schneider & Agras, 1985) as particularly useful techniques for controlling symptoms and increasing self-awareness and self-expression. However, two studies reported that role-playing (Hall, 1985) and diary keeping (Roy-Byrne, et al., 1984) were of little value or were resisted by their patients, respectively. Interestingly, two other cornerstones of behavior therapy, relaxation and assertion training, were not highlighted by investigators or their patients as useful ingredients in group; in fact, Johnson et al. (1983) reported that patients rated these two interventions as least helpful. Cognitive techniques such as cognitive restructuring, self-instruction, and psychoeducation were also favorably implicated in a couple studies (Hornak, 1983; Johnson et al., 1983); however, Freeman et al. (1988) concluded that cognitive interventions added little to the success of behavioral ones, and Huon and Brown (1985) found that only 5% of the patients in their group valued psychoeducation around topics of food and nutrition.

Psychodynamic interventions, particularly interpretations, receive mixed reviews. Interpretations of resistance yielded more resistance (Hendren et al., 1987), and interpretations were too intrusive for a clinical population psychologically allergic to overinvolvement (Hall, 1985). Roy-Byrne et al. (1984) agreed that group-as-a-whole interpretations threatened the autonomy and tenuous identity of eating disordered patients; yet, on the other hand, observed that such interventions minimized privatization of negative group events. Shisslak et al. (1986) described how interpretations of transference reactions promoted reality testing and personal boundaries in group members. Interpretations also have been found to help eating disordered patients make connections between their group life and everyday life (Hall, 1985; Moreno & Hileman, 1991), as well as help patients "put words to" behaviors that otherwise are acted out (Moreno & Hileman, 1991). Roth and Ross (1988), however, reported that patients in their group resisted making connections between group and everyday life. Overall, leader interpretations and other dynamic interventions in the eating disorders group is a neglected area of investigation compared to other cognitive, behavioral, and psychoeducational techniques.

Clinical support for some less traditional leader interventions is not very favorable. For instance, Hinz and Ragsdell (1990) reported that an eating disorder group of 9 months deteriorated with respect to attendance, attrition, and cohesion following the introduction of a mask-making/videotaping exercise. Similarly, Lafeber and Lansen (1967) found attendance to drop considerably after the introduction of puppet-making and play therapy in an otherwise talk-therapy group for anorexics. Over time, however, a few patients in this group were able to make better use of this therapeutic medium. Hall (1985) asserted that gestalt techniques were unhelpful in group therapy with anorexics, although Kearney-Cooke (1988) reported various experiential exercises to be of use to incested bulimics. Reed and Sech (1985) observed that the feedback eating disordered patients gave to themselves following observation of their group on videotape was more valuable to them than feedback from other patients in the group. Finally, several studies concluded that flexibility with respect to leader technique was particularly helpful to patients (Brotman et al., 1985; Fernandez, 1984; Hall, 1985). Brotman et al., however, found that leader technical flexibility was particularly confusing and frustrating for patients when not used in an integrated and well-orchestrated fashion.

Therapeutic Factors

Controlled research on therapeutic factors (Yalom, 1985) in group therapy with eating disorders is virtually nonexistent. However, a number of retrospective observations of curativeness provided by patients, therapists, and investigators in a variety of controlled as well as uncontrolled studies have been reported in the literature (Berry & Abramowitz, 1989; Block & Llewelyn, 1987; Bohanske & Lemberg, 1987; Brisman & Siegel, 1985; Dixon & Kiecolt-Glaser, 1984; Edmands, 1986; Franko, 1987; Gary, 1986; Gray & Hoage, 1990; Hendren et al., 1987; Hobbs, Birtchnell, Harte, & Lacey, 1989; Hornak, 1983; Inbody & Ellis, 1985; Kearney-Cooke, 1988; Lacey, 1983; Lieb & Thompson, 1984; Loganbill & Koch, 1983; Marner & Westerberg, 1987; Moreno & Hileman, 1991; Moreno, Hileman, & Fuhriman, 1992; Reed & Sech, 1985; Roth & Ross, 1988; Shisslak et al., 1986; Yellowlees, 1988). Overall, universality, insight, and cohesion are far and away the most commonly cited reasons why eating disordered patients benefited from group treatment. Given the shame, poor interoceptive awareness, and isolation/alienation that are almost invariably associated with anorexia and bulimia, it is easy to see how hearing others disclose similar problems, identifying one's thoughts, feelings, and needs, and being accepted and fitting-in with others would be of particular value to these patients.

Another cluster of therapeutic factors mentioned fairly frequently include catharsis, imparting information, vicarious learning, and hope. Again, given the emotional restriction, irrational beliefs around food/body/weight, and the hopelessness also commonly associated with these disorders, it is understandable how emotional expression, psychoeducation, and the witnessing of improvement in others would be viewed as beneficial. The frequency with which vicarious or observational learning is mentioned in the literature suggests that despite low levels of interaction in a group, more learning may be occurring in the silent member(s) than meets the eye. In several studies, patients reported that they were largely motivated to improve by observing another member of the group get worse.

Finally, altruism, socialization techniques, existential factors, and recapitulation of the primary family group are rarely mentioned as helpful by patients and/or therapists. This is somewhat surprising given that group affords patients the opportunity to be of use to one another, thereby counteracting common feelings of use/worthlessness. Likewise, this is surprising given the number of cognitive-behavioral groups in the literature where training in assertiveness and other coping skills is a cornerstone of treatment. If one defines many of the interventions described in the cognitive-behavioral literature as "socialization techniques," then the importance of this factor for eating disorder patients would be on par with universality, insight, and cohesion. Several cognitive-behavioral investigators suggested that other factors associated with interaction in group may have promoted outcome *along with* more traditional cognitive and behavioral interventions (e.g., Lee & Rush, 1986).

Anecdotal observations on the development of therapeutic factors also are embedded in the aforementioned studies addressing curativeness in the eating disorders group (Edmands, 1986; Hobbs et al., 1989; Loganbill & Koch, 1983; Moreno & Hileman, 1991; Roth & Ross, 1988). Without a doubt, universality is associated with the earlier stages of group treatment. Food, weight, and body related talk in particular appear to stimulate the development of this factor. Cohesion is also frequently associated with the earlier stages of group, and there is some evidence to suggest that the more frequent and intense the group format, the earlier that cohesion will emerge (Brisman & Siegel, 1985). Several studies, however, found cohesion to emerge later in the group (Loganbill & Koch, 1983), or not at all (Maher, 1984). Moreno and Hileman (1991) found the cohesion level in their mixed eating disorder group to fluctuate considerably even after one year of treatment. Imparting information and socialization techniques also appear to be associated with earlier stages of treatment, particularly in the short-term, cognitive-behavioral, and psychoeducational studies. Otherwise, socialization techniques, catharsis, and interpersonal learning seem to emerge later in treatment, particularly for the less structured eclectic or psychodynamic groups.

Age or developmental level, patient and therapist perceptions of curativeness, and factors found not to be helpful are also addressed. For instance, Hendren et al. (1987) reported that older groups were better at generating insight around group dynamics and giving and receiving feedback than younger ones. Hobbs et al. (1989) found patients and therapists differed in their perceptions of curativeness, with patients valuing self-understanding, vicarious learning, universality, and hope, and therapists valuing self-understanding, acceptance, self-disclosure, interpersonal learning, and catharsis. Differences in patient and therapist perceptions of significant events also have been reported by Hall (1985) and Moreno, Fuhriman, and Hileman (1993). Shisslak et al. (1986) found universality lowered denial, increased anxiety, and precipitated attrition to some degree in their group, while Moreno and Hileman (1991) reported that some patients in their group did not always benefit by universality because it threatened their need to be special or different. Overall, attention to what is not therapeutic to the eating disorder patient in group is conspicuously absent in the literature, and may be another avenue for furthering our understanding as to how group does or does not help this difficult population.

Other Features of the Eating Disorders Group during Treatment

In addition to the above comments on treatment setting, duration, modality, and techniques, some investigators have made some interesting observations on the topical, emotional, and interpersonal climate of the eating disorder group. The following discussion summarizes some of these notations in the spirit of generating additional insight into the process, as well as outcome of eating disorder groups.

Content

A number of studies describe the process of an eating disorder group with respect to themes around content (Bauer, 1984; Hall, 1985; Hendren et al., 1987; Lieb and Thompson, 1984; Loganbill and Koch, 1983; Roth and Ross, 1988; Roy-Byrne et al., 1984; Vanderlinden and Vandereycken, 1988; Weber and Gillingham, 1984; Weinstein and Richman, 1984). In reviewing these descriptions, food, weight, eating disorder symptoms and functions, and body dissatisfaction were the most commonly reported topics in the eating disorder group. Moreover, these themes appeared to be more pronounced in the early stages of the group, and returned to periodically later in the group when members were under stress. "Food talk," in fact, is described by several investigators as a particularly useful metaphor for understanding the eating disordered person's feelings about self and others throughout the tenure of the group.

Other commonly reported themes in the literature include parent-family issues, perfectionism, fear of rejection, need for approval, low self-esteem, men/sex, and relationship difficulties in general. Thoughts and feelings about relationships outside the group (e.g., family/friends) also seemed to precede group members' discussion of thoughts and feelings about relationships in the group. Also, feelings about other members of the group (especially the therapists) were described by several investigators as embedded in discussions of other persons outside the group. This sequence of content development (food talk, out-group relationship talk, in-group relationship talk) appeared similar in both short-term and long-term groups. In other words, groups as brief as several months and as long as a year or more, evidenced similar patterns of content development. Finally, there is some evidence to suggest that anorexic groups spend more time on food and family topics, while bulimic ones devote more time to relationships. Other evidence suggests that the content of the eating disorder group varies with respect to developmental level, with older groups focusing more on work, sex, and relationships, and younger ones focusing more on school and family issues.

Affect

The presence of affect in the eating disorder group is another subject receiving much attention (Edelstein & Moguilner, 1986; Edmands, 1986; Hall, 1985; Loganbill & Koch, 1983; Lonergan, 1991; Moreno et al., 1992; Reed & Sech, 1985; Roy-Byrne et al., 1984; Shisslak et al., 1986). In general, there is wide agreement that eating disordered patients avoid the identification and expression of feelings in group, particularly in the earlier stages of group development. However, in the later stages of group, affect is oftentimes still not well tolerated as evidenced by food talk, silence, topic jumping, intellectualization, tardiness, absences, and other distractions in or following its presence. Anger appears to be the most frequently cited feeling that patients wrestle with in group, with guilt and fears of retaliation, rejection, and/or abandonment in its wake. When anger is dealt with in the group, it is often after the emergence of other feelings like guilt, shame, fear, and sadness. In addition, most observers found that eating disordered persons will express anger at the therapist(s) before venting at other members. No evidence exists to suggest that certain feelings are more pronounced in anorexic versus bulimic groups; however, there is some agreement that bulimic groups, in general, are more affectively charged than anorexic ones.

Interaction

In addition to content and affect themes, some observers comment on interaction patterns in the eating disorder group (Brisman & Siegel, 1985; Hall, 1985; Hendren et al., 1987; Inbody & Ellis, 1985; Moreno & Hileman, 1991). In general, interaction appears to be less frequent and less spontaneous than interaction in groups with other populations; moreover, interaction in the anorexia group is more restricted than that reported in the bulimia group, where patient participation is much more inconsistent or labile. It appears that the eating disordered person uses the group and food much in the same way: the anorexic restricts (doesn't participate), and the bulimic binges (engages group) and then purges (rejects group) or starves (avoids group). Therapist exploration of patients' resistance to interacting has elicited fears of attachment, dependency and rejection, engulfment, the belief that others (especially the therapist) already know (or should know) what they are thinking, a wish to avoid negative affect, the wish to be special, fears of being selfish or greedy, and an inability to attend to others because of one's preoccupation and concern for oneself.

Controlled comparisons in the literature have not consistently demonstrated the superiority of one treatment approach over any other. Outcome data across controlled and uncontrolled studies, however, suggest that cognitive-behavioral procedures are slightly more clinically significant than psychodynamic, educational, or eclectic ones. This observation notwithstanding, experimenters are still unclear on exactly what leader, patient, and group behaviors account for most of the changes evidenced in group members. Post-treatment observations by patients, therapists, and investigators suggest that therapist activity, structure, and empathic attention to the identification, experience, and expression of emotions are particularly useful during the course of the group. Likewise, cognitive-behavioral procedures such as goal setting, contracting, menu planning, identification of alternative coping skills, cognitive restructuring, self-instruction, and psychoeducation also appear to be quite useful. Psychodynamic interpretations receive mixed reviews, as have other interventions with more of an experiential flavor. Universality, cohesion, insight, and socialization techniques appear to be the most operative therapeutic factors in group, with universality emerging almost immediately and the others following later during the course of the group. Finally, eating disordered persons spend a fair amount of time discussing food and symptoms in group, and seem to have more difficulty interacting with one another—especially around affectively charged topics—than patients in other types of groups.

METHODOLOGICAL CONSIDERATIONS

A host of methodological limitations in the empirical literature on group therapy for eating disorders may interfere with the digestion of the presentation above. For instance, small sample sizes, overrepresentation of university students, variable diagnostic criteria, overreliance on self-report assessment and outcome measures, therapist inexperience, poorly operationalized treatment strategies, inappropriate statistical analyses, liberal alpha levels, and inadequate follow-up periods are some of the more common problems observed across studies. Likewise, control for subject/experimenter bias, concurrent treatment, crossover (e.g, anorexia to bulimia or bulimia to substance abuse), pretreatment differences among subjects, and other extraneous factors influencing outcome is frequently absent in the empirical literature. Finally, there is wide variability in reporting styles across investigators and journals, thereby adding to the confusion of how a group may have affected its members. As others (e.g., Strupp & Binder, 1992; Yalom, 1985) have intimated, we may never reach the point where we can identify all the factors operative when two or more people gather and interact with one another over time. Future attention to some of the empirical problems noted above, however, may bring us closer to this goal than is currently the case.

A MENU FOR CLINICIANS

Methodological problems notwithstanding, there is much to be consumed in the empirical literature for the group therapist in clinical practice. First and foremost, there is no substitute for thoughtful and thorough assessment and preparation. Multiple assessment procedures conducted over a two- or three-week period may provide the practical, diagnostic, and motivational information necessary to determine patient suitability for group. Pregroup preparation will give the opportunity to predict future difficulties in group (among other things), and explore and identify alternatives to absenteeism, withdrawal, premature termination, and other forms of acting out. Such attention to assessment and preparation of the patient for group should do much to minimize attrition and potentiate outcome in members.

Patients with severe characterological disturbances and precariously low body weight, among other things, are generally not good candidates for group, particularly short-term experiences. Previous success in treatment, a capacity for attachment, rapport with the pregroup interviewer, some modicum of insight, and a willingness to commit to group for a significant period of time, however, may be good prognostic signs for all patients, regardless of symptom severity. In general, a larger group (e.g., 8 to 10 members) consisting of anorexics and bulimics similar in age may provide the interpersonal, observational, and developmental resources conducive to outcome over time. With respect to duration, the longer the group the better, unless one has the time and resources to offer a brief *intensive* outpatient group. Treatment results should find roughly one-third of the membership dramatically improved, with another third mildly-moderately improved following termination from the group. One-third of one's patients may show little or no improvement and, consequently, may benefit from additional treatment. Treatment of more recalcitrant patients may best be provided concurrently, where the group therapist is also the individual therapist.

In treatment, one may need to intervene more actively and flexibly in the eating disorders group than in other group populations. A fair amount of activity is particularly warranted in the beginning of the group in order to contain the anxiety that otherwise might be acted out by absenteeism or premature termination. On the other hand, one must be careful not to be too active, lest one threaten the patient's already precarious sense of identity and autonomy. With respect to specific techniques, probing, clarification, empathy, acceptance, and warmth may be most useful in exploring, identifying, expressing, and tolerating patient affect. Collectively, these techniques should also serve as the tray upon which all other leader interventions are served.

Some other methods one may elect to use during the course of treatment are psychoeducational, cognitive, behavioral, and psychodynamic in nature.

Psychoeducational strategies (e.g., literature, lectures) may be especially helpful in modifying unhealthy attitudes about food, body, and weight, as well as facilitate normalization of eating. Confrontation of discrepancies in members' appraisal of events *inside as well as outside* of the group may promote more reasonable ways of evaluating self and others. Self-monitoring, goal-setting, and contracting may promote self-awareness as well as potentiate further control of eating disorder symptoms. The identification and application of alternatives to binging, purging, and/or restricting (e.g., assertion training) may be another behavioral strategy worth employing, particularly if practiced within the context of the group. Finally, one may elect to interpret individual or group events in order to help patients "put words to" behaviors that heretofore have been expressed symbolically in eating disordered and other self-defeating activity. Food associations, tardiness, absenteeism, and dramatic changes in eating, symptoms, and other behaviors within and/or between groups are just some of the things worthy of interpretation. To the extent the patient can verbalize these feelings, the interpretation, too, may be instrumental in the promotion of "alternative behaviors" that lend themselves to symptom control and cognitive modification.

Developmentally, group members are likely to focus on food and weight-related issues earlier in the tenure of the group, and more on personal and interpersonal issues as the group matures. Affective expression, especially anger, will probably be particularly difficult for patients, but ambivalence around intimacy and dependence is likely to be problematic for members as well. Self-disclosure and interaction in the group may vary considerably, as members are likely to binge, purge, and restrict in the group the same way they do with food. The therapist is likely to be puzzled, frustrated, and drained oftentimes over the life of the group, because of the difficulties this population has with affect, engagement, and maintenance of treatment gains. Consequently, one is best advised to conduct the group with a cotherapist where the opportunity for normalization and management of negative self-experience is maximized. At times the services of a supervisor may be indicated, especially if one is a relatively inexperienced group and/or eating disorder therapist.

CONCLUSION

Group therapy is a common approach to the treatment of anorexia and bulimia nervosa. Empirical research suggests that it is certainly superior to no-treatment, and that it may be more cost effective than other treatment modalities. There remains more to know about how, precisely, talking in a group helps this patient population. Future case and experimental investigations should explore and test additional hypotheses designed to develop this nascent body of research.

REFERENCES

American Psychiatric Association. (1987). *Diagnostic and statistical manual of mental disorders* (3rd ed., rev.). Washington, DC: Author.

Asner, J. (1990). Reworking the myth of personal incompetence: Group psychotherapy for bulimia nervosa. *Psychiatric Annals, 20,* 395–397.

Barth, D., & Wurman, V. (1986). Group therapy with bulimic women: A self-psychological approach. *International Journal of Eating Disorders, 5,* 735–745.

Bauer, B. G. (1984). Bulimia: A review of a group treatment program. *Journal of College Student Personnel, 25,* 221–227.

Berry, D. M., & Abramowitz, S. I. (1989). Educative/support groups and subliminal psychodynamic activation for bulimic college women. *International Journal of Eating Disorders, 8,* 75–85.

Block, E., & Llewelyn, S. (1987). Leadership skills and helpful factors in self-help groups. *British Journal of Guidance and Counselling, 15,* 257–270.

Bohanske, J., & Lemberg, R. (1987). An intensive group process-retreat model for the treatment of bulimia. *Group, 11,* 228–237.

Boskind-Lodahl, M., & White, W. C. (1978). The definition and treatment of bulimarexia in college women—A pilot study. *Journal of the American College Health Association, 27,* 84–86, 97.

Brisman, J., & Siegel, M. (1985). The bulimia workshop: A unique integration of group treatment approaches. *International Journal of Group Psychotherapy, 35,* 585–601.

Brotman, A. W., Alonso, A., & Herzog, D. B. (1985). Group therapy for bulimia: Clinical experience and practical recommendations. *Group, 9,* 15–23.

Brotman, A. W., Herzog, D. B., & Hamburg, P. (1988). Long-term course in 14 bulimic patients treated with psychotherapy. *Journal of Clinical Psychiatry, 49,* 157–160.

Browning, W. N. (1985). Long-term dynamic group therapy with bulimic patients: A clinical discussion. In S. W. Emmett (Ed.), *Theory and treatment of anorexia nervosa and bulimia: Biomedical, sociocultural, and psychological perspectives.* New York: Brunner/Mazel.

Chelton, L. G., & Bonney, W. C. (1987). Addiction, affects and selfobject theory. *Psychotherapy, 24,* 40–46.

Connor-Greene, P. A. (1987). An educational group treatment program for bulimia. *Journal of American College Health, 35,* 229–231.

Connors, M. E., Johnson, C. L., & Stuckey, M. K. (1984). Treatment of bulimia with brief psychoeducational group therapy. *American Journal of Psychiatry, 141,* 1512–1516.

Cox, G. L., & Merkel, W. T. (1989). A qualitative review of psychosocial treatments for bulimia. *Journal of Nervous and Mental Disease, 177,* 77–84.

Dedman, P. A., Numa, S. F., & Wakeling, A. (1988). A cognitive behavioral group approach for the treatment of bulimia nervosa—A preliminary study. *Journal of Psychosomatic Research, 32,* 285–290.

452   Group Treatment for Eating Disorders

Dixon, K. N., & Kiecolt-Glaser, J. (1984). Group therapy for bulimia. *The Hillsdale Journal of Clinical Psychiatry, 6,* 156–170.

Edelstein, E. L., & Moguilner, E. (1986). Homogeneous groups as treatment modality for anorectics. *Psychotherapy and Psychosomatics, 46,* 205–208.

Edmands, M. S. (1986). Overcoming eating disorders: A group experience. *Journal of Psychosocial Nursing, 24,* 19–25.

Fernandez, R. C. (1984). Group therapy of bulimia. In P. S. Powers & R. C. Fernandez (Eds.), *Current treatment of anorexia nervosa and bulimia.* New York: Karger.

Franko, D. L. (1987). Anorexia nervosa and bulimia: A self-help group. *Small Group Behavior, 18,* 398–407.

Freeman, C., Sinclair, F., Turnbull, J., & Annandale, A. (1985). Psychotherapy for bulimia: A controlled study. *Journal of Psychiatric Research, 19,* 473–478.

Freeman, C. P. L., Barry, F., Dunkeld-Turnbull, J., & Henderson, A. (1988). Controlled trial of psychotherapy for bulimia nervosa. *British Medical Journal, 296,* 521–525.

Freeman, C. P. L., & Munro, K. M. (1988). Drug and group treatments for bulimia/bulimia nervosa. *Journal of Psychosomatic Research, 32,* 647–660.

Frommer, M. S., Ames, J. R., Gibson, J. W., & Davis, W. N. (1987). Patterns of symptom change in the short-term group treatment of bulimia. *International Journal of Eating Disorders, 6,* 469–476.

Garner, D. M., Fairburn, C. G., & Davis, R. (1987). Cognitive-behavioral treatment of bulimia nervosa: A critical appraisal. *Behavior Modification, 11,* 398–431.

Garner, D. M., & Garfinkel, P. E. (1985). Introduction. In D. M. Garner & P. E. Garfinkel (Eds.), *Handbook of psychotherapy for anorexia nervosa and bulimia* (pp. 3–6). New York: Guilford Press.

Gary, J. M. (1986). A problem-solving workshop on eating disorders. *Journal of College Student Personnel, 27,* 182–183.

Gerstein, L. H., & Hotelling, K. (1987). Length of group treatment and changes in women with bulimia. *Journal of Mental Health Counseling, 9,* 162–173.

Glassman, J. N. S., Rich, C. L., Darko, D., & Clarkin, A. (1990). Some correlates of treatment response to a multicomponent psychotherapy program in outpatients with eating disorders. *Annals of Clinical Psychiatry, 2,* 33–38.

Gordon, K., & Ahmed, W. (1988). A comparison of two group therapies for bulimia. *British Review of Bulimia and Anorexia Nervosa, 3,* 17–31.

Gray, J. J., & Hoage, C. M. (1990). Bulimia nervosa: Group behavior therapy with exposure plus response prevention. *Psychological Reports, 66,* 667–674.

Griffiths, R. A., Touyz, S. W., Mitchell, P. B., & Bacon, W. (1987). The treatment of bulimia. *Australian and New Zealand Journal of Psychiatry, 21,* 5–15.

Hall, A. (1985). Group therapy for anorexia nervosa. In D. M. Garner & P. E. Garfinkel (Eds.), *Handbook of psychotherapy for anorexia nervosa and bulimia.* New York: Guilford Press.

Hamilton, S. A. (1988, August). Group therapy for bulimia: The role of evaluation. In *evaluating group therapy outcome in university counseling centers.* Symposium conducted at the meeting of the American Psychological Association, Atlanta, GA.

Hendren, R. L., Atkins, D. M., Sumner, C. R., & Barber, J. K. (1987). Model for the group treatment of eating disorders. *International Journal of Group Psychotherapy, 37,* 589–602.

Hinz, L. D., & Ragsdell, V. (1990). Using masks and video in group psychotherapy with bulimics. *The Arts in Psychotherapy, 17,* 259–261.

Hobbs, M., Birtchnell, S., Harte, A., & Lacey, H. (1989). Therapeutic factors in short-term group therapy for women with bulimia. *International Journal of Eating Disorders, 8,* 623–633.

Hornak, N. J. (1983). Group treatment for bulimia: Bulimics anonymous. *Journal of College Student Personnel, 24,* 461–463.

Hudson, J. I., & Pope, H. G., Jr. (1986). Treatment of bulimia: A review of current studies. In F. E. F. Larocca (Ed.), *New directions for mental health services* (No. 31, pp. 71–85). San Francisco, CA: Jossey-Bass.

Huon, G. F., & Brown, L. B. (1985). Evaluating a group treatment for bulimia. *Journal of Psychiatric Research, 19,* 479–483.

Inbody, D. R., & Ellis, J. J. (1985). Group therapy with anorexic and bulimic patients: Implications for therapeutic intervention. *American Journal of Psychotherapy, 39,* 411–420.

Johnson, C., & Connors, M. E. (1987). *The etiology and treatment of bulimia nervosa: A biopsychosocial perspective.* New York: Basic.

Johnson, C., Connors, M., & Stuckey, M. (1983). Short-term group treatment of bulimia: A preliminary report. *International Journal of Eating Disorders, 2,* 199–208.

Kearney-Cooke, A. (1988). Group treatment of sexual abuse among women with eating disorders. *Women & Therapy, 7,* 5–21.

Kirkley, B. G., Battaglia, L., Earle, L., Gans, K., & Molloy, M. E. (1988). Health education as a component of campus bulimia treatment programs. *Journal of American College Health, 37,* 40–43.

Kirkley, B. G., Schneider, J. A., Agras, W. S., & Bachman, J. A. (1985). Comparison of two group treatments for bulimia. *Journal of Consulting and Clinical Psychology, 53,* 43–48.

Lacey, J. H. (1983). Bulimia nervosa, binge eating, and psychogenic vomiting: A controlled treatment study and long term outcome. *British Medical Journal, 286,* 1609–1613.

Laessle, R. G., Waadt, S., & Pirke, K. M. (1987). A structured behaviorally oriented group treatment for bulimia nervosa. *Psychotherapy and Psychosomatics, 48,* 141–145.

Laessle, R. G., Zoettl, C., & Pirke, K. M. (1987). Meta-analysis of treatment studies for bulimia. *International Journal of Eating Disorders, 6,* 647–653.

Lafeber, C., & Lansen, J. (1967). *A group therapy with anorexia nervosa patients.* Paper presented at the International Congress of Psychotherapy, Wiesbaden, West Germany.

Lansen, J. (1986). Group therapy with anorexia nervosa patients. *International Journal of Group Psychotherapy, 36,* 321–322.

Laube, J. J. (1990). Why group therapy for bulimia? *International Journal of Group Psychotherapy, 40,* 169–187.

454 Group Treatment for Eating Disorders

Lee, N. F., & Rush, A. J. (1986). Cognitive-behavioral group therapy for bulimia. *International Journal of Eating Disorders, 5,* 599–615.

Leitenberg, H., Rosen, J. C., Gross, J., Nudelman, S., & Vara, L. S. (1988). Exposure plus response-prevention treatment of bulimia nervosa. *Journal of Consulting and Clinical Psychology, 56,* 535–541.

Lenihan, G. O., & Sanders, C. D. (1984). Guidelines for group therapy with eating disorder victims. *Journal of Counseling and Development, 63,* 252–254.

Lieb, R. C., & Thompson, T. L., II (1984). Group psychotherapy of four anorexia nervosa inpatients. *International Journal of Group Psychotherapy, 34,* 639–642.

Loganbill, C., & Koch, M. (1983). Eating disorder group. *Journal of College Student Personnel, 24,* 274–275.

Lonergan, E. C. (1991, November). *Using group therapy to foster the psychosexual development of patients with eating disorders.* Paper presented at the Group Therapy Symposium, University of California, San Francisco. CA.

MacKenzie, K. R., Livesley, W. J., Coleman, M., Harper, H., & Park, J. (1986). Short-term group psychotherapy for bulimia nervosa. *Psychiatric Annals, 16,* 699–708.

Maher, M. S. (1984). Group therapy for anorexia nervosa. In P. S. Powers & R. C. Fernandez (Eds.), *Current treatment of anorexia nervosa and bulimia.* New York: Karger.

Malenbaum, R., Herzog, D., Eisenthal, S., & Wyshak, G. (1988). Overeaters anonymous: Impact on bulimia. *International Journal of Eating Disorders, 7,* 139–143.

Marner, T., & Westerberg, C. (1987). Concomitant group therapy with anorectics and their parents as a supplement to family therapy. *Journal of Family Therapy, 9,* 255–263.

McNamara, K. (1989). A structured group program for repeat dieters. *The Journal for Specialists in Group Work, 14,* 141–150.

Merrill, C. A., Mines, R. A., & Starkey, R. (1987). The premature dropout in the group treatment of bulimia. *International Journal of Eating Disorders, 6,* 293–300.

Mitchell, J., Fletcher, L., Pyle, R., Eckert, E., Hatsukami, D., & Pomeroy, C. (1989). The impact of treatment on meal patterns in patients with bulimia nervosa. *International Journal of Eating Disorders, 8,* 167–172.

Mitchell, J. E., Hatsukami, D., Goff, G., Pyle, R. L., Eckert, E. D., & Davis, L. E. (1985). Intensive outpatient group treatment for bulimia. In D. M. Garner & P. E. Garfinkel (Eds.), *Handbook of psychotherapy for anorexia nervosa and bulimia.* New York: Guilford Press.

Mitchell, J. E., Pyle, R. L., Eckert, E. D., Hatsukami, D., Pomeroy, C., & Zimmerman, R. (1990). A comparison study of antidepressants and structured intensive group psychotherapy in the treatment of bulimia nervosa. *Archives of General Psychiatry, 47,* 149–157.

Mitchell, J. E., Pyle, R. L., Eckert, E. D., Pomeroy, C., Hatsukami, D., & Zimmerman, R. (1987). Antidepressants versus group therapy in the treatment of bulimia. *Psychotherapy Bulletin, 23,* 41–43.

Mitchell, J. E., Pyle, R. L., Hatsukami, D., Goff, G., Glotter, D., & Harper, J. (1988). A 2 to 5 year follow-up study of patients treated for bulimia. *International Journal of Eating Disorders, 8,* 157–165.

Moreno, J. K., Fuhriman, A. J., & Hileman, E. (1993, February). *Patient and therapist perceptions of significance in an outpatient eating disorders group.* Presented at the meeting of the American Group Psychotherapy Association, San Diego, CA.

Moreno, J. K., & Hileman, E. (1991, February). *Outpatient group therapy for persons with eating disorders.* Paper presented at the meeting of the American Group Psychotherapy Association, San Antonio, TX.

Moreno, J. K., Hileman, E., & Fuhriman, A. J. (1992, February). *Significant events in an outpatient eating disorders group.* Paper presented at the meeting of the American Group Psychotherapy Association, New York, NY.

Oesterheld, J. R., McKenna, M. S., & Gould, N. B. (1987). Group psychotherapy of bulimia: A critical review. *International Journal of Group Psychotherapy, 37,* 163–184.

O'Neil, M. K., & White, P. (1987). Psychodynamic group treatment of young adult bulimic women: Preliminary positive results. *Canadian Journal of Psychiatry, 32,* 153–155.

Piazza, E., Carni, J. D., Kelly, J., & Plante, S. K. (1983). Group psychotherapy for anorexia nervosa. *Journal of the American Academy of Child Psychiatry, 22,* 276–278.

Piran, N., Langdon, L., Kaplan, A., & Garfinkel, P. E. (1989). Evaluation of a day hospital program for eating disorders. *International Journal of Eating Disorders, 8,* 523–532.

Polivy, J. (1981). Group therapy as an adjunctive treatment for anorexia nervosa. *Journal of Psychiatric Treatment and Evaluation, 3,* 279–283.

Pyle, R. L., Mitchell, J. E., Eckert, E. D., Hatsukami, D., Pomeroy, C., & Zimmerman, R. (1990). Maintenance treatment and 6-month outcome for bulimic patients who respond to initial treatment. *American Journal of Psychiatry, 147,* 871–875.

Pyle, R. L., Mitchell, J. E., Eckert, E. D., Hatsukami, D. K., & Goff, G. (1984). The interruption of bulimic behaviors: A review of three treatment programs. *Psychiatric Clinics of North America, 7,* 275–286.

Reed, G., & Sech, E. P. (1985). Bulimia: A conceptual model for group treatment. *Journal of Psychosocial Nursing, 23*(5), 16–22.

Richards, R. L., Burlingame, G. M., & Fuhriman, A. (1990). Theme-oriented group therapy. *The Counseling Psychologist, 18,* 80–92.

Roth, D. M., & Ross, D. R. (1988). Long-term cognitive-interpersonal group therapy for eating disorders. *International Journal of Group Psychotherapy, 38,* 491–510.

Roy-Byrne, P., Lee-Benner, K., & Yager, J. (1984). Group therapy for bulimia: A year's experience. *International Journal of Eating Disorders, 3,* 97–116.

Rubel, J. A. (1984). The function of self-help groups in recovery from anorexia nervosa and bulimia. *Psychiatric Clinics of North America, 7,* 381–394.

Scheuble, K. J., Dixon, K. N., Levy, A. B., & Kagan-Moore, L. (1987). Premature termination: A risk in eating disorder groups. *Group, 11,* 85–93.

Schneider, J. A., & Agras, W. S. (1985). A cognitive behavioral group treatment of bulimia. *British Journal of Psychiatry, 146,* 66–69.

Shisslak, C. M., Crago, M., Schnaps, L., & Swain, B. (1986). Interactional group therapy for anorexic and bulimic women. *Psychotherapy, 23,* 598–606.

Smead, V. S. (1982). Other possible strategies for dealing with eating disorders. *Psychological Reports, 51,* 348–350.

Stevens, E. V., & Salisbury, J. D. (1984). Group therapy for bulimic adults. *American Journal of Orthopsychiatry, 54,* 156–161.

Strupp, H. H., & Binder, J. L. (1992). Current developments in psychotherapy. *The Independent Practitioner, 12,* 119–124.

Stuber, M., & Strober, M. (1987). Group therapy in the treatment of adolescents with bulimia: Some preliminary observations. *International Journal of Eating Disorders, 6,* 125–131.

Swift, W. J., Ritholz, M., Kalin, N. H., & Kaslow, N. (1987). A follow-up study of thirty hospitalized bulimics. *Psychosomatic Medicine, 49,* 45–55.

Telch, C. F., Agras, W. S., Rossiter, E. M., Wilfley, D., & Kenardy, J. (1990). Group cognitive-behavioral treatment for the nonpurging bulimic: An initial evaluation. *Journal of Consulting and Clinical Psychology, 58,* 629–635.

Vanderlinden, J., & Vandereycken, W. (1988). Perception of changes in eating disorder patients during group treatment. *Psychotherapy and Psychosomatics, 49,* 160–163.

Weber, K. J., & Gillingham, W. H. (1984). Group counseling for anorexic and bulimic students. *Journal of College Student Personnel, 25,* 276.

Weinstein, H. M., & Richman, A. (1984). The group treatment of bulimia. *Journal of American College Health, 32,* 208–215.

Weiss, L., & Katzman, M. (1984). Group treatment for bulimic women. *Arizona Medicine, 41,* 100–104.

White, B. C., & Kaczkowski, H. (1983). Anorexia nervosa: A study of psychiatrists and psychologists opinions and practices. *International Journal of Eating Disorders, 2,* 87–92.

White, W. C., & Boskind-White, M. (1981). An experiential-behavioral approach to the treatment of bulimarexia. *Psychotherapy: Theory, Research, and Practice, 18,* 501–507.

Wilson, G. T., Rossiter, E., Kleifield, E. I., & Lindholm, L. (1986). Cognitive-behavioral treatment of bulimia nervosa: A controlled evaluation. *Behavior Research and Therapy, 24,* 277–288.

Wolchik, S. A., Weiss, L., & Katzman, M. A. (1986). An empirically validated, short-term psychoeducational group treatment program for bulimia. *International Journal of Eating Disorders, 5,* 21–34.

Yager, J. (1988). The treatment of eating disorders. *Journal of Clinical Psychiatry, 49* (9, Suppl.), 18–25.

Yager, J., Landsverk, J., & Edelstein, C. K. (1989). Help seeking and satisfaction with care in 641 women with eating disorders: I. Patterns of utilization, attributed change, and perceived efficacy of treatment. *The Journal of Nervous and Mental Disease, 177,* 632–637.

Yalom, I. D. (1985). *The theory and practice of group psychotherapy* (3rd ed.). New York: Basic Books.

Yates, A. J., & Sambrailo, F. (1984). Bulimia nervosa: A descriptive and therapeutic study. *Behavior Research and Therapy, 22,* 503–517.

Yellowlees, P. (1988). Group psychotherapy in anorexia nervosa. *International Journal of Eating Disorders, 7,* 649–655.

Yudkovitz, E. (1983). Bulimia: Growing awareness of an eating disorder. *Social Work, 28,* 472–478.

CHAPTER 13

Group Therapy for Substance Abuse: A Review of the Empirical Research*

RANDY STINCHFIELD, PATRICIA L. OWEN, and KEN C. WINTERS

This chapter reviews the empirical literature, and provides a clinical perspective, concerning group therapy as a treatment for substance abuse.

PREDOMINANCE OF AND RATIONALE FOR TREATING SUBSTANCE ABUSE WITH GROUP THERAPY

Counseling or psychotherapy is invariably a part of every type of comprehensive substance abuse treatment regimen (McLellan, Woody, Luborsky, & Goehl, 1988; Onken & Blaine, 1990a) and group therapy is often the central component of multimodal treatment programs, such as therapeutic communities and Minnesota model Alcoholics Anonymous (AA)-based programs (Hubbard et al., 1989; Price et al., 1991; Schuckit, 1989; Spitz, 1987). Group therapy is the most common form of treatment for substance abusers, having surpassed individual therapy as the psychotherapeutic treatment of choice (Baekeland, 1977; Baekeland, Lundwall, & Kissin, 1975; Cooper, 1987; Miller, 1991; Vannicelli, 1982). It has become such a standard practice in the treatment of substance abuse that it is assumed to be practiced in virtually identical forms across different settings and to be essential for the successful treatment of substance abuse.

Two recent surveys of substance abuse treatment programs in The United States and the United Kingdom indicated that group was the predominant treatment modality. Group therapy is provided in 94% of U.S. outpatient programs (Price et al., 1991) and by the majority of U.K. inpatient programs (Ettorre, 1984). Furthermore, group work theory is Britain's most influential theoretical orientation within the alcoholism treatment services network (Ettorre, 1984).

*This work was partially supported by research grants from the National Institute on Drug Abuse (DA05104) and the National Institute on Alcohol Abuse and Alcoholism (AA08764).

Why Treat Substance Abuse with Group Therapy?

Because substance abusers have historically been one of the most difficult populations to treat with individual therapy, group therapy moved to the forefront as a promising alternative (Ashery, 1985; Yalom, 1975; Yalom, Bloch, Bond, Zimmerman, & Qualls, 1978). Its appeal was bolstered by the fact that group therapy showed success in treating other disorders and was cost effective (Flores, 1988; Kanas, 1982). Accordingly, in the 1970s and 1980s, many adaptations for substance abuse group therapy were developed (Annis, 1979; Brown & Yalom, 1977; Vannicelli, 1982; Yalom, 1974).

There are a number of therapeutic rationales for treating substance abusers with group therapy. Many of these rationales are the same reasons why group therapy is used to treat other disorders. Of primary importance is the basic notion that people in distress often seek out and benefit from the help of others with similar problems. It is comforting for a client to know that they are not alone in their suffering and that others share similar experiences. Other interpersonal benefits of group therapy include opportunities to: disclose personal information to others; actively give and receive support from others with similar problems and experiences; learn about oneself and identify with others by interacting with them on an emotional level; learn to communicate needs and feelings more effectively; make sense of one's story through interaction with others who have had similar experiences; develop interpersonal relationships with other recovering substance abusers; confront problematic behaviors such as denial, manipulativeness and grandiosity; and test new behaviors (Flores, 1988; Institute of Medicine, 1990; Vannicelli, 1982).

Furthermore, the group process can serve as a vital agent in breaking down client denial about the drug abuse problem. The group influence is one of the most potent forces to break through an addict's denial system, particularly when the group is composed of fellow addicts (Galanter, Castaneda, & Franco, 1991). Peer pressure in this context can reduce denial of addiction and of interpersonal difficulties, as well as promote positive behavioral changes (Pfeffer, Friedland, & Wortis, 1949). Even when individuals are not directly confronted about their behavior, a group setting allows them to learn vicariously through others' stories and interactions. When denial is particularly strong, this is a relatively nonthreatening form of confrontation.

REVIEWS OF THE EMPIRICAL LITERATURE

Despite the popularity of group therapy as a treatment for substance abuse, reviews have found the literature wanting on a number of topics. At a basic level, there is neither a systematic description of group therapies for substance abuse, nor a method or taxonomy for classifying group styles (Annis, 1979; Cartwright, 1987). Clinicians themselves vary widely in how they use group therapy in substance abuse treatment. In most settings, inpatient or outpatient, group therapy is not the sole form of treatment. From a clinical point of view, the treatment of substance abuse usually consists of many components, of which group therapy is only one. Education, individual therapy, family therapy, and medical management may be provided in conjunction with group therapy. Further, even within a treatment program, the work that is done within a group setting varies widely. Group therapy may vary from indepth exploration of interaction styles to simply having group members report about their progress in completing behavioral homework assignments. While the latter may appear mundane, deeper therapeutic material may surface. Therefore, in actual practice, it is difficult to isolate and describe the active components of group therapy in a substance abuse population.

Previous reviews note that the effectiveness of group psychotherapy with substance abusers has not been rigorously studied. For example, Parloff and Dies (1977) reviewed the empirical group therapy outcome literature from 1966 to 1975 and found only five studies involving the treatment of substance abuse. Limitations in these studies included small sample sizes, short durations of treatment, and, for the most part, a failure to measure post-treatment substance use. More recent reviews generally come to the same conclusion, that is, the extant evidence is inconsistent regarding the effectiveness of group therapy (Annis, 1979; Brandsma & Pattison, 1985; Emrick, 1982; Galanter et al., 1991; Gwinner, 1979; Miller & Hester, 1980; Miller & Hester, 1986; Onken, 1991; Onken & Blaine, 1990a; Solomon, 1983). Nevertheless, a thorough review of existing empirical research on the process and outcome of group therapy as a treatment for substance abuse is provided next.

GROUP THERAPY OUTCOME AND PROCESS RESEARCH

Outcome research addresses the end rather than the means, whereas process research focuses on the means to the end. This review is limited to articles that satisfied specific criteria regarding the definitions of group therapy and substance abuse, as well as criteria for technical and empirical standards.

Criteria for including outcome studies in the literature review were: (1) the group therapy method must involve a group of clients with a substance abuse problem meeting on a regular basis with an identified therapist or leader for the primary purpose of treating their substance abuse. Studies needed to exhibit more than just the occurrence of group meetings. Inclusion required that a primary therapeutic process was the facilitation of interpersonal interaction and group development. Studies excluded from this review include: treatments conducted in a group setting, but which did not focus on processes of group development and interpersonal interaction, for example, behavioral coping skills training conducted in a group setting (e.g., Miller & Taylor, 1980), general evaluation of a multimodal treatment program, of which group therapy was one modality (e.g., Stephenson, Boudewyns, & Lessing, 1977), self-help or peer-support groups (this topic is covered in another chapter of this book), and couples/marital/family group therapy; (2) although it would have been optimal to include only those articles that formally describe the nature of patients' substance abuse in terms of diagnostic criteria based on data from a structured interview, it was not possible because so few articles did this. It was only possible to use a rather global definition of problem use of any substances including alcohol and other drugs; (3) controlled research, that is, the study included either random assignment or subject matching designs with a control or comparison group (a comparison group refers to a group of substance abuse clients receiving an alternative type of treatment for substance abuse); (4) the study measured substance use frequency or consumption as an outcome variable; (5) external validity, that is, the study used real clients who had a substance abuse problem and real treatment procedures; and (6) reports were written in English. Criteria for selecting process studies were limited to items 1, 2, 5, and 6.

These selection criteria attempted to identify studies with sufficient empirical rigor to allow a fair degree of confidence in the reliability and validity of the results. Because most of these studies are conducted in clinical settings, complete control is not possible. Many, if not all, of the studies included in this review are not immune to alternative explanations for their results. The purpose of the selection criteria was to select those studies which implement general guidelines for conducting empirical research, and which attempt to control those variables which are known to be confounds and which can be controlled. Therefore, these studies have fewer alternative explanations than studies which do not follow these guidelines.

A caveat to the selection criteria is that some studies were included in the review even though it is not completely clear whether they satisfy the definitions of group therapy and substance abuse. Because of the lack of detailed descriptions of group therapy methods and subject characteristics it was difficult to determine whether the study satisfied inclusion criteria. Therefore, some studies are included if they *appear* to satisfy the criteria from their cursory description of the group therapy method.

The literature was searched by three methods: (a) computer-assisted database searches of PsycInfo, Medline, and the University of Minnesota Drug Information Service database, for literature published between 1980 and 1991, (b) a computer-assisted search of the holdings of the University of Minnesota library system for monographs, and (c) examination of reference lists of obtained literature.

Outcome Studies

Outcome research examines the effectiveness of treatment and focuses on whether the client has changed. Generally, the designs of outcome studies are largely influenced (and limited) by the settings in which the studies are conducted. Most clinical settings are not amenable to modifying their programs to allow for the manipulations required to conduct controlled research. Therefore, investigators have attempted to adapt research designs to existing clinical settings. Unfortunately, most of these adaptations create significant confounds that permit alternative explanations of results.

Eight comparative outcome studies were found that satisfied our criteria for group therapy. These eight studies may be categorized into three design types: (1) group therapy is the primary treatment, (2) group therapy is a concurrent supplement to a primary treatment program, and (3) group therapy is a post-treatment supplement to primary treatment. The latter two designs may be considered an additive research strategy because the specific question being addressed is whether group therapy produces an incremental effect beyond that achieved by primary treatment alone. In these additive research designs, subjects participate in primary treatment with or without supplemental group therapy.

Group Therapy as the Primary Treatment

In practice, treatment of substance abuse rarely consists of group therapy alone. Usually, these primary group treatment studies are conducted in order to isolate the effects of group therapy and avoid the confounding effects of other treatment components of treatment programs. Three studies exist with group therapy as the primary treatment. One investigation compared behavioral treatment to group encounter therapy in a university-based outpatient setting (Pomerleau & Adkins, 1980; Pomerleau, Pertschuk, Adkins, & Brady, 1978). The sample of 32 subjects consisted primarily of adult male alcoholics. Groups of 6 or 7 subjects were randomly assigned to either encounter group therapy or behavior therapy. Behavioral therapy groups were conducted by either a psychologist or psychiatrist (both had several years of experience) and one of a number of master's level nurses as a co-therapist. Encounter group therapy was run by a psychiatrist (with several years of group therapy experience) and a master's-level social worker. The treatment goal for the behavior therapy clients was moderation of alcohol use. Treatment strategies included positive reinforcement techniques of shaping, stimulus control, and contingency management. Encounter group therapy included both psychodynamic and insight-oriented techniques and had a treatment goal of abstinence. Both approaches had weekly 90-minute sessions for 3 months and 5 more sessions spread over 9 months. Outcome was measured by treatment completion and alcohol consumption (both self-report and liver enzyme function test). At one-year follow-up, 24 (75%) subjects were contacted. Both groups were similar in that drinking was significantly reduced, but there was no significant difference between the two treatments in alcohol consumption at follow-up.

However, encounter group therapy had more dropouts than the behavioral group. The authors speculate that the treatment goal of abstinence in the encounter group therapy approach may have been too rigid for clients who were not amenable to an abstinence goal. This difference in dropout rate is an important finding because attrition is a significant problem in substance abuse treatment, particularly in outpatient programs. In part, the difference in dropout rates in this study may also be attributed to the fact that clients in behavioral treatment received monetary incentives for continued involvement. However, the authors point out that the pattern and timing of attrition was different in the two groups. Clients in the encounter therapy treatment tended to drop out far later in the treatment process, that is, during the ninth week. This was during the phase of most intense confrontation. It may be that if confrontational methods are used as a matter of course, some participants will leave. It is important to continuously assess an individual's ability to tolerate and benefit from confrontation, and to time it appropriately in the treatment process.

The second study in this category (Telch, Hannon, & Telch, 1984) compared three treatment groups in a public outpatient clinic: (1) covert sensitization, (2) supportive group therapy, and (3) nonspecific control group (relaxation training). Again, the sample size was small (n = 28) and primarily consisted of adult, white male alcoholics. The covert sensitization and nonspecific control groups were conducted by a second-year graduate student in psychology with one year of previous training in administering covert sensitization and progressive muscle relaxation. Group size ranged from 4 to 6 subjects. The covert sensitization and nonspecific control groups involved two 45-minute sessions a week for 6 weeks. Supportive group therapy was an ongoing treatment approach at the clinic and was run by one of several staff therapists. Each of the 9 subjects assigned to the supportive group therapy condition were assigned to one of the ongoing therapy groups made up of 10–15 alcoholics who were not subjects in the study. Supportive group therapy involved 6 weekly 90-minute sessions. A weakness in this study was a lack of control over the supportive group therapy condition, in which subjects were scattered among ongoing supportive therapy groups and therefore, the effects of unspecified therapists and unspecified group members confound the results. Twenty-six subjects were contacted two weeks after treatment. Outcome was measured by blood alcohol concentration obtained from a breath test, self-reported mean daily drinking frequency and daily urges to drink. While there were no significant differences between groups on blood alcohol concentration and urges to drink, supportive group therapy was significantly more effective in reducing subjects' reported drinking two weeks after treatment than either covert sensitization or relaxation training. However, these results are difficult to apply to clinical settings because there was no significant difference in average daily drinking level between the three groups. Simply reducing alcohol intake may not produce the desired effect of reducing problems associated with alcohol.

The third study in this category was conducted by Joanning, Quinn, Thomas, and Mullen (1992) who compared three outpatient treatment groups for adolescent substance abuse. Families (n = 134) were randomly assigned to one of three treatment conditions: (1) family systems therapy (n = 40), (2) group therapy (n = 52), and (3) family drug education (n = 42). Family systems therapy was an integration of Structural and

Strategic family therapies and was conducted in 60 to 90 minute weekly sessions by two doctoral-level family therapy students and a supervisor. The total number of sessions ranged from 7 to 15. The group therapy was process-oriented, involving discussions among group members to examine the effect of drugs on the adolescents' lives and to promote a drug-free lifestyle, which was intended to be representative of outpatient group therapy. Adolescents were seen without their families in group therapy. Group therapy was conducted by a family therapy doctoral student on a weekly basis for 12 sessions of 90 minutes each. The family drug education group involved presentations of information about the effects of drugs on adolescent and family functioning. Education groups consisted of 3 to 4 families that met for two and a half hours every other week for a total of 6 sessions.

Outcome was measured by drug use (using versus not using) and family functioning. Post-test data were collected from 31, 23, and 28 participants from family therapy, group therapy, and family drug education, respectively. Family systems therapy had significantly more drug-free adolescents at post-test (n = 19) than either group therapy (n = 4) or family drug education (n = 8). There were no statistically significant differences between conditions on measures of family functioning. Group therapy had the highest dropout rate of the three conditions (n = 29). This study suggests that family systems therapy is superior to both group therapy and drug education in achieving abstinence in adolescents.

This apparently negative result for group therapy needs to be considered in light of several methodological factors. First, treatment conditions were not equivalent. Family therapy and family drug education included the adolescent's family, while group therapy did not. The high dropout rate for the group therapy condition is likely related to the lack of family participation. Indeed, the authors note that parents were less invested in bringing their adolescent to the group therapy sessions. Furthermore, treatment was confounded with therapist effect in the following ways: (1) each treatment approach was conducted by a unique set of therapists, (2) all of the therapists in the family therapy and group therapy conditions were family therapy students and were likely to have had a family therapy bias, and (3) family therapy was conducted by doctoral students plus a faculty supervisor, while group therapy did not include a supervisor. Finally, treatment conditions were confounded with family type. In spite of random assignment, there were more single parent families in the group therapy condition and single parent families overall had a higher rate of continued drug use at the end of treatment.

These three studies give mixed results for group therapy. On the one hand, both Pomerleau et al. (1978) and Telch et al. (1984) found that group therapy was effective as a primary treatment for substance abuse when compared to behavioral strategies. These findings are relatively compelling evidence for the efficacy of group therapy, in that the group treatment approach compared favorably with behavioral treatments that specifically targeted drinking behavior. On the other hand, Joanning et al. (1992) found group therapy to be inferior to family systems therapy in terms of achieving abstinence in an adolescent sample by the end of treatment. These studies provide an initial understanding of the effectiveness of group therapy for treating substance abusers. However, given the complexity of methodological issues, clear conclusions cannot be drawn. From a clinical point of view, the treatment of choice probably includes a combination of group therapy, behavioral methods, and family involvement.

Group Therapy as a Concurrent Supplement to Primary Treatment

In the three studies in this category, some clients are exposed to primary treatment alone while other clients are exposed to both primary treatment and group therapy. The control group in this type of design is the group exposed to primary treatment alone.

Ends and Page (1957) compared four groups in an inpatient state hospital setting: (a) learning theory based on Mowrer, (b) nondirective, client-centered, (c) psychoanalytic based on Alexander and French, and (d) social discussion control group. All three experimental groups appear to satisfy the criteria for group therapy. The treatment goal was improved social functioning. The 96 subjects were all adult male alcoholics. A latin square design employed four therapists conducting one of each type of group resulting in 16 groups with six subjects in each group, thus controlling for therapist effect. It is not reported if the subjects were randomly assigned to groups. Therapists had at least 2 years of experience and training in psychotherapy. Therapy consisted of three sessions a week for five weeks. Outcome was measured by official records regarding drinking episodes and rehospitalization. At one-and-a-half-year post-treatment, 63 (66%) subjects were contacted. Client-centered and psychoanalytic groups showed significantly more successes than either the learning theory or control groups, and the client-centered group significantly outperformed all other groups in terms of hospital readmission rates. The relative ordering of groups in terms of success rates reported in this study are client-centered, psychoanalytic, control, and learning theory.

In a second study, Annis (1979) compared three groups in a rehabilitation clinic for prison inmates: (1) confrontational group therapy with video feedback, (2) confrontational group therapy without video feedback, and (3) control group that involved primary treatment alone. Subjects were randomly assigned to groups. The sample of 150 subjects were all adult male substance abusers. The primary treatment program was a multimodal milieu approach. Group therapy consisted of intensive confrontation groups of five men each, conducted in two-hour sessions, four days a week for 8 weeks. Outcome was measured by self-report and official records regarding substance use, employment status, and involvement with the law. One year follow-up data on 128 subjects (85%) indicated there were no significant differences between experimental and control groups in post-treatment functioning. In fact, most of the subjects in the study were doing poorly, with only 11% attending Alcoholics Anonymous meetings and having an average daily alcohol intake of 6.2

ounces. Over half (54%) were arrested during the follow-up year. Because it appears that none of the methods had a significant effect clinically, more basic work needs to be done with offenders to find any methods that are helpful in breaking the cycle of addiction.

A third study (Olson, Ganley, Devine, & Dorsey, 1981) conducted in an inpatient hospital setting compared four groups: (1) control group involving primary treatment alone, (2) behavioral treatment, (3) insight-oriented group therapy, and (4) combined behavioral and insight-oriented group. The insight-oriented group appeared to satisfy the definition of group therapy.* The randomly assigned sample of 137 subjects were primarily adult male alcoholics. Primary treatment was an AA-based highly structured multimodal inpatient program lasting four weeks and conducted by staff alcohol counselors. The behavioral treatment consisted of four one-hour sessions a week for four weeks of training in covert sensitization and relaxation. The insight-oriented group therapy was transactional analysis (TA) oriented and was conducted by a certified TA instructor for three one-hour sessions a week for 4 weeks. The combined behavioral and insight-oriented group ran 6 hours a week for four weeks. Outcome was measured by self-reported drinking and clinical adjustment at five points in time over a four year follow-up period. The follow-up sample size was 113 (82%). All four groups significantly reduced drinking and the combined, control, and behavioral groups exhibited significantly less drinking than the TA group.

The three studies in this group also provide a mixed picture. Ends and Page (1957) found that two of the three group treatments (i.e., client-centered and psychoanalytic groups) exhibited greater improvement rates than the control group. This study indicated that the addition of group therapy (particularly client-centered group therapy) enhanced the overall treatment outcome. In contrast, Annis (1979) and Olson et al. (1981) found no differences between primary treatment alone and primary treatment plus group therapy, which suggests that no incremental improvement is obtained from adding group therapy to an existing primary multimodal treatment program.

For the clinician, how group therapy is used as an adjunct method in a treatment program is critical. If the principles that are taught and practiced in group therapy are consistent with the other treatment components, clients will benefit from the multimodal program. But, if group therapy is not seen as important or its principles are inconsistent with other treatment components, clients are likely to become confused and may react against this lack of harmony among treatment components.

---

* The inclusion of the Olson et al. (1981) study is questionable. Due to the brief description of the characteristics of this group therapy approach it is not completely certain whether this study satisfies the definition of group therapy presented earlier. It was included, however, because one of the treatment conditions was titled an insight-oriented Transactional Analysis group, which was characterized as a combination of psychodynamic, interpersonal, and communications principles. This condition appears to emphasize interpersonal interaction.

' EXTEND TEAM '

Group Therapy as a Post-Treatment Supplement to *Primary Treatment*

There were two studies where group therapy was a post-treatment supplement, occurring subsequent to primary treatment. This type of treatment is commonly referred to as "aftercare" in substance abuse treatment jargon. Most clients completing a primary treatment program are referred to aftercare, making this a particularly relevant area of research. Furthermore, it is critical that gains made in primary treatment be maintained to promote ongoing recovery. In a recent congressional hearing on the efficacy of drug treatment, Maxine Stitzer, medical research chief in the Department of Psychiatry at Francis Scott Key Medical Center in Baltimore, stated that the addict's performance in treatment is often not nearly as important as what happens after discharge from treatment. She stated, "'Anybody can stop using drugs. The trick is to keep them off.'" (Buie, 1990, p. 21).

The first study was conducted in a VA Hospital outpatient setting. Ito, Donovan, and Hall (1988) compared a cognitive-behavioral relapse prevention program (RP) to an interpersonal process program (IP). The interpersonal process program appeared to satisfy the definition of group therapy. Again, all subjects (n = 49) were adult male alcoholics. Subject assignment to groups was approximately, but not completely, random. There were three co-therapy teams made up of a male and female therapist. Each team conducted one group in each treatment condition, thus controlling for therapist effect. Therapists included three doctoral-level therapists with experience in cognitive-behavioral therapy and three master's-level staff therapists with a minimum of 5 years experience. Therapists were trained in four 90 minute sessions, two on RP and two on IP. Each group had 8 weekly 90 minute sessions and was then referred to the standard ongoing VA aftercare program for weekly sessions for an additional 4 months. Outcome was measured by treatment completion, alcohol use, and psychological measures. At six-month follow-up, 34 subjects (69%) were contacted. More RP clients completed treatment (80%) than IP (58%), but this was not statistically significant. In terms of drinking outcome, subjects in both treatments significantly reduced their alcohol consumption, but there were no significant differences between treatment groups. This study included co-therapist teams. Many therapists prefer working with a co-therapist because group dynamics are often complex and a team approach allows exchanging roles as observer and responder.

The second study* (Cooney, Kadden, Litt, & Getter, 1991; Kadden, Cooney, Getter, & Litt, 1989) compared behavioral coping skills training to interactional group therapy in an outpatient setting. The sample of 118 subjects were recruited from an inpatient alcoholism treatment program and

---

* The purpose of the study reported by Kadden et al. (1989) was to examine a patient-treatment matching hypothesis—not to conduct an outcome study comparing behavioral versus interactional group therapies. However, the design allows for review as an outcome study, hence its inclusion.

were primarily adult male alcoholics. Subjects were randomly assigned to aftercare groups. There were nine behavioral therapists and eight interactional therapists. Therapists included five doctoral-level clinical psychologists, one psychiatrist, four postinternship doctoral candidates in clinical psychology, four advanced graduate students in psychology, and three master's-level therapists with several years experience. Five coping skills and five interactional groups were conducted, with each group led by two co-therapists who were blind to the experimental hypothesis. Groups met for one 90-minute session a week for 26 weeks. Coping skills training was based on cognitive-behavioral principles, and interactional group therapy was based on facilitating insight and interpersonal functioning. Outcome was measured by drinking and psychological measures at the end of treatment (n = 86) and at 12 (n = 85) and 24 months (n = 76) follow-up. There was a significant main effect for time, but there was no statistically significant difference between treatment groups.

These two aftercare studies indicate that clients in both behavioral and interactional group therapy treatments improved and neither type of treatment proved superior. Both studies had methodological issues that prevented clear conclusions. The lack of a no-aftercare-control group is particularly compromising for these two studies because the effect of the experimental aftercare treatment is confounded with the effect of primary treatment. A no-aftercare-control group would control for the effect of primary treatment alone. Along these same lines, the Ito et al. study was further confounded by the fact that the experimental aftercare treatment occurred after primary treatment and was a substitute for the first two months of a standard 6-month aftercare program. Upon completing the two-month experimental aftercare treatment, subjects were then referred to the standard aftercare program for the remaining four months of this program. Therefore, subjects received an additional four months of the standard aftercare treatment before follow-up measures were administered.

To summarize the outcome literature, the fact that there were only two studies where group therapy was the exclusive treatment indicates that very little research attention has been devoted to this area. These outcome studies, while demonstrating that group therapy is related to improvement, have not answered the fundamental question of whether group therapy for substance abuse is better than no treatment. The lack of empirical rigor and control in existing studies prevents us from concluding that group therapy causes substance abusers to improve.

Studies Relating Process to Outcome

Therapy process research addresses the means to the end, by asking the question: What happens in therapy to effect a change in the client? This type of research attempts to elucidate the relationships among variables and the causal directions of these relationships. The studies reviewed were divided into four subsections: (1) therapist variables related to outcome, (2) client variables related to outcome, (3) interaction of client and therapist variables with outcome, and (4) therapy variables related to outcome.

Therapist Variables Related to Outcome

Therapist characteristics and their relationship to outcome have been virtually unstudied in the substance abuse treatment field (Cartwright, 1981; Onken, 1991). Thus, little is known as to the role played by therapist characteristics in client attrition, compliance, and outcome. Treatment program administrators are often reluctant to compare outcomes between therapists because of the risk of creating unproductive competition or ill-will among therapists. However, if positioned as an opportunity for learning, it could enhance the skills of all clinicians. While systematic studies of the relationship between therapist characteristics and outcome do not exist, related findings on this topic are reviewed.

In a preliminary report, Kleinman et al., (1990) found that the therapist to whom the subject was assigned was the strongest predictor of whether the client would stay in therapy. In a second study (LaRosa, Lipsius, & LaRosa, 1974), professional therapists were compared to paraprofessional therapists in terms of client retention in group therapy. After one year, groups conducted by professional therapists retained more clients (68%) than groups conducted by paraprofessional therapists (40%). This study had a major flaw in that the therapist characteristic of interest, professional versus paraprofessional, was confounded by both therapist substance abuse history and race. The professional therapists had no substance abuse history and were white, while the paraprofessionals were both ex-addicts and black. This confound severely limits the conclusions from this study. Both of the above studies highlight the possible effect of therapist characteristics in retaining clients, yet much work is needed to clarify what therapist characteristics are important for client retention and outcomes.

Client Variables Related to Outcome

Providing group therapy to clients who will not benefit from the experience is a waste. The challenge is determining which clients will benefit from group therapy and which will not. Some authors stated that the client variable of substance abuse itself indicates a poor prognosis for group therapy (Yalom, 1975; Yalom, Bloch, Bond, Zimmerman, & Qualls, 1978). This raises the question whether substance abuse clients can participate in group therapy in a therapeutic manner.

Yalom et al. (1978) evaluated the outcome of interactional group therapy for alcoholics and used a group of neurotic patients receiving similar treatment as a comparison group. There were no differences on a measure of curative factors between alcoholic and neurotic groups, suggesting that both alcoholic and neurotic groups were experiencing similar types of therapeutic factors within group therapy. Furthermore, both types of patients improved and there were no significant differences between groups.

Albrecht and Brabender (1983) studied the effects of short-term interactional group therapy on mixed groups of psychiatric patients with and without a secondary diagnosis of substance use disorder. At post-treatment, patients with a secondary diagnosis of substance use disorder fared as well as patients without a secondary diagnosis of substance use disorder on outcome measures. Thus, interactional group therapy appeared to be effective for members with or without a substance use disorder. Furthermore, the presence of patients with a substance use disorder in a group did not appear to disrupt the therapeutic effect of interactional group therapy. As there is a high prevalence of clients with dual disorders (i.e., substance abuse and one or more psychiatric disorders) in substance abuse treatment, this finding is particularly encouraging because it is often not feasible to separate clients into homogeneous groups.

Page (1982) conducted a linguistic analysis of group member speech. He audiotaped and rated a 16-hour group marathon session with substance abusers on the Hill Interaction Matrix. Group members exhibited interpersonal relating patterns that are therapeutic as measured by the Hill Interaction Matrix. This study suggests that substance abusers can participate in group therapy in a therapeutic manner.

Kilmann and Howell (1974) examined the interaction between client's locus of control and the structure of marathon group therapy (i.e., nondirective versus directive) in a sample of institutionalized female drug addicts. Marathon group therapy refers to a single group therapy session conducted over six or more hours in one day. Subjects with an internal locus of control exhibited greater pre- to post-therapy gains in terms of their level of involvement in therapy, regardless of type of marathon group. The authors concluded that subjects with an internal locus of control are more likely to benefit from marathon group therapy than subjects with an external locus of control.

Studies reviewed earlier are relevant to the discussion of the relationship between client characteristics and outcome: Annis and Chan's (1983) retrospective analysis of an outcome study (Annis, 1979); and Kadden et al. (1989) and Cooney et al.'s (1991) prospective study of a patient-treatment matching strategy. Annis and Chan (1983) compared the effects of primary multimodal treatment plus confrontive group therapy to primary multimodal treatment alone among subjects varying on measures of self-esteem and interpersonal behavior patterns. Subjects were classified into either positive or negative self-image groups based on a cluster analysis of 11 personality measures. Clients with positive self-image in the group therapy condition had fewer reconvictions and less severe offenses upon reconviction than clients with positive self-image in the control condition. The opposite situation was true for clients with negative self-image. Patients with a negative self-image and low interpersonal warmth did not appear to benefit from the addition of confrontive group therapy to primary treatment.

An excellent prospective study examining a client-treatment matching hypothesis was conducted by Kadden et al. (1989) and Cooney et al. (1991).

This study examined the relationship of selected client characteristics (sociopathy, global psychopathology, and cognitive impairment) with two different types of aftercare treatments, one of which was interactional group therapy. Clients were first treated in a 21-day inpatient alcoholism treatment program and then were randomly assigned to aftercare treatments. An interaction between these client characteristics and treatment type was found to effect drinking relapse. Subjects with more sociopathy did better in coping skills training, while subjects with less sociopathy did better in interactional group therapy. Subjects with more psychopathology did better in coping skills training while low psychopathology subjects did better in interactional group therapy. Subjects classified as cognitively impaired appeared to do better in interactional group therapy while cognitively intact subjects showed no difference in outcome between the two treatment types. The finding that clients with greater psychopathology did worse in interactional group therapy is a good reminder to clinicians that confrontation and uncovering of intrapersonal conflict may be contraindicated in these types of clients. There are some alcoholics for whom abstinence, without significant insight, is a success in itself. It may be that these individuals can become more amenable to intrapersonal therapy after a longer period of abstinence.

A weakness of this study relevant to the issue of client variables is the timing of the measurement of sociopathy, psychopathology, and neuropsychological impairment. These characteristics were measured early in primary inpatient treatment, but it would have been better to measure them immediately before the experimental treatment. While these characteristics may be temporally stable, the suggested procedure would help control for the possible effect of inpatient substance abuse treatment on these client variables, particularly psychopathology.

Interaction of Client and Therapist Variables with Outcome

McLachlan (1972) examined the effect of client and therapist conceptual levels on the outcome of group therapy. Conceptual level is a complex construct regarding cognitive and personality development and is measured on a scale with a label of "dependent" at the low end and "independent" at the high end. Therapist conceptual level was related to their style in group therapy, in that, the higher the therapist conceptual level the less directive the therapist style, and vice versa. McLachlan also found an interaction between patient and therapist conceptual level and outcome. Specifically, patients with conceptual levels similar to their therapist fared better than patients with conceptual levels discrepant from their therapist. This study suggests that the effect of group therapy appears to be optimized when client and therapist conceptual levels are similar, and the effect is attenuated when conceptual levels are dissimilar.

Therapy Variables Related to Outcome

The relationship of therapy characteristics to outcome focuses on the effect of specific or nonspecific therapy characteristics. Two studies were reviewed that examined the therapy characteristic of length of therapy session. First, Page (1986) found that prison inmates in substance abuse treatment who had experienced a 16-hour marathon group rated counseling more favorably than matched control subjects who had not experienced a marathon group. Second, Ross, McReynolds, and Berzins (1974) compared a 17-hour marathon group therapy experience to daily group therapy. Pre-post scores indicated that both groups reduced MMPI neurotic triad scale scores, but the marathon group reportedly was more effective at improving specific attitudes about criminal and drug involvement behavior.

To summarize the process literature, there are indications that therapist, client, and therapy variables are related to outcome. There is preliminary evidence that different therapists have varying rates of retaining clients in therapy, although it is not known what therapist characteristics are associated with client retention rates. It follows that therapists may also differ on client outcome success rates. There is also evidence that criminal offenders and other clients with high levels of sociopathy or psychopathology, or low levels of interpersonal warmth may not benefit from interactional group therapy. Perhaps if we knew more about what therapist characteristics and treatment approaches are best suited for these types of clients, their poor prognosis could be addressed. Client-therapist match on conceptual level also appears to be related to outcome, the idea being that the more similar the client and therapist, the better the outcome. Finally, marathon group therapy appears to have differential effects on some measures of outcome as compared to typical-length session group therapy.

CLINICAL KNOWLEDGE

In light of the lack of a substantial empirical knowledge base, it is necessary to turn to conceptual and clinical descriptions of group therapy, as well as reports on individual therapy, concerning treatments for substance abuse. This conceptual and clinical information has great potential for providing clinical insights and for generating research questions and hypotheses to be examined by empirical investigation. This literature addresses a number of themes, including: different theoretical/therapeutic approaches; therapeutic group factors; client effect; therapist effect; and the client-therapist relationship.

Theoretical/Therapeutic Approaches

Group treatment for substance abuse grew out of several different historical paths. As professionals began to recognize their limitations in working with individual addicts (Cooper, 1987), grassroots self-help groups began to develop, leading to the widespread establishment and influence of Alcoholics Anonymous. Treatment programs borrowed the model of alcoholics helping each other, and consequently incorporated group therapy into their treatment programs. At the same time, more advanced methods of group therapy theory and practice were developing (e.g., Yalom, 1974). Group therapy appeared to have a unique set of therapeutic factors, and the intent was to bring the therapeutic factors of group therapy to bear on substance abusers (Yalom, 1974).

There are a number of proposed group therapy approaches with substance abusers (e.g., Ellis, McInerney, DiGuiuseppe, & Yeager, 1988; Khantzian, Halliday, & McAuliffe, 1990; Vannicelli, 1982; Yalom, 1974). Galanter et al. (1991) have identified five distinct group modalities: (1) interactional, (2) modified interactional, (3) behavioral, (4) insight-oriented, and (5) supportive. No single approach has *consistently* demonstrated greater effectiveness than another in the treatment of drug abusers (Onken, 1991). As Emrick (1975) noted, therapeutic technique may not be as important as developing efforts to engage alcoholics in some form of treatment, since most approaches appear to be helpful to the majority of participants.

Amidst the background of mixed results, lies some advice from the literature regarding theoretical approaches. Pomerleau et al. (1978) found that interactional and insight-oriented group therapy treatments have higher dropout rates than behavioral treatments, and Joanning et al. (1992) found that group therapy had a higher dropout rate than either family systems therapy or family drug education. Kaufman (1989) concluded that psychodynamic therapy is contraindicated early in the treatment of the drug abuser and should not be attempted until after abstinence is achieved. For many addicts, abstinence is a prerequisite prior to embarking on intrapsychic exploration. The psychic pain of experiencing intense emotions without the ameliorative effect of drugs may be too difficult, and could jeopardize newly developing sobriety.

It is doubtful that one specific group therapy approach, alone, can produce successful outcome for all clients. In some settings where cost containment is a major concern, there may be a temptation to use the rudiments of group therapy, without fully considering what is needed to maximize the likelihood of recovery. While it may be more efficient to treat clients in a group than in individual therapy, thoughtful consideration needs to be given regarding the therapeutic approach, intensity, and group composition.

Therapeutic Group Factors

In general, success in group therapy depends on the presence of therapeutic factors such as cohesion, trust, willingness of members to disclose information about themselves and to support others' disclosure, and the development of group norms (Bond & Lieberman, 1978). Specific to substance abuse, Vannicelli (1982) identifies three change factors: (1) to share and identify with others who have similar problems, (2) to understand one's own attitudes and defenses pertaining to alcoholism by confronting similar attitudes and defenses in others, and (3) to learn to communicate needs and feelings more effectively. Other therapeutic factors mentioned in the literature include: "making sense" of one's experiences through interaction with others who have had similar experiences, developing relationships with other recovering addicts, and testing new coping behaviors.

A unique therapeutic factor of group therapy with substance abusers is the use of peers (i.e., fellow addicts) to break through an addict's denial system and to promote behavioral changes (Galanter et al., 1991; Pfeffer et al., 1949). Denial may be reduced by direct confrontation by peers, or indirectly by identification and modeling. Furthermore, because substance abusers often have their "drug lifestyle" reinforced by other addicts, the group therapy experience affords an opportunity for the client to replace the "old" peer group with recovering addicts who can support a new drug-free lifestyle.

Some clients may need to be educated about the difference between group therapy and self-help groups (Vannicelli, 1982). Two areas of concern may arise. First, some clients may not understand that the expectations for participation are different for the different types of groups. Second, clients who are accustomed to Alcoholics Anonymous may feel threatened or confused by the emphasis on process and analysis in group therapy. At times in the group therapy process, clients may feel greater emotional pain and turmoil than when they started, leading them to believe that their group participation is threatening their sobriety. This may contrast in their minds with AA, whose main function is to support sobriety. Conversely, they may denigrate the importance of AA because it does not involve active therapeutic methods. By educating the client about the differences and purposes of each type of group experience, the client can learn to use each group to help support gains achieved in the other.

Groups can be designed to have natural phases in the treatment of substance abuse (Kanas, 1982). In the initial phase, newcomers need basic support and information about their new state of abstinence, and clear examples of denial. In the next phase, clients are ready to address the consequences of their addiction, looking at their new lifestyle and how they can make changes. The group serves the purpose of increasing awareness and providing support. Finally, the client may be ready to deal with intrapsychic factors that may have predisposed him or her to the addiction, and most certainly would be predisposing factors for relapse. In primary treatment, most patients can address issues in the first two phases, but may not be ready to address third-stage issues until aftercare.

Finally, seemingly simple factors such as size and composition may have a therapeutic effect. Typically, suggested group size ranges between 6 and 12 clients. Groups larger than this may inhibit participation by all members. Groups smaller than this can lack the richness of diversity, and decrease the opportunities for varied interactions.

Client Characteristics Related to Outcome

Emrick (1975) found in his review of the literature that client characteristics are related to outcome. In fact, client characteristics have proven better predictors of treatment outcomes than have treatment factors (Solomon, 1983). One important client variable already discussed is mental health status. McLellan and colleagues found that psychiatric severity is related to the effect of additional individual psychotherapy beyond paraprofessional drug counseling. Patients with low psychiatric severity did just as well without psychotherapy; mid-severity made extra gains with psychotherapy; and high severity did not improve much with drug counseling alone, but improved significantly with additional psychotherapy (McLellan, Luborsky, Woody, O'Brien, & Druley, 1983; Woody et al., 1984). Furthermore, antisocial personality disorder was found to be related to poor treatment outcome (Woody, McLellan, Luborsky, & O'Brien, 1985). Finally, Kissin, Platz, and Su (1970) reported that successful responders to psychotherapy were more intelligent and field independent.

It may be that many clients with psychiatric disorders, in addition to addiction, are not good candidates for interactional group therapy. Kaufman (1989) states that clients with significant psychiatric disorders do not do well in therapeutic communities due to their inability to tolerate confrontation. Lawton (1982) suggests delaying interactional group therapy with depressed, psychotic, or confused clients until they are more stable.

Several therapists have pointed out the need for caution in uncovering painful internal conflicts with addicts in general. Yalom (1974) states, "the alcoholic patients in the group are capable of tolerating only small degrees of anxiety before resorting to old well-ingrained patterns of anxiety relief, especially alcohol and avoidance (leaving the group)" (p. 93). Vannicelli (1982) points out, however, that alcoholics in general are particularly adept at avoiding or diffusing direct focus on important intrapsychic or interpersonal issues. Given the possibility that addicts may, on the one hand, over-react to emotional discomfort by relapsing, or conversely, raise their defenses in order to ignore the information, the group therapist must continually assess the emotional status of each member. While it is impossible to control the amount and intensity of feedback each client will receive in a group, a skilled therapist can modulate this process.

In any group work with addicts, the question inevitably arises of how to handle the client who lapses into substance use. Several therapists (Vannicelli, 1982; Vogel, 1957; Yalom, 1974) point out that a return to substance use in this context is not a failure, and in fact, can be an important learning experience. If the group therapist sets the group norm as a commitment to abstinence, rather than abstinence itself, group members will be able to return to the group and continue to strive toward recovery and improved quality of life. When a "slip" occurs, a group analysis of the precursors and consequences related to the "slip" can provide rich therapeutic material for all members of the group. Sometimes the group may blame itself for the client's relapse, especially if the "slip" occurs after a group session that focused on the individual. Yalom (1974) describes just such a situation, and methods for resolving it. In general, if the individual can return to the group, it is likely that the therapist will be able to elicit predisposing factors (e.g., preoccupation, planning to use, association with other substance abusers) that played a significant role in precipitating a relapse. The therapist needs to accept responsibility for controlling the group experience as much as is reasonable for each individual, and evaluating each member's ability to continue. At the same time, the therapist, and group, cannot assume an inordinate amount of responsibility for the client's recovery.

Clients vary greatly in their readiness and motivation for treatment, and these factors will have an effect on progress and outcome of treatment. For example, Yalom (1974) describes a situation where one group member was overbearing or unwilling to adapt to group norms and expectations. The person's behavior seemed to affect the progress of other group members negatively, particularly as the group was initially forming. Because having a common purpose is important for group formation and maintenance, group therapists may need to make decisions about accepting or retaining an individual in the group not only on the basis of that individual's needs, but on the needs of the group as a whole.

Therapist Effect

As reported earlier, there is evidence that different therapists yield different rates of both retention of clients in treatment and improvements in outcome variables (Miller, 1991; Onken, 1991). Kleinman et al. (1990) reported tremendous variability in retention rate among therapists but not among therapies. The particular therapist to which a patient was assigned was the best predictor of subject attrition.

Little is known about what therapist variables, in particular, produce good results among addicts in group therapy. Vannicelli (1982) describes the importance of therapist skill and technique in dealing with six predictable group issues: (1) client questions about the therapist's substance use history, (2) therapist's willingness to actively reach out to clients who miss sessions, (3) establishing expectations about attendance at self-help groups and how group therapy is different, (4) dealing with confidentiality, (5) making abstinence a clear goal and handling the drinking/using client, and (6) recognizing when the group's discussions about drinking serve to avoid group process rather than to advance it.

Two other therapist variables worth mentioning are substance use history and level of self-disclosure. Both clients and staff generally place importance on a therapist's alcohol and other drug use history. Therapist substance abuse history may not matter as much as how questions regarding their own history are handled (see Vannicelli, 1982). However, it is an important factor for clinicians to be comfortable in addressing the issue. Second, a greater degree of therapist self-disclosure in the substance abuse field is more often expected than in traditional psychiatric settings. Managing this takes a great deal of skill, and no doubt therapists vary greatly in the amount and appropriateness of material they disclose to clients.

Client-Therapist Interaction

Some client and therapist variables have been found to interact. As mentioned previously, McLachlan (1972) reported that client-therapist pairs matched on conceptual level had better outcomes than mismatched pairs. Also, Luborsky, McLellan, Woody, O'Brien, and Auerbach (1985) found that an early treatment measure of the client-therapist relationship, the Helping Alliance Questionnaire, was significantly correlated with outcome. The Helping Alliance Questionnaire purports to measure the extent to which the client found the therapist to be helpful. Thus, the therapist's ability to develop a therapeutic or helping relationship early in treatment appears to be a predictor of outcome.

Process research is especially important in understanding group therapy with substance abusers, because there is so much diversity among clients with this diagnosis. Clients vary not only in drug of choice, but in severity of addiction, environmental support, presence of additional psychopathology, and motivation to change, to name a few. A substance abuser, therefore, may range from being a depressed upper-class suburban housewife addicted to minor tranquilizers, to a young person living on the streets committing crimes to obtain narcotics. A group therapist may be a psychiatrist with 20 years of experience or an uneducated, but enthusiastic recovering addict. Some would say that the addiction itself is the main factor which overrides all other client characteristics. However, this assumption is untested. An even greater unknown is the effect on outcome of the mix of different types of clients within a particular group. In the absence of empirical knowledge, clinicians must rely on judgment and experience in taking these factors into considerations for making clinical decisions.

In summary, clinicians have amassed a wealth of experience-based information they use to guide their practice of group therapy. This has been necessary in the relative vacuum of empirical research. No single therapeutic approach proves to be superior over another. However, intensive intrapsychic or interpersonal group therapy may be best employed after sobriety is achieved. Clinicians need to be attentive, in general, to matching the group therapy experience to an individual's progress in recovery. A unique problem in working with substance abusers is one's response to relapses. Skilled therapists may be able to convert many of these episodes into respectful learning experiences for the entire group.

Limitations of Existing Research

The studies reviewed in this chapter have a number of recurring and potentially avoidable methodological problems. These problems pose significant barriers to drawing clear, unambiguous conclusions and to future attempts to replicate or compare across studies.

One of the most significant problems in the outcome studies reviewed was a general lack of experimental control. For example, there was a lack of

standardization of treatment conditions, that is, few studies trained therapists, provided manuals, or monitored adherence to a treatment protocol.
Furthermore, most outcome studies did not include a control group. This
weakness prevents a test of the hypothesis that treatment is better than no
treatment. It would be unethical to purposefully withhold treatment, but in
light of the fact that some treatments are brief (e.g., some primary treatments last only four weeks), and the fact that treatment programs often
have waiting lists longer than four weeks, the inclusion of a wait-list (or at
least minimal treatment) control group may not be unreasonable.

The group therapy conditions in most studies were confounded with other
variables, particularly other treatments that occurred either before, during,
or after the experiment. Often these other confounding treatments have more
potential for therapeutic impact than the experimental condition. For example, the group therapy condition was often confounded with primary
treatment which was typically a residential, highly structured, multimodal
program including group therapy, individual therapy, AA/NA meetings and
"12-step work," educational activities such as films and lectures, recreational and occupational therapy, and invited presentations from community
members. The difference in amount of time spent in the group therapy condition (e.g., a few hours/week) versus primary treatment (structured therapeutic activities for 12 or more hours/day), is quite a mismatch. This puts
the group therapy condition at a marked disadvantage in the comparison. Although there are practical advantages to conducting a study where the experimental treatment is a supplement to a standard treatment program, one
cannot draw clear conclusions in the absence of adequate controls.

Furthermore, some studies compared treatment conditions that had different or unspecified treatment goals. For example, the treatment goal
of some conditions was moderation while the comparison condition had a
treatment goal of abstinence. To compare two approaches with differing
treatment goals is somewhat unfair.

Group therapy conditions were frequently confounded with the therapist
variable. This confound occurred because each group therapy condition was
conducted by a different therapist, that is, the therapist variable was nested,
rather than crossed, with treatment conditions. Therefore, it is unknown
how much of the effect is due to the group therapy condition and how much
is attributable to the particular therapist conducting the group. In a related
issue, most studies failed to report whether therapists were blind to the experimental hypothesis being tested. As just described, therapists wield an
effect in treatment and therapists are often personally invested in particular
therapeutic approaches. To avoid the potential confound of therapists influencing the outcome of a study because of personal convictions about a therapeutic approach, they should be blind to the hypothesis being tested.
Therapists exert powerful effects in the treatment process and they must be
taken into consideration in study designs. Failing to recognize the effect of
the therapist variable jeopardizes the ability to draw valid conclusions
(Crits-Christoph, Beebe, & Connolly, 1990).

Most studies failed to describe specifically the client, therapist, and therapy characteristics; this oversight is noted in other reviews (e.g., Miller & Hester, 1986). Such detail is essential to allow replication and comparison across studies. McLellan and Alterman (1991) made this point when they argued that studies should include *well-specified* interventions for *well-specified* patient populations. Indeed, group therapy is a heterogeneous intervention as practiced in substance abuse treatment. It varies across treatment programs by theoretical orientation and training of therapists and by the therapeutic philosophy of the treatment program (Institute of Medicine, 1990). Furthermore, group treatment is utilized at different points along the substance abuse treatment continuum and has different treatment goals at these varying points (Cartwright, 1987). As such, it is relatively meaningless to describe a group treatment with only the adjectives of "standard" or "traditional" group therapy.

Finally, many studies included only white adult males, thus limiting the generalizability of research findings. Furthermore, most studies had small sample sizes, which restrict statistical power. Without sufficient statistical power, it is more difficult to find a significant difference if, in fact, one exists. Investigators should conduct power analyses prior to conducting the study in order to determine what sample size is required in order to find a difference. The magnitude of difference between various treatment approaches appears to be rather small. The smaller the difference, the larger the sample size required to find a statistically significant difference.

RECOMMENDATIONS FOR FUTURE RESEARCH

In addition to correcting the limitations noted above, the field needs to address other pressing research needs. First, there are so few empirical studies on group therapy for substance abuse (Brandsma & Pattison, 1985; Hill & Blane, 1967; Onken & Blaine, 1990a; Woody, Luborsky, McLellan, & O'Brien, 1985) that we know little about the process and outcome of this predominant treatment modality. There are only a handful of outcome studies, and the process of group therapy for substance abuse has been virtually unstudied. As is true for many psychological treatments, when research lags behind practice, clinicians rely on tradition, experience, and other clinicians, to guide practice. This situation is problematic in that a clinician's confidence in a treatment's efficacy is not necessarily a reliable indicator of its effectiveness (Institute of Medicine, 1989).

Therefore, group therapy as a treatment for substance abuse needs to be systematically examined with a number of strategies. An important starting point is careful observation and description of the phenomenon, leading to more careful descriptions of group processes and outcomes. Pre- and quasi-experimental research designs (Campbell & Stanley, 1966) also are appropriate for accomplishing these goals. Careful descriptions of group processes could lead to the development of a method of classifying the range of existing group therapy procedures for substance abuse treatment. From this description, it would be possible to: (a) develop a multidimensional classification system that will serve as a common language of identifying group therapy procedures, and (b) derive testable hypotheses to be evaluated in controlled experimental studies. It would also be possible to examine the relationships between different group therapy procedures and outcome, particularly for different client groups (Cartwright, 1987; Kaul & Bednar, 1986).

Careful consideration must be given to the guiding research questions in this inquiry. How a research question is phrased is important both for the method employed to answer it and for the type of answer obtained from the study. In terms of treatment outcome studies, the question "Does treatment work?" is too simplistic and ambiguous (Miller, 1992). This question assumes that group therapy is a homogeneous treatment and that substance abusers are a homogeneous population—neither of which are true (Gwinner, 1979; Miller, 1992). Also, when the research question is too broad, research designs tend to be broad and nonspecific, which leads to ambiguous results. About all that can be concluded from studies of this type is that some clients benefit from therapy, and others do not. Therefore, *advocates* of treatment view the proverbial glass as half full, while *critics* claim that it is half empty.

Similarly, there is little theoretical dividend from general outcome studies. More knowledge about group therapy will be gained from highly specified, standardized, and controlled studies examining specific questions regarding the relationship between process and outcome, than from large outcome studies of unspecified, unstandardized, and unmonitored interventions provided by unspecified therapists to unspecified clients under unspecified circumstances (Annis, 1973; Garfield & Bergin, 1986; Institute of Medicine, 1990; Pattison, 1966). If this field of inquiry follows a similar path as psychotherapy research, it will be more informative to identify what approach is most beneficial for what type of substance abuse client, conducted by what type of therapist, than from comparing one therapeutic model to another. Some promising client variables already examined include conceptual level, locus of control, psychopathology, sociopathy, and cognitive functioning. It will be useful to identify additional client and therapist variables that are related to outcome.

In order to answer the empirical question of the effectiveness of group therapy, it is necessary to conduct controlled research. Although this type of research is difficult to conduct, it is essential for answering the question of the effectiveness of group therapy with confidence. Lest we forget the risk of being misled by uncontrolled research, recall Viamontes (1972) who reviewed 89 studies of pharmacological treatment of alcoholic patients and found that 95% of the uncontrolled studies reported positive effects, whereas only 6% of the studies employing control groups reported positive effects.

The studies reviewed in this chapter also indicate a lack of consensus on outcome variables and measures and timing of administration of outcome assessments, a problem identified by others (Galanter et al., 1991; Lambert, 1990). Outcome assessments were conducted at varying times, ranging from as early as the end of treatment to as late as four years after treatment. Both the content of the outcome assessment and the timing of administration demands standardization. The comparison of studies would be facilitated if a common battery of outcome measures were employed across studies. For example, the American Group Psychotherapy Association (1980) proposed a core battery of instruments to be used in group therapy outcome research. Development of a "substance abuse" battery may be warranted. Outcome batteries should include reliable and valid measures of addiction severity and substance use frequency, such as the Addiction Severity Index (McLellan et al., 1985) for adults, and the Personal Experience Inventory (Winters & Henly, 1989) for adolescents. These tools have applicability for both clinical as well as research purposes.

This topic of a standardized outcome battery brings us to the issue of abstinence as an outcome. Substance use is often dichotomized as either abstinence or nonabstinence. Abstinence is a common outcome criterion in studies involving treatment programs for which abstinence is a treatment goal. But this dichotomous outcome variable is too simplistic in terms of the actual behavior of substance use following treatment. It ignores pretreatment substance use and the value of comparing post-treatment to pretreatment measures to obtain an index of change. Furthermore, it fails to recognize that clients display a variety of post-treatment behaviors. Some clients may significantly reduce their substance use compared to pretreatment levels; this reduction should not be ignored or interpreted as a treatment failure. For example, clients may have one or more slips, but use these in a positive way to learn better methods of maintaining their recovery. Using a dichotomous outcome criterion tied to an absolutistic treatment goal is less than optimal. Given that most human behavior is best represented by a continuum, we recommend that outcome be assessed in terms of increments of improvement.

In this review, we have separated process and outcome research. While this distinction is quite standard in the treatment literature, one should be aware that the ideal is to study process and outcome variables conjointly. Outcome studies that ignore the relationship of process variables to outcome relegate treatment to a black box. That is, clients may show improvement from pretreatment to post-treatment, but if process is ignored, then it is unknown what factors and influences played a role in these changes.

One strategy in examining the process of change is to begin by evaluating proposed theoretical models of change. To date, a number of group therapy approaches with substance abusers have been proposed (e.g., Ellis et al., 1988; Khantzian et al., 1990; Vannicelli, 1982; Yalom, 1974). These approaches advocate specific mechanisms of change that should be put to empirical test, to determine if the results are consistent with the theoretical model. Within a particular group therapy approach, investigators may test a theoretical model of group therapy by operationalizing and measuring those variables that are purported to be therapeutic and then correlate these measures with outcome. Future studies should seek to clarify proposed change agents within specific group therapy approaches and to build stronger theoretical models of treatment efficacy.

The study of group therapy requires the consideration of the group climate or interpersonal atmosphere. Groups are more than the sum of the individual members and have a climate and atmosphere of their own. From a clinical perspective, it would be helpful to understand what effect, both positive and negative, individual members have on group climate. This information could be used to make important clinical decisions about retaining clients in ongoing groups.

In terms of measurement, rapid growth characterizes the development of psychotherapy process and outcome measures in the general psychotherapy literature (e.g., Greenberg & Pinsof, 1986; Lambert, Christensen, & DeJulio, 1983). Much of this work may be applicable to substance abuse group therapy. These measures would help describe the nature of group therapy and allow comparisons between different substance abuse group therapy approaches. Such existing measures of group process may help address questions pertaining to what effect will a specific intervention have on a particular client at a particular point in the group development. For example, group therapy with substance abusers in therapeutic communities and Minnesota Model AA-based programs is characterized as directive and confrontational. An interesting strategy would be to conduct a linguistic study of the speech of group therapists and substance abusers within these two treatment approaches. This type of study would test the hypothesis that these group therapy approaches for substance abusers are directive and confrontational. Next, sequential analysis studies could measure both immediate and longer term effects of these directives and confrontations. Verbal response patterns of therapist and client speech could be measured with existing instruments of directive speech (e.g., Hill, 1986; Stiles, 1986; Stinchfield & Burlingame, 1991) and compared to the speech patterns of other therapy models.

CONCLUSIONS

In a review of psychotherapy research 40 years ago, Eysenck (1952) found a lack of highly controlled experiments of psychotherapy and, not surprisingly, concluded that there was no real evidence for the effectiveness of psychotherapy. Sadly, Eysenck's conclusion is appropriate for the substance abuse group therapy literature. Outcome research has not answered the fundamental question of whether substance abuse group therapy is better than no treatment.

Yet research evidence, like human behavior, can be represented on a continuum. At one end, are anecdotal descriptions, followed next by quasi-experimental studies in the middle position, with highly controlled experiments at the rigorous end of the continuum. Although there are no highly controlled experiments evaluating the effectiveness of group therapy for substance abuse, extant quasi-experimental outcome studies suggest that participation in group therapy is *related* to client improvement. Quasi-experimental studies do not clarify specifics about the causal relationship, but they do serve as a promising launching pad from where more rigorous research can begin.

Most of the treatment research on substance abuse that includes group therapy is not conducted out of a direct interest in group therapy. The intent of most of the studies reviewed was to compare the effectiveness of a specific intervention against the "standard" group therapy. Thus, group therapy was often relegated to the status of control or comparison group (e.g., Ito et al., 1988). This pattern may be due to the belief that group therapy is accepted as a treatment dogma and is rarely questioned (Gwinner, 1979). Ironically, it may be the general popularity and widespread acceptance of group therapy that has prevented its empirical investigation.

We can only speculate about the future of substance abuse group therapy research. Eysenck's (1952) challenge 40 years ago was the impetus for a tremendous surge of psychotherapy research effort. Given that group therapy is the backbone of contemporary substance abuse treatment, it is critical to understand this important treatment modality. The burden to prove the effectiveness of group therapy for a substance abuse clientele and to advance conceptual and theoretical models, awaits researchers, treatment providers, and funding agencies.

REFERENCES

Albrecht, J., & Brabender, V. (1983). Alcoholics in inpatient, short-term interactional group psychotherapy: An outcome study. *Group, 7,* 50–54.

American Group Psychotherapy Association. (1980). *The CORE Battery.* New York: AGPA.

Annis, H. (1973). Directions in treatment research. *Addictions, 20,* 50–59.

Annis, H. (1979). Group treatment of incarcerated offenders with alcohol and drug problems: A controlled evaluation. *Canadian Journal of Criminology, 21,* 3–15.

Annis, H., & Chan, D. (1983). The differential treatment model: Empirical evidence from a personality typology of adult offenders. *Criminal Justice and Behavior, 10,* 159–173.

Ashery, R. S. (Ed.).(1985). Issues in the brief treatment of drug abusers. *Progress in the development of cost-effective treatment for drug abusers: NIDA Research Monograph 58* (pp. 1–8). Rockville, MD: National Institute on Drug Abuse.

Baekeland, F. (1977). Evaluation of treatment methods in chronic alcoholism. In B. Kissin & H. Begleiter (Eds.), *Treatment and rehabilitation of the chronic alcoholic* (pp. 385–440). New York: Plenum Press.

Baekeland, F., Lundwall, L., & Kissin, B. (1975). Methods for the treatment of chronic alcoholism: A critical appraisal. In R. J. Gibbins, Y. Israel, H. Kalant, R. E. Popham, W. Schmidt, & R. G. Smart (Eds.), *Research advances in alcohol and drug problems* (pp. 247–327). New York: Wiley.

Bond, G. R., & Lieberman, M. A. (1978). Selection criteria for group therapy. In J. Brady (Ed.), *Controversy in psychiatry* (pp. 679–702). Philadelphia, PA: Saunders.

Brandsma, J. M., & Pattison, E. M. (1985). The outcome of group psychotherapy alcoholics: An empirical review. *American Journal of Drug and Alcohol Abuse, 11,* 151–162.

Brown, S., & Yalom, I. (1977). Interactional group therapy with alcoholics. *Journal of Studies on Alcohol, 38,* 426–456.

P 467 Buie, J. (1990, February). Message for hill staff: Drug treatment works. *APA Monitor,* p. 21.

Campbell, D. T., & Stanley, J. C. (1966). *Experimental and quasi-experimental designs for research.* Chicago, IL: Rand McNally.

Cartwright, A. K. (1981). Are different therapeutic perspectives important in the treatment of alcoholism? *British Journal of Addiction, 76,* 347–361.

Cartwright, A. K. (1987). Group work with substance abusers: Basic issues and future research. *British Journal of Addiction, 82,* 951–953.

P. 471, 472 Cooney, N., Kadden, R., Litt, M., & Getter, H. (1991). Matching alcoholics to coping skills or interactional therapies: Two-year follow-up results. *Journal of Consulting and Clinical Psychology, 59,* 598–601.

Cooper, D. E. (1987). The role of group psychotherapy in the treatment of substance abusers. *American Journal of Psychotherapy, 41,* 55–67.

Crits-Christoph, P., Beebe, K. L., & Connolly, M. B. (1990). Therapist effects in the treatment of drug dependence: Implications for conducting comparative treatment studies. In L. S. Onken & J. D. Blaine (Eds.), *Psychotherapy and counseling in the treatment of drug abuse: NIDA Research Monograph 104* (pp. 39–49). Rockville, MD: National Institute on Drug Abuse.

Ellis, A., McInerney, J. F., DiGuiuseppe, R., & Yeager, R. J. (1988). *Rational-emotive therapy with alcoholics and substance abusers.* New York: Pergamon Press.

Emrick, C. D. (1975). A review of psychologically oriented treatment of alcoholism: II. The relative effectiveness of different treatment approaches and the effectiveness of treatment versus no treatment. *Journal of Studies on Alcohol, 36,* 88–108.

Emrick, C. D. (1982). Evaluation of alcoholism psychotherapy methods. In E. M. Pattison & E. Kaufman (Eds.), *Encyclopedic Handbook of Alcoholism* (pp. 1152–1169). New York: Gardner Press.

Ends, E. J., & Page, C. W. (1957). A study of three types of group psychotherapy with hospitalized male inebriates. *Quarterly Journal of Studies on Alcohol, 18,* 263–277.

Ettorre, E. M. (1984). A study of alcoholism treatment units: I. Treatment activities and the institutional response. *Alcohol and Alcoholism, 19,* 243–255.

Eysenck, H. J. (1952). The effects of psychotherapy: An evaluation. *Journal of Consulting Psychology, 16,* 319–324.

Flores, P. J. (1988). *Group psychotherapy with addicted populations.* New York: Haworth Press.

Galanter, M., Castaneda, R., & Franco, H. (1991). Group therapy and self-help groups. In R. J. Frances & S. I. Miller (Eds.), *Clinical textbook of addictive disorders* (pp. 431–451). New York: Guilford Press.

Garfield, S. L., & Bergin, A. E. (Eds.). (1986). *Handbook of psychotherapy and behavior change* (3rd ed.). New York: Wiley.

Greenberg, L. S., & Pinsof, W. M. (Eds.). (1986). *The psychotherapeutic process.* New York: Guilford Press.

Gwinner, P. (1979). Treatment approaches. In M. Grant & P. Gwinner (Eds.), *Alcoholism in perspective* (pp. 113–121). Baltimore, MD: University Park Press.

Hill, C. E. (1986). An overview of the Hill Counselor and Client Verbal Response Modes Category Systems. In L. S. Greenberg & W. M. Pinsof (Eds.), *The psychotherapeutic process* (pp. 131–160). New York: Guilford Press.

Hill, M. J., & Blane, H. T. (1967). Evaluation of psychotherapy with alcoholics: A critical review. *Quarterly Journal of Studies on Alcohol, 28,* 76–104.

Hubbard, R. L., Marsden, M. E., Rachal, J. V., Harwood, H. J., Cavanaugh, E. R., & Ginzburg, H. M. (1989). *Drug abuse treatment: A national study of effectiveness.* Chapel Hill, NC: The University of North Carolina Press.

Institute of Medicine. (1989). *Prevention and treatment of alcohol problems: Research opportunities.* Washington, DC: National Academy Press.

Institute of Medicine. (1990). *Broadening the base of treatment for alcohol problems.* Washington, DC: National Academy Press.

Ito, J. R., Donovan, D. M., & Hall, J. J. (1988). Relapse prevention in alcohol aftercare: Effects on drinking outcome, change process, and aftercare attendance. *British Journal of Addiction, 83,* 171–181.

Joanning, H., Quinn, W., Thomas, F., & Mullen, R. (1992). Treating adolescent drug abuse: A comparison of family systems therapy, group therapy, and family drug education. *Journal of Marital and Family Therapy, 18,* 345–356. ?463

Kadden, R. M., Cooney, H. L., Getter, H., & Litt, M. D. (1989). Matching alcoholics to coping skills or interactional therapies: Posttreatment results. *Journal of Consulting and Clinical Psychology, 57,* 698–704.

Kanas, N. (1982). Alcoholism and group psychotherapy. In E. Kauffman & M. Pattison (Eds.), *Encyclopedic handbook of alcoholism* (pp. 1011–1021). New York: Gardner Press.

Kaufman, E. (1989). The psychotherapy of dually diagnosed patients. *Journal of Substance Abuse Treatment, 6,* 9–18.

Kaul, T. J., & Bednar, R. L. (1986). Experiential group research: Results, questions, and suggestions. In S. L. Garfield & A. E. Bergin (Eds.), *Handbook of psychotherapy and behavior change* (3rd ed., pp. 671–714). New York: Wiley.

Khantzian, E. J., Halliday, K. S., & McAuliffe, W. E. (1990). *Addiction and the vulnerable self: Modified dynamic group therapy for substance abusers.* New York: Guilford Press.

Kilmann, P., & Howell, R. (1974). Effects of structure of marathon group therapy and locus of control on therapeutic outcome. *Journal of Consulting and Clinical Psychology, 42,* 912.

Kissin, B., Platz, A., & Su, W. (1970). Social and psychological factors in the treatment of chronic alcoholism. *Journal of Psychiatric Research, 8,* 13–27.

Kleinman, P. H., Woody, G. E., Todd, T., Millman, R. B., Kang, S., Kemp, J., & Lipton, D. S. (1990). Crack and cocaine abusers in outpatient therapy. In L. S. Onken & J. D. Blaine (Eds.), *Psychotherapy and counseling in the treatment of drug abuse: NIDA Research Monograph 104* (pp. 24–35). Rockville, MD: National Institute on Drug Abuse.

Lambert, M. J. (1990). Conceptualizing and selecting measures of treatment outcome: Implications for drug abuse outcome studies. In L. S. Onken & J. D. Blaine (Eds.), *Psychotherapy and counseling in the treatment of drug abuse: NIDA Research Monograph 104* (pp. 80–90). Rockville, MD: National Institute on Drug Abuse.

Lambert, M. J., Christensen, E. R., & DeJulio, S. S. (1983). *The assessment of psychotherapy outcome.* New York: Wiley.

LaRosa, J. C., Lipsius, J. H., & LaRosa, J. H. (1974). Experiences with a combination of group therapy and methadone maintenance in the treatment of heroin addiction. *International Journal of the Addictions, 9,* 605–617.

Lawton, M. (1982). Group psychotherapy with alcoholics: Special techniques. *Journal of Studies on Alcohol, 43,* 1276–1278.

Luborsky, L., McLellan, A. T., Woody, G. E., O'Brien, C. P., & Auerbach, A. (1985). Therapist success and its determinants. *Archives of General Psychiatry, 42,* 602–611.

McLachlan, J. F. (1972). Benefit from group therapy as a function of patient-therapist match on conceptual level. *Psychotherapy: Theory, Research and Practice, 9,* 317–323.

McLellan, A. T., & Alterman, A. I. (1991). Patient treatment matching: A conceptual and methodological review with suggestions for future research. In R. W. Pickens, C. G. Leukefeld, & C. R. Schuster (Eds.), *Improving drug abuse treatment: NIDA Research Monograph 106* (pp. 114–135). Rockville, MD: National Institute on Drug Abuse.

McLellan, A. T., Luborsky, L., Cacciola, J., Griffith, J., McGahan, P., & O'Brien, C. P. (1985). *Guide to the Addiction Severity Index.* Rockville, MD: National Institute on Drug Abuse.

McLellan, A. T., Luborsky, L., Woody, G. E., O'Brien, C. P., & Druley, K. A. (1983). Predicting response to alcohol and drug abuse treatments: Role of psychiatric severity. *Archives of General Psychiatry, 40,* 620–625.

McLellan, A. T., Woody, G. E., Luborsky, L., & Goehl, L. (1988). Is the counselor an "active ingredient" in substance abuse rehabilitation? An examination of treatment success among four counselors. *Journal of Nervous and Mental Diseases, 176,* 423–430.

Miller, W. R. (1991). Emergent treatment concepts and techniques. In P. E. Nathan (Ed.), *Annual review of addictions research and treatment* (pp. 283–296). New York: Pergamon Press.

Miller, W. R. (1992). The effectiveness of treatment for substance abuse. *Journal of Substance Abuse Treatment, 9*, 93–102.

Miller, W. R., & Hester, R. K. (1980). Treating the problem drinker: Modern approaches. In W. R. Miller (Ed.), *The addictive behaviors: Treatment of alcoholism, drug abuse, smoking, and obesity* (pp. 11–141). Oxford: Pergamon Press.

Miller, W. R., & Hester, R. K. (Eds.).(1986). The effectiveness of alcoholism treatment: What research reveals. *Treating addictive behaviors: Processes of change* (pp. 121–174). New York: Plenum Press.

Miller, W. R., & Taylor, C. A. (1980). Relative effectiveness of bibliotherapy, individual and group self-control training in the treatment of problem drinkers. *Addictive Behaviors, 5*, 13–24.

Olson, R. P., Ganley, R., Devine, V. T., & Dorsey, G. C. (1981). Long-term effects of behavioral versus insight-oriented therapy with inpatient alcoholics. *Journal of Consulting and Clinical Psychology, 49*, 866–877.

Onken, L. S. (1991). Using psychotherapy effectively in drug abuse treatment. In R. W. Pickens, C. G. Leukefeld, & C. R. Schuster (Eds.), *Improving drug abuse treatment: Research Monograph 106* (pp. 267–278). Rockville, MD: National Institute on Drug Abuse.

Onken, L. S., & Blaine, J. D. (1990a). Psychotherapy and counseling research in drug abuse treatment: Questions, problems, and solutions. In L. S. Onken & J. D. Blaine (Eds.), *Psychotherapy and counseling in the treatment of drug abuse: NIDA Research Monograph 104* (pp. 1–5). Rockville, MD: National Institute on Drug Abuse.

Page, R. C. (1982). Marathon group therapy with users of illicit drugs: Dimensions of social learning. *International Journal of the Addictions, 17*, 1107–1116.

Page, R. C. (1986). The effects of marathon groups on the ways illicit drug users perceive counseling. *International Journal of the Addictions, 20*, 1675–1684.

Parloff, M. B., & Dies, R. R. (1977). Group therapy outcome research: 1966–1975. *International Journal of Group Psychotherapy, 27*, 281–319.

Pattison, E. M. (1966). A critique of alcoholism treatment concepts with special reference to abstinence. *Quarterly Journal of Studies on Alcoholism, 27*, 49–71.

Pfeffer, A. Z., Friedland, P., & Wortis, S. B. (1949). Group psychotherapy with alcoholics. *Quarterly Journal of Studies on Alcohol, 10*, 198–216.

Pomerleau, O., & Adkins, D. (1980). Evaluating behavioral and traditional treatment for problem drinkers. In L. C. Sobell, M. B. Sobell, & E. Ward (Eds.), *Evaluating alcohol and drug abuse treatment effectiveness: Recent advances* (pp. 93–108). New York: Pergamon Press.

Pomerleau, O. F., Pertschuk, M., Adkins, D., & Brady, J. P. (1978). A comparison of behavioral and traditional treatment for middle-income problem drinkers. *Journal of Behavioral Medicine, 1*, 187–200.

Price, R. H., Burke, A. C., D'Aunno, T. A., Klingel, D. M., McCaughrin, W. C., Rafferty, J. A., & Vaughn, T. E. (1991). Outpatient drug abuse treatment services, 1988: Results of a national survey. In R. W. Pickens, C. G. Leukefeld, &

C. R. Schuster (Eds.), *Improving drug abuse treatment: NIDA Research Monograph 106* (pp. 63–92). Rockville, MD: National Institute on Drug Abuse.

Ross, W. D., McReynolds, W., & Berzins, J. (1974). Effectiveness of marathon group psychotherapy with hospitalized female narcotics addicts. *Psychological Reports, 34,* 611–616.

Schuckit, M. A. (1989). *Drug and alcohol abuse: A clinical guide to diagnosis and treatment* (3rd ed.). New York: Plenum Press.

Solomon, S. D. (1983). Individual versus group therapy: Current status in the treatment of alcoholism. *Advances in Alcohol and Substance Abuse, 2*(1), 69–86.

Spitz, H. I. (1987). Cocaine abuse: Therapeutic group approaches. In H. I. Spitz & J. I. Rosecan (Eds.), *Cocaine abuse: New directions in treatment and research* (pp. 156–201). New York: Brunner/Mazel.

Stephenson, N. L., Boudewyns, P. A., & Lessing, R. A. (1977). Long-term effects of peer group confrontation therapy used with polydrug abusers. *Journal of Drug Issues, 7,* 135–149.

Stiles, W. B. (1986). Development of a taxonomy of verbal response modes. In L. S. Greenberg & W. M. Pinsof (Eds.), *The psychotherapeutic process* (pp. 161–200). New York: Guilford Press.

Stinchfield, R., & Burlingame, G. (1991). Development and use of the Directives Rating System in group therapy. *Journal of Counseling Psychology, 38,* 251–257.

Telch, M. J., Hannon, R., & Telch, C. R. (1984). A comparison of cessation strategies for the outpatient alcoholic. *Addictive Behaviors, 9,* 103–109.

Vannicelli, M. (1982). Group psychotherapy with alcoholics: Special techniques. *Journal of Studies on Alcohol, 43,* 17–37.

Viamontes, J. A. (1972). Review of drug effectiveness in the treatment of alcoholism. *American Journal of Psychiatry, 128,* 1570–1571.

Vogel, S. (1957). Some aspects of group psychotherapy with alcoholics. *International Journal of Group Psychotherapy, 7,* 302–309.

Winters, K., & Henly, G. (1989). *Personal Experience Inventory (PEI) Manual.* Los Angeles, CA: Western Psychological Services.

Woody, G. E., Luborsky, L., McLellan, A. T., & O'Brien, C. P. (1985). Psychotherapy for opiate dependence. In R. S. Ashery (Ed.), *Progress in the development of cost-effective treatment for drug abusers: NIDA Research Monograph 58* (pp. 9–29). Rockville, MD: National Institute on Drug Abuse.

Woody, G. E., McLellan, A. T., Luborsky, L., & O'Brien, C. P. (1985). Sociopathy and psychotherapy outcome. *Archives of General Psychiatry, 42,* 1081–1086.

Woody, G. E., McLellan, A. T., Luborsky, L., O'Brien, C. P., Blaine, J., Fox, S., Herman, I., & Beck, A. T. (1984). Psychiatric severity as a predictor of benefits from psychotherapy: The Penn-VA study. *American Journal of Psychiatry, 141,* 1172–1177.

Yalom, I. D. (1974). Group therapy and alcoholism. *Annals New York Academy of Sciences, 233,* 85–103.

Yalom, I. D. (1975). *The theory and practice of group psychotherapy* (2nd ed.). New York: Basic.

Yalom, I. D., Bloch, S., Bond, G., Zimmerman, E., & Qualls, B. (1978). Alcoholics in interactional group therapy. *Archives of General Psychiatry, 35,* 419–425.

CHAPTER 14

The Self-Help, Mutual-Support Group*

GERALD GOODMAN and MARION K. JACOBS

Future studies see the ubiquitous mutual support group (MSG) (i.e., self-help group) as America's major method for delivering psychological comfort and repair by 1999 (Borkman, 1990; Prochaska & Norcross, 1982; Zinman, 1986). The growth curve appears stunningly steep. For better or worse, the number of people in public mutual support groups (MSGs) now rivals those in individual and group therapy combined (Jacobs & Goodman, 1989). The picture is blurred by the fact that formats for MSGs sometimes resemble formats for classical group therapy, and private, informal MSGs are hidden from the scholar's view. Definitions are confounded as professionals become consultants, leaders, co-leaders, members, and even founders of MSGs. Frequent professional involvement probably represents or predicts a national pattern and signals an alert to group therapists that (1) their scholarship and practice skills should be applied to MSG methods, (2) MSG activity is now encroaching, competing, and is being confused with group therapy by the public, and (3) therapist migration toward MSG work may be a symptom of a de facto mental health system that is failing (Kiesler & Morton, 1988).

This chapter introduces recent theory and research on MSGs to group therapists and group therapy scholars. We intend to demonstrate the massive scope of such activity, and offer a new picture of professional involvement. Our goal is to illustrate the variety of MSG needs that can be addressed by group therapy specialists along with the ideological reframing required for successful professional intervention and research. But first, by way of vignettes, we introduce four specific groups. Collectively, they highlight the difficulties inherent in trying to identify the generic features, parameters, and essential properties of MSGs. To provide a context for understanding the state of MSG phenomena, it is useful to conceive a continuum of all help-intended interventions, bounded on one end by everyday acts of social

* Thanks to J. T. Blackledge for his contributions to our thinking and his help in organizing the literature along with Laura McIntosh and Paul Allen. Thanks also to Dr. Steve Shoptaw who helped with the early hammering out of the chapter structure, and Nerissa Leonardo and Lucia Hodgson who typed and worried through the manuscript beyond the call of duty.

support (like friends or family trying to help someone ill or hurt) and on the other end by the methods of group therapy. The difficulty lies in the fact that MSGs exist throughout the space between these two poles.

The four vignettes provide a context for examining the nature of these help-intended groups; they do not fit current conceptions of help oriented groups. The intent is to expand the small-group professional's perspective and give substance to the problem of parameters.

REPRESENTATIVE VIGNETTES

A Meeting of Middle Managers

Passing acquaintances, a man and a woman peer into their newspapers at a lunch table in the company cafeteria. They are reading the same story with worried faces—their company just laid off 80 managers. Would they be next? Noticing each other reading, they talk. It starts with a dispassionate discussion of the layoffs, then moves to more emotional matters of fair play, the terrible job market, and mutual worries. Their feelings are quite similar. It is a good talk in bad times. The next day, they meet at the same table. Talk turns to estimating how long before the ax falls on them. They exchange confessions of fear. The pair leave lunch feeling like new friends, bonded by their common predicament. Over the following four months, they happen to meet once or twice a week, discussing new job possibilities and rumors about their company's financial prospects. Increasingly, their random lunches become more mutually helpful. They prepare contingencies for several scenarios, share job leads, provide each other "middle manager therapy" and become confidants. Eventually, the layoff threat abates and the working lunches are abandoned. At this writing, they remain friendly, share an occasional lunch, but no longer engage in intense conversation.

This man and woman exchanged help over dozens of lunches. It wasn't romantic. After the first few meetings, an implicit contract maintained commitment to fairly regular meetings, confidentiality, and a problem-solving conversation. That is, this accidental pairing caused by a common concern evolved toward mutual expectations of reciprocal, private help. Expectations ended as their problem ended.

The discovery of a common problem by a pair of people at their workplace, school, clinic, or other setting that leads to further conversation must occur millions of times each year. How should social scientists address such phenomena? When the help is exchanged around a common problem, are current concepts of informal social support sufficient for understanding these pairings?

The Technicolor Mothers' Group

Because they live in the same housing project, three new mothers acquire the habit of having phone conversations at their babies' nap time. Just like the previous dyad, they talk of common concerns: articles on single mothers, getting too much or too little support from families, coping with their babies' fathers, relating to new boyfriends, managing welfare budgets, and so on. Empathy is easy. Phone chats are random, but their "spontaneous" dinners together are almost always on Tuesdays or Thursdays in one of the apartments, while babies hopefully sleep. One mother, who works as a social worker's assistant, slowly becomes the group's guide, taking over whenever the conversation addresses touchy topics. Sometimes someone cries. They are frequently surprised about their similarity because their backgrounds are so diverse: African-American, Pakistani, and New England Caucasian. Such diversity, contrasted with their similar experiences as single mothers, is openly important to them. That's why they playfully took the name "Technicolor Mothers" during one of their dinners, and why it remains ten months later. Lately, they've ritualized their dessert time with a round-robin to see who should lead off their serious conversation after light dinner talk. At the moment, they are trying to decide about inviting another mother who asked to join them. Somehow it feels like an intrusion. Then again, they know she could use their help.

These three mothers seem to have formed a quasi-formal, instrumental *group*—not just a social gathering. But if not just a social group, what are they? What do they become if a new member enters and she follows their rituals? Occasionally, they skip a few weeks because of other demands or lack of an initiator. Gathering for dinner when it pleases them does not show the commitment generally found in MSGs or therapy. On the other hand, they clearly exchange emotional and cognitive support. Such groups that develop beyond typical social interaction probably come and go in large numbers, unnoticed and uncounted by social scientists.

Alcoholics Obvious

Near Clinch Mountain, Tennessee, four high school seniors and a college drop-out make beautiful bluegrass music. It's 1992. They're into their Sunday ritual—pizza for lunch, then plenty of beer as they practice. People in town know these kids are serious talents; they also know they have serious drinking problems. Beautiful music, ugly behavior. After two years of heavy drinking and dozens of shouting matches, the townsfolk are surprised the boys are still together. The cohesion comes from the group's shared frustration and disorganized attempts at making it in the music business. They've said it many times, but now they have come to believe that the "only way out of town" is to stop drinking. So one Sunday, after pizza and practice, they call an "Alcoholics Obvious" meeting. Their mocking name is actually apt because the group's alcoholic antics around town are far from anonymous, and their plans for "fighting the filthy bottle" differ from the sometimes somber 12-step AA method. Somehow they manage to laugh a lot while still being sensitive to each other's trepidations. Sunday meetings continue, starting with a ritual "round of small solos" so current moods and progress can be disclosed. Then, there are a couple of "long songs" in the form of "all for one" episodes focused on the members who are feeling most pressed. The college drop-out frequently introduces cognitive reframing techniques learned at Rational Recovery meetings during his year at East Tennessee State. After 11 months and a few relapses, all five are sober. Their progress is monitored via town gossip and three new members are allowed into meetings during the year. They contact a clinical psychologist who drives in from a nearby city once a month to lead a three-hour session. She charges $30 per hour which is divided among the eight members ($11.25 each). She has helped them apply client-centered theory and methods. They use many of her suggestions but continue to resist her proposal for twice-a-week meetings. It's clear this group belongs to the members. At last report, one of the original five quit after a session of serious criticism, but he is reconsidering a return. The group voted to allow town alcoholics to drop in the first Sunday of each month. Avoiding constant seriousness is still a group rule. Meetings end with a raucous singing of the irreverent Alcoholics Obvious Anthem accompanied by two guitars, a five-string banjo, a mandolin, and a bass.

If this group were in California and asked to be listed on our referral service, they would qualify as a clear-cut MSG because (1) control of the process, recruitment, selection, leadership, and ideology belongs to the membership, (2) the group theme is restricted to a single common concern, (3) members alternate roles as helper and help seeker, and (4) dues or fees are moderately inexpensive. However, some observers might question the systematic and commercial use of a psychologist, and the employment of cognitive restructuring methods and client-centered therapy. They might classify Alcoholics Obvious as some sort of quasi-therapy.

A Classical Group

These struggling people suffer from serious personal problems: panic disorder, severe agoraphobia, "anger attacks," recovering schizophrenia, obsessive-compulsive disorder, chronic phobias, and clinical depression. The experienced woman who runs the show is tired tonight. She just flew back from meetings on national mental health issues with social scientists at a major university. Tonight's group session starts with an orienting talk that settles the eight ex-mental patients and gets them ready for initial self-disclosures about distresses during their week. A young woman details "almost falling apart," having to wait 20 minutes at the check-out of a short-handed supermarket. She describes the ordeal as amplified because she was already late for an appointment. Others offer encouragement as she relates how she successfully reframed the situation and calmed her mounting panic—something she could not have accomplished six months ago. The group is quite sophisticated in addressing such vulnerable disclosures. Its work is tightly organized and theory driven. Almost everyone has done some serious reading on the theory and method that shapes their process.

Tonight, a gray-haired man quotes some scholarly notion from their founding psychiatrist. The founder began his work in the 1930s and polished his theory over 15 years of working with patients before producing a formal publication. The woman guiding the group (i.e., offering interpretations, encouraging disclosure) can criticize the method, but her devotion shows when she talks of the early days. She is masterful at teaching others the theory and techniques of symptom management. The current psychological research literature contains convincing support for this approach to treatment. Some sophisticated scholars see the founder's work as the forerunner of current cognitive therapy.

This particular vignette makes a point. The severity and apparent heterogeneity of problems, the sophisticated theory, long experience, and national scholarly connections of the woman in charge, the group size, and the controlled weekly meetings suggest group therapy. But this mutual support group is eager to distinguish itself from therapy. It's called Recovery, Inc. and was established and shaped between 1937 and 1950 by psychiatrist Abraham Low. After writing a book on his cognitively oriented theory and method, Low gave control of everything to his patients. In this case, the skilled leader is a former patient without professional credentials. Today, 800 Recovery chapters run tightly controlled, theory-driven sessions led by former patients. These groups have many parameters that parallel group therapy. Recovery, Inc., with its complex theory and precise process, belongs near the group therapy end of the help-intended group continuum. Yet it deliberately retains essential features of the MSG model: group leaders are (or have been) fellow sufferers; members enter free or make donations; there is one common concern (serious psychological problems); and the groups are organized around a dual-role process where all members give and take help. Therapists never run sessions but may refer patients, see some members individually, or attend as regular members.

A Problem of Parameters

These four vignettes illustrate the problem of parameters confounding the important task of defining mutual support group activity in America. The pair of middle managers developed a process that could be designated as social support or, perhaps, a mutual support group, depending upon the observer's bias and definition of "group." Recovery, Inc., with its professionally developed theory and sophisticated practice, could be viewed as overlapping with elements of the group therapy model. Yet when Technicolor Mothers and Alcoholics Obvious are included, it becomes clear that all four of these help-intended enterprises operate with the essential structures of the current MSG model: (1) similarity of presenting problem, (2) an expectation of *reciprocal* help among members, (3) indigenous leadership, and (4) no fees, modest charges, or voluntary contributions. The ideologies or change theories across MSGs are both more varied and more problem specific when compared with group therapy theories.

Whether affiliated or free standing, these MSGs bear similarity to therapy groups in their "public" recruitment policy. The California Self-Help Center alone, with its 4,600 group database, referred about 120 people a day to such public groups in 1993. But a segment of MSGs are closed to the public. Technicolor Mothers is an example. Alcoholics Obvious is another because they are ambivalent about new members. We suspect there may be a surprisingly large number of such free-standing, problem-specific groups that meet informally within neighborhoods, churches, organizations, corporations, colleges, and other avenues of propinquity that are "private." Because there is no public recruitment, they escape notice of scholarly investigators, self-help clearinghouses, and the media. That is, there is probably a massive underground of MSG activity that remains unexamined in the professional literature. Informal observations and anecdotal evidence repeatedly point to the existence of a large varied, unstudied, free-standing set of MSGs that meet with indigenous leaders to reciprocate help for specific personal concerns.

These private groups, with their shared predicament and reciprocal help, appear different from everyday acts of social support where a sick relative is visited or a bereaved friend is taken to dinner. Private MSGs are characterized by reciprocal help for a common problem. They may also use an implicit or explicit agreement (contract) for scheduling meetings, leadership process, meeting length, or confidentiality. Nobody knows the true scope, variety, methods, and typical size of such groupings. We imagine that most are small groups (e.g., two to four people) that meet irregularly with unexpressed intentions to reciprocate help for a "shared problem." Maybe a natural division of labor and leadership evolves—something like the Middle Managers, Technicolor Mothers, and the original members of Alcoholics Obvious. An historic example of such a private mutual support dyad was formed in 1935 by two self-diagnosed "drunks," Dr. Bob and Bill W., who gave each other empathy, confession, and a group process plan that grew into Alcoholics Anonymous. That is, the granddaddy of modern, public MSGs, which now claims 1.1 million members, was born as a tiny private MSG.

THE PASSING OF PURE MUTUAL SUPPORT GROUPS

The essential psychology of the MSG process is suggested by the metaphor: miniature mental health democracy. Group ideologies consistently emphasize that power resides in the membership, that leadership rises from the membership and serves at its will (Emerick, 1990; Rosenberg, 1984). Egalitarianism is the ideal and fosters equal rights within a group process. A sometimes fierce autonomy, zeal, and even chauvinism colors MSG sentiment. Public MSGs tend to resist external rule (professional takeover), but seem to shift from early isolationism toward cautious collaboration with foreign powers (usually mental health professionals) (Black, 1988; Stewart,

1990). Some of these MSG miniature democracies evolve into oligarchies, dictatorships, advocacy campaigns, laissez-faire social clubs, or simply homogeneous therapy groups or "theme groups."

The remarkably rapid growth of public MSG activity over the past 10 to 15 years is often noted in the professional literature and demonstrated by the increasing frequency of member appearances on TV talk shows (Madara, 1990; Madara, Kalafat, & Miller, 1988; Zinman, 1986). Evangelism, docudramas, advice column publicity, and thousands of public service announcements are making MSGs into an obvious aspect of our culture (Leerhsen, 1990). Less obvious is the increased involvement of professionals in these "grass roots," "member managed" groups. Traditionally, the appeal of MSGs has come from the nonprofessional cost effectiveness, fierce independence, and do-it-yourself empowerment.

This picture of a generic MSG ideology and method that works across a variety of problems has colored the professional literature and public view. The public picture of MSGs that help themselves (self-help groups) has been most strongly shaped by media coverage over the past five years, in particular, the Oprah and Donahue talk shows and various dramas displaying group members that function as experientially qualified help givers and help receivers. The images of self-sufficient, grass-roots, nonprofessional groups suggest an inspiring, do-it-yourself purity. But the public and the professionals have been misinformed. The indigenous purity of MSGs seems exaggerated. An incidental finding at the California Self-Help Center led to some discoveries that have recently altered our view of the typical American MSG.

It began early in 1985 with a routine survey of the 2,000 MSGs on the California Self-Help Center's (CSHC) statewide database. We were assessing the needs for external services requested by a variety of groups scattered across California. The answer to one of the demographic questions suggested 84% had professional involvement (Burstein, 1985). This was puzzling, but because needs assessment was the main mission, the peculiar finding was put aside as a possible error. Later that year, the issue of professional involvement arose again. Ted Gradman was studying differential perception between MSG leaders and members in 253 random groups. One of his secondary findings revealed 83% of the sampled groups had some form of professional "involvement" in their MSG (Gradman, 1985). Once again the deviant finding was disregarded, perhaps because both findings were so contradictory to the "purist" model of member-managed MSGs. The characterization of MSGs in the professional literature and years of correspondence with MSGs on the CSHC referral service led to the belief that most groups functioned without professional intervention. A small study of 43 groups suggested that 72% had "involvement" with one or more professionals, but the sample was not representative (Toseland & Hacker, 1982). There was evidence that many groups would welcome a bit of professional help (Knight, Wollert, Levy, Frame, & Padgett, 1980) and indirect help with referrals and consultation (Gottlieb, 1985), but the bulk of the literature depicted member-managed MSGs. Eventually the significance of the findings from Toseland and Hacker, the California Self Help Center survey, and Gradman's study was persuasive: there must be substantial professional involvement in MSG affairs. Did professional involvement mean mental health professionals, and did "involvement" mean leadership? Gradman's findings suggest that in about half the cases the word "involvement" meant leadership. He also found that "professional leadership" referred to mental health specialists in 32% of the groups, and other professionals (administrators, teachers, etc.) for 11% of the groups. "Trained nonprofessionals" led 18% of the groups, and regular group members led about 36%. It is unclear if leadership was full-time, part-time, shared (co-leader) or solo, but two-thirds of the professionals were paid; the remainder volunteered.

These initial studies not only disturb the traditional concept of the member-managed MSG, but raises pressing questions about the specific roles professionals take in MSG settings. Jennifer Lotery (1985) decided to address the matter with a study focusing on the specific nature of professional involvement in MSGs. She sent detailed questionnaires on leadership structure to a random sample of 850 MSGs of the 3,000 listed in the California Self-Help Center's database. It was the largest comprehensive MSG survey ever conducted, and represented every category of MSG in every California county. The 426 responding groups reported that 83% were somehow involved with professionals. This figure was the same as Burstein's (1985) and Gradman's (1985) findings drawn from earlier and smaller samples. There was little doubt that the picture of the typical MSG needed revision to include some sort of professional participation—at least in California. It also became painfully apparent that much of the professional literature was probably interpreting results and making generalizations about an American MSG model that usually excluded professional involvement.

THE ROLES PROFESSIONALS PLAY IN MUTUAL SUPPORT GROUPS

Some evidence about the surprising variety of professional involvement came out of Lotery's work. Professionals participated in, at least, thirteen roles! About 14% of the groups "frequently" had professionals in the role of solo leader. Another 35% used professionals as co-leaders along with, or alternating with a member. So, almost half the groups frequently experienced a professional as part-time, full-time, or as a co-leader. This finding should not be confused to mean half the MSGs are simply led by professionals. Most groups had several professional leaders, with physicians and nurses most common in the medical MSGs.

The most common form of professional involvement is referring new members (57%), but professionals also recruit/accept clients for their practice (39%). Another surprise: In 38% of the MSG sample, professionals participated as regular members. Close to 35% of Lotery's sample frequently brought in professionals as speakers—probably specialists in the specific common concern of a group. Another 35% used professional consultants or advisors, perhaps for problems in group process. Professionals that help locate meeting places or financial aid and other resources worked with 29% of the sample. These may be mostly agency professionals. In some cases (25%), a professional originated, established, organized, or coordinated an entire group or network of groups. Specialists in small group communication, helping methods, and management of meetings frequently intervened in 18% of the sample, and intervened "sometimes" for 46% of the groups. Professionals sat in as observers for 17% of the groups; 14% took tutorial or workshop instruction. Finally, Lotery found that program "evaluators" were involved with about 12% of the sample.

Most of these professional activities are welcomed with a desire for even more involvement, especially as a referral source, speaker, teacher, student, and co-leader. Respondents were least interested in having professionals serve as solo leaders or coordinators/organizers. Lotery's careful work should alter current conceptions of the typical MSG. It seems time for both MSG separatists and purists to recognize that when AA groups are separated out, most MSGs welcome professionals in a variety of roles. At first glance, the image of professionals performing many roles for satisfied MSGs might suggest that the typical group includes a professional at every meeting. Lotery's findings warn us away from that impression. With a 75% response rate, her data suggest that for 37% of the groups, professionals intervene less than two hours a month. Involvement is between two and ten hours a month for 20% of the groups, and over ten hours of contact each month for 10% of the sample. Clearly, we need more research to understand more clearly how much time professionals spend with MSGs.

Unfortunately, the newly emerging picture impairs the representativeness of some past research and theory publications. Yet, accepting the significant professionalization of American MSG activity, and the existence of a large but uncounted set of "underground" private groups, frees the field to bring new insight to a very complex phenomenon. Hybrid groups that amalgamate professional, indigenous, and programmed leadership seem poised to become the fastest growing format. Private groups guided by public programs are another logical combination with prospects for widespread activity. We may even be catching a glimpse of major mental health coping methods for the next century. Our prediction is that the MSG will become the nation's de facto "treatment of choice" for many psychopathologies and nonpsychiatric life predicaments by the year 2010 or 2020.

Early findings seem to indicate that professional involvement in MSGs will become widespread. This new view also points to the existence of many "private" miniature MSGs shaped by methods learned through the media or packaged programs, and distributed by researchers and practitioners. It looks like the efficacy, empowerment, low cost, psychological safety, flexibility, and member dignity usually offered by the basic MSG method will be combined with the psychological sophistication, research and development capacity, and networked knowledge of professionals. This blending of "natural" and professional methods, supplemented with future forms of interactive media, could even create the foundation for a new image of psychotherapeutics. Maybe it will be common to speak of something like "Mutual Support Therapy."

These interpretations about the extent of private MSGs and the degree of professional involvement have radically changed our view of the MSG in America. It appears that the spectrum of MSG methods spans from private, informal miniature groups to sessions that look like group therapy. The available literature reviewed in this chapter only covers the public, formal MSG. Though some articles address specific issues of professional involvement, none reflects an awareness of the widespread use of professionals as consultants and leaders.

SCOPE AND VARIETY OF MUTUAL SUPPORT GROUPS IN AMERICA

Our best empirical estimate conservatively shows 7.6 million adults will be involved in public self-help, mutual-support groups during 1993 (Jacobs & Goodman, 1989, pp. 536–537). Lieberman (see this edition) has generated an almost identical estimate using a different approach. This massive phenomenon is poorly understood and disregarded by many professionals because: (1) MSGs are typically quiet, small, and local (Gottlieb, 1985). They blend unnoticed into city and small town cultures (AA type groups are a vivid exception, but represent less than eight percent of all MSG participants). Most mental health professionals rarely see MSGs in action. (2) The accelerating growth curve of MSG activity over the past decade is just starting to be discussed in the literature of group therapists and general psychology. (3) Apparently, many professionals are unfamiliar with the vast array of MSGs or erroneously believe such groups reject professional involvement. (4) The millions of MSG participants are camouflaged when outside of their groups because they identify with their predicament and not with the generic phenomenon of MSGs. They are unlike people in therapy who refer to themselves as "patients" or "clients."

In the small, private, free-standing groups, members remain unnoticed and uncounted by professionals and are probably unaware that what they do is called self-help/mutual support. If we cautiously assume the scope of private, informal MSGs to be only half of the public groups, then the 1993 incidence of total MSG activity becomes 11.4 million—easily outnumbering all forms of therapy.

The range of problems addressed by public MSGs is vast, covering almost every serious medical problem and a range of psychological problems beyond the practices of group and individual therapists. The list is larger than the psychopathologies described in the DSM-IIIR. To convey an impression of the variety and specificity, an alphabetical list of 48 problems from MSGs addressed in the professional literature (1975–1992) follows. It is but a modest sample of active groups: Adolescent Children of Alcoholics, Adult Children of Alcoholics, Agoraphobia, AIDS Support, Alcoholism, Anorexia Nervosa, Caregivers of the Demented Elderly, Children with Eye Cancer, Family Members, Cocaine Dependence, Co-Dependency, Diabetes, Divorce, Drug Abusing Teens, Epilepsy, Gay Alcoholics, Hearing Impaired Adults, Hypertension Treatment Patients, HIV Support, Homicide Survivors, Hospice Staff Volunteers, Incest Survivors, Individuals Who Have Lost a Family Member to Drunk Driving, Juvenile Offenders, Late Deafened Adults, Manic Depression, Mastectomy Patients, Multiple Sclerosis, Obsessive Compulsive Disorder, Older Divorced Women, Bereaved Children, Parents of Children with Cancer, Perinatal Bereavement, Imprisoned Men, PTSD and Vietnam Veterans, Rape (Victims and Perpetrators), Schizophrenia and Substance Abuse, Sexual Addiction, Sickle Cell Anemia, Spouses of Head Injury Survivors, Stroke, and Widows.

This list of problems shows the concerns of groups discussed in the literature. It does not represent the wider variety of groups now operating in California, and probably America. That is, the 48 problems discussed in the literature are less than a quarter of the 212 problems addressed by active groups on the California Self-Help Center's referral database. Some examples from that database are listed here to round out the picture and point to the sometimes extreme specificity of problems that characterize MSG activity: A New Beginning (Divorce), Adolescent Deaf Children of Alcoholics, Alternatives to Domestic Violence (Battered Women), Bread of Life (Anorexia), Cafe Europa '45 (Holocaust Survivors), Circle of Friends (Friends of Suicide Victims), Crack Prevention Program, Go-Go Stroke Club, Hipsters Club Support Group (Aged), Life Goes On (Friends and Relatives of Homicide Victims), Men Overcoming Violence (Men Who Batter), Moms in Recovery (Alcoholism), One Step at a Time (Widows), Open Arms (Co-Dependency), Panic Assistance League (Agoraphobia), Parents of Murdered Children, Parents Without Partners, People Assisting Violence Victims, Perpetrators Support Group (Physical Abusers), Senior Crime Victims, Sex Addicts Anonymous, Stress and Black Women, Survivors of Incest, Together Expecting a Miracle (Adoption Support), Ups and Downs (Manic Depression).

THE ESSENTIAL PROCESS OF MUTUAL SUPPORT GROUPS

The literature on self-help/mutual support groups reveals an active identity struggle from 1975 to 1993. Articles often begin by quoting several definitions by social scientists like Katz (1976), Killilea (1976), Kurtz and Powell (1987), Lieberman (1990), Lieberman and Borman (1979), Rootes and

Aanes (1992), Van der Avort and Van Harberden (1985), or Wollert (1986), and then offering a newer definition or taxonomy of goals, processes, and populations. The diffused expansion of group frequency and variety over the past 18 years has increased the range of ideologies, techniques, recruiting and selection procedures, and ways of networking. Perhaps the field's preoccupation with definition is stimulated by the remarkable changes in MSG scope, variety, technique, ideology, and networking styles. Assessing such changes with accuracy is impossible, and frustrating for scholars. How can such a massive, sometimes seclusive, and unstable phenomenon be defined? And without a sturdy definition, there is little hope of building a body of knowledge. The lack of a sound generic MSG model has rendered this form of helping, used by many millions, to suffer a meager research literature.

Some of the difficulty in establishing a durable MSG picture can be overcome by focusing on the essential group processes that seem to remain constant across the variety of problems, goals, ideologies, and techniques of MSGs (Kurtz, 1990). With some exceptions (e.g., Biegel & Yamatani, 1987; Jacobs & Goodman, 1989; Levy, 1979; Rappaport et al., 1985; Rosman & Berkman, 1986; Shoptaw, 1990), the literature rarely addresses the basic elements of interpersonal process or specific communication behavior during group meetings. It lacks a psychology of its intimate method. However, there are frequent indirect, incidental, and partial descriptions of communication behavior described in competing definitions and research findings. These help us to create an initial picture of a generic MSG process. The following two propositions are intended to isolate essential parameters and serve as a "starter kit" toward a formal model.

Each *member* will *give and get help* for *similar life-disrupting predicaments*.   *"Member,"* not patient or client. Participants describe themselves in a significantly egalitarian setting compared to psychotherapy patients. They rate their current or potential status as equal to almost any member. The universal choice of the term "member" for MSG participants reflects a widespread measurable experience of mutuality, fidelity, or constituency somewhat parallel to club member, team member, or even family member.

"Give and get" refers to the eventual exchange of psychological, informational, or material resources over the group's life. Members enter the group with an expectation to provide help as well as to obtain it. They expect to perform in both the roles of helper and help seeker.

"Help" is given in seven communication behaviors: (1) expressed empathy, (2) advice, (3) explanation, (4) generalization, (5), factual information, (6) self-disclosure ("sharing"), and (7) attentive silence. Material help is given in the form of books, tapes devices, programs, and so on.

"Similar life-disrupting predicaments" means that members are intimate with many aspects of the group's designated problem. Individual self-descriptions are familiar and easily recognizable to most members. Members frequently attribute their similarities of experience as a cause or stimulant for the extreme openness and empathic understanding in group

meetings. They see their similarity creating psychological safety and personal change.

Group process is characterized by *less skeptical response to each other's disclosures; fewer interpretations of character;* **and** *more empathic responses* **when compared with group or individual therapies.** *"Less skeptical response to each other's disclosures"* originates in the presentation of self as coping with the group's common problem. Such presentation (confession, self-diagnosis, or obvious condition of impairment) is a requirement for membership. As "members," there is a de facto acceptance of each other's affliction. This diminishes the typical denial and avoidance stages of the self-discovery process in psychotherapy. Insights are usually about coping failures with the group's common concern. Resistance to trying new coping strategies can be met with criticism. Rationalization or denial of obvious coping failures may stimulate group skepticism, but the typical process tends to be bland, patient, and instructional. Skeptical experience and expression are uncommon in MSG interaction.

"Fewer interpretations of character" because the typical MSG mission is to gain relief through better coping with a specific problem. Broad self-disclosure of life histories are not expected (and sometimes not tolerated). Instead of evaluating personalities through the measure of character, these groups can obsess over details of a particular addiction, medical condition, existential loss, phobia, or life transition. Creation of new meaning about a member's personality may come from such narrow discussion, but the personal interpretation of neuroses is a rare part of the process. However, interpretations about generic aspects of the group's common concern are very common. Such "general interpretations" (as opposed to "personal" interpretations) create meaning about every member's experience and condition, for example, "People like us are wrong when we expect others to understand what we experience," "Losing a kid to suicide is way beyond anything on those human stress scales," "Most people can't even put themselves in our shoes for five minutes!"

"More empathic responses" in the form of (1) self-disclosures that display parallel experience ("me-too" disclosures), or (2) questions based on empathic understanding, or (3) "reflections" that mirror an expressed emotion. Me-too disclosures are a particularly prominent part of MSG interaction. Similarity of suffering from a specific common problem creates environments with a high frequency of expressed empathy. Members describe their received empathy as "really being known" or talking to "someone in the same boat" and attribute its existence to some aspect of member similarity. That is, they recognize a connection between similarity and the abundance of group empathy.

These two propositions describe a peculiar psychological safety generated by similarity of suffering, reciprocity of roles as helper (therapist) and helpseeker (patient), an unskeptical audience, minimum coping with negative personal interpretation (confrontation), and a flow of expressed empathy. These hypotheses specify a dynamic process starting with member similarities and eventually creating a protective interpersonal arena.

Other speculations on essential processes that occur in the typical MSG that could be expanded into formal hypotheses toward a generic model include:

1. The typical group compensates for the lack of full-time professional leadership by protecting or "overprotecting" the psychological vulnerabilities of its members. This sense of responsibility for each other's self-concepts, coping methods, and defenses should appear in their measured attitudes and views on group ideology. They "take care of their own" in the absence of a professional caretaker.

2. The frequent generalizations (general interpretations) about common concerns that MSGs use are generated by at least six measurable sources: (a) lessons learned by actually coping with the group's problem and experiencing success and failure, (b) ideas, attitudes, and techniques gleaned from television and print mass media, (c) direct experience with a professional caregiver, (d) familiar customs and practices learned in an ethnic or other subculture i.e. folk wisdom, (e) special self-help programs packaged as books, audio tapes, and pamphlets, and (f) the group's idiosyncratic ideology evolved through an amalgam of member contributions.

3. Because the basis of MSG membership is clear acknowledgment, i.e. admission, self-diagnosis, confession, etc. of a personal problem, not much group time is devoted to this subject. MSG ideologies are biased toward accepting presenting problems. The typical group's process centers on tension relief, specific problem solving, and sometimes advocacy. Discussion of individual pathogenesis is uncommon.

4. MSG process is characterized by a more active coping style, a greater display of personal agency, more emotionally expressive talk, and more resource exchange when compared to their matched cohorts in a typical therapy group.

5. The MSGs' propensity to use generalizations that create new meaning about its common concern serve to (a) reframe the members' methods of thinking about their problems, (b) restructure the members' beliefs about their problems, and (c) generate behavioral prescriptions for coping with the problem. That is, MSG ideologies, methods, and frequent use of general interpretations stimulate cognitive restructuring in members.

SELECTED CONTRIBUTIONS FROM LITERATURE

Much of the literature is limited to (1) promotion of a single group, program, or ideology; (2) descriptive studies; (3) attempts to generalize from research on a single common concern; and (4) conceptual work that assumes most MSG activity occurs with little or no professional involvement, and is consistent from session to session and chapter to chapter. On the other hand, several writers have made substantive and integrative contributions to the extant literature. Lieberman (1986) characterizes the weak body of empirical knowledge and points to the severe dilemmas facing investigators of MSGs that usually cannot be controlled, nor subject assignment randomized. Experimental research is rare and typically focuses on unrepresentative, time-limited groups that are created and controlled by professionals. In addition, the measurement of outcome bumps into another dilemma: MSGs frequently conceive their goals differently from professional concepts of mental health. Lieberman's chapter is a landmark contribution on MSG history, scope, research, and theory of change mechanisms that defines the field much as Mary Killilea's encompassing overview did a decade earlier (1976). At that time, Killilea used the terms "self-help group therapy" and "mutual-help psychotherapy." She wanted to delineate this new form of psychological help by contrasting it to "orthodox psychotherapy." Her table of parameters characterizes self-help therapy as non-authoritative, non-professional, non-commercial, without appointments or records; meeting in non-clinical settings with peers that identify with each other and serve as role models; where self-disclosure is bilateral and members must help; and where there is more concern with behavior change than with underlying cause. Sometimes she mistakenly used the well-known "12-step" parameters (representing a minor percentage of all MSGs) to describe the entire body of MSG methods.

Although many of Killilea's generic, and sometimes idealized, conceptions have shown us that most MSG parameters such as parity, reciprocity, modeling, bilateral disclosure, and behavior emphasis still stand as essential features of current MSGs, others are called into question. For example, "non-authoritative" no longer fits the atmosphere of some 12-step programs with tightly organized procedures and a full set of behavioral rules monitored by leaders. "Non-professional" is another questionable parameter because it appears at least half of the current California MSGs sometimes have professionals as occasional co-leaders or solo leaders.

The years of struggle toward defining a generic and representative MSG model have hampered development of a coherent body of findings. In addition to the problems of contriving control groups, employing randomization, and coping with a variety of non-traditional outcome goals that Lieberman describes, investigators face resistance to collecting on-site data; the field is saturated with dubious questionnaire findings. And now we must contend with a serious influx of professionals involved in a variety of roles. But the cruelest blow of all is what Levy (1988) terms the "intrinsic positive bias effect." He argues that drop-out patterns create group compositions of more socially competent, adjusted, and active members. That is, MSGs evolve systematically toward more effective instruments of change. Because members are both "therapists" and "clients," the quality of helping covaries with group composition. Levy makes the point with elegance:

And herein lies the dilemma. For in contrast to any other intervention, SHG's [self-help groups] do not exist as interventions apart from their members who are both the instrumentality and the objects of the intervention: change the characteristics of their membership and the intervention is changed as well. (p. 23)

In another contribution toward a generic model, Lieberman (1990) offers a framework for examining all help-intended groups where MSGs are conceived as social microcosms that vary along continua of technological complexity, psychological closeness between helper and helpee, differentiation among participants, and specificity of helping methods. Compared to group therapy, MSGs can be seen as more of a social microcosm than psychotherapy. They have their own ideologies and subcultural values, less psychological distance between leader and member, greater specificity of methods, and less differentiation among participants. Riessman sees the essential method of MSGs as operating on the "helper-therapy" principle, thus avoiding the problematic, dependent, asymmetrical, inadequate role of the "help receiver" (patient, client). That is why he argues for a deemphasis of the "professional-centered" model in the 1990s.

Other efforts toward identifying essential parameters or initiating a generic model frequently employ unspecific or even vague concepts along with some fairly obvious generic parameters. In the following examples, most of the "soft" or vague descriptors relate to the specific process parameters presented earlier in the two propositions. Four values inherent in all MSGs are self-determination, authenticity, hope, and solidarity according to Van der Avort and Van Harberden (1985). Shulman (1985–1986) evokes ten basic processes in the psychology of "mutual-aid" that include sharing data in a dialectical conversation, exploring taboo topics, experiencing the "all in the same boat" phenomenon, modifying mutual expectations, and recognizing the "strength in numbers" phenomenon. A similar set of characteristics came from investigating anorexia and bulimia MSGs. Barbara Kinoy (1985) found that members felt a gradual erosion of isolation in suffering as they demythologized their health misconceptions. Additional support for the earlier hypotheses in this chapter come from a longitudinal survey of 10 MSGs for families of the mentally ill (Biegel & Yamatani, 1987). They also found "nondirective" processes occurred most frequently and confrontation activities (usually involving negative personal interpretations) least frequently. Member satisfaction after six months showed some correlation with nondirective processes.

The basic set of MSG characteristics discussed by Rootes and Aanes (1992) is an effort to reduce professional confusion in medical mental health systems that see MSGs as important, but fail to understand their methods. Such attempts to illuminate the MSG to populations of professionals are scattered throughout the literature. MSG-process descriptions are often limited to poetic language like "shared experience," "the gifting of experiential learning," and "the deep ambiance of support." Descriptions of specific process behaviors or communication acts are uncommon, with some notable exceptions (e.g., Rappaport et al., 1985). But, poetic or not, almost all the articles characterize MSGs as having members with similar life disrupting predicaments, employing help-intended communication, showing infrequent skepticism, eliciting frequent empathic responses, and most of the other parameters listed earlier in this chapter.

Linda Kurtz and Thomas Powell (1987) reason that professionals can better understand MSGs by applying three conceptual frameworks: social networks, social learning, and cognitive theory. They attempt to persuade the reader to use these frameworks to help their clients realize the full benefits of MSG membership. Lemberg (1984) developed an entertaining but serious set of techniques for insuring a MSG's failure. Lack of communication skills, group organization experience, and methods for enhancing commitment are major concerns. Klass (1984–1985) used a participant-observation method to study the entrance process into a MSG for coping with the severe bereavement after the death of a child (the Compassionate Friends). He suggests the process involves major decisions to attend, affiliate, and transform oneself into a helper for the group. Klass does not generalize beyond bereavement groups. A generic model for describing the integration of members might explain patterns of MSG stability, levels of member commitment, success in recruiting, and attendance. Deciding to become a helper is the key for Klass because it allows a reinvestment of energy from grieving.

Maton's (1988) study of 144 members of Compassionate Friends, multiple sclerosis groups, and Overeaters Anonymous suggests that group organization characteristics affect outcome. MSGs with a high level of role differentiation, "capable leadership," and order were positively associated with the members' sense of well-being and satisfaction with the group. Lieberman (1990) examined 36 MSGs that failed to benefit most of their members. Pre- and one-year post-measures found these unsuccessful groups to be low on cohesiveness, saliency of discussion, methods for reframing common concerns, and range of "therapeutic experiences."

Studies of MSG leadership appear to be largely disconnected and are difficult to integrate because they frequently fail to distinguish between full-time, part-time, solo leader, co-leader, and type of professional: mental health, non-mental health, and former members that have become professionals. Few investigators attend to pertinent variables such as medical versus non-medical common concerns, group size, meeting length, and change theory (for example, 12-step ideology, Recovery Inc. theory).

Conceptual work on the meaning of leadership for the MSG method is needed to differentiate between activities that (1) actually guide group conversation, (2) develop procedures for training facilitators, (3) provide influential consultation, (4) develop media programs, and (5) speak only to the group's common concern as someone else contrives group process. Stewart (1990) attempted to integrate 19 studies on leader activities but stumbled over sampling problems, noncomparable measures, and conceptual inconsistencies. She also noted an absence of minorities and low SES populations, but managed to formulate a few general interpretations about the MSG member's perspective compared to the professional's perspective on leadership. Members tend to want consultation and referrals without much control or protectionism from professionals. They frequently describe professionals as making inappropriate referrals, failing to follow up, not investing enough time and energy, and being naive about MSG methods and values. On the other hand, professionals see their appropriate roles as initiators of processes, group trainers, and networkers who create some ambivalence in members. Professionals also saw themselves as referral resources and speakers on the group's common concern. They worry about MSGs providing false information to their members. Stewart believes the studies show that both members and professionals desire some interaction, but the barriers remain: professionals' lack of information and preparation for helping MSGs. Members want indirect, nonauthoritarian help.

Toro et al. (1988) compared actual group processes for professionally led and member led GROW groups (mental patients). When members led, the groups perceived more cohesion, emotional expression, and self-discovery. When professionals led, members saw themselves giving fewer self-disclosures, agreements, small talk, and information. Members also showed less small talk and mutual agreements. The authors believe professionals may be prone to "professionalize" MSGs. In another study, contrasting 33 MSGs for the mentally ill with psychodynamic therapy groups, Toro, Rappaport, and Seidman (1987) found some instructive social climate/group process differences. Members saw their leaders as more active, their groups as more cohesive, structured, task oriented, and independent than did patients in therapy who saw their groups encouraging more expression of negative feelings and with more flexibility for changing activities.

MSG mortality appears associated with professional involvement and affiliation to a national organization according to Maton, Leventhal, Madara, and Julien's (1989) survey of 3,152 groups over a two-year period. When professionals attend meetings (probably for less than two hours a month as co-leader, consultant, lecturer, etc.) and the group is free from the ideology, method, and control of a bureaucracy, the MSG has good odds of surviving. But when a group is attached and influenced by both a bureaucracy and direct professional involvement, it seems at risk for failure. The investigators suspect too much external support is counterproductive because members may lose their sense of group ownership, or because of existing conflict between the methods of an organization or professional. However, a complete lack of organizational or direct professional influence leaves an MSG at high risk for disbanding. It seems groups weaken with too much or too little technical assistance.

Toseland, Rossiter, Peak, and Hill (1990) found no differences in the long-term effectiveness of peer and professionally led MSGs for stressed caregivers of frail elderly persons. Both formats produced better outcomes involving reduced stress and increased interpersonal competence than no treatment. There is a bit of evidence suggesting parallel processes and outcomes for the MSG method across cultures (Israel and United States) and problems (parenting a child with cancer or a mentally ill child). Gidron, Chesler, and Chesney (1991) are convinced comparative international research could reveal universal characteristics of MSG process.

In one of the rare studies of actual verbal behavior of MSG leaders, Tracey and Toro (1989) compared their helping styles with mental health professionals and divorce lawyers. Leaders met independently with a coached client presenting marital problems. A rating system allowed leaders to be classified as successful and less successful. Successful helpers tended to offer acts of non-critical guidance following their "clients'" emotional disclosures more than when reports of factual events were made. This pattern occurred across the three types of helpers.

Cancer patients not receiving satisfying support from family, friends, and medical caregivers are the ones who appear to join MSGs (Taylor, Falke, Shoptaw, & Lichtman, 1986). These joiners are mostly white middle-class females. The investigators in this study then explore outreach to a wider range of cancer patients.

Overall, outcome research on MSGs generally paints a positive picture. That trend is captured in "Selected Highlights of Research on Effectiveness on Self-Help Groups" (Medvene, 1987), a sampling of twenty-two positive outcome studies done for the California Self-Help Center. Among people coping with acute and chronic physical problems, MSG members coping with airway obstructions were less likely to be hospitalized and to be hospitalized for shorter periods of time than high-risk controls (Jensen, 1983); smokers participating in support groups as compared to nonparticipants had higher quit rates and maintained higher cessation rates (Jason et al., 1987); surgery and bracing patients in a scoliosis support group, as compared to similar but nonparticipating patients, had fewer psychosomatic symptoms, higher feelings of mastery, fewer feelings of shame and estrangement, higher self-esteem, a more positive outlook, and better patient-physician relationships (Hinrichsen, Revenson, & Shinn, 1985); women with metastasized breast cancer who were in a support group had lower mood disturbances, fewer maladaptive coping responses, and were less phobic when compared to similar patients who did not join a group (Speigel, Bloom, & Yalom, 1981); participants as compared to non-participants with rheumatoid arthritis showed greater improvement in joint tenderness (Shearn & Fireman, 1985); ostomy patients who served as visitors for other ostomy patients, as compared to those who were not visitors, were more accepting of their own ostomies, which is associated with better health and greater ability to maintain social relationships (Trainor, 1982); mastectomy patients who were visited by other mastectomy patients returned to normal activities earlier than similar others (Rogers, Bauman, & Metzger, 1985); laryngectomized cancer patients reported in interviews that attending a group helped them improve their communication abilities, function well socially, and not experience serious post-surgical depression (Richardson, 1980); cancer patients who had lengthy cancer therapy and joined a self-help group reported that they benefited significantly in terms of their knowledge about cancer, their ability to talk with people, their friendships and family life, and their coping with cancer (Maisiak, Cain, Yarbro, & Josof, 1981); and multiple sclerosis patients felt a support group helped them care for themselves (Spiegelberg, 1980).

For people participating in groups to deal with stressful life events or life transitions, parents of premature infants visited their infants more often in the hospital, touched, talked, and looked at their infants more often than did controls, and rated themselves as more competent infant care givers (Minde et al., 1980); new parents who participated in a group reported feeling more positive and less alone in their new role as well as showing greater skill in caring for their children and understanding their developmental process (Kagey, Vivace, & Lutz, 1981); widows paired with other widows who provided supportive contact, when compared to nonpaired widows, felt better, were less likely to anticipate difficulties in adjusting, made new friends more, and began new activities more (Vachov, Lyall, Rogers, Reedman-Letofsky, & Freeman, 1980); members of a group for recently widowed people, as compared to similar nonmembers, showed less anxiety, less use of psychotropic medications, and had an increased sense of well-being and mastery (Lieberman & Videka-Sherman, 1986); bereaved parents in a group, particularly the most active ones, as compared to nonparticipants, experienced more personal growth in the areas of feelings, personal strength, and resiliency (Videka-Sherman, 1982); and pediatric ICU nurses who participated in a support group had a lower turnover rate (Weiner & Caldwell, 1983–1984).

Finally, in groups dealing with mental health issues, patients discharged from a state psychiatric hospital who participated in groups, required less rehospitalization and far fewer days than non-participants (Gordon, Edmunson, & Bedell, 1979); participation by patients with a history of psychiatric problems resulted in less nervousness, tension and depression, and for longer-term members they had less need for professional psychotherapy and took less medication (Galanter, 1988); children of parents with drinking problems who participated in a group for such teenagers suffered less emotional and physical disturbance than nonmembers (Hughes, 1977); groups for the families of psychiatric patients had a reduced sense of burden, more information, and better coping strategies as a result of MSG membership (Potasznik & Nelson, 1984); child abusers gained insight into their own reactions to abuse as children and learned new ways of expressing love and affection to their own children (Comstock, 1982); and parents of young drug and alcohol abusers reported that their group participation was associated with improvement in their children's drug problems. A literature review of the period 1990–1992 (Goldstein, 1992) also generally showed positive effects for MSG membership across a variety of concerns except smoking problems.

Nevertheless, as MSG activity blended into the scene during the early 80s and ended the decade as a more visible institution of American life, along with visibility came an increase in criticism. Some professionals worried about the blind leading the blind in MSGs and their lack of helping skills. Other concerns centered on the need for ethical guidelines, professional consultation, and responsibility for damaged drop-outs.

Beyond professional fears about MSGs in general, there were specific concerns about Alcoholics Anonymous ("AA") and the 12-step ideology. Stanton Peele argued that AA was out of control in interpreting alcoholism as a disease attacking powerless victims (1989). He saw their claims of successful outcome as distorted and unscrupulous. Ragge (1990), in an analysis of the 12-step method, views the procedure as a somewhat deceptive indoctrination into a religious sect. He describes AA procedures as essentially coercive and driven by an evangelical ideology that is publicly mistaken for a mental health program. Media attacks on 12-step programs probably influence some public opinion about MSGs in general, even though 12-step activity represents only a minor proportion of the American MSG scene. Realizing the necessity of seriously examining criticism levelled at MSGs, Riessman, a major voice in MSG thinking, brought much of it together in an article on the "new self-help backlash" (1990). He summarizes the critique as (1) participants can become addicted to attending meetings to the point of disabling other aspects of their lives, (2) some MSGs have become brazenly profit oriented, (3) MSG professionals exaggerate the number of people that need them, (4) spontaneous remission and self-controlled recovery is disregarded by many MSGs, (5) MSGs overestimate their success rate, and (6) the focus of some MSGs diverts members from addressing community and social factors that cause or contribute to their predicament or illness. Riessman interprets some motivation for the criticism as coming from the threat they pose to professionals, such as potential for financial encroachment and melting the prestige and mystique of therapies.

There is a dramatic difference in focus between the literatures of MSGs and group therapy. MSG articles and books are more contextual as they address organizational phenomena, sociological matters, public health concerns, and social work issues. Investigation seems to stop at the borders of group meetings. The inner workings of group interaction that involve language behavior, cognitive intricates, and process patterns which constitute the leading edge of personal change, represent only a tiny portion of MSG research and theory work. The field needs an influx of new scholars to make sense of how the internal dynamics of MSGs produce their effects. The interested group therapy investigator can learn more about what is being done and left undone by reading Thomas Powell's influential book (1987) on MSGs and professional practice. Powell sees parallels and complimentarity between the two, and argues that the explosive growth of MSGs is stimulating the growth of professional programs. A public health/social work bias appears in his choice of theoretical frameworks for understanding the essentials of MSGs: organizational theory, reference group theory, and social network theory. Powell also adds yet another taxonomy of MSG types to the dozens extant (habit-disturbance, lifestyle, general purpose, significant other, and physical handicap organizations), but his is used to explore the quality of interaction between groups and professionals. Powell's work will have even more utility when we can also examine differences in the intimate helping environments created by "pure" MSGs and those influenced by professional theory, technique, ambition, and ethics. In a broader perspective, the public health/social work focused literature on MSGs should gain much utility when it becomes more interdisciplinary.

SUMMARY

This chapter invites group therapy professionals to participate in the American self-help, mutual-support phenomenon. The concern remains that most professionals are misinformed or unfamiliar with the scope, variety, and basic processes of mutual support groups (MSGs). Opportunities for involvement in research, conceptual work, group establishment, co-leadership, consultation, program development, referral exchange, specialty instruction, policy, and administrative guidance appear more extensive than in the group therapy field. Research indicates that appropriate professional intervention is now widely welcomed by a large majority of MSGs.

Parameters of help-oriented small support groups are examined via vignettes that illustrate issues of process control, recruitment, selection, leadership, theory, ideology, group theme, source of help, fees, group therapy-MSG overlap, and homogeneity of presenting problems. There is a confounding of models for help-intended groups. Besides the public MSG, a large, varied, unstudied, free-standing set of "private" MSGs exists. Taken together, the public and private MSGs will probably involve 11.4 million participants in 1993–1994, outnumbering all forms of psychotherapy clients.

The remarkably rapid recent growth of MSG activity seems to be accompanied by an increase in professional involvement. The traditional picture painted in the literature of a nonprofessional MSG with "do-it-yourself" purity requires revision. Recent findings show professional involvement to be over 80% in California; an earlier, smaller sample midwestern study generated 72%. In any case, it appears that our old image of MSGs must be updated to reflect increasingly frequent professional involvement. Further, it is becoming clear that MSG members are welcoming professionals, especially as speakers, teachers, co-leaders, referral sources, and student-observers. The professional as sole leader seems less frequently desired, but that varies for medical and nonmedical MSGs. So far, over a dozen roles for professionals are known, including referral source, therapist for some individual members, co-leader, regular member, speaker, consultant, resource, locator, coordinator, establisher of new groups, communication specialist, observer, researcher, and solo leader.

MSG theory and research are in sore need of a general model. A handful of scholars have struggled toward that goal, but it is clear that additional help is needed to establish parameters for what promises to be a major method for delivering mental health services. Offered herein is a general model "starter kit," with parameters describing participants' perceived status as "member," reciprocity of helping, dimensions of communication behavior, the functions of similar life-disrupting predicaments, the relative infrequency of skeptical responses and interpretations of character, the high-frequency of empathic responses, compensatory "overprotection" of members in lieu of full-time professional control, a process rich in generalizations about the group's common concern (drawn from coping experience, media, professional guidance, subcultural custom, packaged MSG programs, and idiosyncratic ideologies generated by group interaction), focus on tension relief and problem-solving more than individual pathogenesis, more personal agency and resource exchange than in psychotherapy, and a propensity to reframe thinking and believing about the group's common concern.

MSG literature over the past 20 years is dominated by articles that simply promote a program, descriptive studies, overgeneralization from research on single common concerns, and conclusions based on the false assumption of little or no professional involvement and consistency of leadership and practice from session to session. The weak body of empirical knowledge points to severe dilemmas facing investigators because of their inability to control or randomize representative MSGs. Also outcome criteria frequently used in therapy research is often at odds with MSG ideology. In addition, the peculiar and essential method of many MSGs causes members to be both the instrumentality and the objects of intervention. That is, members are both "therapists" and "clients," so changes in group composition change the nature and quality of the intervention.

The selected sampling of MSG research in this review appears of special interest to group therapy scholars. Some of the innovative work contributes to the building of a generic model and begins to establish a small, fascinating base of knowledge. Leadership studies are difficult to integrate because the field lacks a usable model. Unfortunately, gross underestimation of professional involvement at the national level has weakened the contribution of many early studies. There are some scattered solid findings that should stimulate the adventuresome group therapy scholar. The steeply accelerating growth curve of MSG activity and its predicted prominence in national mental health policy makes it difficult for professionals, and hence, researchers to disregard. New funding patterns, shifts in public preference, and the dilution of therapies are likely to draw new workers in to the arena. Hopefully, some will be group therapy scholars uniquely equipped to bring a new generation of MSGs into the next century.

REFERENCES

Biegel, D. E., & Yamatani, H. (1987). Help-giving in self-help groups. *Hospital and Community Psychiatry, 38,* 1195–1197.

Biegel, D. E., & Yamatani, H. (1987). Self-help groups for families of the mentally ill: Roles and benefits. *International Journal of Family Psychiatry, 8,* 151–173.

Black, M. E. (1988). Self help groups and professionals—What is the relationship? [Editorial]. *British Medical Journal Clinical Research Edition, 296,* 1485–1486.

Borkman, T. (1990). Self-help groups at the turning point: Emerging egalitarian alliances with the formal health care system. *American Journal of Community Psychology, 18,* 321–332.

Burstein, B. (1985). *Needs assessment of California mutual support groups.* Unpublished manuscript, California Self-Help Center, Department of Psychology, UCLA.

Comstock, C. M. (1982). Preventive processes in self-help groups: Parents Anonymous. *Prevention in Human Services: Helping People Help Themselves, 1*(3).

Dean, K. (1989). [Review of *Self-help organizations and professional practice.*] *Social Science and Medicine, 29*(2), 263–264.

Emerick, R. E. (1990). Self-help groups for former patients: Relations with mental health professionals. *Hospital and Community Psychiatry, 4,* 401–407.

Galanter, M. (1988). Zealous self-help groups as adjuncts to psychiatric treatment: A study of Recovery, Inc. [139th Annual Meeting of the American Psychiatric Association (1986, Washington, DC)]. *American Journal of Psychiatry, 145,* 1248–1253.

Gidron, B., Chesler, M. A., & Chesney, B. K. (1991). Cross-cultural perspectives on self-help groups: Comparison between participants and nonparticipants in Israel and the United States. *American Journal of Community Psychology, 19*(5), 667–681.

Goldstein, M. S. (1992). *Self-help groups: A review of the literature, 1990–1992.* Unpublished manuscript, California Self-Help Center, Department of Psychology, UCLA.

Gordon, R. E., Edmunson, E., & Bedell, J. (1979). Peer mutual aid networks reduce rehospitalization of mental patients. *Self-Help Reporter, 3.*

Gottlieb, B. H. (1985). Assessing and strengthening the impact of social support on mental health. *Social Work, 30,* 293–300.

Gradman, T. (1985). *Leader and member perception of communication problems in self-help groups.* Unpublished manuscript, Psychology Clinic, UCLA.

Hinrichsen, G. A., Revenson, T. A., & Shinn, M. (1985). Does self-help help? An empirical investigation of scoliosis peer support groups. *Journal of Social Issues, 41,* 65–87.

Hughes, J. M. (1977). Adolescent children of alcoholic parents and the relationship of Alateen to these children. *Journal of Consulting and Clinical Psychology, 45*(5), 946–947.

Jacobs, M. K., & Goodman, G. (1989). Psychology and self-help groups: Predictions on a partnership. *American Psychologist, 44,* 536–545.

Jason, L. A., Gruder, C. L., Martino, S., Flay, B. R., Warnecke, R., & Thomas, N. (1987). Work site group meetings and the effectiveness of a televised smoking cessation intervention. *American Journal of Community Psychology, 15*(1), 57–72.

Jensen, P. S. (1983). Risk, protective factors and supportive interventions in chronic airway obstruction. *Archives of General Psychiatry, 40*(11), 1203–1207.

Kagey, J. R., Vivace, J., & Lutz, W. (1981). Mental health primary prevention: The role of parent mutual support groups. *American Journal of Public Health, 71*(2), 166–167.

Katz, A. H. (1976). *The strength in us: Self-help groups in the modern world.* New York: New Viewpoints.

Kiesler, C. A., & Morton, T. L. (1988). Psychology and public policy in the "health care revolution." *American Psychologist, 43*(12), 993–1003.

Killilea, M. (1976). Mutual help organizations: Interpretations in the literature. In G. Caplan & M. Killilea (Eds.), *Support systems and mutual help.* New York: Grune & Stratton.

Kinoy, B. P. (1985). Self-help groups in the management of anorexia nervosa and bulimia: A theoretical base [Special issue: Eating disorders]. *Transactional Analysis Journal, 15,* 73–78.

Klass, D. (1984–1985). Bereaved parents and The Compassionate Friends: Affiliation and healing. *Omega Journal of Death and Dying, 15,* 353–373.

Knight, R., Wollert, R., Levy, L. H., Frame, C. L., & Padgett, V. P. (1980). Self-help groups: The members perspectives. *American Journal of Community Psychology, 8,* 53–65.

Kurtz, L. F. (1990). The self-help movement: Review of the past decade of research. *Social Work with Groups, 13,* 101–115.

Kurtz, L. F., & Powell, T. J. (1987). Three approaches to understanding self help groups. *Social Work with Groups, 10,* 69–80.

Leerhsen, C. (1990, February 5). Afflicted, addicted? Support groups are the answer for 15 million Americans. *Newsweek,* pp. 49–55.

Lemberg, R. (1984). Ten ways for a self-help group to fail. *American Journal of Orthopsychiatry, 54,* 648–650.

Levy, L. H. (1979). Processes and activities in groups. In M. A. Lieberman & L. Borman (Eds.), *Self-help groups for coping with crises: Origins, members, processes, and impact* (pp. 234–271). San Francisco, CA: Jossey-Bass.

Levy, L. H. (1988). *Self-help groups.* Unpublished manuscript.

Lieberman, M. A. (1986). Self-help groups and psychiatry. *American Psychiatric Association Annual Review, 5,* 744–760.

Lieberman, M. A. (1990a). A group therapist perspective on self-help groups. *International Journal of Group Psychotherapy, 40,* 251–278.

Lieberman, M. A. (1990b). Understanding how groups work: A study of homogeneous peer group failures. *International Journal of Group Psychotherapy, 40,* 31–52.

Lieberman, M. A., & Borman, L. (1979). *Self-help groups for coping with crises: Origins, members, processes, and impact.* San Francisco, CA: Jossey-Bass.

Lieberman, M. A., & Videka-Sherman, L. (1986). The impact of self-help groups on the mental health of widows and widowers. *American Journal of Orthopsychiatry, 16,* 435–445.

Lotery, J. L. (1985). *A review of self-help/mutual support group theory and research with an emphasis on the role of mental health professionals.* Unpublished doctoral dissertation, University of California, Los Angeles.

Madara, E. J. (1990). Maximizing the potential for community self-help through clearinghouse approaches. *Prevention in Human Services, 7,* 109–138.

Madara, E., Kalafat, J., & Miller, B. N. (1988). The computerized self-help clearinghouse: Using "high-tech" to promote "high-touch" support networks. *Computers in Human Services, 3,* 39–54.

Maisiak, R., Caine, M., Yarbro, C. H., & Josof, L. (1981). Evaluation of TOUCH: An oncology self-help group. *Oncology Nursing Forum, 8*(3).

Maton, K. I. (1988). Social support, organizational characteristics, psychological well-being, and group appraisal in three self-help group populations. *American Journal of Community Psychology, 16,* 53–77.

Maton, K. I., Leventhal, G. S., Madara, E. J., & Julien, M. (1989). Factors affecting the birth and death of mutual-help groups: The role of national affiliation, professional involvement, and member focal problem. *American Journal of Community Psychology, 17,* 643–671.

Medvene, L. (1987). *Selected research highlights on the effectiveness of self-help groups.* Unpublished manuscript, California Self-Help Center, Department of Psychology, UCLA.

Minde, K., Shosenberg, N., Marton. P., Thompson, J., Ripley, J., & Burns, S. (1980). Self-help groups in premature nursery—A controlled evaluation. *Journal of Pediatrics, 96*(5), 933–940.

Peele, S. (1989). *The diseasing of America: Addiction treatment out of control.* Lexington, MA: Lexington Books.

Potasznik, H., & Nelson, G. (1984). Stress and social support: The burden experienced by the family of a mentally ill person. *American Journal of Community Psychology, 12*(5), 589–607.

Powell, T. J. (1987). *Self-help organizations and professional practice.* Silver Spring, MD: National Association of Social Workers.

Prochaska, J. D., & Norcross, J. C. (1982). The future of psychotherapy: A Delphi poll. *Professional Psychology, 13,* 620–627.

Ragge, K. (1990). *More revealed.* Henderson, NV: Alert Publishing.

Rappaport, J., Seidman, E., Toro, P. A., McFadden, L. S., Reischl, T. M., Roberts, L. J., Solem, D. A., Stein, C. H., & Zimmerman, M. A. (1985). Collaborative research with a mutual help organization. *Social Policy, 50,* 12–24.

Richardson, J. (1980). *Determinants of adjustment to laryngectomy surgery.* Unpublished doctoral dissertation, UCLA School of Public Health.

Riessman, F. (1990). The new self-help backlash. *Social Policy, 21*(1), 42–48.

Rogers, T. F., Bauman, L. J., & Metzger, L. (1985). An assessment of the reach-to-recovery program. *Cancer Journal of Clinicians, 35*(2).

Rootes, L. E., & Aanes, D. L. (1992). A conceptual framework for understanding self-help groups. *Hospital and Community Psychiatry, 43,* 379–381.

Rosenberg, P. P. (1984). Support groups: A special therapeutic entity. *Small Group Behavior, 15,* 173–186.

Rosman, M. D., & Berkman, I. P. (1986). Application of the normalization principle to support groups for parents with children in residential treatment. *Residential Group Care and Treatment, 3,* 53–63.

Shearn, M. A., & Fireman, B. H. (1985). Stress management and mutual support groups in rheumatoid arthritis. *American Journal of Medicine, 78*(5), 771–775.

Shoptaw, S. (1990). *Functions of risky disclosures in self-help groups.* Unpublished doctoral dissertation, University of California at Los Angeles.

Shulman, L. (1985–1986). The dynamics of mutual aid [Special issue: The legacy of William Schwartz: Group practice as shared interaction]. *Social Work with Groups, 8,* 51–60.

Speigel, D., Bloom, J. R., & Yalom, I. (1981). Group support for patients with metastatic cancer: A randomized prospective outcome study. *Archives of General Psychiatry, 38*(5), 527–533.

Spiegelberg, N. (1980). Support group improves quality of life. *ARN Journal, 5*(6), 9–11.

Stewart, M. J. (1990). Expanding theoretical conceptualization of self-help groups. *Social Science and Medicine, 31,* 1057–1066.

Stewart, M. J. (1990). Professional interface with mutual-aid self-help groups: A review. *Social Science and Medicine, 31,* 1143–1158.

Taylor, S. E., Falke, R. L., Shoptaw, S. J., & Lichtman, R. R. (1986). Social support, support groups, and the cancer patients. *Journal of Consulting and Clinical Psychology, 54,* 608–615.

Toro, P. A., Rappaport, J., & Seidman, E. (1987). Social climate comparison of mutual help and psychotherapy groups. *Journal of Consulting and Clinical Psychology, 55,* 430–431.

Toro, P. A., Reischl, T. M., Zimmerman, M. A., Rappaport, J., Seidman, E., Luke, D. A., & Roberts, L. J. (1988). Professionals in mutual help groups: Impact on social climate and members' behavior. *Journal of Consulting and Clinical Psychology, 56,* 631–632.

Toseland, R. W., & Hacker, L. (1982). Self-help groups and professional involvement. *Social Work, 27,* 341–347.

Toseland, R. W., Rossiter, C. M., Peak, T., & Hill, P. (1990). Therapeutic processes in peer led and professionally led support groups for caregivers. *International Journal of Group Psychotherapy, 40,* 279–303.

Tracey, T. J., & Toro, P. A. (1989). Natural and professional help: A process analysis. *American Journal of Community Psychology, 17*(4), 443–458.

Trainor, M. A. (1982). Acceptance of ostomy and the visitor role in a self-help group for ostomy patients. *Nursing Research, 31,* 102–106.

Vachov, M. L., Lyall, W. A., Rogers, J., Reedman-Letofsky, K., & Freeman, S. J. (1980). A controlled study of self-help intervention for widows. *American Journal of Psychiatry, 137*(11), 1380–1384.

Van der Avort, A., & Van Harberden, P. (1985). Helping self-help groups: A developing theory. *Psychotherapy, 22,* 269–272.

Videka-Sherman, L. (1982). Effects of participation in self-help groups for bereaved parents: Compassionate Friends. *Prevention in Human Services, 1*(3).

Weiner, M. F., & Caldwell, T. (1983–1984). The process and impact of an ICU nurse support group. *International Journal of Psychiatry in Medicine, 13*(1).

Wollert, R. (1986). Psychosocial helping processes in a heterogeneous sample of self-help groups. *Canadian Journal of Community Mental Health, 5,* 63–76.

Zinman, S. (1986). Self-help: The wave of the future. *Hospital and Community Psychiatry, 37,* 213.

ADDITIONAL REFERENCES

Adam, D., & Hoehne, D. (1989). Mutual aid in remote areas: Addressing the obstacles. *Canada's Mental Health, 37,* 18–21.

Adelson, L., & Freeman, L. (1985). On the road to advocacy: Family self-help groups. *Psychosocial Rehabilitation Journal, 8,* 76–82.

Alcoholics Anonymous (3rd ed.). (1976). New York: Alcoholics Anonymous World Service.

Antze, P. (1976). The role of ideologies in peer psychotherapy organizations: Some theoretical considerations and three case studies. *Journal of Applied Behavioral Science, 12,* 323–346.

Balgopal, P. R., Ephross, P. H., & Vassil, T. V. (1986). Self-help groups and professional helpers. *Small Group Behavior, 17,* 123–137.

Battaglino, L. (1987). Family empowerment through self-help groups. *New Directions for Mental Health Services, 34,* 43–51.

Baumgarten, M., Thomas, D., & de Courval, L. P. (1988). Evaluation of a mutual help network for the elderly residents of planned housing. *Psychology and Aging, 3,* 393–398.

Berenson, D. (1990). A systemic view of spirituality: God and Twelve Step programs as resources in family therapy. *Journal of Strategic and Systemic Therapies, 9,* 59–70.

Black, D. W., & Blum, N. S. (1992). Obsessive-compulsive disorder support groups: The Iowa model. *Comprehensive Psychiatry, 33,* 65–71.

Block, E., & Llewelyn, S. P. (1987). Leadership skills and helpful factors in self help groups. *British Journal of Guidance and Counseling, 15,* 257–270.

Bebbington, P. E. (1976). The efficacy of alcoholics anonymous: The elusiveness of hard data. *British Journal of Psychiatry, 128,* 572–580.

Bond, G. R., & de Graaf-Kaser, R. (1990). Group approaches for persons with severe mental illness: A typology [Special issue: Group work with emotionally disabled]. *Social Work with Groups, 13,* 21–36.

Brown, L. N. (1984). Mutual help staff groups to manage work stress. *Social Work with Groups, 7,* 55–66.

Brownell, A., & Shumaker, S. A. (1984). Social support: An introduction to a complex phenomenon. *Journal of Social Issues, 40,* 1–9.

California Self-Help Center (1985). Evolving roles: Self-help and the professional. *The Self-Helper, 2,* 3–4

Castaneda, D., & Sommer, R. (1989). Mental health professionals' attitudes toward the family's role in care of the mentally ill. *Hospital and Community Psychiatry, 40,* 1195–1197.

Cherniss, C., & Cherniss, D. S. (1987). Professional involvement in self-help groups for parents of high-risk newborns. *American Journal of Community Psychiatry, 15,* 435–444.

Chesler, M. A., Barbarin, O. A., & Lebo-Stein, J. (1984). Patterns of participation in a self-help group for parents of children with cancer. *Journal of Psychosocial Oncology, 2,* 41–64.

Chesney, B. K., Rounds, K. A., & Chesler, M. A. (1989). Support for parents of children with cancer: The value of self-help groups [Special issue: Groups in health care settings]. *Social Work with Groups, 12,* 119–139.

Christenson, I. (1984). Self-help groups for depressed elderly in the nursing home. *Physical and Occupational Therapy in Geriatrics, 3,* 39–47.

Coleman, M. T. (1987). Mutual support groups for families of the mentally ill. *Marriage and Family Review, 11,* 77–93.

Collins, G. B., Janesz, J. W., Byerly-Thrope, J., & Manzeo, J. (1985). Hospital sponsored chemical dependency self-help groups. *Hospital and Community Psychiatry, 36,* 1315–1317.

Dean, K. (1986). Lay care in illness [Special issue: Medical sociology and the WHO's programme in Europe]. *Social Science and Medicine, 22,* 275–284.

Dean, S. R. (1970). Self-help group psychotherapy: Mental patients rediscover will power. *International Journal of Social Psychiatry, 17,* 72–78.

Deeble, E. A., & Bhat, A. V. (1991). Women attending a self-help group for anorexia nervosa and bulimia: Views on self-help and professional treatment. *British Review of Bulimia and Anorexia Nervosa, 5,* 23–28.

Diggs, C. (1990). Self-help for communication disorders. *Asha, 32,* 32–34.

Droge, D., Arntson, P., & Norton, R. (1986). The social support function in epilepsy self-help groups. *Small Group Behavior, 17,* 139–163.

Ehrlich, P., & McGeehan, M. (1985). Cocaine recovery support groups and the language of recovery. *Journal of Psychoactive Drugs, 17,* 11–17.

Emrick, C. D. (1989). Alcoholics Anonymous: Membership characteristics and effectiveness as treatment. *Recent Developments in Alcoholism, 7,* 37–53.

Emerick, R. E. (1989). Group demographics in the mental patient movement: Group location, age, and size as structural factors. *Community Mental Health Journal, 25,* 277–300.

Emerick, R. E. (1991). The politics of psychiatric self-help: Political factions, interactional support, and group longevity in a social movement. *Social Science and Medicine, 32,* 1121–1128.

Farrell, D., & Wilner, N. (1986). Mutual help groups for widows: A study of the process. *Israel Journal of Psychiatry and Related Sciences, 23,* 297–305.

Finisdore, M. M. (1984). Self-help in the mainstream. *Volta Review, 86,* 99–107.

Fram, D. H. (1990). Group methods in the treatment of substance abusers. *Psychiatric Annals, 20,* 385–388.

Frew, J. E. (1986). Leadership approaches to achieve maximum therapeutic potential in mutual support groups [Special issue: Support groups]. *Journal for Specialists in Group Work, 11*, 93–99.

Friedlander, S. R., & Watkins, C. E. (1985). Therapeutic aspects of support groups for parents of the mentally retarded. *International Journal of Group Psychotherapy, 35*, 65–78.

Frustaci, J. (1988). A survey of agoraphobics in self-help groups. *Smith College Studies in Social Work, 58*, 193–211.

Fuehrer, A., & Keys, C. (1988). Group development in self-help groups for college students. *Small Group Behavior, 19*, 325–341.

Galanter, M., Gleaton, T., Marcus, C. E., & McMillen, J. (1984). Self-help groups for parents of young drug and alcohol abusers. *American Journal of Psychiatry, 141*, 889–891.

Gartner, A., & Riessman, F. (1979). *Self-help in the human services.* San Francisco, CA: Jossey-Bass.

Gartner, A., & Riessman, F. (1985). *Self-help revolution.* New York: Human Services Press.

Gates, J. C. (1980). Comparison of behavior modification and self-help groups with conventional therapy of diabetes. *Dissertation Abstracts International, 40*, 3084-B.

Gidron, B., Guterman, N. B., & Hartman, H. (1990). Stress and coping patterns of participants and non-participants in self-help groups for parents of the mentally ill. *Community Mental Health Journal, 26*, 483–496.

Gilden, J. L., Hendryx, M. S., Clar, S., Casia, C., & Singh, S. P. (1992). Diabetes support groups improve health care of older diabetic patients. *Journal of the American Geriatrics Society, 40*, 147–150.

Gitterman, A. (1985/1986). The reciprocal model: A change in the paradigm [Special issue: The legacy of William Schwartz: Group practice as shared interaction]. *Social Work with Groups, 8*(4), 29–37.

Gitterman, A. (1989). Building mutual support in groups. *Social Work with Groups, 8*, 5–21.

Glosser, G., & Wexler, D. (1985). Participants' evaluation of educational/support groups for families of patients with Alzheimer's Disease and other dementias. *Gerontologist, 25*, 232–236.

Goetzel, R. Z., Croen, L. G., Shelov, S., Boufford, J. I., & Levin, G. (1984). Evaluating self-help support groups for medical students. *Journal of Medical Education, 59*, 331–340.

Goldstein, M. Z. (1990). The role of mutual support groups and family therapy for caregivers of demented elderly. *Journal of Geriatric Psychiatry, 23*, 117–128.

Goodman, C. (1990). Evaluation of a model self-help telephone program: Impact on natural networks. *Social Work, 35*, 556–62.

Goodman, G., & Esterly, G. (1988). *The talk book: The intimate science of communicating in close relationships.* New York: Ballantine.

Goodman, G., & Jacobs, M. J. (1985). *The Common Concern program: For forming and enhancing self-help support groups.* Sacramento, CA: Mental Health Promotion Division of the California Department of Mental Health.

Goodman, G., Jacobs, M. J., Medvene, L., & Burney, L. (1988). *The programmed self-help group: A feasibility study with older divorced women.* Unpublished manuscript, UCLA.

Gould, E., Garrigues, C. S., & Scheikowitz, K. (1975). Interaction in hospitalized patient-led and staff-led psychotherapy groups. *American Journal of Psychotherapy, 29,* 383–390.

Gressard, C. F. (1986). Self-help groups for Vietnam veterans experiencing post traumatic stress disorder [Special issue: Support groups]. *Journal for Specialists in Group Work, 11,* 74–79.

Grimsmo, A., Helgesen, G., & Borchgrevink, C. (1981). Short-term and long-term effects of lay groups on weight reduction. *British Medical Journal, 283,* 1093–1095.

Grodin, D. (1991). The interpreting audience: The therapeutics of self-help book reading. *Critical Studies in Mass Communication, 8,* 404–420.

Hall, R. P., Kassees, J. M., & Hoffman, C. (1986). Treatment for survivors of incest [Special issue: Support groups]. *Journal for Specialists in Group Work, 11,* 85–92.

Halperin, D. (1987). The self-help group: The mental health professional's role. *Group, 11,* 47–53.

Hamm, M. S. (1988). Current perspectives on the prisoner self-help movement. *Federal Probation, 52,* 49–56.

Hartley, P., & Newton, T. (1991). Self-help groups for eating disorders. *British Review of Bulimia and Anorexia Nervosa, 5,* 65–72.

Hasegawa, Y. (1988). Morita-based self-help learning groups in Japan. *International Bulletin of Morita Therapy, 1,* 52–57.

Hatfield, A. B. (1984). The family consumer movement: A new force in service delivery. *New Directions for Mental Health Services, 21,* 71–79.

Henry, S. (1978). The dangers of self-help groups. *New Society, 22,* 654–656.

Hildebrand, J. F. (1986). Mutual help for spouses whose partners are employed in stressful occupations [Special issue: Support groups]. *Journal for Specialists in Group Work, 11,* 80–84.

Howe, M., & Graham, B. (1990). The importance of captioning for late deafened adults. *International Journal of Technology and Aging, 3,* 121–131.

Howlett, M., & Archer, V. E. (1984). Worker involvement in occupational health and safety. *Family and Community Health, 7,* 57–63.

Humphreys, K., Mavis, B., & Stofflemayr, B. (1991). Factors predicting attendance at self-help groups after substance abuse treatment: Preliminary findings. *Journal of Consulting and Clinical Psychology, 59,* 591–593.

Hunt, R. W., Bond, M. J., & Pater, G. D. (1990). Psychological responses to cancer: A case for cancer support groups. *Community Health Studies, 14,* 35–38.

Hurvitz, N. (1976). The origins of the peer self-help psychotherapy group movement. *Journal of Applied Behavioral Science, 12,* 283–294.

Hutchinson, C. H., & McDaniel, S. A. (1986). The social reconstruction of sexual assault by women victims: A comparison of therapeutic experiences [Special issue: Women and mental health]. *Canadian Journal of Community Mental Health, 5,* 17–36.

Jason, L. A. (1985). Using the media to foster self-help groups. *Professional Psychology Research and Practice, 16,* 455–464.

Jason, L. A., Greiner, B. J., Naylor, K., Johnson, S. P., et al. (1991). A large-scale, short-term, media-based weight loss program. *American Journal of Health Promotion, 5,* 432–437.

Jason, L. A., La Pointe, P., & Billingham, S. (1986). The media and self-help: A preventive community intervention. *Journal of Primary Prevention, 6,* 156–167.

Jason, L. A., Tabon, D., Tait, E., Iacono, G., Goodman, D., Watkins, P., & Huggins, G. (1988). The emergence of the inner-city self-help center. *Journal of Community Psychology, 16*(3), 287–295.

Johnson, N. P., & Phelps, G. L. (1991). Effectiveness in self-help groups: Alcoholics Anonymous as a prototype. *Family and Community Health, 14,* 22–27.

Katz, A. H. (1979). Self-help health groups: Some clarifications. *Social Science and Medicine, 13,* 491–494.

Katz, A. H. (1981). Self help and mutual aid: An emerging social movement? *Annual Review of Sociology, 7,* 129–155.

Katz, A., & Bender, E. (Eds.). (1976a). *The strength in us: Self-help groups in the modern world.* New York: Franklin Watts.

Katz, A. H., & Bender, E. (1976b). Self-help groups in western society: History and prospects. *Journal of Applied Behavioral Science, 12,* 265–282.

Kelley, P., & Kelley, V. R. (1985). Supporting natural helpers: A cross-cultural study. *Social Casework, 66,* 353–366.

Kendall, J. (1992). Promoting wellness in HIV-support groups. *Journal of the Association of Nurses in Aids Care, 3,* 28–38.

Khantzian, E. J., & Mack, J. E. (1989). Alcoholics Anonymous and contemporary psychodynamic theory. *Recent Developments in Alcoholism, 7,* 67–89.

Kielman, M. A., Mantel, J. E., & Alexander, E. S. (1976). Collaboration and its discontents: Their perils of partnership. *Journal of Applied Behavioral Science, 12,* 403–409.

Kiesler, C. A., & Morton, T. (1987). Responsible public policy in a rapidly changing world. *The Clinical Psychologist, 40,* 28–31.

Klass, D. (1987). The self-help process and the resolution of parental bereavement. *International Journal of Family Psychiatry, 8,* 9–24.

Knight, B., Wollert, R. W., Levy, L. H., Frame, C. L., & Padgett, V. P. (1980). Self-help groups: The members' perspectives. *American Journal of Community Psychology, 8,* 53–65.

Korte, C. (1991). The receptivity of older adults to innovative mutual-aid arrangements. *Journal of Community Psychology, 19,* 237–242.

Kowaz, A. M., Roesch, R., & Friesen, W. J. (1990). Personal needs and social goals: Issues in professional involvement with victims' self-help groups. *Canadian Journal of Community Mental Health, 2,* 63–73.

Kurtz, L. F., Mann, K. B., & Chambon, A. (1987a). Comparison of self-help groups for mental health. *Health and Social Work, 12,* 275–283.

Kurtz, L. F., Mann, K. B., & Chambon, A. (1987b). Linking between social workers and mental health mutual-aid groups. *Social Work in Health Care, 13,* 69–78.

Kus, R. J. (1987). Alcoholics Anonymous and gay American men [Special issue: Psychotherapy with homosexual men and women: Integrated identity approaches for clinical practice]. *Journal of Homosexuality, 14,* 253–276.

Lazar, E. (1984). Logotherapeutic support groups for cardiac patients. *International Forum for Logotherapy, 7,* 85–88.

Lenihan, G. O. (1985). The therapeutic gay support group: A call for professional involvement. *Psychotherapy, 22,* 729–739.

Leon, A. M., Mazur, R., Montalvo, E., & Rodrieguez, M. (1984). Self-help support groups for Hispanic mothers. *Child Welfare, 63,* 261–268.

Levens, H. (1968). Organizational affiliation and powerlessness: A case study of the welfare poor. *Sociological Problems, 16*(1), 203–217.

Leventhal, G. S., Maton, K. I., & Madara, E. J. (1985). *Systemic organizational support for self-help groups.* Paper presented at the meeting of the American Orthopsychiatric Association.

Leventhal, G. S., Maton, K. I., & Madara, E. J. (1988). Systemic organizational support for self-help groups. *American Journal of Orthopsychiatry, 58,* 592–603.

Levy, L. H. (1976). Self-help groups: Types and psychological processes. *Journal of Applied Behavioral Science, 12,* 310–322.

Levy, L. H. (1978). Self-help groups viewed by mental health professionals: A survey and comments. *American Journal of Community Psychology, 6,* 305–313.

Levy, L. H. (1982). Mutual support groups in Great Britain. *Social Science and Medicine, 16,* 1265–1275.

Levy, L. H. (1985). Issues in research and evaluation. In A. Gartner & F. Riessman (Eds.), *The self-help revolution* (pp. 155–172). New York: Human Services Press.

Lieberman, M. A. (1983). Comparative analyses of change mechanisms in groups. In H. H. Blumberg, A. P. Hare, V. Kent, & M. Davies (Eds.), *Small groups in social interaction* (Vol. 2, pp. 239–252). San Francisco, CA: Wiley.

Lieberman, M. A. (1986). Self-help groups and psychiatry. *American Psychiatric Association Annual Review, 5,* 744–760.

Lieberman, M. A. (1989a). Group properties and outcomes: A study of group norms in self-help groups for widows and widowers. *International Journal of Group Psychotherapy, 39,* 191–208.

Lieberman, M. A. (1989b). Mutual-aid groups: An underutilized resource among the elderly. *Annual Review of Gerontology and Geriatrics, 9,* 285–320.

Lieberman, M. A., & Bliwise, N. G. (1985). Comparisons among peer and professionally directed groups for the elderly: Implications for the development of self-help groups. *International Journal of Group Psychotherapy, 35,* 155–175.

Lieberman, M. A., & Bond, G. R. (1976). The problem of being a woman: A survey of 1,700 women in consciousness-raising groups. *Journal of Applied Behavioral Sciences, 12,* 363–379.

Lincoln, R., & Janze, E. (1988). The process of recovery: Its impact on adult children and grandchildren of alcoholics. *Alcoholism Treatment Quarterly, 5,* 249–259.

Litwak, E. (1985). Complementary roles for formal and informal support groups: A study of nursing homes and mortality rates [Special issue: The future administration of human services]. *Journal of Applied Behavioral Science, 21,* 407–425.

Llewelyn, S. P., & Haslett, A. V. (1986). Factors perceived as helpful by the members of self-help groups: An exploratory study. *British Journal of Guidance and Counseling, 14,* 252–262.

Lodl, K. D., McGettigan, A., & Bucy, J. (1984–1985). Women's responses to abortion: Implications for post-abortion support groups [Special issue: Feminist perspectives on social work and human sexuality]. *Journal of Social Work and Human Sexuality, 3,* 119–132.

Lukas, E. (1990). Self-help and crisis intervention. *International Forum for Logotherapy, 13,* 24–31.

Lund, D. A., Dimond, M. F., & Juretich, M. (1985). Bereavement support groups for the elderly: Characteristics of potential participants. *Death Studies, 9,* 309–321.

Lyon, E., & Moore, N. (1990). Social workers and self-help groups for transitional crises: An agency experience [9th Annual Symposium on Social Work with Groups (1987, Boston, Massachusetts)]. *Social Work with Groups, 13,* 85–100.

Madara, E. J., Kalafat, J. M., & Bruce, N. (1988). The computerized Self-Help Clearinghouse: Using "high tech" to promote "high touch" support networks. *Computers in Human Services, 3,* 39–54.

Maharaj, K. (1990). Life-stress events, depression and purpose-in-life in first admission alcoholics and members of Alcoholics Anonymous. *West Indian Medical Journal, 39,* 161–165.

Makela, K. (1991). Social and cultural preconditions of Alcoholics Anonymous (AA) and factors associated with the strength of AA. *British Journal of Addiction, 86,* 1405–1413.

Malekoff, A., Levine, M., & Quaglia, S. (1987). An attempt to create a new "old neighborhood": From suburban isolation to mutual caring. *Social Work with Groups, 10,* 55–68.

Manne, S., Sandler, I., & Zautra, A. (1986). Coping and adjusting to genital herpes: The effects of time and social support. *Journal of Behavioral Medicine, 9,* 163–177.

Marmar, C. R., Horowitz, M. J., Weiss, D. S., Wilner, N. R., et al. (1988). A controlled trial of brief psychotherapy and mutual-help group treatment of conjugal bereavement. *American Journal of Psychiatry, 145,* 203–209.

Maton, K. I. (1989a). Community settings as buffers of life stress? Highly supportive churches, mutual help groups, and senior centers. *American Journal of Community Psychology, 17,* 203–232.

Maton, K. I. (1989b). Towards an ecological understanding of mutual-help groups: The social ecology of "fit" (1989). *American Journal of Community Psychology, 17,* 729–753.

Mayers, R. S., & Souflee, F. (1990–91). Utilizing social support systems in the delivery of social services to the Mexican-American elderly [Special issue: Applications of social support and social network interventions in direct practice]. *Journal of Applied Social Sciences, 15,* 31–50.

Mays, V. M. (1985). Black women working together: Diversity in same sex relationships [Special issue: Rethinking sisterhood: Unity in diversity]. *Women's Studies International Forum, 8,* 67–71.

Mays, V. M. (1985–1986). Black women and stress: Utilization of self-help groups for stress reduction. *Women and Therapy, 4,* 67–79.

McCown, W. (1989). The relationship between impulsivity, empathy and involvement in Twelve Step self-help substance abuse treatment groups. *British Journal of Addiction, 84,* 391–393.

McLatchie, B. H., & Lomp, K. G. (1988). Alcoholics Anonymous affiliation and treatment outcome among a clinical sample of problem drinkers. *American Journal of Drug and Alcohol Abuse, 14,* 309–324.

McWhirter, B. T., McWhirter, E. H., & McWhirter, J. J. (1988). Groups in Latin America: Comunidades Eclesial de Base as mutual support groups [Special issue: Group work and human rights (Volume 1)]. *Journal for Specialists in Group Work, 13,* 70–76.

Meissen, G. J., Gleason, D. F., & Embree, M. G. (1991). An assessment of the needs of mutual-help groups. *American Journal of Community Psychology, 19,* 427–442.

Michael, S., Lurie, E., Russell, N., & Unger, L. (1985). Rapid response mutual aid groups: A new response to social crises and natural disasters. *Social Work, 30,* 245–252.

Moore, T. (1991). The African-American church: A source of empowerment, mutual help, and social change. *Prevention in Human Services, 10,* 147–167.

Naisbitt, J. (1984). *Megatrends.* New York: Warner Books.

Nash, K. B. (1989). Self-help groups: An empowerment vehicle for sickle cell disease patients and their families [Special issue: Groups in health care settings]. *Social Work with Groups, 12,* 81–97.

Nicholaichuk, T. P., & Wollert, R. (1989). The effects of self-help on health status and health-services utilization. *Canadian Journal of Community Mental Health, 8,* 17–29.

Newton, G. (1984). Self-help groups: Can they help? *Journal of Psychosocial Nursing and Mental Health Services, 22,* 27–31.

Nwuga, V. C. (1985). A study of group-self identification among the disabled in Nigeria: A case for support groups. *International Journal of Rehabilitation Research, 8,* 61–67.

Parry, J. K. (1989). Mutual support groups for hospice staff: Planned or ad hoc? *Journal of Palliative Care, 5,* 34–36.

Priddy, J. M. (1987). Outcome research on self–help groups: A humanistic perspective. *Journal for Specialists in Group Work, 12,* 2–9.

Priest, P., Wagner, H., & Waller, G. (1991). Psychological characteristics of anorexic and bulemic women who attend self-help groups. *British Review of Bulimia and Anorexia Nervosa, 5,* 77–84.

Quinn, G. (1989). A multiple sclerosis self-help group. *Canada's Mental Health, 37,* 13–14.

Rhoades, C. M., Browning, P. L., & Thorin, E. J. (1986). Self-help advocacy movement: A promising peer-support system for people with mental disabilities. *Rehabilitation Literature, 47,* 2–7.

Richardson, A. (1991). Health promotion through self-help: The contribution of self-help groups. *WHO Regional Publications European Series, 37,* 467–475.

Riessman, F. (1985). New dimensions in self-help. *Social Policy, 50,* 2–5.

Riessman, F. (1990). Restructuring help: A human services paradigm for the 1990s [Invited address to Division 27 of the American Psychological Association (1989, Atlanta, Georgia)]. *American Journal of Community Psychology, 18,* 221–230.

Riordan, R. J., & Beggs, M. S. (1987). Counselors and self-help groups. *Journal of Counseling and Development, 65,* 427–429.

Riordan, R. J., & Beggs, M. S. (1988). Some critical differences between self help and therapy groups. *Journal for Specialists in Group Work, 13,* 24–29.

Rivera, J. A. (1987). Self-help as mutual protection: The development of Hispanic fraternal benefit societies. *Journal of Applied Behavioral Science, 23,* 387–396.

Robinson, D., & Henry, S. (1977). *Self-help and health.* London: Martin Robertson.

Roosa, M. W., Sandler, I. N., Beals, J., & Short, J. L. (1988). Risk status of adolescent children of problem-drinking parents. *American Journal of Community Psychology, 16,* 225–239.

Rueveni, U. (1985). The family as a social support group now and in 2001 [Special issue: Critical issues in group work: Now and 2001]. *Journal for Specialists in Group Work, 10,* 88–91.

Salem, D. A., Seidman, E., & Rappaport, J. (1988). Community treatment of the mentally ill: The promise of mutual-help organizations. *Social Work, 33,* 403–408.

Schubert, M. A., & Borkman, T. J. (1991). An organizational typology for self help groups. *American Journal of Community Psychology, 19,* 769–787.

Schultz, S. K. (1984). Use of a support group to aid parental coping with a chronically ill child. *Paedovita, 1,* 22–28.

Seitz, M. (1985). A group's history: From mutual aid to helping others. *Social Work with Groups, 8,* 41–54.

Self-help groups [Special issue]. (1991). *American Journal of Community Psychology, 19,* 643–807.

Shields, S. A. (1985–1986). Busted and branded: Group work with substance abusing adolescents in schools [Special issue: The legacy of William Schwartz: Group practice as shared interaction]. *Social Work with Groups, 8,* 61–81.

Shumaker, S. A., & Brownell, A. (1984). Towards a theory of social support: Closing conceptual gaps. *Journal of Social Issues, 40,* 11–36.

Silverman, P. R. (1986). The perils of borrowing: Role of the professional in mutual help groups [Special issue: Support groups]. *Journal for Specialists in Group Work, 11,* 68–73.

Silverman-Dresner, T. (1989–1990a). Self-help groups for women who have had breast cancer. *Imagination, Cognition and Personality, 9,* 237–243.

Silverman-Dresner, T., & Restaino-Baumann, L. (1989–1990b). Problems associated with mastectomy. *Imagination, Cognition and Personality, 9,* 157–176.

Silverman-Dresner, T., & Restaino-Baumann, L. (1990–1991). Comparison of symptom profiles between postmastectomy patients and normal healthy middle-aged women. *Imagination, Cognition and Personality, 10,* 195–200.

Smart, R. G., Mann, R. E., & Anglin, L. (1989). Decreases in alcohol problems and increased Alcoholics Anonymous membership. *British Journal of Addiction, 84,* 507–513.

Sommer, R. (1990). Family advocacy and the mental health system: The recent rise of the alliance for the mentally ill. *Psychiatric Quarterly, 61,* 205–221.

Storer, J. H., Frate, D. A., Johnson, S. A., & Greenberg, A. M. (1987). When the cure seems worse than the disease: Helping families adapt to hypertension treatment. *Family Relations Journal of Applied Family and Child Studies, 36,* 311–315.

Stunkard, A., Levine, H., & Fox, S. (1970). The management of obesity: Patient self-help and medical treatment. *Archives of Internal Medicine, 125,* 1067–1072.

Suarez de Balcazar, Y., Seekins, T., Paine, A., Fawcett, S. B., & Mathews, R. M. (1989). Self help and social support groups for people with disabilities: A descriptive report. *Rehabilitation Counseling Bulletin, 33*(2), 151–158.

Sutro, L. D. (1989). Alcoholics Anonymous in a Mexican peasant-Indian village. *Human Organization, 48,* 180–186.

Tax, S. (1976). Self-help groups: Thoughts on public policy. *Journal of Applied Sciences, 12,* 448–454.

Thyer, B. A. (1987). Community-based self-help groups for the treatment of agoraphobia. *Journal of Sociology and Social Welfare, 14,* 135–141.

Toro, P. A. (1986). A comparison of natural and professional help. *American Journal of Community Psychology, 14,* 147–159.

Toseland, R. W., & Hacker, L. (1985). Social workers' use of self-help groups as a resource for clients. *Social Work, 38,* 232–237.

Tracy, G., & Gussow, Z. (1976). Self-help groups: A grass-roots response to a need for services. *Journal of Applied Behavioral Sciences, 12,* 381–396.

Trojan, A. (1989). Benefits of self-help groups: A survey of 232 members from 65 disease-related groups [Special issue: Health self-care]. *Social Sciences and Medicine, 29,* 225–232.

Tunnard, J. (1989). Local self-help groups for families of children in public care [Special issue: 1988 International Child and Youth Care Conference]. *Child Welfare, 68,* 221–227.

Turcotte, D. (1990). Intervention based on principles of mutual aid: Process and impact on parents of adolescents. *Canada's Mental Health, 38,* 16–19.

Tyler, L. E. (1980). The next twenty years. *The Counseling Psychologist, 8,* 19–21.

Van den Bergh, N. (1991). Workplace mutual aid and self-help: Invaluable resources for EAPs. *Employee Assistance Quarterly, 6,* 1–20.

Wax, J. (1985). Self-help groups. *Journal of Psychosocial Oncology, 3,* 1–3.

Webb, B. (1990). Mutual support for families of children with eye cancer. *Child Care, Health and Development, 16,* 319–329.

Wilson, J. (1992). Support groups. Ready for take-off. *Nursing Times, 88,* 26–28.

Wintersteen, R. T., & Young, L. (1988). Effective professional collaboration with family support groups. *Psychosocial Rehabilitation Journal, 12,* 19–31.

Wollert, R. (1987). Human services and the self-help clearinghouse concept. *Canadian Journal of Community Mental Health, 6,* 79–90

Wulsin, L., Bachop, M., & Hoffman, D. (1988). Group therapy in manic depressive illness. *American Journal of Psychotherapy, 42,* 263–271.

Yoak, M., & Chesler, M. (1985). Alternative professional roles in health care delivery: Leadership patterns in self-help groups [Special issue: The future administration of human services]. *Journal of Applied Behavioral Science, 91,* 437–444.

Yoak, M., Chesney, B. K., & Schwartz, N. H. (1985). Active roles in self-help groups for parents of children with cancer [Special issue: Active roles of parents]. *Children's Health Care, 14,* 38–45.

Young, J., & Williams, C. L. (1988). Whom do mutual-help groups help? A typology of members. *Hospital and Community Psychiatry, 39,* 1178–1182.

Zeigler, E. A. (1989). The importance of mutual support for spouses of head injury survivors. *Cognitive Rehabilitation, 7,* 34–37.

Zimmer, A. H. (1987–1988). Self-help groups and late-life learning [Special issue: Late-life learning]. *Generations, 12,* 19–21.

Zimmerman, M. A., Reischl, T. M., Seidman, E., Rappaport, J., Toro, P. A., & Salem, D. A. (1991). Expansion strategies of a mutual help organization. *American Journal of Community Psychology, 19*(2), 251–278.

CHAPTER 15

Growth Groups in the 1980s: Mental Health Implications

MORTON A. LIEBERMAN

It is almost 50 years since the first intrepid seekers of personal enlightenment migrated to an obscure, picturesque village in western Maine. These
businessmen, community workers, and members of the armed forces
brought high levels of enthusiasm and equally high levels of apprehension
and puzzlement—Human Relations Training was hardly a household word.
Bethel, Maine, provided the first organized setting for a new type of adult
education, a laboratory in human relations whose center piece was the "T"
group or sensitivity training (Bradford, Gibb, & Benne, 1964). The opportunity to talk about oneself unfettered by the stringent rules of the workplace, and to have perfect strangers tell you "like it is" provided a heady
cocktail for the new seekers of personnel enlightenment. There were few
rules and precedents made to be broken.

Human Relations Training was the spartan first small step of what has
for nearly 50 years provided millions of Americans an opportunity to rediscover themselves. The brainchild of a displaced academic from Nazi Germany, Kurt Lewin, and supported by a cadre of home-grown academics
from M.I.T. and the University of Michigan, these early beginnings provided no hint of the future explosive growth of the hydra headed "human
potential" movement. This chapter examines groups engaged in the "self-
development" business during the 1980s.

The changes in the human potential activities since the 1950s were dramatically brought to my attention when I was invited, in 1984, to talk about
growth groups to a graduate psychology seminar at UC Berkeley. At least
one-half of the students had never heard of, much less participated in an
encounter group. This, on a campus where, in the 1960s and 1970s, bulletin
boards vied for space to announce the latest growth group. Crudely
scrawled notices and slickly printed posters heralded a never-ending supply
of groups for personal change and growth.

Where have encounter groups gone? Were they, like many other "innovative" social institutions, a product of a specific historical time destined to
fade from our culture like the proverbial Hula Hoop. Or have encounter

groups transmuted into a new form, serving similar people with goals identical to those found in encounter groups during the 1960s and 1970s. People still attend groups called encounter, more however participate in their transformed states. Large Group Awareness Training (LGAT) was the principal expression during the 1980s of growth groups. The labels have changed. Human Relations Training, Sensitivity Groups, Encounter, Personal Development, Large Group Awareness Training are but a few of the touchstones for growth groups.

This is not to say that during the nearly 50 years of growth groups only the labels have changed. Substantive alterations in the goals of growth groups are markers to their transformation. The modest raison d'etre of human relations training, to provide a new method of education, experientially based learning about oneself in society, was soon to become the guarantee of encounter groups for a total remake of the mind, body, and soul. The procedures as well as the promises became grandiose; all dissatisfactions in life could be addressed and all of oneself could be remade. The marketplace took over. They offered salvation by proffering to provide a reborn self without edges or scratches, shiny and sleek.

To set the stage for examining the 1980 decade it is useful to think about the stages of growth groups: (1) The Early Days (1945 to 1959); Human Relations Training, Sensitivity Training, and Laboratory Education are the touchstones describing this era, (2) the Explosion, Years of Encounter, and Growth Centers (1960–1980); this era reflected an increased focus on personal development that utilized, in addition to the procedures developed during the 1940s and 1950s, "body work" and ideas borrowed from eastern philosophies, and (3) decade of the 1980s, High-Tech Growth Groups; increasing commercialization and the growth of business organizations to provide "growth services"; the flourishing of Large Group Awareness Training organizations.

THE SEEKERS: HOW MANY? WHO ARE THEY? WHAT DO THEY SEEK?

With unfailing regularity, the media will quote a well-known pundit of American culture announcing the eminent demise of the human potential movement. Such opinions are apparently based on, "Not one of my friends has attended a growth group in years." "Esalen's (the California mecca during the 1960s and 1970s for growth groups) registration is down." "Hollywood released a picture about growth groups (*Bob and Carol and Ted and Alice*), a reliable indicator of a social movement's decline." But are these predictions true? Answers to the question are not resolved by the musing of experts. They become known by straightforward survey research.

How many people go to growth groups? An analysis by the chapter's author of a national survey on getting help when faced with "emotional" difficulties (Mellinger & Balter, 1983) provides some information on the demographic and psychological status of growth group participants compared to other "help proving" settings. The survey of 3,000 Americans in 1980 reports that during one year 3.5 million people participated in some type of human potential activity. What kind of groups were they attending? The most frequently mentioned were meditation, yoga, assertiveness training, EST, human awareness courses, workshops in interpersonal relationships, self-confidence courses, past life reincarnations, hypnosis seminars, stewardship training, think-positive courses, self-improvement programs, anger seminars, career goal, and ambition classes.

A useful comparison to this report on attenders of growth groups are the number who sought help for emotional problems. During the same 12-month period, 9 million adults used a mental health professional and 4.8 million Americans sought out a self-help group to deal with emotional or physical problems or feelings of discrimination. Information about specific growth group organizations during the 1980's decade supports this survey findings. Finkelstein, Weinegrat, and Yalom (1982) estimated by 1982 that 450,000 had participated in EST, and based on recent membership reports, well over 1 million entered EST or FORUM (the current designation of EST) and another 300,000, Lifespring.

Who were these people? Again, turning to the national survey, we see that they were disproportionately separated and divorced, overwhelmingly Caucasian, and those who had never married. A recent survey of Lifespring respondents (Ross & Vallone, 1989) reported that participants are young (between 20 and 40) (74%), single or divorced (69%), educated (only 12% had not attended college), users of psychotherapy (28%), have self-stated motivations that emphasize better interpersonal relationships (69%), insight (87%), desire for a "happier" life (71%), and want help with immediate personal problems (41%). Figure 15.1 graphically shows the different participant composition of three help-providing settings: growth groups, self-help groups, and professional mental health providers.

Do people seek out growth groups because they are deeply troubled? To answer this question, the survey data were used to compare the growth group participants with those who sought out mental health specialists (Lieberman, 1992). The comparisons were based on measures of psychiatric distress (number of current psychiatric symptoms); life stress (the number of negative life events encountered during the past 12 months); role impairment (an index of how well individuals were functioning in the ordinary roles of parent, husband or wife, student, worker, etc.); degree of emotional upset during the past year; and diagnostic information about major categories of common mental illnesses.

The survey found that approximately 22% of all adult Americans experienced high psychic distress. Figure 15.2 compares the levels of psychological symptoms across the three settings. Based on psychic distress (symptoms) and impairment measures, those who sought out growth

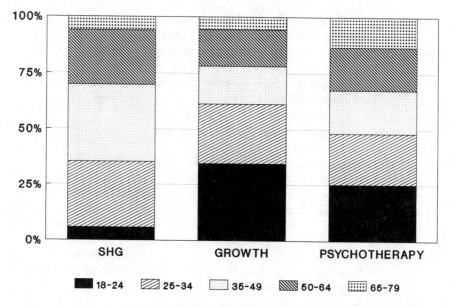

Figure 15.1. Age and help settings.

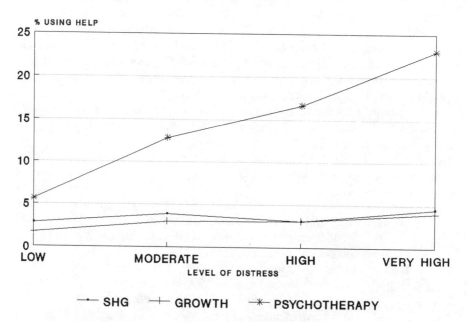

Figure 15.2. Symptoms and help settings (Source: Mellinger-Balter survey).

groups were *not* overly represented by those who were particularly disturbed or impaired in their lives. There is no evidence based upon these analyses that human potential settings are attracting disproportionately those who suffer from psychiatric problems.

Why, then, did they seek out growth groups? One clue can be found in the national survey. Nearly one-half of the growth group participants reported significant life events during the year they sought out such groups. Job changes, problems in their marriages, losses of people, and changes in important relationship are piled up in these people at the time they turned to a growth group. Those who seek out self-change learning settings do so when they are experiencing in the normal course of life, events that they define as stressful. They come to re-address who they are, what they are, and how they should change, stimulated by life events that have challenged them during the year. Figure 15.3 summarizes these comparisons, showing the increases of participation with total levels of life stress.

But contemporary society provides many alternatives for relieving stress—why a growth group? Several studies suggest that other factors play a role in this choice. Fisher, Grant, Hall, and Keashly (1990) report that both higher levels of psychological stress, as well as more recent negative life events, and values that include self-responsibility and self-awareness are the major characteristics that distinguish growth group participants from their peers.

The available evidence does not support the perception that there has been a precipitous decline in growth group participation. The form and perhaps

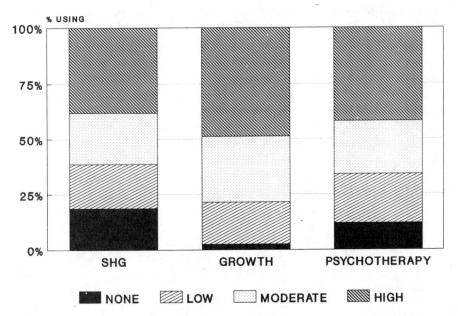

Figure 15.3. Level of stress and helping sources (Source: Mellinger-Balter survey).

the goals represent a different era; the decade of the 1980s was not identical to those that preceded it, and there would be no reason to expect that the presentation of growth would be identical with earlier decades.

Despite evidence that participation in growth groups has increased since their inception in the late 1940s, and that large numbers of Americans have sought out such experiences in the 1980s, an examination of the research productivity in the past decade tells a different story. The following section provides an overview of research productivity investigating the various manifestations of growth groups.

RESEARCH ON "GROWTH" GROUPS: OVERVIEW 1972–1992

The research literature was searched for studies and theoretical treatises on personal change groups (sensitivity training, encounter, growth, large group awareness training, and so forth). During the past 20 years, a total of 944 articles and dissertations were published: 1972–1976, n = 545; 1977–1981, n = 172; 1982–1986, n = 153; 1987–1992, n = 80. These studies were categorized into nine general categories, and each category was further subdivided into areas of study. Figure 15.4 shows the distribution of research areas by time; Figure 15.5 displays the same information by percentages of total studies during the four, 5-year periods.

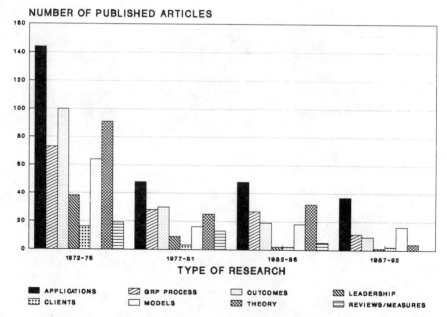

Figure 15.4. Research activity growth groups 1972–1992.

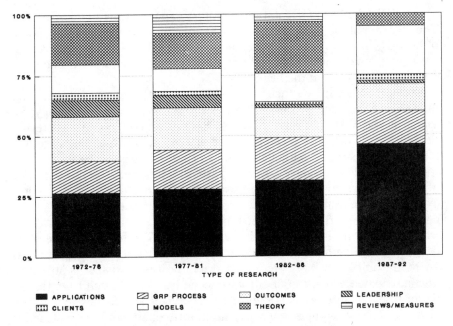

Figure 15.5. Type of research 1972–1992.

There has been a substantial decrease in the number of published studies during the 1980s; the past five year rate is only ¹/₇ of the 1972–1976 time period. Not only has the absolute number of studies declined, but an examination of Figure 15.5 indicates that more recent research is primarily applied (50%) compared to the comparable figures for the earlier time period. Other areas of inquiry have nearly disappeared from the literature, for example, the present small number of theoretical publications as well as studies of leadership. An analysis of the details on research interests (not shown) show similar patterns, overall decline with some areas of inquiry disappearing. Process research studies show that the exploration of interpersonal relationships in growth groups is no longer a major area in the recent research literature; studies of group development and feedback currently predominate the small number of process studies.

A sampling of 1980s, studies reveals several common themes: the study populations were mostly college undergraduates; analog research strategies were dominant (illustrated by Stokes, Fuehrer, & Childs, 1983); explorations of processes focusing on cohesiveness and its enhancement (Hurley, 1989; Roark-Sharah, 1989; Wright & Duncan, 1986) were plentiful. Prepreparation of participants (Muller & Scott, 1984), leader behavior and orientation (Shoemaker, 1987), leaders' personality (McWhirter & Frey, 1987), and amount of structure (Caple & Cox, 1989) were representative of studies in the 1980s. Outcome evaluations varied widely from enhanced social skills (McNamara & Blumer, 1982) to traditional tests such as the POI (Personal Orientation Inventory) and measures of self-esteem. The research in the 1980s may represent an actual regression in the quality of investigation. We are no further along in understanding the processes nor the unique conditions linked to learning in growth groups at the end of the 1980s than we were at the beginning.

The almost exclusive focus on college students and the limited range of both outcome and process measures did not provide a rich legacy. Research in the 1980s on growth groups has not grown beyond the previous decades. Little evidence could be found of a vigorous, expanding field with innovative constructs. Although studies of cohesiveness, a basic construct for indexing group adequacy, were typical, this construct was characteristic of studies when growth groups first appeared. It still provides a potent explanation for outcome differences. The frequent employment of this construct, however, has not been matched by an enhanced conceptual framework nor an improvement in measurement. The increasing use of experimental analog has been heralded by some reviewers as a sign for optimism; the ability for more precise control of process variables is attractive. The anticipated expansion of our knowledge base anticipated from this superior research strategy is not apparent. The vigor and expansiveness, coupled with growth group's longevity, has unfortunately not been matched by an comparable increment in the quality of research findings. These comments do not imply the total absence of quality studies over the nearly five decades of inquiry. They are sporadic, occur over the decades, and give little evidence that growth group research in the 1980s represents a meaningful progression in methodological quality and conceptual clarity.

Why? If the epidemiological data available correctly reflect a still lively interest in growth groups, why the relative lack of investigator interest and the absence of substantial progress in conceptualization and measurement? The reasons for this are complex. In part, the almost complete demise of a vigorous and variegated research community of scholars interested in small groups truncated the development of the basic conceptual and methodological input required for the continued growth of a research subspecialty. Perhaps the limitations of growth group research in this decade may be the unfortunate outgrowth of the collapse of small group research as an academic discipline. The 1980s were characterized by a decrease in the number of students small group research attracted, the disappearance of academic centers of excellence, and lowered productivity (if measured by the volume of publications). It is beyond the scope of this chapter to discuss some of the reasons for this collapse. The interested reader may find an early publication portending the fate of small group research as a useful starting point (*Journal of Applied Behavioral Science,* whole issue, 1976). The basic science of small group and the role it previously served for investigators of growth groups has ceased to be a dominant theme. Attendant with this academic decline is, of course, the absence of critical masses of investigators at any given institution, limiting the likelihood that graduate students will enter the field. An analysis of dissertations during the past 20 years echoes the previous analysis of published studies [Dissertation Productivity: 1972–1979 = 117 (52% of total dissertations), 1977–1981 = 44 (19%), 1982–1986 = 33 (15%), 1987–1992 = 32 (14%)]. Analysis of the areas addressed in the dissertations mirrors the previously cited one. For example, in the 1972–1976 period, 15% addressed applied issues, next five-year period, 23%, then 52%; and in the most recent time period, 69% of the dissertations represent practical topics. Finally, the payoffs of the earlier research on growth groups and the noncumulative buildup of a substance knowledge base may have contributed to the present state of affairs. Little that was new or that moved the enterprise forward could be found in the 1980s studies reviewed.

LARGE GROUP AWARENESS TRAINING

This section examines "growth groups" in the 1980s, focusing on Large Group Awareness Training (LGAT), the largest and most prevalent expression of the human potential movement in that decade. Asked are: (1) What are they? (2) What are their risks? (3) What role, if any, do they play in delivering services traditionally provided by mental health professionals? and (4) What is their impact on participants as assessed by measures of attitudes, belief, role functioning, self-concept, and personality dimensions.

WHAT IS LARGE GROUP AWARENESS TRAINING?

LGATs focus on philosophical, psychological, and ethical issues related to personal effectiveness, decision-making, personal responsibility, and commitment. These issues are examined through lectures, demonstrations, dialogue with participants, structured exercises, and participants' testimonials of personal experiences relevant to the themes presented. Participants are encouraged to apply the insights they obtain to improving their own lives. The two largest LGAT organizations are EST and Lifespring; a detailed description of EST is provided by Finkelstein et al. (1982). Lifespring and EST share many similarities, although aspects of their philosophy and resultant prescriptive cognitive structures are distinct. Both use structured settings with sharp and specific ground rules of appropriate behavior and demeanor and a philosophy or cognitive structure that is distinct and articulate, emphasizing personal responsibility and high levels of control over one's destiny. They differ in that Lifespring uses the interactional mode typical of the encounter groups that proceeded LGATs. Lifespring relies on a series of emotionally toned experiences that involve role playing, guided group interaction, dyadic, and small group exercises. Unlike sensitivity training and encounter groups, LGATs are less open to leader differences, since there is a detailed written plan which is followed with little variation from one training to another.

Risk and Negative Effects of LGAT

Since the development in the mid-1940s of growth groups, critics have charged that they may be dangerous to participants' mental health. Mental health professionals' interest in the effects of growth groups stems from two concerns: clinical experiences with patients who were distraught and, at times, seriously psychiatrically ill subsequent to their participation, and perceptions that many of the prominent methods used in growth groups are similar to the tools used by psychotherapists. They question the use of such "powerful processes" by "untrained" people. Some of the growth-group seekers are the same people, with similar motivations, who enter psychotherapy. Lieberman and Gardner (1976) found that 81% of their growth center sample were currently, or had recently been in psychotherapy. From a public health perspective, the combination of large numbers of participants and possible toxic effects merits investigation.

In the 1940s and 1950s, critical publications in professional journals attacked sensitivity training; in the 1960s and 1970s, publications with similar criticisms were directed toward encounter groups; the cycle was repeated in the 1980s with almost identical "criticisms" of LGATs.

What is the evidence for toxic effects? During most of these nearly 50 years, much of the evidence has been anecdotal: reports of mental health professionals treating people who, subsequent to growth group, were psychologically ill. Patients or their therapists attributed this illness to their group participation (Gottschalk & Pattison, 1969; Jaffe & Scherl, 1969). In 1969, the American Psychiatric Association appointed a task force to survey the field (Encounter Groups and Psychiatry, 1970). The report's bottom line was that, despite strongly held opinions, there was virtually no controlled research in the field. With the publication in 1973 of a controlled, comparative study of encounter groups (Lieberman, Yalom, & Miles, 1973), reliable evidence of measurable psychological harm (casualty rate among participants was 9.8%) associated with encounter groups led by charismatic and highly stimulating leaders became available.

The development of LGATs in the late 1970s and their near explosive popularity in the 1980s stimulated a renewed concern of the potential for psychological harm. A review of the status of research in 1982 (Finklestein et al., 1982) aped the finding of the APA task force; aside from isolated case reports and analysis based on the supposition of noxious psychological processes (e.g., Adams & Haaken, 1987), systematic research on the risks of LGAT participation was almost nonexistent.

During the nearly five decades of growth group research, the handful of systematic studies assessing risk rely on two approaches for its assessment: negative effects and casualty. Negative effects is a term borrowed from psychotherapy; it implies a worsening of a patient's symptoms or functioning as a result of the therapy. It commonly refers to increases on some test scores assessing psychiatric symptoms and decreases in self-esteem. In contrast, a judgment of casualty is based on a clinical finding that the person has deteriorated in major adult role functioning. Casualty usually implies that the person is suffering from a psychiatric illness. Another commonly used indicator of the growth group's negative impact is seeking psychotherapy after group participation. This way of assessing risk is useless. People enter psychotherapy for a variety of reasons. Discovering in a growth group that psychotherapy may be useful to you is more often a sign of success rather than failure. For example, the increased sensitivity to personal problems and the motivation for changing it are positives that may occur in a growth group.

Discovering some people that were psychiatrically ill after a growth group, what could we conclude about the "cause" of their difficulties? Could we say that their group experience was the culprit? During my studies of various growth groups, I was constantly surprised by participants' responses. Yes, we both agreed that they were in serious psychological trouble and needed help. Often our concordance stopped there. Detailed knowledge, based on observations of the group and person suggested a direct link between the experience and the current difficulties. Not so for the participants. They often did not view the growth group as contributing to their problem. The reverse could and did occur.

Such differences in perspective signal the complexity of assessing risk. If the researcher were able to assign people randomly in a strict experiment to participants and controls, much of the ambiguity about risk would evaporate. Opportunities for this kind of research are rarely available. In its absence, the only method (with all its imperfections) is the development of accurate knowledge of the person before and after the growth group, combined with detailed information about their group experience.

Two series of studies have examined the risks involved in LGAT based on adequate measurement and reasonable sampling strategies: studies of EST by Fisher et al., (1990) and on Lifespring (Lieberman, 1986b; Lieberman, 1992). The studies differ not only in the obvious target of study, the particular LGAT they chose to examine, but in their operational definitions of risk. Fisher et al. studied negative effects by examining changes in self-report inventories such as symptoms, self-esteem, well-being, and the accumulation of negative life events subsequent to the experience; Lieberman examined casualty rates by using clinical evaluations in one study, and in a second study, a diagnostic interview (DIS) assessing psychopathology (ECA public use wave 1 codebook, 1989) to provide DSM-III diagnosis.

Casualty Assessment in Lifespring (Lieberman, 1986b)

One basic Lifespring training session (60 hours) was studied. Of the 299 participants, 289 returned useable forms. Three methods were used to identify *potentially* vulnerable Ss for further clinical study: (1) direct observations during the training. (Risk cues included high conversion, physical and psychological stress responses, bizarre or erratic behavior, and trainer-induced incidents that might be experienced as demeaning or ridiculing.)

Fifteen participants were identified, (2) a series of scales administered prior to training that had previously been found to be associated with high risk (Lieberman et al., 1973) (Psychological profiles—perceived danger and phoniness of the upcoming training; extreme scores on values about experiential education; a negative self-concept and low self-esteem; and a misanthropic world view). Fourteen participants had four or more positive signs, and (3) peer-nomination (other participants' judgments that the person had been overly distressed, hurt, harmed, or disturbed). Seventeen were nominated by three or more people; four others nominated themselves.

In all, 30 participants (10%) were selected for further study. They were contacted within 1 week and interviewed during the following 3 to 4 weeks. Three refused to be interviewed; four others moved out of the area. The interview covered the participants' view of their participation; a review of specific behavior during the first week following training, including physiological symptoms indicative of distress; dreams and other fantasy material; and areas of psychological and social functioning in the major role areas, including marital, parental, and occupational.

Casualty criteria were identical to those developed in the encounter study: the person is "functioning significantly poorer than [he or she] had prior to the training, . . . the decrement in functioning has some enduring implications in the person's life," and the poor functioning was associated with the group experience. Within the limitations of our methodology, no positive evidence was found that permanent psychological harm to the participants occurred. Five people showed behaviors indicative of high stress. For example, one who had a history of ulcers developed bleeding directly linked to the training; another experienced what can best be described as a transitory psychotic episode lasting 1½ days; others experienced milder states of disorientation and depression. All of these states, however, were transitory, and within a week or less after training all of the affected participants had reorganized themselves and resumed their previous level of functioning.

Incidence of Psychopathology after Lifespring Participation (Lieberman, 1986b)

All 38 participants who entered a single advanced Lifespring training group were studied. After six months, of the 37 who completed, 33 were again interviewed (two people refused, and two others moved out of the area). A clinical interview (similar to that used in study 1) and the Diagnostic Interview Schedule (DIS), a 263-item questionnaire validated to produce a DSM-III diagnosis, were administered. The DIS was scored using the standard computer routing provided by the National Institute of Mental Health.

Prior to participation, six subjects met the criteria for current psychiatric disorders; three showed patterns of depressive illness, and three were classified as demonstrating phobic illnesses. All six subjects who met DSM-III criteria 6 months after participation demonstrated an identical disorder over their lifetime; there is no evidence that they became psychiatric casualties as a result of their participation. Simply put, those who had experienced psychiatric disorders throughout their adult lifespan manifested those disorders both before and after their participation.

Negative Effects of EST (Fisher et al., 1990)

One hundred and thirty-five participants and 72 comparable peer-nominated controls were assessed 4 to 6 weeks prior to training, 4 to 6 weeks later, and then again, 1½ years later. Nineteen percent were living alone, 60% were woman, 95% were Caucasian; the mean educational level was 14.9 years. Measures included: Affect Balance Scale (Derogatis, 1975a), General Health Measure, and the Brief Symptom Inventory (Derogatis & Melisartos, 1983).

Negative effects in the EST study used changes in the scores based upon the brief symptom inventory. No significant differences between the experimental and control were noted. Negative effects could also have been revealed on a variety of other indicators (reduced self-esteem, reduced life satisfaction, etc.). Such results were not observed. Other potential indicators of negative outcomes were the participants' listing of negative events occurring in the year following EST (being fired from work or experiencing a significant failure), or finding negative changes in a participant's social network (e.g., losing network members who are experiencing increased psychological distance from them). No evidence of negative effects were found on any of the measures. The authors concluded that they could not find any evidence of negative effects on the measures they used.

The findings from these studies do not provide positive evidence that large group awareness training settings are inherently risky, even when participants with previous diagnosable psychopathology are considered. The processes used in large group awareness training can be emotionally arousing to some participants; the impact of such emotions was shown in the results of the initial Lifespring study previously described. What is clearly lacking, however, is a coherent theory for linking a set of experiences ordinarily encountered in LGATs to the development, exacerbation, or intensification of psychopathology. Emotional intensity, which is a dominant causal element reflected in the literature critical of growth groups, is not of itself a known pathogenic factor. Neither precise measurement nor a well-articulated conceptual base exists for linking the psychology of defense and coping strategies to the processes used in large group awareness training. In summary, based on the evidence currently available, no compelling evidence exists suggesting that participation in LGATs presents an unusual or unacceptable risk.

PSYCHOTHERAPEUTICS IN GROWTH GROUPS

Throughout the often controversial history of growth groups, mental health professionals have charged that group leaders and attendant organizations practice psychotherapy without a license. Growth group advocates have just as vigorously claimed that their activities are not psychotherapeutic. What is the evidence?

Do people join growth groups to achieve solace for serious psychological problems? Studies of participants' motivations and goals have found some do so to find relief and help for psychic distress. For example, about half of the participants in Lifespring cited as important goals: "to deal with a current life problem," "to solve long-term personal hang-ups," "to obtain relief from feelings I have that trouble me," and to "get help." When asked, prior to participation, to indicate how they would characterize their lives during the past year, 65% indicated major life changes, such as separation, divorce, and career changes. On a scale of 1 to 10 assessing the importance of these changes, compared to other past events, the median score was 7.

Studies of Therapeutics: Effects on Symptoms and Pathology

Early LGAT studies are typified by the Ornstein, Swencionis, Deikman, and Morris (1975) report on a post participation study of 1,200 EST participants using Ss evaluation of their physical and mental health as compared to a year prior to participation. Such studies fail to meet even the rudimentary levels of methodology. Pre-post designs such as the Tondow, Teague, Finney, and LeMaistre (1973) study, using the California Psychological Inventory and comparing EST participants to a comparable matched control group, offer a modest improvement in methodology. They reported that EST participants exhibited improved self-image and lower anxiety, guilt, and dependency. Unfortunately, the pre and post measures of the control group were never directly compared to those of experimental groups. Weiss's (1977) study using a small wait-control group provided a more sophisticated design. The study reported that participants (the female members) decreased in their self status concept in congruity and had decreased average levels of distress. For a more detailed review of the LGAT literature, see the Finkelstein, Weinegrat, and Yalom (1982) research, as well as the more recent monograph by Fisher, Silver, Chinsky, Goff, Klar, and Zagieboylo (1989). Collectively, these early studies do not provide clarifications of the findings reported in this chapter.

Due to these limitations, the bulk of the evidence to be presented in this and subsequent sections on benefits relies on findings from studies of Lifespring by the chapter's author and those of Fisher and his colleagues (1990) on EST. These studies will be briefly described prior to discussions of specific results. Table 15.1 shows the characteristics of the samples studied; Table 15.2 indicates the outcome measures used in each of the studies.

Both studies administered symptom inventories several weeks prior to their participation and then again one year later. No significant changes were found in either study. The second Lifespring study examined all participants who entered one advanced LGAT. Of the 37 who completed, 33 were interviewed prior to, and again 6 months after the training via a clinical

TABLE 15.1.   The Studies—Demographic Characteristics

	Lifespring		EST
Sample Size	Study 1	77	135
	Study 2	38	
Refuser	Study 1	36%	69%
	Study 2	—	
Control Group	Study 1 matched Normative (50) Study 2 wait controls (16)		Snowball, friends like you (72)
Age	33.5		—
Gender	55% women		60% women
Education	84% college		Mean yrs. 15.0
Married	18%		Status not given 19.7% Living alone
Sep/Div/Wid	30%		—
Never married	52%		—
Psychotherapy	53%		—

interview and the Diagnostic Interview Schedule (DIS) (a 263-item questionnaire validated to provide a DSM-III diagnosis). Fifteen Ss showed a classifiable DSM-III diagnosis present during the 6 months proceeding participation.

Will LGATs help resolve the symptoms associated with emotional problems? The studies just described found no convincing evidence that participation provides measurable improvement in either symptoms associated with mental illness or a diminution of the manifestations of the illness. Participants who manifest, prior to participation, psychopathological signs rarely show mitigation after participation. Psychic distress levels failed to show shifts over time. Such symptoms almost always show significant decreases in studies of psychotherapy outcomes; this despite the observations that a significant minority of those sampled show signs and symptoms and goals equivalent to populations studied in psychotherapy. Seeking relief from serious psychological problems in LGAT is rarely successful.

The Lifespring risk studies also determined that psychopathology as measured by the DIS did not affect level of benefit; outcomes assessed by measures of role functioning and self concept found that outcomes were similar when the pathology (DSM-III criteria) and nonpathology groups were compared. Those whose level of emotional distress mirror psychotherapy users are able to utilize LGAT in the same way as those who do not show such deficits. On the other hand, the processes characteristic of LGAT do not directly address these emotional problems. Participants who, prior to participation, manifest psychopathological signs may improve in their role functioning and their feelings about their self, but their symptoms are rarely mitigated.

TABLE 15.2. The Studies—Measures

	Lifespring	EST
Mental Health	Hopkins symptoms (Derogatis et al., 1974) Self-esteem (Rosenberg, 1965)	General health measure (Rotter, 1966) Symptom inventory (Derogatis & Melisartos, 1983)
Affect Measures	Control mastery (Pearlin & Lieberman, 1979)	Affect balance (Derogatis, 1975) Locus of control (Rotter, 1966) Satisfaction life (Andrews & Crandall, 1976) Life stress (Sarason, Johnson, & Siegel, 1978)
Role Measures	Single role, marriage parenting and occupation stress and strain (Pearlin & Lieberman, 1989)	Occupational stress (House et al., 1979)
Coping	Role coping (Pearlin & Schooler, 1979)	Daily hassles (Wortman & Silver, 1981)
Attitudes-Values	Personality dimensions (Leary, 1957) Adaptation (Lieberman & Tobin, 1983) Values of self and significant others (Lieberman, 1992) Attitudes towards growth groups (Lieberman et al., 1973) 25 items; four areas: 1. *Views about interpersonal relationship:* unconditional positive regard, the role of criticism from others, being alone vs. being with others, honoring commitments, and the importance of looking good to others. 2. *Control over one's destiny vs. chance or fate:* the past represents our future, beliefs restrict our ability, self-reliance vs. dependence on others for help, confronting problems vs. letting things take their due course, the ease or difficulty of making changes, and the role of risk taking. 3. *Beliefs about the nature of people:* their predictability and non-predictability, their trust-worthiness, their honesty (intrinsic to people vs. honesty because they feared getting caught), altruism, the ease or difficulty of understanding others, the influence others have on decision making, whether people are unique or basically alike, and the degree to which people understand themselves. 4. *Aspiration/achievement values:* the role of achievement in feeling good about oneself, levels of aspiration, and the degree to which people value growth.	Social desirability (Crowne & Marlow, 1960) Self-improvement (Sarason et al., 1978)
Social Support/Social Network	Perceptions of interpersonal world, friends, and family (Lieberman, 1992)	Social support (Norbeck et al., 1981) Social density (Hirsch, 1979)
Self-Image/Esteem Measures	Self-esteem (Rosenberg, 1965) Self-sort (Lieberman & Tobin, 1983) Items like and unlike self examples from current life supporting self-image items, coded for quality of evidence (Rosner, 1968)	Self-esteem (Rosenberg, 1965)

Direct measure of the mental illness manifestations were not mitigated by participation in LGATs. Both the Lifespring and EST studies examined a variety of other than direct measures of mental health to test the impact of LGATs. Some of these areas assessed have implications for the question about LGAT's benefits to mental health. Effects are discussed in four heuristic "outcome" categories: (1) self-image, (2) values/beliefs, (3) role behaviors, and (4) personality (see Table 15.2 for a list of measures).

Self-Transformations

Growth groups reflect society's concerns with personal identity. They began when Americans were shifting from a preoccupation with "what am I" to "who am I?" The search for answers provides the "common concern" that unites the diverse activities that characterize growth groups. How successful has the 1980s form been in responding to participants' search for self? Is self change an unabashed good?

How our self-image is organized and how it changes has been a topic of scientific interest since the beginning of psychology. Formal studies of psychotherapy outcome that began in earnest during the 1940s renewed interest in the psychology of the self. For many, the core of psychotherapy is a reexamination of the self. Change is intrinsically linked to the self. The most prominent and early proponent of this view was Carl Rogers, the originator of client centered psychotherapy. He and his students, beginning in the 1950s, examined intensively the direction, amount, and type of self-image changes that resulted from client centered therapy. Emphasis was on the correspondence between the self and each person's image of an ideal or wished-for self. Other investigators focused on positive and negative feelings about themselves. Still others examined the various "selves" representing any single person. Underlining these variations is the assumption that changes in the self-image connote progress and lead directly to other positive benefits. An unchanging self is t. ,ught to represent failure in psychotherapy; those who fail to accomplish this task often are viewed as less psychologically healthy than those who are able to accomplish changes in the self.

Many people enter growth groups at a point in their lives when they question their lives and who they are. They often are beset with feelings of dissatisfaction. They expect and desire revisions in their self-image. This section reviews studies on the impact of LGATs on changes in how people think about themselves and they way they use this new "self-knowledge." To place the impact of growth groups on the self in perspective, changes in the self for participants is compared to the impact on the self of life transitions-expectable and eruptive life crises—for example, marriage, the birth of a child, divorce, and so forth.

Prior to participation, Ss selected, on average, 30 self-sorted descriptive items, with five cited as new characteristics and 4.5 as old characteristics having been previously part of the respondent's self-image. One year after Lifespring, participants increased in seeing the self as having changed, evidenced by adding additional new elements (x = 6.7) and excluding old elements (x = 7.0) at a higher frequency. The content of the self-image changed radically in the direction of presenting a more dominant self. These findings fit expectations; growth groups confront participants with new information and new ways of thinking that may require self-image restructuring.

Ordinarily, the research inquiry would stop here having reported positive and significant findings. However, findings from a previous longitudinal study (Lieberman, 1992) on self change, using a large probability sample, raised questions about the positive meaning usually attached to self-concept changes. In that study, Ss who proved to be less well-adapted were more likely to perceive themselves as changing in response to impactful life events; those who proved to be better adapted perceived the event as having impact on their lives, but did not take it as a signal to revise how they thought about themselves.

Would the same relationship between self-perceived change be found in a population who migrate to formal settings in search of change? An analysis of the Lifespring data based on the self-sort is more fully described in Lieberman (1992). Results found were that: (1) One year after Ss' participation in a growth group, a highly malleable, changing self was related to prior psychopathology based on DSM-III diagnosis, and (2) an analysis based on pre-post scores on symptoms and self-esteem (controlling for self-image content and time 1 scores in a hierarchal regression) found changes in mental health and self-esteem. It makes a difference when individuals see their current self-concept as being a stable one consistent with the past, as opposed to those who see their current self-concept as being, in some important aspects, inconsistent with their past selves. *Revisions of the self prior to training and subsequent to the training (1 year later) are linked to decrements to positive mental health scores (increases in anxiety and in depression).*

How useful is a changing self? Alterations in how participants construe their self-image is something people expect and accomplish in growth groups. Perplexing was the finding that the more the self-image changed, the less likely they were to reap other benefits from the group experience such as increased well-being and happiness. High self-changers were also more likely, prior to the growth group, to be psychologically disabled. There appears, therefore, to be some advantages in perceiving a relatively immutable self-image in the face of adversity or in maintaining a stable self-image while seeking change. Although flexibility may be a desired adaptive characteristic, such a characteristic when expressed through an ever changing self-image appears to constitute a psychological burden.

Both the EST and Lifespring studies examined the impact of the experience on self-esteem using the Rosenberg Self-Esteem scales. A significant effect (p = .01) compared to the normal control groups was observed in the Lifespring study; Fisher et al. (1990) reported no systematic changes in self-esteem compared to their control group. As will be discussed in the final section of this chapter, the differences in outcomes between these two major studies of LGATs whose current procedures differ markedly, provides some insights to relevant change processes. It should, however, be noted that the two studies relied on different control samples for their contrasts and also experienced different sample retention rates. Such method factors must caution the discussion of differences in outcomes noted in the two LGAT settings.

Values and Beliefs

Education and psychotherapy's impact and success in providing a setting for change is accomplished, in large part, because they challenge a person's basic beliefs about self, relations to others, and the larger society. Despite the classical and perhaps outmoded stance of early psychoanalysis of value neutrality, most mental health practitioners have come to recognize that they are deeply and inextricably involved in values transformations. Since their inception, growth groups have trafficked in value challenge and change. The decade of the 1980s and the ascendancy of LGATs brought to center stage the concern with value challenges. LGATs are about changing beliefs; they believe that they are successful to the extent they challenge participants' prior values and beliefs and produce changes in them.

To examine values in the Lifespring studies, 25 bipolar beliefs were developed, based on the dominant values espoused by growth groups: People are burdened with old views and perceptions or false beliefs about what happened to them and how others acted in the past; change or improvement is possible; change comes about through an understanding of a person's belief system; when confronting problems, the best thing is to take some kind of action to overcome them; others are capable of love, warmth, and trust; fulfilling commitments is a central aspect of all social relationships; and self-responsibility must be taken for what happens in life.

In the Lieberman study, participants, when compared to wait controls at Time 2 (T2), significantly differed on 5 of the 25 value items. Six months after, participants were significantly more trusting of people; they saw people as acting on altruistic motives; they believed that it is better to confront problems and take some action; they espoused beliefs as more restricting possibilities in life and believed that other people are an important source of support in difficult times. Some items that did not discriminate between the experimental and controls at T2, did show statistically significant changes between T1 and T2. There was a movement by the participants, but not controls, to emphasize control over what happens to them compared to chance or fate; they viewed the world of people as being intrinsically honest rather than being controlled by external sanctions; they increased valuing the taking of risks in life, and they increasingly emphasized following-through on commitments.

The finding, that subsequent to participation in Lifespring there are significant shifts in certain attitudes and beliefs in the direction consistent with the overt values of the LGATs, appears to support the influence of the setting. However, referent group theory might suggest an alternative explanation for value change and the maintenance of such values long after the LGAT experience. The social context influence may be particularly salient for LGAT participants because of the frequent post LGAT experience activities in which some engage. To test the question, a new analysis compared the relative weight of LGAT participation to social network influence.

Each participant and control was asked at both T1 and T2 (6 months later) to think of four people whom they consider to be their closest friends, which could include family members. The type of relationship, how much time they spend with them per week, the denseness (known to one another) or looseness (unknown to one another) of their networks, and the number of years they have known them were noted. We also asked how many of these people had attended a Lifespring training. Prior to the basic training, 48% of Lifespring participants had at least one close friend who at some time in the past had participated in a LGAT. The comparable wait control group figures were 32%. These differences were not statistically significant. After training, participants had increased the number of close friends drawn from LGAT participants: 71% had at least one friend; the controls, 38%. This was a statistically significant difference, p = 0.03.

A significant linear relationship was found between the number of close friends in Lifespring and the degree of value change when the participants and the controls were compared at T2. Multivariate analyses of covariance revealed that Lifespring friendships were considerably more influential than participation or nonparticipation in the basic training in shaping values over time.

Although participation may serve as a stimulus to value changes, the maintenance of such changes was found to be linked to alterations in their social networks. The more their friends included people similar to themselves (e.g., friends who had also participated in the growth group), the greater the values changed. Growth groups act as a stimulus, making belief change possible. To maintain these new ways of thinking about their world, requires a recasting of who is important to the person.

The EST studies concentrated their examination of values and beliefs on the values and beliefs towards self improvement and change. The ASIS is a 10-item scale designed to measure how strongly people believe in the utility of achieving self awareness, and their solving problems through participation and activities designed to enhance self awareness. The beliefs about change instrument assesses the expectations that people have about the occurrence of personal change in their lives. The test consists of 13 pairs of adjectives describing people's "attitudes about significant change." For example, people can make significant changes ranging from anything to nothing: I believe change is possible for none—possible for all. No significant differences were found on these measures when comparing the experimental and control groups.

Work, Marriage, and Parenthood

The success and ease people encounter in the central adult roles is a sensitive indicator of how well they are doing. Many enter "growth groups" with a strong desire to change their marriages, the problems they experience in their careers, and how they relate to their parents. How well do growth groups serve these objectives? Both series of LGAT studies examined some of the major adult roles: work, marriage, and parenting. The Lifespring studies assessed role strains in: (1) occupation, (2) relationships (single or marital strain by assessing the amount of reciprocity and affection-fulfillment provided by the relationship) (Pearlin & Lieberman, 1979), (3) parenting strain based on two dimensions (worries and problems) (Mullen, 1981), and (4) coping strategies indexed for occupation and marriage. The Perceived Occupational Stress Scale (House et al., 1975) was used in the EST studies.

T-tests on difference scores revealed that the Lifespring sample showed significant decrements in the role strains from T1 to T2; the control groups showed statistically significant increases. (The component tests of each index found that all displayed the same pattern, except for singles' strain, on which there were no significant effects.) No significant changes, comparable to those observed in the Lifespring study, were found for EST participants.

Lifespring participants, one year after the growth group experience, demonstrated measurable improvements in their central adult roles, reporting less stress and strain in their jobs and their marriages, and alterations in the way they approach and solve problems in these areas. No comparable outcomes were observed in the study of EST participants.

Personality and Effectiveness

"I want to be different," "I want to be more effective in life," is a common refrain of the growth group seekers. Do they succeed in this quest? Do they become more effective in life? Have they changed their personalities? Information on personality traits was not available from the EST studies; the results of the analysis on Lifespring participants are briefly reviewed in this section.

Before attending a growth group and then again one year later, participants were asked to describe themselves on a standard personality trait measure assessing eight traits (Leary, 1957). The number of Ss classified by personality types pre and post LGAT participation were as follows: Managerial (T1 = 11%, T2 = 31%), Competitive (14% to 20%), and Responsible (8% to 14%) increased. Sixty-five percent, at T2, can be characterized by these three personality types. There was a marked reduction in Aggressive (28% to 9%), Docile (14% to 9%), and Cooperative (14% to 9%) personality types. Fewer changes were observed for Rebellious (8% to 6%) and Self-effacing (5% to 2%). Figure 15.6 shows the distributions at T1 and one year later, T2.

In general, there was a move over the year towards becoming a person who expresses strength, force, energy, and leadership, as well as communicating a clear love and approval of the self. They appear to others as people who are independent and confident. One year after, personality types who communicate messages of hard-boiled toughness and who are made anxious in situations which call for tender, agreeable or docile feelings, as well as those who rely on skeptical alienation from conventions and from

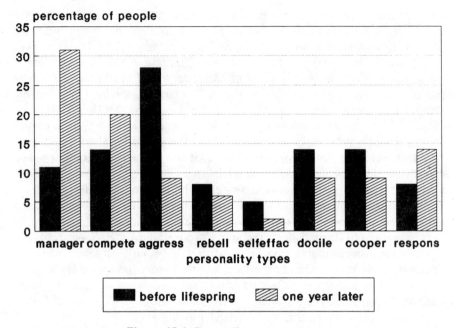

Figure 15.6. Personality types—pre/post.

acceptance of others, are less frequently found. We also found that participants whose personality styles emphasize communications of weakness and meekness are less characteristic of those afterwards than they were prior to the experience. The amount of change appears substantial, however comparable control data were not available for this study of personality, suggesting caution in interpreting these findings.

Participant Characteristics and Benefit

A variety of subject characteristics have been hypothesized to effect both the experience and the resultant outcomes. Among the best studied is the influence of expectations, attitudes, goals and personality. Findings from the LGAT studies are briefly reviewed.

At T1, Ss were asked their views of Lifespring. These attitude scales (Lieberman et al., 1973) assess expectations of benefit, danger, and genuine-phoniness. Participants showed a moderately positive view at T1, and their positive perceptions increased over time. These perceptions could be interpreted as expectations; they were weak predictions of individual differences in outcomes. For each of the four major outcome areas, multiple hierarchical regressions were computed on all three T1 attitude measures together. First the corresponding T1 outcome index was entered as a covariate. Prior attitudes, in combination, predicted only 2% of the variance for Roles, and 8%, for Self-image. The strongest relationship found was between benefit and T2 Self-image, 7% of the remaining variance in Self-image when entered last. Perceptions of danger predicted worse T2 Mental Health scores.

Ss were asked at T1 to choose the most applicable goal from a set of four statements reflecting curiosity, a specific problem/solutions, inner change, and general change. This forced-choice format was used to avoid "ceiling effects" (Lieberman et al., 1973). The relationship between goals and outcomes was tested by a multiple regression analysis of each of the T2 outcome areas. T1 outcome scores were entered as a covariate. Neither T2 role strain nor self-image outcomes were appreciably predicted by the goals measures (3% and 2% of the variance in Role Strain and Self-image, respectively). Goals did a slightly better job of predicting Mental Health, 12%. The best subset of three predictors (multiple $R^2 = 22\%$) included "Curiosity," "General Change," and "Inner Change." Of these, "Inner Change" was the best single predictor, accounting for 7% of the variance; improvement in Mental Health at T2 was characteristic of Ss who emphasized inner change goals. Participants' goals did not account for most of the observed T1 − T2 changes in Self-image and Role Strain. However, the desire for inner change as a motivation to take Lifespring did seem to account for more of the individual differences in Mental Health changes.

Overall, participants did better if they showed a certain degree of cynicism about the experience and emphasized more modest goals (the difference between a goal seeking increased meaning or self awareness as opposed to those emphasizing doing away with long-term problems or becoming a new person). More limited expectations and the sense of healthy skepticism appear to "mitigate" negative changes (increases in mental illness signs and role strain disturbance).

This section was organized around two major studies of large group awareness training; as is so often the case in the history of growth group research, these studies yielded contradictory effectiveness findings. Variations are often a function of method differences, particularly in how outcomes are conceptualized and measured. Another major problem interfering with the accumulation of empirical knowledge about growth groups is the specification of what constitutes a growth group. Absent herein is a set of both process and structural operations that would enable investigators to define precisely the comparisons among growth groups.

This all too common problem is dramatically portrayed in the outcome findings presented in this chapter. The two LGATs compared yielded starkly different outcomes. Although methods differences cannot be ruled out as an explanation, neither can it explain all of these discrepancies. Studies of LGATs are at a disadvantage compared to earlier studies on encounter groups. The most successful studies of encounter groups were able to capitalize on powerful process variables such as differences in leader behaviors and style. Variations (Lieberman et al., 1973) provided a meaningful "experimental" difference which could be exploited to understand the fluctuations in outcomes. Large group awareness training within a particular organization does not differ markedly from one group to another. Both Lifespring and EST have standard protocols that the group leaders follow down to rather minute details. There are no major variations within Lifespring or within EST that provide the leverage for looking at process variations and outcomes.

Nevertheless, there is some value in speculatively comparing Lifespring and EST processes. Both LGAT organizations share many features. Common are the settings, several hundred people and one central leader with assistants for logistical help. Both emphasize sharp and distinct boundaries, specified rules for interacting, and lengthy massed time sessions. Furthermore, they share a common philosophical orientation. Despite these similarities, they differ markedly in process procedures. The revised format of EST, Forum, relies on a lecture format and exclusively emphasizes cognitive restructuring through the challenge of participants' belief system. Lifespring, on the other hand, is a process cafeteria offering a large number of different experiences; from challenge of participant's beliefs about themselves and their world, to small group interaction and a variety of "exercises" borrowed from previous growth group technologies. Lifespring, in contrast to EST, is interpersonally focused and provides mechanisms for interactive experiences; it resembles, more than EST does, the encounter groups of the 1960s and 1970s. The marked outcome differences this chapter reports may be a function of these "process" distinctions. Unfortunately, no meaningful process information on the LGATs studied is available that would enable us to move beyond interesting speculations.

THE FUTURE OF GROWTH GROUPS

To recap the major findings on growth groups in the 1980s, survey data suggest that a substantial number of people participated in growth groups, most of whom attended LGATs. They do so at points in their lives when they experience discomfort, distress, and unhappiness, often stimulated by high levels of life stress. Growth groups in the 1980s did not attract disproportionately large number of participants who manifest serious mental disorders. For those who had a previous history of mental disorders, large group awareness training did not provide repair and alleviation of troublesome psychiatric symptoms.

The transformations of growth groups over the five decades have more to teach us about the nature of our society and the needs of its members. Over time, although both growth group goals and procedures have altered, the function they serve remains constant. There is no reason to assume, based upon the information presented here on the demographics of participation, that we are rapidly approaching an end to the claim they have on the American Psyche. The death of the growth group has been heralded by many, and certainly the popular press' attention to this area has waned considerably.

This inattention should certainly not be taken as a meaningful clue that it no longer exists. Scholarly work such as the important monograph, *Beyond Words: The Story of Sensitivity Training and the Encounter Movement,* by Kurt W. Back, originally published in 1972 and revised in 1987, traces the origins of sensitivity training and their later day derivative, encounter groups. It is Back's view that the context of major social trends in our society have altered, heralding the death of growth groups. He does not, however, examine the rapid transformations of these activities into new forms and new labels. In contrast to Back's thesis, the chapter's author sees the desire for self-transformation as inexhaustible; begetting a never-ending supply of growth groups based on a common set of processes that are poured into differently shaped and labeled vessels.

How will the future be shaped? The predominance of LGATs that characterized the 1980s is unlikely to continue. Several important recent trends in the people changing—people helping professions suggest that the 1990s will be characterized by new and distinctive forms of growth groups, representing a break with the traditions that have held sway for nearly five decades. Historically, investigators divided the universe of helping groups, addressing repair and growth into three separate activities: growth groups, self-help groups, and psychotherapy. They represent distinct entities in our society with their own unique history. Each provided a different view of the nature of man and his ills and how these "ills" are to be addressed. Although such distinctiveness has not always been clear in the consumer's mind, purveyors of these services, and researchers alike, described specific and different activities servicing different people, or at least people at different points in their life span.

Mental health professionals have always recognized that such clear distinctions were not reflected in the minds of consumers. Many clients who sought us out for psychotherapy had at some point in the past, or even concurrent with treatment, involved themselves in other help providing self-transforming settings. For example, studies of self-help groups (Lieberman & Bond, 1976; Lieberman, Solow, Bond, & Reibstin, 1979; Lieberman & Videka-Sherman, 1986; Videka-Sherman & Lieberman, 1985) found that many of the participants in both consciousness raising groups and self-help groups dealing with specific afflictions (widowhood and loss of a child) were much more likely, compared to controls sharing the same problem, to be involved in other helping activities (including the services of mental health professionals). However, based on survey analysis described in this chapter, the majority of participants in growth groups would not be designated as psychiatrically ill.

Strikingly, the converse is closer to truth: nonpatients in psychotherapy are likely to be more frequent. A substantial number of people seek out psychotherapy to address problems of living or to examine issues of the self and are not, at the time they present themselves for psychotherapy, suffering from a significant psychiatric disorder (defined in terms of a DSM-III diagnosis). To illustrate, in preparing this chapter, I examined the Epidemiologic Catchment Area (Robins & Regier, 1991) data, the best and most thorough source of the incidence of mental disorder in the United States. The ECA survey also provides information on the use of a variety of helping sources to address these disorders. Found was that close to half of those who seek out psychotherapy (in the previous 6 months) did not manifest symptoms at a level used for DSM-III diagnosis. Almost 5% of the 20,000 adults, age 18 through 98 studied, sought out a mental health specialist in a clinic or through a health plan; 50% of them had no current DSM-III diagnosis; 13.1% sought out a mental health professional in private practice, 51% had no current DSM-III diagnosis; 4% turned to mental health center, 40% of them had no DSM-III diagnosis. As I believe is clear from these illustrations of the ECA (Epidemiologic Cutchment Area) (Eaton & Kessler, 1985) findings, many individuals who seek out psychotherapy do so for problems other than addressing a specified mental disorder.

What I have described so far is a state of affairs that has been going on for many decades and should come as no surprise to the reader of this chapter. However, recently, there has been substantial social and professional practice changes that diminish the conceptual and practical distinctions we make between activities designated as psychotherapy, from those labeled self-help groups and growth groups.

The Diseasing of Growth Groups

The history of sensitivity training, its evolution into encounter groups, and the more recent development of LGATs, as well as the countless variations and flavors of growth groups representing the growth industry, shared a common and fundamental assumption about the nature of humans and their goals. They were not interested in illness and did not see their activity as addressing repair. Early sensitivity training focused on the individual's relationship to society and how it could be enhanced through the use of the small group setting. It began with a belief that democratic institutions in our society could be enhanced through people altering how they worked with and related to society's diverse social structures. The evolution to the encounter moved the center of focus to enhancement of the person's potential and self development. The belief was that these goals could be achieved through increased access to and expression of emotions, coupled with an unfettered temporary relationship in a group setting. Neither sensitivity training nor encounter groups involved a view that their clients suffered from a common illness or a fatal flaw intrinsic to the human condition. Illness or disease was not addressed or assumed.

Recent years are characterized by a new, and in this author's mind, distinct claimant to the throne of growth groups. The labels are numerous, but all view people as suffering from a fundamental and common flaw that needs to be addressed before growth can occur. Most typical is the mass movement surrounding the notion that the flaw is associated with an up-bringing in a dysfunctional family; a term that connotes much emotional baggage, but little precision. It provides nearly everyone who wants to find a basis for unhappiness and difficulty in living to be located in one's earlier childhood. The core belief illuminating this movement is only the "coming to terms" with this common problem that then permits and unleashes growth. I think this represents a new and rapidly growing theme of growth groups and will, certainly in the 1990s, represent the setting for the self-enhancement, self-improvement movement in our society.

It should of course be noted that talking about modal trends, some of these practitioners of encounter contained in their view of people, their troubles, and source of troubles, and the pathways for salvation as similar to the current pre-occupation with dysfunctional families. The work of Eric Berne and the transformation of a therapeutic modality to encounter groups contained many of the seeds of what we see today. There has always been borrowing, which encourages blurring of the boundaries between growth and psychotherapy. A careful examination, however, suggests that despite such borrowing, growth groups and psychotherapy maintained a separation; they still represent distinct activities serving unique functions in society. In fact, it is probably more reasonable to assume that the exchanges of procedures between growth activities and psychotherapy have mostly occurred in the direction of psychotherapy borrowing from growth groups. For example, the increasing closing of the psychological distance between the psychotherapist and the client and the creation in a therapeutic transaction of a more human, realistic person, were more a product of the influence of the growth culture than psychotherapy. One can find many techniques commonly used by psychotherapists to have had their origins in the growth group. However, the diseasing of the growth groups does serve to alter fundamentally the boundaries of what is therapy and what are growth groups.

The Professionalization of Self-Help Groups

Since the inception of Self-Help Groups (SHGs), their images have been shaped by a few simple, yet powerful ideas: ordinary people with a common problem come together, share their problems and learn from one another without benefit of professionals, in settings which they own and control. As attractive as this populist view may be, a recent study of over 3000 California SHGs (Lieberman, 1993) found that as many as 60% (omitting substance abuse groups) were led, or directed by professionally trained leaders, many of whom were paid (see Goodman and Jacobs chapter in this book, for details on this issue). The ideal portrait of SHGs presented in texts does not match empirical reality. The classical picture of such groups, often based on Alcoholics Anonymous is misleading; diversity and change over time is the rule. Some groups begin as small face-to-face support systems, but soon develop into complex, multifaceted client run social agencies; others start as social protest or social action movements that evolve into quasi-therapeutic settings; still others, whose origin was face-to-face help and support, move in the opposite direction, becoming social action settings more intent on changing society than in changing themselves.

The traditional definition of SHGs as those led by the clients themselves is an appealing one since it provides a conceptual basis for a boundary. Professional leaders operate from a specific set of perspectives and utilize behaviors that are different from nonprofessionals. Professional leaders manifest greater psychological distance between themselves and their participants. They have an organized and, at times, distinctive view of the cause of illness. They believe, despite variations in theory, that the curative powers of therapeutic groups are derived from their social microcosm characteristics; examination of the interaction among members is the central therapeutic task. SHGs do not commonly emphasize such examinations. From this perspective, professionalization of SHGs may have profound impact in how such SHGs provide help to their members and the resulting types of outcomes (e.g., participant feelings of mastery, control, and empowerment). A definition of SHGs based on nonprofessional leaders sharing the common problem of the group, although appealing conceptually, does not match current practice.

The penetration by mental health professionals into an activity with its own procedures and belief system about the cause and cure of peoples' difficulties, erodes further the boundaries of three distinct helping-changing settings: self-help, growth groups, and psychotherapy. These rearrangements present us with the possibility that the growth groups, as we have known them over nearly five decades, are the proper concern of the social historian. I believe, but do not know, of course, the details, that this massive blurring of boundaries portends new arrangements and new structures in our society, representing the same fundamental needs for a temporary attachment, mechanisms of self-transformation, and the enhancement of living and relationships. Seeking has not gone out of business, and probably what is constant over these five decades and in the decade before us is the all too American belief that one can find meaning and purpose through involving oneself in structured activities with others, and do it in a relatively brief period of time. Shared across all variants of growth groups is the consumers' hope that the group will provide the necessary changes so devoutly and intensely sought.

REFERENCES

Adams, R., & Haaken, J. (1987). Anticultural culture: Lifespring's ideology and its roots in humanistic psychology. *Journal of Humanistic Psychology, 27*(4), 501–517.

American Psychiatric Association Task Force. (1970). *Encounter groups & psychiatry*.

Andrews, F. M., & Crandall, R. (1976). The validity of measures of self-reported well-being. *Social Indicators Research, 3,* 1–19.

Back, K. W. (1987). *Beyond words: The story of sensitivity training and the encounter movement* (rev. ed.). New York: Sage Foundation.

Bond, G. R., Borman, L. D., Bankoff, L., Lieberman, M. A., Daiter, S., & Videka, L. (1979). The growth of mended hearts—a medical self-help group. *Social Policy,* 50–57.

Bond, G. R., & Lieberman, M. A. (1981). The role and function of women's consciousness-raising: Self-help psychotherapy or political activation. In C. L. Heckerman (Ed.), *Women and psychotherapy, changing emotions in changing times.* New York: Basic Books.

Borman, L., & Lieberman M. A. (Eds.). (1976). Special issue/self-help groups. *Journal of Applied Behavioral Science, 12*(3).

Bradford, L., Gibb, J., & Benne, K. (1964). *T-Group theory and laboratory method: Innovation in re-education.* New York: Wiley.

Caple, R. B., & Cox, P. L. (1989). Relationships among group structure, member expectations, attraction to group and satisfaction with group experience. *Journal for Specialists in Group Work, 14,* 16–24.

Crowne, D. P., & Marlowe, D. (1960). A new scale of social desirability independent of psychopathology. *Journal of Consulting Psychology, 24,* 349–354.

Derogatis, L. R. (1975a). Social class, psychological disorder, and the nature of the psychopathologic indicator. *Journal of Consulting and Clinical Psychology, 43*(2), 183–191.

Derogatis, L. R. (1975b). *The Affects Balance Scale (ABS).* Baltimore, MD: Clinical Psychometric Research.

Derogatis, L. R., Lipman, R. S., Rickles, K., Uhlenhuth, E. H., & Covi, L. (1974). The Hopkins symptoms checklist (HSCL): A self-report symptom inventory. *Behavioral Science, 19,* 1–15.

Derogatis, L. R., & Melisaratos, N. (1983). The brief symptom inventory: An introductory report. *Psychological Medicine, 13,* 595–605.

Eaton, W. W., & Kessler, L. (Eds.). (1985). *Epidemiology field methods in psychiatry: The NIMH epidemiologic attachment area program.* Orlando, FL: Academic Press.

Finkelstein, P., Weinegrat, B., & Yalom, I. (1982). Large group awareness training. *Annual Review of Psychology, 33,* 515–539.

Fisher, R. J., Grant, P. R., Hall, D. G., & Keashly, L. (1990). The development and testing of a strategic simulation of intergroup conflict. *Journal of Psychology, 124*(2), 223–240.

Fisher, J. D., Silver, R. C., Chinsky, J. M., Goff, B., Klar, Y., & Zagieboylo, C. (1989). Psychological effects of participation in a large awareness training. *Journal of Consulting and Clinical Psychology, 57*(6), 747–755.

Gottschalk, L. A., & Pattison, E. M. (1969). Psychiatric perspectives on T-groups and the laboratory movement: An overview. *American Journal of Psychiatry, 126,* 823–39.

Haaken, J., & Adams, R. (1983). Pathology as personal growth: A participant-observation study of lifespring training. *Psychiatry, 46,* 270–280.

Hirsch, B. J. (1979). Psychological dimensions social networks: A multi-method analysis. *American Journal Community Psychology, 7,* 263–272.

House, J. S., McMichael, A. J., Wells, J. A., Kaplan, B. H., & Landerman, L. R. (1975). Occupational stress and health among factory workers. *Journal of Health and Social Behavior, 20,* 139–160.

Hurley, J. R. (1989). Self-acceptance and other-acceptance scales for small groups. *Genetic, Social and General Psychology Monograph, 115*(4), 483–503.

Jaffe, S. L., & Scherl, D. L. (1969). Acute psychosis precipitated by T-group experiences. *Archives of General Psychiatry, 21*(4), 443–448.

Lakin, M. (Ed.). (1987). What happened to small group research? *Journal of Applied Behavioral Sciences, 12*(3).

Leary, T. (1957). *Interpersonal diagnosis of personality.* New York: Ronald Press.

Lieberman, M. A. (1976). Change induction in small groups. *Annual Review of Psychology, 27,* 217–250.

Lieberman, M. A. (1986a). Self-help groups: Comparisons to group therapy. *American Psychiatric Association in Annual Review, 5.*

Lieberman, M. A. (1986b). The effect of large group awareness training on participants' psychiatric status. *The American Journal of Psychiatry, 144,* 460–464.

Lieberman, M. A. (1989). Mutual aid groups: An underutilized resource among the elderly. *Annual Review of Gerontology and Geriatrics, 9,* 285–320.

Lieberman, M. A. (1992). Perceptions of changes in the self: The impact of life events and large group awareness training. In Y. Klar, J. D. Fisher, J. M. Chinsky & A. Nadler (Eds.), *Self change* (pp. 43–62). New York: Springer-Verlag.

Lieberman, M. A. (1993, February). Prevalence and membership characteristics of self help group participants. Ann Arbor Conference, Center in Self Help Research, Ann Arbor, MI.

Lieberman, M. A., & Bliwise, N. G. (1985). Comparison among peer and professional directed groups for the elderly: Implications for the development of self-help groups. *International Journal of Group Psychotherapy, 35*(2), 155–175.

Lieberman, M. A., & Bond, G. R. (1976). The problem of being a woman: A survey of 1700 women in consciousness-raising groups. *Journal of Applied Behavioral Science, 12*(3), 363–379.

Lieberman, M. A., & Borman, L. (1979). *Self-help groups for coping with crises: Origins, members, processes, and impact.* San Francisco, CA: Jossey-Bass.

Lieberman, M. A., & Gardner, J. A. (1976). Institutional alternatives to psychotherapy: A study of growth center users. *Archives of General Psychiatry, 33,* 157–162.

Lieberman, M. A., Solow, N., Bond, J. R., & Reibstein, J. (1979). The psychotherapeutic impact of women's consciousness-raising groups. *Archives of General Psychiatry, 36,* 161–168.

Lieberman, M. A., & Tobin, S. (1983). *The experience of old age: Stress, coping, and survival.* New York: Basic Books.

Lieberman, M. A., & Videka-Sherman, L. (1986). The impact of self-help groups on the mental health of widows and widowers. *American Journal of Orthopsychiatry, 16,* 435–445.

Lieberman, M. A., Yalom, I. D., & Miles, M. B. (1973). *Encounter groups: First facts.* New York: Basic Books.

McNamara, J. R., & Blumer, C. A. (1982). Role playing to assess social competence: Ecological validity considerations. *Behavior Modification, 6*(4), 519–549.

McWhirter, J. J., & Frey, R. E. (1987). Group leader and member characteristics and attraction to initial and final group sessions and to the group and group leader. *Small Group Behavior, 18*(4), 533–547.

Mellinger, G., & Balter, M. (1983). *Collaborative project* (GMIRSB Report). Washington, DC: National Institute of Mental Health.

Muller, E. J., & Scott, T. B. (1984). A comparison of film and written presentations for pre-group training experiences. *Journal for Specialists in Group Work, 9*(3), 122–126.

Mullen, J. (1981). *Parental distress and marital happiness: The transition to the empty nest.* Unpublished doctoral dissertation, University of Chicago.

Norbeck, J. S., Lindsey, A. M., & Carrieri, V. L. (1981). The development of an instrument to measure social support. *Nursing Research, 30,* 264–269.

Ornstein, R., Swencionis, C., Deikman, A., & Morris, R. (1975). A self report survey: Preliminary study of participants in Erhard Seminars Training. est Found., San Francisco, CA.

Pearlin, L. I., & Lieberman, M. A. (1979). Social sources of emotional distress. In R. G. Simmons (Ed.), *Research in Community and Mental Health* (pp. 217–248). Greenwich, CT: JAI Press.

Pearlin, L. I., & Schooler, C. (1978). The structure of coping. *Journal of Health and Social Behavior, 19,* 2–21.

Roark-Sharah, E. (1989). Factors related to group cohesiveness. *Small Group Behavior, 20,* 62–69.

Robins, L. N., & Regier, D. A. (1991). *Psychiatric disorders in America.* New York: The Free Press.

Rosenberg, M. (1965). *Society and the adolescent self-image.* Princeton, NJ: Princeton University Press.

Rosner, A. (1968). *Stress and maintenance of self concept in the aged.* Unpublished doctoral dissertation, University of Chicago.

Ross, L., & Vallone, R. (1989). *Perceptions and evaluation of Lifespring participants.* Unpublished manuscript, Stanford University.

Rotter, J. B. (1966). Generalized expectancies for internal versus external control of reinforcement. *Psychological Monographs, 80* (Whole No. 609).

Sarason, I. G., Johnson, J. H., & Siegel, J. M. (1978). Assessing the impact of life changes: Development of the life experiences survey. *Journal of Consulting and Clinical Psychology, 46,* 932–946.

Shoemaker, G. (1987). A study of human relations training groups: Leadership style and outcome. *Small Group Behavior, 18*(3), 356–367.

Stokes, J. P., Fuehrer, A., & Childs, I. (1983). Group members self disclosures: Relation to perceived cohesion. *Small Group Behavior, 14,* 63–76.

Tondow, D. M., Teague, R., Finney, J., & LeMaistre, G. (1973). *Abstract of the Behaviordyne report on psychological changes measured after taking the Erhard seminars training.* Palo Alto, CA: Behaviordyne.

Videka-Sherman, L., & Lieberman, M. A. (1985). The effects of self-help groups on child loss: The limits of recovery. *American Journal of Orthopsychiatry, 55,* 70–81.

Weiss, J. A. (1977). *Reported changes in personality, self-concept, and personal problems following Erhard seminars training.* Unpublished doctoral dissertation, California School of Professional Psychology, San Diego.

Wortman, C. B., & Silber, R. L. (1981). *SIDS loss: Psychosocial impact and predictors of coping.* (Grant No. PHS MCH260470). U.S. Public Health Service.

Wright, T. L., & Duncan, D. (1986). Attraction to group, group cohesiveness, and individual outcome: A study of training groups. *Small Group Behavior, 17*(4), 487–492.

Epilogue

Only to a magician is the world forever fluid, infinitely mutable and eternally new. Only he knows the secret of change, only he knows truly that all things are crouched in eagerness to become something else, and it is from this universal tension that he draws his power.

PETER BEAGLE

In retrospect, several broad themes emerge from reading the "book as a whole"—themes that might go unnoticed except that one sees the whole as greater than the sum of its parts. This phenomenon parallels group theory: all the parts and their relationship must be seen, or the overall meaning of the whole may be overlooked. The following themes, then, stand as sightings from the whole.

An unsettling theme that appears across a large number of chapters is one of definition. After nearly 90 years of practice, leading thinkers in group psychotherapy are still grappling with definitions: What is structure? What is development? What is self-help versus professional help? For example, in the former, a refinement of a past construct is proffered. Conceptual parameters are adjusted as another author wrestles with the construct of development and how it has been empirically studied. A new definition of mutual support is tendered based on emergent trends over the past decade. It is clear that a careful examination of empirical evidence facilitates the conquest of definitional difficulties; emerging empirical boundaries require new conceptual definitions. However, it is also apparent that complacency in our past understanding of group psychotherapy holds some risk. That is, in light of the continual calibrations that occur in the literature, empirical and conceptual understandings of the mechanisms of change in group therapy have shown themselves to be dynamic.

The significance of structure and its place and form in the process of therapy is woven throughout the book. In a more formal sense, structure emerges as treatment boundaries are established for inpatient, eating disordered, and time-limited outpatient psychotherapy groups. In a more subtle fashion, structure arises as authors search for a paradigm to understand the interactional dynamics and developmental changes noted across the life of a therapy group. Given the nearly universal acknowledgment regarding the complexity of therapeutic process in group treatment, it is not surprising that group writers have regularly tired of simple structural interventions or explanations. In response to this, some have recently applied nonlinear dynamics theory on both a conceptual and empirical front to explore the underlying complexity of therapeutic processes operative in group therapy. The potential of these models for successfully plotting the serpentine evolution of small groups stands in bold relief to the past utility of linear or stage models reflected in group therapy models. These methods (nonlinear dynamic models) plus other emerging, time-sensitive methodologies may be the harbingers of structure paradigms available to future group therapy models and conceptualizations.

The long-time interplay of small group psychology and group therapy is also evident throughout the book. Quite unexpectedly, dual contributions that both of these fields have made to the conglomerate nature of the group therapy literature are independently recognized, separated, and documented by several authors. For instance, the confluence of the two fields unfolds in the conceptual modeling offered in the area of group development and structure. Integration also emerges in the review of therapeutic aspects of member interactions and the application of group therapy principles to specific populations (mutual support and large group awareness). In spite of the wide array of outlets for group therapy research during a 12-year review period, it is refreshing to see the authors refrain from parochial review practices. Given that general scientific advances often follow coordinated, interdisciplinary conceptual and empirical efforts, the aforementioned incorporation of relevant conceptual and empirical advances found in the small group psychology literature is promising. Collaboration among the participants of these overlapping and interactive fields of inquiry and practice would stand group therapy in good stead.

The acknowledgment of and call for a more collaborative relationship between the scientist and the practitioner weds many of the chapters. This issue is reflected in the applied dual standard of rigor and relevance. When empirical rigor seems higher, prescriptive recommendations are found in clinical matters such as which client variables to consider more carefully in composing and structuring groups. When the clinical relevance appears stronger, authors are more prescriptive methodologically, making recommendations for how therapeutic factors, substance abuse, and child and adolescent groups should be studied in future investigations. In some cases, the dual standard is evident by the intertwining of research and practice considerations, as in the review of group therapy for eating disorders. It is encouraging to see several reviewers abstaining from unduly harsh inclusion standards in their review of the group research. The multistep standard of rigor noted in several chapters (i.e., single case versus multigroup experiment criteria) demonstrates an empathic understanding of the exponentially complex logistics involved in group therapy as opposed to dyadic treatment research. We need to continue to encourage practitioners to adopt a "scientific" attitude toward the efficacy of group treatments offered. This may mean establishing a legitimate scientific position for small n studies. In doing so, we will need to maximize rigor in small n studies by suggesting methodological standards that accommodate practical limitations. For instance, if a small n study were a systematic replication (Kazdin, 1980) of previous research, then it should be viewed as cumulative rather than limited knowledge. This stance assumes that the small n study meets minimal standards for systematic replication studies. Other creative alternatives are also possible.

A persistent petition from reviewers during the last 40 years has been the call for increased conceptual modeling. This theme is echoed in several of the chapters in this volume. However, a subtle and paradoxical observation can be found in a number of the chapters. That is, the preponderance of articles in the group literature falls into conceptual rather than empirical categories. For instance, in the first two chapters, more than 2,000 group therapy abstracts were recovered for a period spanning 1980–1992. However, only 400 of these articles met a generous inclusion criteria for empirical studies, including single group case studies. This pattern is essentially replicated in the substance abuse, mutual support, large group awareness, child and adolescent, client variable, and short-term group therapy literatures.

Have the majority of conceptual articles in the literature been ignored by reviewers, or do reviewers have a particular type of conceptual model in mind when they make that call? We believe the latter to be true. That is, the vast majority of nonempirical papers reviewed in the first two chapters were very limited in scope, especially with respect to the extant literature. It is the painstaking integration of empirical work scattered across diverse journals and disciplines that has gone unheeded in virtually all of the conceptual papers in the literature. On the other hand, various chapters herein provide us with examples of new conceptual vistas based on a careful integration of previous empirical findings. At times this is accomplished by tracing an evolutionary trail as in the development, mutual support, and large group awareness reviews. At other times, we find authors recasting old conceptual models in new ways, such as in the pregroup training and interactional chapters. Although far from complete, the conceptual modeling efforts begin to meet the demands of the continual voice from the empirical wilderness that has pled for an increase in such modeling over the years.

Threaded throughout the chapters is evidence of clinical and methodological diversity and maturity. At times, these phenomena coexist and explain the attendant breadth and depth in methodological practices, as exemplified in the therapist characteristic chapter. In other instances, clinical maturity seems unrelated to method, as illustrated in the substance abuse and child and adolescent reviews. The client variables chapter demonstrates the reciprocal interplay between the complexity of methods and the interpretation of findings. Finally, the development and therapeutic factor chapters confront us with the relevance of context in explaining variables and their interaction.

The themes from the whole lay out the direction for our inquiry and practice; that is, the need for recognition and delineation of the individual components, of their relationship to and impact on one another, and of the dynamic influence of the group as a whole. Hopefully, the individual contributions, as well as the aforementioned thematic patterns, will lend insight to both clinicians and researchers and assist them in navigating the shoals surrounding empiricai inquiry.

There is nothing worse for mortal men than wandering.

Homer, The Odyssey

For the history that I require and design, special care is to be taken that it be of wide range and made to the measure of the universe. For the world is not to be narrowed till it will go into the understanding (which has been done hitherto), but the understanding is to be expanded and opened till it can take in the image of the world.

Francis Bacon, The Parasceve

Author Index

Fleiss, J., 63
Fleming, B. M., 133
Fletcher, J. M., 257
Flick, A., 375, 377, 378, 382, 383
Flohr, R., 90, 91
Flores, P. J., 459
Flowers, J. V., 126, 133–134, 250, 280, 284, 385, 401
Flynn, H. R., 372
Follette, V. M., 90, 94, 125, 143
Follette, W., 61, 90, 94
Fornes, G., 90, 93, 102
Forth, A., 132, 357
Foss, T., 194, 199, 245
Foulkes, 3, 270
Fox, S., 475
Foxx, R. M., 385
Frame, C. L., 495
Francis, D. J., 257
Franco, H., 459, 473, 474, 481
Frank, J., 17, 41, 44, 45, 160
Frank, J. D., 97, 101, 102, 329–330
Frank, M., 125, 126, 131, 132, 143, 374, 377, 378, 382, 383, 391
Franklin, C., 360
Franko, D. L., 419, 422, 430, 431, 434, 438, 439, 442, 444
Freeman, A., 395, 396
Freeman, C., 13, 15, 17
Freeman, C. P. L., 418, 420, 438, 443
Freeman, E. M., 360, 374
Freeman, S. J., 508
Freud, S., 5, 224, 232–233
Freudenberg, W., 180–181
Freudenheim, M., 319
Frey, R. E., 533
Friedland, P., 459, 474
Friedlander, M. L., 193, 197, 199, 208
Friedman, S., 293, 330
Fritz, G., 377, 378, 396, 399
Froelich, I., 279
Fromme, D. K., 132, 135, 140, 377, 378
Frommer, M. S., 418, 421, 425, 435
Frosh, S., 357
Fuehrer, A., 129, 178, 243, 294, 533
Fuhriman, A. J., 3, 13, 15, 33, 45, 64, 73, 118, 129, 136, 138–139, 191, 193, 206, 209–210, 211, 250, 272, 302–303, 324, 329, 386,

387, 388, 419, 431, 444, 446, 447, 559–562
Furia, R., 397
Futoran, G. C., 197

Gaines, J., 125, 126, 131, 132, 139, 142, 143, 374, 377, 378, 382, 383, 391
Galanter, M., 459, 460, 473, 474, 481, 508
Galinsky, M. J., 391
Galkigher, D., 65, 75
Gallagher, E. B., 142
Ganley, R., 466
Gans, J., 20
Gans, K., 419, 422, 438
Garant, J., 92, 163–166, 168, 169, 323
Gardner, J. A., 536
Garfield, S. L., 86, 173, 321, 480
Garfinkel, P. E., 416, 419, 420, 421, 439
Garland, J. A., 234
Garner, D. M., 416, 418, 425
Garrison, J., 168, 174
Gary, J. M., 419, 439, 444
Gazda, G. M., 194, 207, 340, 341, 363, 377, 391
Gendlin, E. T., 194, 201
Gerber, G. J., 382, 383
Gerler, E. R., 346
Gershaw, M. J., 399
Gersick, C. J. G., 251, 252
Gerstein, L. H., 418, 434
Getter, H., 90, 93, 98, 124, 125, 126, 132, 168, 193, 197, 208, 467, 470
Ghuman, H. S., 393, 394
Gibb, J., 527
Gibb, J. R., 244
Gibbard, G., 193, 214, 235–237, 240, 248, 257, 258
Gibbs, B., 183
Gibhard, M. E., 384, 385
Gibson, J. W., 418, 421, 425, 435
Gidron, B., 507
Giedt, F. H., 95
Gilbert, M., 132, 133, 357
Gilbride, T. V., 375
Gillespie, C. R., 132, 385, 398
Gillingham, W. H., 419, 422, 423, 432, 439, 446
Gilmore, J. B., 89, 90, 288
Gilner, F. G., 383, 384, 389, 396
Gilner, R. H., 287
Gilson, M., 374, 395, 396

Ginzburg, H. M., 458
Girling, A. J., 102
Gist, M., 244
Gitzinger, I., 246
Glad, D. D., 277
Glaser, K., 246
Glasgow, R. E., 396
Glass, G. V., 15–16, 18, 88, 173
Glassman, J. N. F., 419, 421, 427
Gleser, G. C., 194, 198, 207, 247, 329
Gliedman, L. H., 97, 101, 103
Glotter, D., 418, 421, 433
Godfrey, A. B., 319
Goehl, L., 458
Goettelmann, K., 115, 125, 131, 133, 138, 139, 140
Goff, B., 540
Goff, G., 418, 421, 433
Gold, E., 360
Gold, M., 323, 360
Goldberg, D. A., 327
Goldstein, A. P., 377, 385, 396, 397, 398, 399
Goldstein, J. A., 389
Goldstein, M. J., 194, 198, 202, 207, 211
Goldstein, M. S., 508
Goldstein, N., 384
Goldwasser, A. N., 132, 143
Goodman, G., 489, 498, 500, 553
Gordon, K., 419, 434, 440
Gordon, R. E., 508
Gorham, D. R., 385
Gotestam, G., 379, 391, 395, 397
Gottlieb, B. H., 496, 498
Gottman, J., 73
Gottschalk, L. A., 193, 198, 207, 247, 536
Gould, N., 13, 15
Gould, N. B., 417, 418
Graber, S., 360
Gradman, T., 495, 496
Graff, R. W., 130
Graham, J. W., 257
Grant, P. R., 531, 537, 539, 541, 544
Gray, J. J., 418, 421, 430, 435, 442, 444
Greenberg, D. J., 384, 385
Greenberg, L. S., 192–193, 482
Greenberg, R. L., 327
Greene, L. R., 141, 373, 377, 378, 389, 394
Greenwood, V. B., 375

Subject Index